Feature Review Papers in Chemical/Bio-Sensors and Analytical Chemistry in 2024

Feature Review Papers in Chemical/Bio-Sensors and Analytical Chemistry in 2024

Guest Editors

Nicole Jaffrezic-Renault
Camelia Bala
Marco Frasconi
Jose V. Ros-Lis

MDPI

Basel • Beijing • Wuhan • Barcelona • Belgrade • Novi Sad • Cluj • Manchester

Guest Editors
Nicole Jaffrezic-Renault
Institute of UTINAM
University of Franche-Comté
Besançon
France

Camelia Bala
Department of Analytical Chemistry
University of Bucharest
Bucharest
Romania

Marco Frasconi
Department of Chemical Sciences
University of Padova
Padova
Italy

Jose V. Ros-Lis
Inorganic Chemistry Department
Universitat de València
Valencia
Spain

Editorial Office
MDPI AG
Grosspeteranlage 5
4052 Basel, Switzerland

This is a reprint of the Special Issue, published open access by the journal *Chemosensors* (ISSN 2227-9040), freely accessible at: https://www.mdpi.com/journal/chemosensors/special_issues/QIK79MF4R2.

For citation purposes, cite each article independently as indicated on the article page online and as indicated below:

Lastname, A.A.; Lastname, B.B. Article Title. *Journal Name* **Year**, *Volume Number*, Page Range.

ISBN 978-3-7258-4193-6 (Hbk)
ISBN 978-3-7258-4194-3 (PDF)
https://doi.org/10.3390/books978-3-7258-4194-3

Contents

Preface

This Special Issue, "Review Articles on Chemical Sensors/Biosensors and Analytical Chemistry in 2024", includes ten review articles that fall within *Chemosensors'* scope.

Six review articles explore the use of sensors in health monitoring as follows:

- Humidity sensors for monitoring respiratory status and skin humidity;
- Optical neuroimaging techniques to study sepsis-associated delirium;
- Various origami-based biosensor techniques and their applications;
- Electrochemical sensors based on dual/multi-matrix molecularly imprinted polymers for various targets;
- Emerging technologies in HCV (hepatitis C virus) detection;
- Nanomaterial-based electrochemical sensors for drug detection.

Two review articles investigate the following applications of sensors in environmental monitoring:

- Biopolymer-based sensors for the detection of heavy metals;
- Micro/nanorobots for environmental monitoring.

The final two review articles cover their use in food safety as follows:

- The detection of mycotoxins using biosensors;
- The detection of biogenic amines in aquatic products.

Nicole Jaffrezic-Renault, Camelia Bala, Marco Frasconi, and Jose V. Ros-Lis
Guest Editors

chemosensors

MDPI

Review

Biosensors for Food Mycotoxin Determination: A Comparative and Critical Review

Aurelia Magdalena Pisoschi [1,*], Florin Iordache [1], Loredana Stanca [1], Elena Mitranescu [1], Liliana Bader Stoica [1], Ovidiu Ionut Geicu [1,2], Liviu Bilteanu [3] and Andreea Iren Serban [1,2]

[1] Department Preclinical Sciences, Faculty of Veterinary Medicine, University of Agronomic Sciences and Veterinary Medicine of Bucharest, 105 Splaiul Independentei, 050097 Bucharest, Romania; florin.iordache@fmvb.usamv.ro (F.I.); loredana.stanca@fmvb.usamv.ro (L.S.); elena.mitranescu@fmvb.usamv.ro (E.M.); liliana.bader@fmvb.usamv.ro (L.B.S.); ovidiu-ionut.geicu@fmvb.usamvb.ro (O.I.G.); andreea-iren.serban@fmvb.usamv.ro (A.I.S.)

[2] Department Biochemistry and Molecular Biology, Faculty of Biology, University of Bucharest, 91–95 Splaiul Independentei, 050095 Bucharest, Romania

[3] Molecular Nanotechnology Laboratory, National Institute for Research and Development in Microtechnologies, 126A Erou Iancu Nicolae Street, 077190 Bucharest, Romania; liviu.bilteanu@imt.ro

* Correspondence: aurelia-magdalena.pisoschi@fmvb.usamv.ro

Abstract: The need for performant analytical methodologies to assess mycotoxins is vital, given the negative health impact of these compounds. Biosensors are analytical devices that consist of a biological element for recognizing the analyte and a transducer, which translates the biorecognition event into a signal proportional to the analyte concentration. The biorecognition elements can be enzymes, antibodies, or DNA fragments. The modalities of detection can be optical, electrochemical, thermal, or mass-sensitive. These analytical tools represent viable alternatives to laborious, expensive traditional methods and are characterized by specificity given by the biorecognition element, sensitivity, fast response, portability, multi-modal detection, and the possibility of in situ application. The present paper focuses on a comprehensive view, enriched with a critical, comparative perspective on mycotoxin assay using biosensors. The use of different biorecognition elements and detection modes are discussed comparatively. Nanomaterials with optical and electrochemical features can be exploited in association with a variety of biorecognition elements. Analytical parameters are reviewed along with a broad range of applications.

Keywords: mycotoxins; enzyme sensors; immunosensors; aptasensors; fluorescence; electroanalysis

1. Introduction

Mycotoxins are natural products that occur as a result of the metabolism of some fungi and are found in some foods like cereals, dried fruits, dried beans, coffee, animal feed, various agricultural products, and many others. The toxicity of mycotoxins has been largely documented [1–6], and as a result, international legislation was introduced [7,8] as well as at the national level [9,10]. Legislation requires mycotoxin contents in food products to be as low as possible to protect consumers from the risk of illness (establishing tolerable daily intakes). The main mycotoxins are as follows:

- Aflatoxins (AFB1, AFB2, AFG1, AFG2, and AFM1) produced by certain *Aspergillus* molds;
- Ochratoxin A (OTA), produced by certain *Aspergillus* and *Penicillium* molds, is the most active of the nine ochratoxins;
- Patulin toxin produced by *Penicillium*, *Aspergillus*, and *Byssochylamys* molds;
- Fumonisins produced by *Fusarium* molds;
- Trichothecenes (mainly nivalenol-NIV, deoxynivalenol-DON, T-2, and HT-2 toxin) produced by different species belonging to the genera *Fusarium*, *Myrothecium*, *Trichoderma*, *Trichothecium*, *Cephalosporium*, *Verticimonosporium*, and *Stachybotrys*;

- Zearalenone (ZEN) produced by some species of *Fusarium* and *Gibberella;*
- Ergot alkaloids, citrinin (CIT), sterigmatocystin (STC), *Alternaria* toxins, etc.

The most representative mycotoxins are illustrated in Scheme 1.

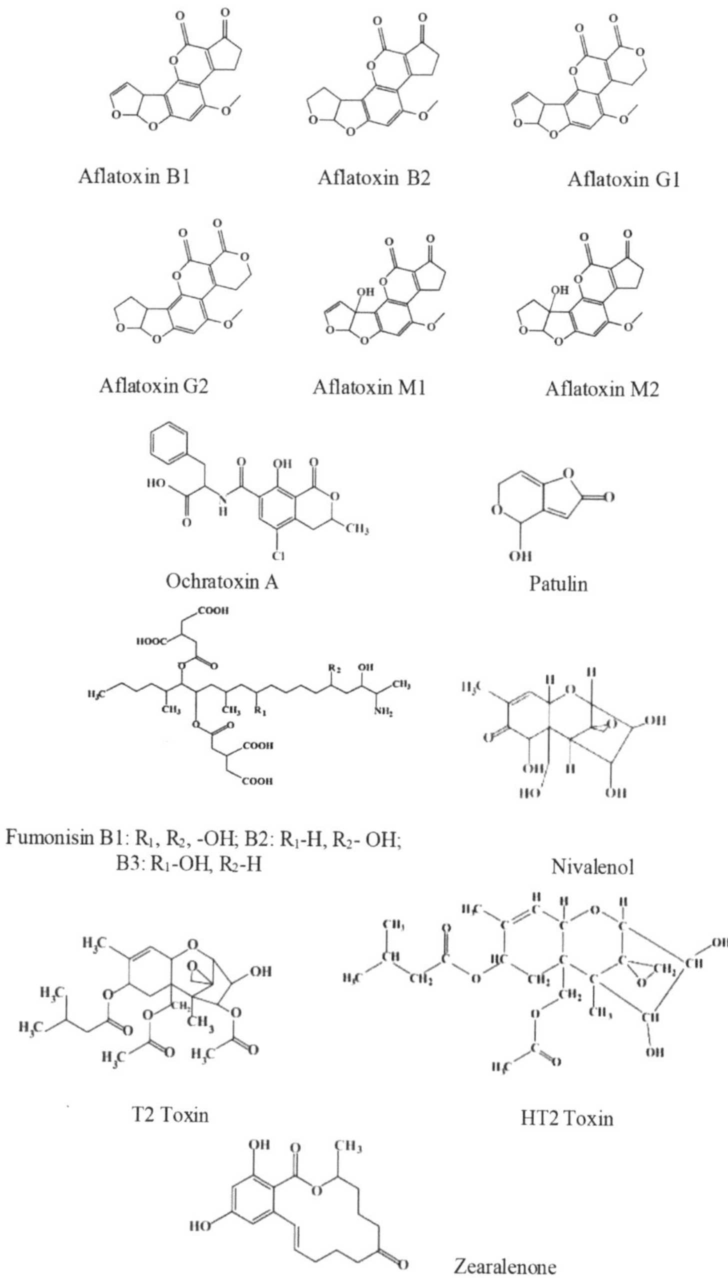

Scheme 1. The structures of some of the most representative mycotoxins.

More than 500 mycotoxins have been identified, and new mycotoxins are expected to be discovered [11].

The lethal dose (LD50, as milligrams of substance per kilogram of body weight) is defined as the amount of an ingested compound inducing the death of one-half of a tested sample (population). The LD50 values for aflatoxins are found within the range of 0.5 to 10 mg/kg. The liver is mainly affected, with centrilobular necrosis, bile duct proliferation, fatty acid infiltration, and hepatic lesions, which can result in liver cancer [12]. For most animal species, the oral LD50 value for aflatoxin B1 ranges between 0.3 and 17.9 mg/kg body weight. Oral LD50 values of 78 and 46 mg/kg body weight have been reported for deoxynivalenol in B6C3F1 and DDY mice, respectively [13]. The oral LD50 of patulin in rodents ranges between 29 and 55 mg/kg body weight [14].

Mycotoxins have been investigated for their genotoxic, mutagenic, and carcinogenic potential. Aflatoxin B1, due to the presence of a double bond at the 8,9 position, can be converted to the reactive AFB1-8,9-epoxide, which interacts with key biomolecules including DNA. The main DNA adduct resulted is AFB1-N7-guanine, and this pro-mutagenic insult leads to a G $\rightarrow$ T transversion mutation [15]. This mutation will impact the cell cycle by affecting the P53 gene, which encodes a tumor suppressor protein that counteracts tumorigenesis and carcinogenesis [16].

In the case of FB1, the DNA damage was assigned to the stimulation of oxidative decay and lipid peroxidation. In vitro genotoxicity studies revealed micronuclei and chromosomal aberrations [15]. It inhibits protein synthesis and DNA synthesis at elevated concentrations. Its carcinogenic potential was ascribed to its potential to stimulate ^{3}H thymidine incorporation. Following animal studies, it was reported as an inductor of liver, oesophageal, kidney cancer, and neurodegeneration [16].

Ochratoxin A inhibits protein and nucleic acid synthesis due to competitive inhibition of phenylalanine-tRNA ligase. Co-administration of phenylalanine in animals could lower the acute toxic effects of OTA. The formation of DNA adducts induced by OTA was linked to its carcinogenic potential. It was found that the OTA phenoxy radical resulted from metabolic activation, and the associated DNA damage resulting from reactive oxygenated species represents the source of adduct formation [15]. Moreover, Ochratoxin A is considered strong hepatotoxic and nephtotoxic and was reported as a promoter of lipid peroxidation and an inhibitor of mitochondrial ATP synthesis [16].

Deoxynivalenol exerts toxicity via its epoxide moiety without necessitating metabolic activation. Trichothecene exposure at low doses led to the modulation of the expression of several cytokines and chemokines, hence immune function, in animal studies. DON is involved in the modulation of physiological processes controlled by mitogen-activated protein kinases: control of cell growth, differentiation, and apoptosis, which are essential for signal transduction in the immune response. Along with alterations in cytokine expression, alterations in MAPK expression also result in the immune imbalance and toxicity linked to DON and other trichothecenes [15].

Zearalenone represents a competitive substrate for enzymes present in steroid synthesis pathway and metabolism and, therefore, has the potential to act as an endocrine disruptor. So, it was stipulated that ZEA could exert intense effects on gene expression as a result of the altered activity of nuclear transcription factors [15]. Zearalenone is genotoxic, induces DNA alterations, is reported as carcinogenic in mice, and is an inductor of hepatocellular adenomas and pituitary tumors [16].

Patulin was characterized as carcinogenic, mutagenic, and teratogenic and as an inductor of intestinal injuries. Its involvement in carcinogenesis and tumorigenesis was ascribed to its ability to impair cellular DNA. The inactivation of the active site of protein tyrosine phosphatase, a regulator of intestinal epithelial barrier function, was considered the source of patulin toxicity for intestinal cells [16].

The toxicity of aflatoxins is also proved by EFSA, which evaluated over 200,000 analytical results, assessing that the risk of poisoning with AFM1 comes from milk and fermented milk products and the risk for AFB1 comes from the consumption of grains and grain-based products [17].

Because of their toxicity, the levels allowed in food products are very low (as shown in Table 1) [7,8], especially in milk and baby food products.

Table 1. Maximum mycotoxin levels allowed for some food products [7,8].

Aflatoxin	Food Product	Level (μg Kg^{-1})
Aflatoxins total	Almonds (ready to eat)	10
	Hazelnuts (ready to eat)	
	Pistachios (ready to eat)	
Aflatoxin M1	Milk	0.5
Aflatoxin B1	Cereals and processed cereal products. Exceptions: rice and maize meant to be sorted or to undergo other physical treatments prior to their placing on the market to reach the consumer, or before employing as food ingredients, baby food, food meant for particular medical purposes for young children and infants, food based on processed cereals for young children and infants	2.0
	Food meant for particular medical aims, for young children and infants	0.1
Sum of aflatoxins B1, B2, G1 and G2	Dried fruits meant to be sorted or to undergo other physical treatments prior to their placing on the market to reach the consumer or before employing as food ingredients. Exception: dried figs	10.0
	Groundnuts (peanuts) and other oilseeds meant to be sorted or to undergo other physical treatments prior to their placement on the market to reach the consumer or before employing as food ingredients. Exceptions: groundnuts (peanuts) and other oilseeds to be crushed to obtain refined vegetable oil	15.0
Ochratoxin A	Raw wheat	5.0
	Barley	
	Rye	
Deoxynivalenol	Pasta	750
	Bread, pastries, biscuits	500
Patulin	Fruit juices	50.0

Biosensors approached in this review, by their analytical parameters, show their ability to detect such low levels in the analyzed food products.

There are numerous recent articles on the determination of aflatoxins (B1, B2, G1, G2, M1) from different food products [18–27]. Among the determination methods, the immunochemical and chromatographic techniques in tandem with mass spectrometry are mentioned. Immunochemical methods are fast and, therefore, used in routine controls and on-site detection. Chromatographic methods ensure a sensitive and selective analysis [28].

Traditional techniques such as HPLC, gas chromatography, mass spectrometry, and enzyme-linked immunosorbent assay, though accurate and sensitive, require training, accessibility, costs, and the sample pre-treatment is time-consuming.

Biosensors, as broadly used analytical tools for determining the quality of food products, aim at circumventing these drawbacks [29–37]. They consist of two important parts: a biological element for recognizing the analyte and a transducer, which translates the biorecognition event into a signal proportional to the analyte concentration. Therefore, biosensors are classified according to the biological recognition element and according to the type of transducer [38]. The recognition element is either a biomolecule or a molecular assembly capable of recognizing an analyte (a substrate). According to the biological element of recognition (bioreceptor), they are the following [39]:

- Enzyme sensors [40];
- Immunosensors, which use antibodies, antibody fragments, antigens, or antigen conjugates as biorecognition elements [41];
- Aptasensors (DNA-based biosensors), which use nucleic acid molecules as biorecognition elements [42];

- Biomimetics [43];
- Sensors using synthetic biorecognition elements (molecularly imprinted polymers) [44].

So, biosensors can be developed by incorporating a variety of biorecognition elements, including enzymes, aptamers, antibodies, nucleic acids, cells, tissues, and molecularly imprinted polymers [39].

According to the type of transducer, the biosensors can be classified as follows [45]:

- Electrochemical—based on the variation of electrochemical properties [46];
- Optical—based on the variation of optical properties [47];
- Thermal biosensors—based on thermal energy variation [48];
- Mass sensitive biosensors—based on mass variation [49];
- Acoustic biosensors—the target analyte is detected through the induced variations in the frequency, velocity, or amplitude of the acoustic waves generated by piezoelectric materials [50].

M. Ramesh et al. [51] developed an illustrative general scheme regarding the components and the functioning of biosensors.

The general scheme of a biosensor, encompassing various biorecognition elements and transduction principles, is shown in Figure 1 [45,51].

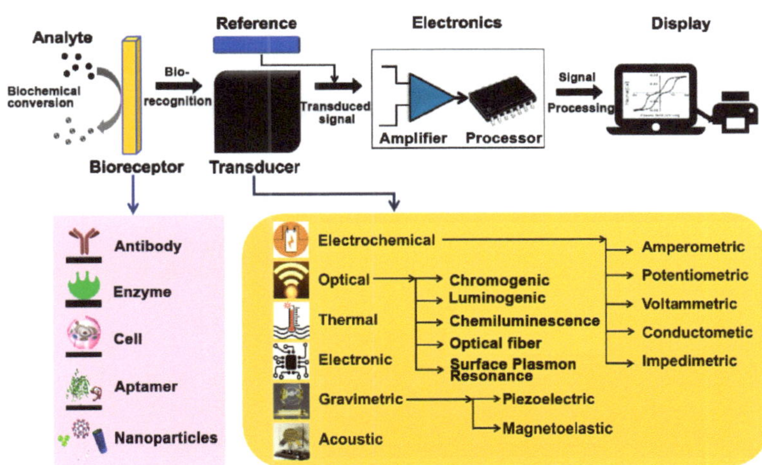

Figure 1. General diagram of a biosensor from [45,51], MDPI 2021, 2023.

The number of articles published yearly and indexed in Clarivate Analytics-Web of Science Core Collection related to the use of biosensors in the analysis of mycotoxins is presented in Figure 2. The search dealt with the last 15 years and was performed according to the keywords "biosensors for mycotoxins" (271 indexations in total). These keywords gave the most results when compared to "biosensors for analysis of mycotoxins" (126 indexations in total) or "biosensors for determination of mycotoxins" (84 indexations in total). The data were collected on 26 January 2024.

As can be seen, the tendency to use biosensors for mycotoxins is increasing, demonstrating the potential and viability of this analytical method.

The proposed paper aims to present an overview enriched by a critical perspective on biosensing techniques using various biorecognition elements and modes of detection. Enzyme sensors, immunosensors, and aptamers with different transduction modes are comparatively reviewed and critically discussed. The databases accessed for collecting information were Web of Science Core Collection, ScienceDirect Freedom Collection Elsevier, Springer Journals, Wiley, Google Scholar, etc.

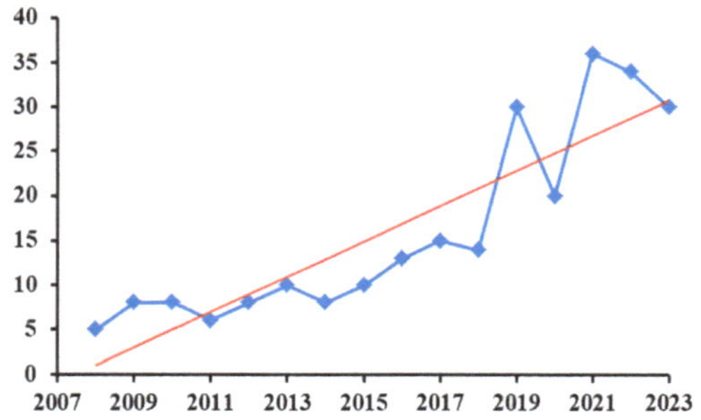

Figure 2. Number of articles indexed yearly in Clarivate Analytics-Web of Science Core Collection database.

Sections 2 and 3 present the most relevant development and detection principles relying on different kinds of transducers, as well as methods of immobilizing bioelements. The applications of food assay (presented in Table 2), as well as the recent developments depicted in the section dealing with the comparative overview and future perspective, are focused on the last five years.

The present paper is distinguished by a quasi-exhaustive analytical approach, which integrates the comprehensive view that details the variety of biorecognition elements (antibodies, enzymes, aptamers) and transducers (electrochemical, optical, thermal, piezoelectrical). The critical, comparative perspective deals with the advantages and disadvantages of each biosensor type, as well as recent trends and authors' views.

2. Types of Transducers

In this section, the biosensing applications are analyzed depending on the type of transducer that transforms the recognition reaction into a measurable signal proportional to the concentration value.

2.1. Electrochemical Biosensors

These sensors are characterized by the fact that the biochemical reaction between the analyte and the substrate is transformed into an electrical signal; the latter can be measured by several techniques [52,53].

- Potentiometric, by measuring potential or charge accumulation; this mode of detection includes, as transducers, ion-specific electrodes or field-effect transistors; the latter rely on measuring the current as a result of a potentiometric effect at a gate electrode;
- Amperometric, by measuring the current intensity at a fixed potential value;
- Voltammetric, by measuring the current—potential dependence at the controlled variation of the potential in time;
- Impedimetric, by measuring impedance (both resistance and reactance);
- Conductometric, by measuring the conductive properties of a medium.

Electrical measurements are performed with the use of electrodes, their name deriving from the role played in the measurement, working electrode, reference electrode, and counter electrode. The most common reference electrode is Ag/AgCl, which has the role of maintaining a stable (fixed) and known (established) potential. The working electrode converts the biochemical reaction into an electrical signal and is made of Au, Pt, carbon, or silicon. Working electrodes should impart good conductivity and be chemically stable. The counter electrode establishes a connection to the electrolytic solution so that a current can pass through the working electrode [53]. Mehrvar and Abdi [54] described the biosensor types depending on the afore-mentioned transduction modes. For the first-generation biosensors, the reaction product of the biocatalyzed reaction directly diffuses to the transducer. The second-generation or mediated biosensors make use of specific mediators between the biorecognition reaction and the transducer, enhancing sensitivity [54].

Potentiometric biosensors are based on measuring the potential between the working electrode and the reference electrode and use ion-selective electrodes (ISE) and ion-sensitive field effect transistors (ISFET). These biosensors involve ion-selective electrodes in the detection of an electrical signal determined by the reaction of the biological element with the analyte. The biological recognition element (enzyme) is immobilized on a semi-permeable membrane that surrounds the working electrode (for instance, the glass membrane electrode) or is immobilized with gels (ion-selective electrodes).

Rameil et al. [55] developed a potentiometric biosensor for the determination of Aflatoxin M1, composed of a polypyrrole-surface-working electrode coated with a polyclonal anti-M1 antibody (20 μg mL^{-1}) and an HRP-aflatoxin B1 conjugate. 3-(4-hydroxyphenyl)propionic acid functioned as an electron-donating compound for the enzyme. Ag/AgCl electrode served as a reference. The limit of detection (LOD) was 40 pg mL^{-1}. The working time was less than 10 min without sample treatment in different milk matrices. Aflatoxin B1 was determined from real samples of sesame, walnut, and pea with a potentiometric biosensor based on pH-sensitive field-effect transistors and acetylcholinesterase. The obtained calibration curve was between 0.2 μg mL^{-1} and 40 μg mL^{-1} [56].

Field-effect transistor biosensors are semiconductor electronic devices with a general structure consisting of three components—source, gate, and drain—which represent the three electrodes (Figure 3). The biosensor has an insulating layer and a semiconductor layer. The gate on which the biorecognition element is fixed is placed between the drain and the source. It interacts with the analyte, transforming the chemical information into a charge change, recorded as a measurable electrical signal [57–59].

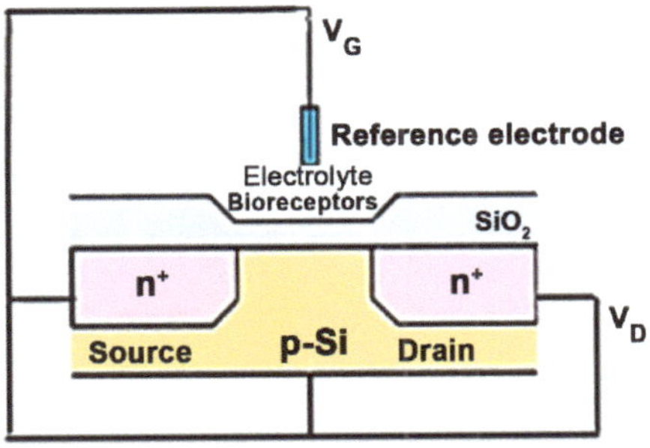

Figure 3. Schematic representation of an ISFET-based biosensor (V_D-voltage drain-source, V_G-voltage gate-source).

Ochratoxin A was determined from white and red wines using a biosensor based on a graphene field-effect transistor integrated into a single silicon chip. A specifically designed aptamer against ochratoxin A was chosen as a biorecognition element. 1-pyrenebutyric acid N-hydroxysuccinimide ester was employed to covalently attach the aptamer to the graphene surface. An electric field stimulation was employed to induce more efficacious π-π stacking of pyrenebutanoic acid succinimidyl ester to graphene. The G-rich aptamer exhibited π-π stacking on graphene and reconfiguration in G-quadruplex arrangement in the presence of OTA. The real aptamer behavior became sensitive to the ionic force of the analyte solution. Hence, a specific, sensitive, and fast assay was achieved. The LOD was 1.4 pM, and the response time was as low as 10 s [60]. It should be mentioned that electrochemical methods can be combined with gravimetric techniques (like quartz crystal microbalance with dissipation monitoring) or microscopic techniques (like scanning probe microscopies and fluorescent microscopies). These methods promote increased sensitivity in the proximity of the surface of the electrochemical/optical transducer (electrode, waveguide, sensing tip, etc.), enabling delineation of the interfacial phenomena, acquiring a broader range of information and exerting control on the biosensing environment [53].

Amperometric and voltammetric biosensors are based on the measurement of current intensity at controlled, for amperometry, or variable potential, in the case of voltammetry. Pt, Au, Ag, Hg, graphite, glassy carbon, carbon paste, carbon nanotubes, screen-printed electrodes, metallic oxide nanoparticles, boron-doped diamond, and composites are used as electrodes. The recognition biomolecules are fixed on the surface of the transducer.

Second-generation biosensors make use of mediators (functioning as electron acceptors) instead of molecular oxygen to perform electron transport to the electrode and to hamper oxygen dependence of the analytical signal. In voltammetric or amperometric assay, mediators allow diminution of the working potential versus bare electrodes, minimizing the influence of interferent species. Mediators are represented by low-molecular-weight redox active molecules (e.g., ferrocyanide, ferrocene derivatives, quinones, or conducting organic salts). They react at the enzyme active site and then at the electrode's surface, transferring electrons. For instance, if the biocatalyzed reaction is an oxidation one, the mediator is reduced following the enzyme reaction, is subsequently transported to the electrode, and converted to its oxidized form. So, it gives rise to electron transfer at the electrode's surface and yields a measurable current proportional to the analyte's concentration [61].

Aflatoxin B1 was determined by cyclic voltammetry with aflatoxin-oxidase as a biorecognition element, which is embedded in sol-gel, coupled with a multiwalled carbon nanotubes-modified Pt transducer. The modification resulted in optimized surface area, electrocatalytic effect, and sensitivity. The linearity ranged between 3.2 nmol L^{-1} and 721 nmol L^{-1} with a detection limit of 1.6 nmol L^{-1}. The silica sol-gel afforded stabilization of the enzyme activity, prevented biocatalyst leakage, and ensured a biocompatible environment [62]. Vidal et al. [63] describe the determination of mycotoxins by amperometry based on electrodes made of inert metals (Pt, Au), carbon (graphite, glassy-carbon), or screen-printed electrodes.

For the determination of Ochratoxin A (OTA), an amperometric microfabricated biosensor was used, employing the immobilized synthetic peptide NFO4 as a biorecognition element, characterized by enhanced affinity and enabling OTA molecular recognition by simulation of the specific toxin antibody. Horseradish peroxidase-conjugated OTA was added to the free toxin solutions, followed by incubation on the specific biotransducer. The amperometric responses versus hydrogen peroxide were taken after 5 min of enzyme reaction, post H_2O_2/luminol addition. Simultaneously, the recording of light emission signals enabled a direct comparison of the amperometric and luminescence assay modes of the biochip. OTA concentrations up to 10 µg L^{-1} were measured, the authors reporting a broader dynamic range in amperometry [64].

Impedimetric biosensors [65] are based on the measurement of circuit impedance. Electrochemical impedance biosensors measure the current passing through a cell to which an alternating current potential, a sinusoidal potential, and a small excitation signal that causes an impedance response are applied. The biorecognition elements are fixed on the surface of the electrode. Electrochemical impedance spectroscopy (EIS) is an effective technique employed for the analysis of interfacial features connected to bio-recognition events occurring at the surface of the electrode, such as antibody-antigen interaction, substrate-enzyme interaction, or whole-cell capture [66].

Electrochemical impedance spectroscopy relies on a perturbation induced in an electrochemical system found in equilibrium. A sinusoidal signal (*ac* voltage or *ac* current) is applied on a wide frequency domain, and the sinusoidal response (current or voltage) of the system is eventually recorded as a consequence of the induced perturbation [67]. The applied frequency can vary from less than 1mHz to over 1 MHz, and the impedance of the circuit is measured in ohms [66]. The technique is non-destructive and sensitive, obtaining a detection limit of 0.5 ng mL^{-1} for ochratoxin A [68].

For the determination of OTA, Malvano et al. [69] applied an alternating sinusoidal potential of 10 mV in the frequency range from 0.1 to 10^4 Hz, which was superimposed on 0.00 mV DC potential (considered vs. reference electrode). They obtained a LOD value between 0.37 and 5.42 ng mL^{-1}, depending on the biosensor used, with 5 or 10 µg mL^{-1}

OTA monoclonal antibody for biorecognition. The linear range of analytical response was between 0.3–20.0 and 5.0–40.0 ng mL^{-1}, depending on the biosensor used, with 5 μg mL^{-1} anti-OTA or 10 μg mL^{-1} anti-OTA, respectively.

Conductometric biosensors [70,71] are based on measuring, using two electrodes, the conductivity of a solution, which is directly dependent on the amount of ions in the solution. The biosensitive element can be embedded in a film that is deposited on the surface of the electrode. An ohmmeter measures the conductance change caused by the biorecognition reaction [72]. Soldatkin et al. [73] determined Aflatoxin B1 using acetylcholinesterase immobilized onto the surface of a conductometric transducer. The detection error was less than 7%, and the minimum limit of detection was 0.05 μg mL^{-1}. Patulin was determined with a conductometric biosensor, with urease being used as a biorecognition element, and it was co-immobilized with bovine serum albumin by cross-linking with glutaraldehyde. The linear range was 1–50 μM [74].

Characterized as novel electrochemical analytical tools, *photoelectrochemical biosensors* integrate the benefits of biological and optical analysis [32]. The biorecognition event takes place under illumination and induces a signal variation in the photoactive nanomaterial. The reduction of the background signal and the increased sensitivities were ascribed to the thorough separation between the source of excitation (light) and the detected signal (current) [32].

2.2. Optical Biosensors

These analytical tools are viewed as the most widespread and frequently used class of biosensors. The property measured following the reaction of the biomolecule with the analyte is of optical nature. These sensors were divided into two general classes: label-free and label-based. In label-free sensors, the quantified signal is directly produced by the interaction between the analyte and the transducer. Label-based sensors employ labels, and the analytical signal is quantified via a colorimetric, fluorescent, or luminescent technique [75].

Optical sensing makes use of surface plasmon resonators, interferometers, optical waveguides, and photonic crystals, quantifying various properties like absorption, refraction, phosphorescence, fluorescence, and Raman scattering [76,77].

An optical fiber biosensor comprises a fiber core, a metal coating, and a layer containing the bioelement. Part of the covering region will encompass the metal coating and the bioelement, thus enabling the immobilization of the biocatalytic component on the fiber core and its integration with the optical transducing system. Optical fiber biosensors are small-sized, cost-effective, and easy to use [77].

In *surface plasmon resonance optical biosensors*, analyte molecules and biomolecules (proteins, bacteria, cells, DNA, etc.) determine the modification of the refractive index of the surrounding medium, which leads to deviation of resonance conditions of the resonator [78,79]. Zearalenone was determined with a relative standard deviation (RSD) of 2.81% [80].

In *interferometric biosensors*, the difference in the change in the refractive index between two light beams is measured. The assay is based on a single input beam and two output beams, one for reference and another influenced by the interaction of biomolecules. The difference in refractive index between the two beams shows the modification brought into the system by the biorecognition reaction [81]. AFB1, OTA, ZON, and B1 were quantified with a polarization interferometer biosensor, with a LOD of 0.002 ng mL^{-1} (estimated by linear extrapolation of the graph) [82].

Optical waveguide biosensors are constituted of a sensitive layer, cladding, and waveguide layers located on a substrate. The evanescent wave scattering results in an optical change in the vicinity of the guiding surface, which is exploited as a mechanism of detection in optical waveguide biosensors [77].

In most cases, planar waveguides are placed on a thin layer of stable substrate and are commonly constituted of low refractive index and glassy materials (e.g., silica or polymers). Relying on their geometrical design, we can classify planar waveguides into slab waveguides and channel waveguides [83].

Figure 4 shows the representation of a waveguide biosensor with an optical alignment platform [84].

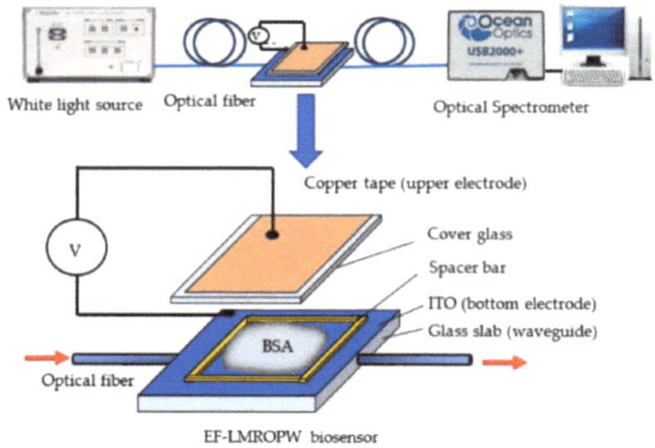

Figure 4. A representation of an electrical field-induced lossy mode resonance-based optical planar waveguide sensor (experimental set-up and photo), from [84] MDPI 2021.

Zearalenone was determined with an immunosensor that functioned as a polarization interferometer with a detection limit of 0.01 ng mL^{-1} [85]. Novel planar waveguide-based sensors operate by relying on the polarization interferometry principle, measuring a phase shift between p- and s-components of the polarized light obtained during analyte binding. The sensor functions similarly to a Mach–Zehnder interferometer, but its principle is much simpler, not requiring the splitting of the waveguide into two arms. The refractive index sensitivity corresponded to 5200 radians per refractive index unit. Ochratoxin A was determined using the optical planar waveguide in a broad concentration range between 0.01 and 100 ng mL^{-1}, corresponding to an analytical response increase [86]. Surface plasmon resonance, evanescent wave fluorescence, and optical waveguide interferometry exploit the evanescent field in the proximity of the surface of the biosensor to detect the biorecognition reaction. Evanescent wave fluorescent and luminescent optical fiber biosensors can be subsequently developed [75].

Chemiluminescence is distinguished from fluorescence or phosphorescence in that the electronic excited state results from a chemical reaction rather than the absorption of a quantum (photon). Figure 5 illustrates the principle and main components of a chemiluminescent assay.

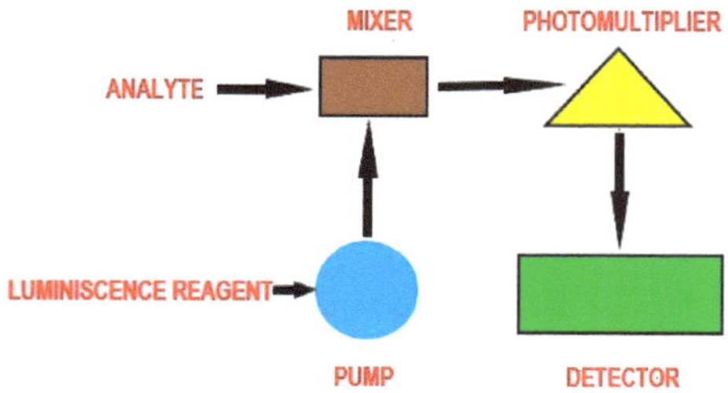

Figure 5. The principle of chemiluminescence—general scheme.

Jia et al. [87] developed a portable chemiluminescence optical fiber aptasensor aiming at the detection of four mycotoxins (aflatoxin B1, FB1, ZEN, and OTA). A single-stranded binding protein was chosen to be responsible for specific biorecognition. The LOD obtained at mycotoxin assay was between 0.015 pg mL^{-1} and 0.423 pg mL^{-1}. The sensor proved successful in the determination of four mycotoxins in infant foods (baby rice flour and baby rice cake) [87].

Fluorescent biosensors are based on the phenomenon of fluorescence, which is considered a form of chemiluminescence. Fluorescence is an emission of photons that occurs when electromagnetic radiation of a certain wavelength is absorbed by molecules (fluorophores or fluorescently labeled). An immunochromatographic assay for the quantitative detection of AFB1 in foodstuffs was developed by Li et al., based on AFB1 antibody and phycocyanin-labeled latex nanospheres. The assay enabled obtaining a LOD of 0.16 ng mL^{-1}. Phycocyanin and anti-AFB1 monoclonal antibodies on the surface of latex nanospheres enhanced the fluorescent signal and sensitivity [88].

In fluorescence resonance energy transfer or Förster resonance energy transfer (based on a non-radiative dipole-dipole coupling), the energy is transferred from an excited fluorophore donor to a fluorophore acceptor, whose excitation spectrum overlaps with the donor's emission spectrum. The donors and acceptors are generally dye molecules. The transfer depends on the distance between the donor and the acceptor, and eventually, the emission of photons from the acceptor can be detected [89,90].

Given the loss of energy through non-radiative processes, the fluorescent photons have lower energy compared to the energy of the photons responsible for the generation of the excited state. So, the wavelength of fluorescent emission is higher than that of the excitation one, the Stokes shift being the difference (in wavenumber, frequency, or energy) between the positions of absorption and emission maxima. The emitted radiation may have a smaller wavelength or the same wavelength as the excitation radiation, and then the phenomenon is called resonance fluorescence [91].

When fluorescent emission occurs, an optical measurable signal is generated from the sample. The signal occurrence relies on the three most commonly encountered mechanisms [89]:

- The bioreceptor recognizes the analyte, so the analytical signal takes into account the presence of analytes and their amount;
- Conformational changes can result following the biorecognition event, so the measured signal reflects specific alterations in the bioreceptor's conformation;
- Biocatalyst activity changes can occur, so the signal can also reflect enzyme activity.

The following methods can be applied to detect the generated analytical signal: FRET (Förster resonance energy transfer, previously detailed), FLIM (fluorescence lifetime imaging, which relies on the differences in the exponential decay rate of photon emission of a fluorophore present in a sample), FCS (fluorescence correlation spectroscopy, which performs correlation analysis of the time-related fluctuations of the fluorescence intensity), or mere change in fluorescence intensity. Figure 6 represents the key components and mechanisms of a fluorescent assay [92].

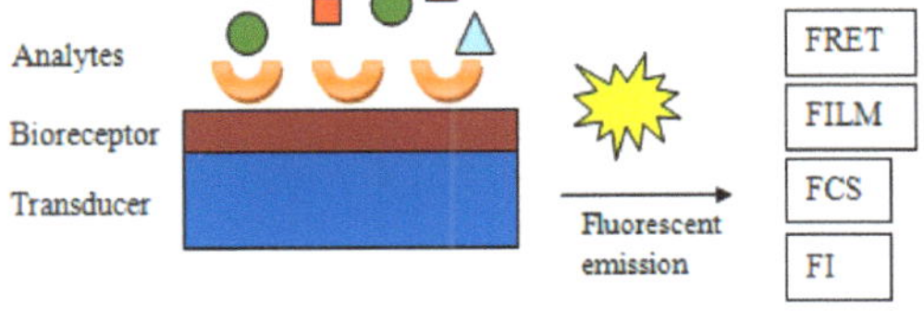

Figure 6. General scheme of fluorescent biosensors and underlying mechanisms from [92], MDPI 2018.

Tan et al. [93] determined Aflatoxin B1 with a detection limit of 0.13 ng mL^{-1}. The linearity range was 0.5–50 ng mL^{-1}. The biosensor was constituted of mesoporous silica nanoparticles, the fluorescence being imparted by the presence of Rhodamine 6G [93].

ELISA (Enzyme-linked immunosorbent assay) was developed as an enzyme-competitive technique for aflatoxin quantitation relying on *fluorescent* or, more often, on *colorimetric* detection. The sample and an enzyme-coupled mycotoxin conjugate are mixed and then added to antibody-coated microtiter wells. After the addition of the enzyme substrate, the blue color develops. Alkaline phosphatase, horseradish peroxidase, β-galactosidase, acetylcholinesterase, and catalase function as bioreceptors for biological recognition [27]. Also, exploiting the rapid and simple colorimetric detection in solution or on paper-based strips, novel DNA aptamers as biorecognition elements were used in combination with the optical transducing properties of gold and silver nanoparticles for AFB1 and AFM1. Thiolated DNA aptamers can be covalently conjugated to the surface of golden nanoparticles via gold–thiol bonds or by physisorption to the surface of the nanoparticles. For non-thiolated DNA aptamers, chemical interaction forces (such as hydrophobic effects and van der Waals forces) between the atoms of the DNA bases lead to strong adsorption on the surface of the nanoparticles [94].

Vibrational spectroscopy can also be applied as a nondestructive analytical detection methodology for assessing mycotoxins. Surface-enhanced Raman scattering as a biosensing method relies on the amplification of the intensity of the vibration signals of a molecule by several orders of magnitude in the proximity of a gold or silver metallic nano-structure surface [75]. The plasmonic resonance frequency influences the choice of the metal. Visible and near-infrared radiation are applied to promote Raman mode excitation. Silver and gold, having particularly their plasmon resonance frequency values placed within these wavelength ranges, enable amplification of visible and near infrared light, so they are considered ideal for use in surface-enhanced Raman scattering spectroscopy. Figure 7 shows the application of surface-enhanced Raman scattering spectroscopy for the detection of contaminants present in a liquid food sample [95,96].

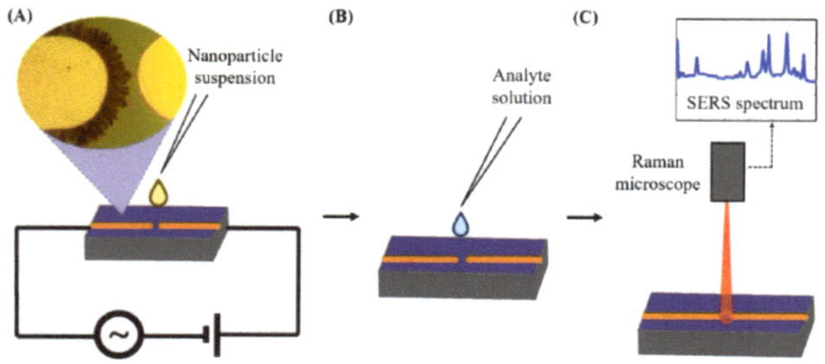

Figure 7. (**A**) Preparation of nanostructures. (**B**) Addition of the analyte solution to the microelectrodes' surface (**C**) Analyte detection by SERS, from [95,96], MDPI 2018, 2021.

2.3. Mass Sensitive Biosensors

These analytical devices use quartz crystal microbalance to record mass variation. They rely on the measurement of the changes occurring in the resonance frequency of a piezoelectric crystal due to mass variations in the crystal structure [97].

To develop these biosensors, the bioelement is coupled with a piezoelectric transducer, usually a gold electrode-coated quartz-crystal. Many types of materials (quartz, tourmaline, lithium tantalate or niobate, oriented zinc oxide, or aluminum nitride) can function as viable piezoelectric transducers. The vibration of these crystals can be induced at a specific frequency by applying an electrical signal of a specific frequency. Consequently, the oscillation frequency depends on the electrical frequency applied to the crystal and on the crystal's mass [98].

Nolan et al. [49] determined several mycotoxins (T2 mycotoxin, Fumonisin B1, and ZEN) with a mass sensitive biosensor. The lowest and highest T2 content in food ranged between 15 and 1000 ppb, for Fumonisin B1 between 200 and 4000 ppb, and for ZEN between 50 and 400 ppb. The most sensitive result obtained with the mass sensitive microarray analytical tool was 1.3 ng mL^{-1} for T2 in singleplex analysis based on the portable microfluidic device [49].

Figure 8 depicts an immunosensor relying on the use of a piezoelectric crystal as a transducer [99].

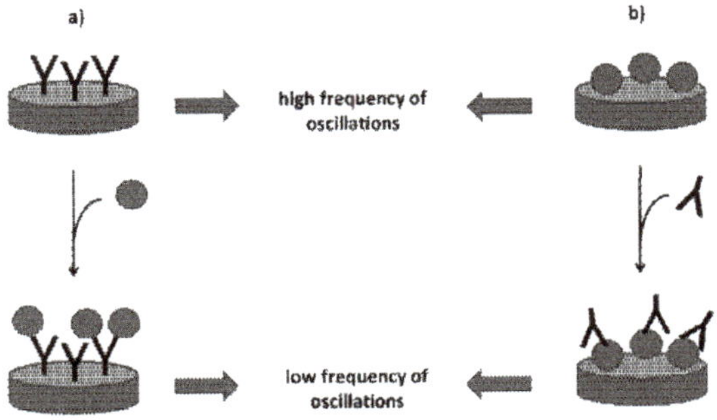

Figure 8. Representation of piezoelectric immunosensors for the determination of an antigen (**a**) or an antibody (**b**). The blue disc represents the piezoelectric crystal. The antibodies are depicted as Y letter, following the typical immunoglobulin shape; the red ball represents the antigen from [99], MDPI 2018.

2.4. Acoustic Biosensors

The functioning of acoustic wave sensors relies on the monitoring of the variations occurring in the physical characteristics of an acoustic wave imparted by the analyte's presence [50]. Piezoelectric materials are constituted of crystals devoid of a centre of inversion symmetry and presenting an intensified coupling between mechanical strain and electrical polarization. Such transducers currently exploited in acoustic sensors generate acoustic waves across solid materials using adequately balanced electrical fields. The acoustic waves are detected by the charge produced through induced mechanical deformation. Quartz is often employed, as it is available in high amounts, amenable to cost-effective manufacturing, and characterized by high mechanical properties and good chemical stability.

The functioning of these devices relies on the modulation of a physical property of the acoustic wave (acoustic velocity, resonant frequency, dissipation) that can consequently be related to the amount of adsorbed analyte. Acoustic wave devices are sensitive analytical tools that can detect a series of physical parameters (mass, pressure, temperature, etc.) [100]. Acoustic waves can be essentially classed into two main types, bulk acoustic waves (BAW) and surface acoustic waves (SAW), relying on the propagation of mechanical waves in piezoelectric materials [50].

In BAW sensors, the acoustic wave is propagated from one crystal surface to another, whereas in SAW sensors, it is propagated along a single crystal face from one location to another. Figure 9 presents a surface acoustic wave-based biosensor [45].

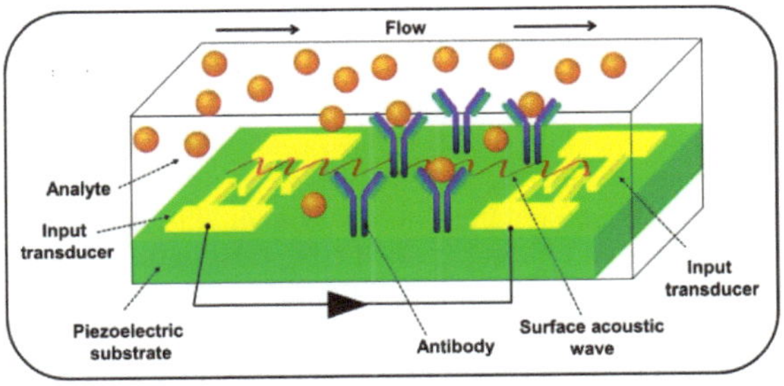

Figure 9. A surface acoustic wave (SAW)-based biosensor, from [45], MDPI 2021.

Juodeikiene et al. [101] used an acoustic spectrometer with transmission and an acoustic impulse spectrometer with transmission and reflection to assess the content of deoxynivalenol. The range of frequencies of 4.95 to 35.70 kHz was applied for the operation of the acoustic spectrometer, and the amplitude of the acoustic signal crossing the sample was monitored. A similar model has been exploited by employing the acoustic impulse spectrometer, where the amplitude of the reflected acoustic signal diminished with increasing DON concentration. The authors determined performance analytical characteristics such as relative standard deviation of repeatability for deoxynivalenol, with results ranging from 4.03 to 16.48%.

2.5. Thermal Biosensors

These sensors are based on the measurement of the temperature variations that occur during the biochemical reaction. Temperature sensors can be of two types: thermistors or thermopiles. Thermistors change their electrical resistance depending on the temperature, while thermopiles (metal or semiconductor-based structures) measure the temperature differences between two distinct areas [102,103].

In Figure 10, an enzymatic thermistor-based sensor is presented [45].

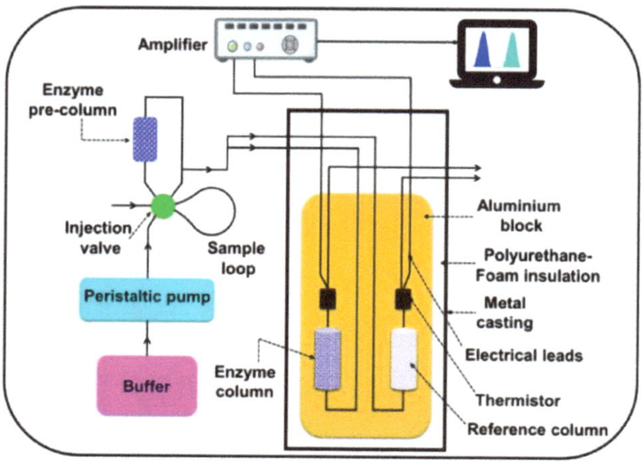

Figure 10. The detailed component parts of an enzyme thermistor-based biosensor, from [45], MDPI 2021.

3. Biomolecule Immobilization

Immobilizing and recognizing biomolecules can be performed directly on the transducer or on a support that is fixed on the transducer. This can be performed reversibly through adsorption, encapsulation, affinity binding, or irreversibly through entrapment, cross-linking, and covalent bonding. Another classification is determined by the method of immobilization: physical or chemical immobilization. The fixation on the surface of the support material must be stable and ensure the diffusion and exchange of electrons. In the case of adsorption, the interactions established can be Van der Waals, electrostatic, or other noncovalent bonds like hydrophobic interactions. Adsorption and encapsulation are classed as physical methods, whereas crosslinking and covalent bonding are chemical immobilization techniques [104]. Covalent binding, cross-linking, and entrapment are irreversible and impart stability, whereas adsorption and bioaffinity binding are reversible and do not bring cross-linker toxicity. Moreover, adsorption binding occurs fast but is less reproducible, and affinity interaction, though highly specific, can involve high costs [105].

Physical immobilization is much weaker than chemical immobilization due to weaker bonds established with the support. The support on which the biological recognition element is fixed can be inorganic (e.g., alumina, silica, zeolites, etc.), organic (polymers like polyketone polymers, acrylic resins, chitosan, cellulose, starch, carrageenans, etc.), or can be represented by nanoparticles (e.g., noble metals, magnetic nanoparticles, etc.). The support must be chemically and mechanically stable and insoluble [53,106]; its nature depends on the type of transducer, the immobilization method, the surface stability, etc. Following the immobilization of the recognition element on the support, an efficient transfer of electrons must be ensured.

Encapsulation is a method that uses the inclusion of the recognition element in a porous polymer network, in a sol-gel [104], or in lipids (liposomes) [106]. Sol-gel matrixes enable the entrapment of large enzyme amonts, are thermally and chemically stable, and are characterized by the easiness of preparation [104,107]. Affinity binding consists in binding the recognition element to a ligand through Van der Waals, hydrogen bridges, or electrostatic bonds [108]. Entrapment is based on the embedding of biomolecules in a polymeric gel network. Polyacrylamide, chitosan, starch, nylon, silastic gel, sol-gel-like polymers, etc. were used as polymers [109]. Cross-linking consists of fixing biomolecules via cross-linking agents, such as glutaraldehyde or hexamethylene diamine. A widely used immobilization technique is the fixation of biomolecules on the surface of the transducer through the layer-by-layer technique, which allows the deposition of a wide range of substances in thin films, layer by layer (alternatively), positively and negatively charged [110,111]. Incorporation of a broad variety of materials (metals, metal oxides, luminescent compounds, dyes) or biocompounds (proteins, aptamers, antibodies, antigens) into the multilayer structure, can lead to optimization of the sensing films' characteristics: selectivity, sensitivity, response time and dynamic range [110]. Essentially, the promotion of biosensing performance needs a transducer material to impart a good signal, and effective communication/connection between the biomolecules and the electrode surface must be obtained to enhance signal processing at the electrode surface [112].

4. Stability and Response Time of Biosensors

The stability of biosensors is a particularly important characteristic; the analyst should make use of reliable instruments, which, among other things, ensure good reproducibility over time, especially when dealing with commercial sensors. It was found that the analytical response of biosensors decreases over time, the stability being considered as shelf-life and as operational stability, depending mainly on the immobilization mode of the biological recognition element. Shelf life is related to the improvement in the activity retention of a biocatalyst under specific conditions of storage. Operational stability refers to the activity retention of a biocatalyst during its usage [113]. In addition to the immobilization method, other factors that determine stability are storage temperature, working environment (acidic or basic), ionic concentration, nature, and degradation of the biological element [114–116].

Improving the immobilization of the biological recognition element leads to an increase in the stability of the biosensor as well as an increase in sensitivity [117,118]. Also, depending on the nature of the biological element, Y. Alhamoud et al. found that the antibody is sensitive to pH, temperature, and ionic strength, with poor stability, the peptides are quite stable, and the aptamer is much more stable and has a longer life at room temperature [117]. These authors consider molecular imprinted polymers to be the most stable at high temperatures and pressures, with a long life.

Some electrochemical semiconductor biosensors have been improved in immobilization and the use of the most suitable mediator. The stability was evaluated for 9 weeks, the variation of the analytical signal in this interval being 6%. It was inferred that the semiconductor manufacturing electrochemical biosensor platform had a 94% stability [119].

Y. Zhang et al. [120], using an electrochemical biosensor based on carboxylated polystyrene nanospheres, an aptamer, and horseradish peroxidase assembled on a carbon nanofiber/carbon felt support for the determination of aflatoxin B1, found that after four weeks, recovery rates were reduced by 10.4% (Figure 11).

Zhao et al., building an evanescent optical fiber aptasensor, checked the reproducibility in 35 cycles that included the sequential injections of the blank (copy DNA only), 0.5%

sodium dodecyl sulfate (regeneration buffer at 1.9 pH value), and toxin sample (1 pM ZEN and copy DNA). The developed sensor was stable for use, undergoing proper regeneration for up to 28 cycles [121].

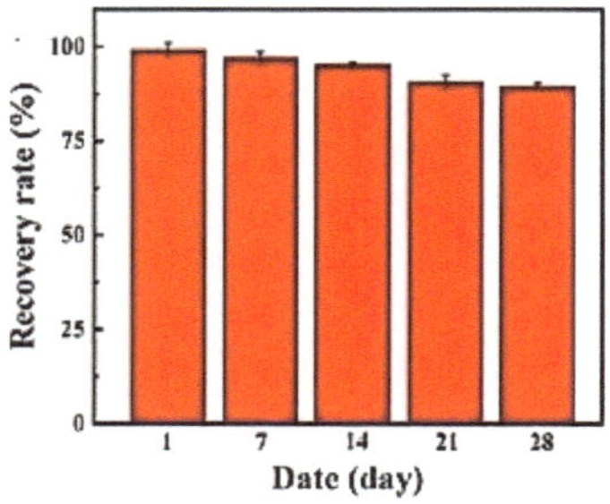

Figure 11. Stability of biosensor as a function of the time, from [120], MDPI 2022.

An aptasensor based on an anti-AFB1 aptamer with a methylene blue redox tag present at the 3′-end immobilized on the surface of a gold electrode allowed for the determination of AFB1 in 20 times diluted beer and in 50 times diluted white wine, the stability determined being one week after storage at 4 °C in phosphate buffer solution pH 7.5, containing $MgCl_2$ [122].

An aptasensor relying on electrochemical impedance spectroscopy as a transduction mode for the quantitation of FB1, AFB1, ZEN, and OTA present in the same corn flour sample was tested at 0, 7, 14, 21, and 28 days, respectively. The biosensing chip's analytical responses to FB1, AFB1, ZEN, and OTA after 28 days were 87.2%, 92.4%, 90.5%, and 92.7%, respectively, of their original levels [123].

Song and collaborators [124] highlighted the dependence of the stability of biosensors on the nature of the interface (the layer between the sensing elements and the electrode's surface), stressing the role of noble metal particles, along with carbon-based materials and polymers. Nanomaterials can mimic the activity of biocatalysts and can substitute bioenzymes, enhancing stability. Nanomaterials based on noble metals and alloys, as well as bimetallic nanocrystals, are endowed with high catalytic activities.

Given the variety of biorecognition elements, support materials, transducers, different immobilization methods, etc., it is very difficult to compare the performances of biosensors with each other, including regarding stability. In addition, the stability of a biosensor depends on storage conditions (dry or wet), the composition of the atmosphere (air or nitrogen), pH, the composition of the buffer, and the influence of matrix components [52]. The stability of the biosensor strongly influences the sensitivity; this is determined, along with the chemical stability of the biomolecules, by the transducer and the electronics of the device (amplification, signal processing) [125].

The response time of a biosensor differs from biosensor to biosensor and is defined as the time in which at least 90% of the value of the signal transmitted to the transducer is reached. The response time is influenced by many parameters related to the analyte, substrate, biological recognition system, hydrodynamic conditions, pH, temperature, etc. [52].

A novel sensitive graphene field effect transistor-aptamer sensor for OTA showed a response time as low as 10 s and proved more than 30 times faster when compared to other reported aptamer-based techniques for mycotoxin analysis [60].

Using a poly(2-hydroxyethyl methacrylate-co-aminoethyl methacrylate) hydrogel and an amperometric bioassay for Ochratoxin A based on NFO4 immobilized synthetic peptide for biorecognition, the maximum inhibition was obtained at 10 μg L^{-1} and the response time was less than one minute (50 s) [64].

An acetylcholinesterase-based conductometric biosensor allowed for the determination of aflatoxin B1 in 5 min, highlighted by the authors as much lower when compared to HPLC, ELISA, or TLC assay time (20, 40, and 60 min, respectively) [73].

Biosensors based on optical planar waveguides operating as polarization interferometers and imparting high sensitivity in the sub-ppt level had the analytical signal reported as a time-dependent phase shift, stabilized after 300 s [82]. Microfluidic paper-based analytical tools relying on specific aptamer-gold nanoparticles nanoconjugates allow for on-site assay of food toxins in less than one minute [126].

5. Analytical Performances of Biosensors Applied to Mycotoxins Quantitation

Table 2 shows the main performances of some biosensors used in the determination of mycotoxins in the last 5 years [49,60,62,68,73,82,85,87,120–123,126–170].

Table 2. Analytical performances at mycotoxin assay in various food matrixes by biosensors with different transduction modes [49,60,62,68,73,82,85,87,120–123,126–170].

No.	Mycotoxin	Matrix	Detection/Bioelement	LOD	RSD%	Linearity	Ref.
1.	AFB1	milk	colorimetric/aptamer	up to10 nM in spiked samples		1 pM–1 μM	[126]
2.	OTA, AFB1	peanut, barley	colorimetric/aptasensor		4.7–8.4 ng mL^{-1}	5–250 ng mL^{-1} (AFB1) 0.5–80 ng mL^{-1} (OTA)	[127]
3.	AFB1	rice, flour, seed, maize, pistachio	colorimetric/aptasensor			0–25 nM	[128]
4.	AFB1	spiked cattle feed samples	colorimetric/aptasensor	0.88 μg mL^{-1} (at 1:10 AuNP:aptamer ratio)		0–10 μg mL^{-1}	[129]
5.	AFB1	maize flour	colorimetric/aptasensors developed through in silico maturation and computational simulation approaches	0.1 and 0.5 ng mL^{-1}		0.1–50 and 0.5–50 ng mL^{-1}	[130]
6.	AFB1	foodstuffs	colorimetric and fluorescence/aptasensor	7.32 ng mL^{-1} (colorimetric) 1.48 ng mL^{-1} (fluorescence)	<13.3	10–320 ng mL^{-1} 3–320 ng mL^{-1}	[131]
7.	AFB1 FB1	whole grain samples (wheat and maize)	light reflectance spectroscopy/immunosensor	0.05 ng mL^{-1} (aflatoxin B1) 1.0 ng mL^{-1} (fumonisin B1)		0.1–5.0 ng mL^{-1} 2.0-50 ng mL^{-1}	[132]
8.	AFB1		optical planar waveguide operating as a polarization interferometer/aptasensor	0.7 pg mL^{-1}	mean standard deviation of phase shift as ± 0.5 rad	0.01–100 ng mL^{-1}	[133]
9.	ZEN		planar waveguide operating as a polarization interferometer/immunosensor	0.01 ng mL^{-1}		0.01–1000 ng mL^{-1}	[85]
10.	AFB1 OTA		optical planar waveguide operating as polarization interferometer/immunosensor	2 pg mL^{-1}		0.01–1111.11 ng mL^{-1}	[82]
11.	OTA	wheat and corn	fluorescence/aptamer	2.28 nM	6.08	10–5000 nM	[134]
12.	AFB1	rice sample extract	fluorescence/aptamer	0.05 nM		0.05–5 nM	[135]
13.	AFM1	milk powder	fluorescence/aptamer	0.05 μg kg^{-1}		0.2–10 μg kg^{-1}	[136]
14.	FB1, OTA	maize	fluorescence/aptamer	0.019 pg mL^{-1} (FB1) 0.015 pg mL^{-1} (OTA)		0.0001–0.5 ng mL^{-1}	[137]
15.	ZEN	cereal samples (maize, wheat, rye flour)	fluorescence/aflatoxin-smartphone-based molecularly imprinted polymer	1 μg mL^{-1}		1–10 μg mL^{-1}	[138]
16.	ZEN	spiked maize samples	fluorescence/immunosensor	20 pg mL^{-1}	3.0-9.0	0.05–0.5 ng mL^{-1} as dynamic range	[139]
17.	T2 toxin	barley sample	fluorescence/immunosensor	0.1 ng mL^{-1}	9.42–15.73	1–100 ng mL^{-1}	[140]
18.	PAT	apple juice samples	fluorescence/immunosensor	8.0 μg L^{-1}		0–150 μg L^{-1}	[141]
19.	OTA	coffee, tea, and corn	fluorescence/aptasensor	8 pg mL^{-1}		0.01–35 ng mL^{-1}	[142]
20.	AFB1	diluted beer and corn flour	fluorescence/aptasensor	61 pM		0.2–31.2 nM	[143]
21.	OTA	grain samples	luminescence/immunosensor	0.045 μg L^{-1}	<4.2	0.1–63 μg L^{-1}	[144]
22.	AFM1, AFB1	peanuts and pure milk	fluorescence/aptasensor	6.24 pg mL^{-1} (AFM1) 9.0 pg mL^{-1} (AFB1)	1.8–8.6	0.01–200 ng mL^{-1} (AFM1) 0.01–150 ng mL^{-1} (AFB1)	[145]
23.	OTA, PAT	apple juice samples	fluorescence/aptasensor	0.06 ng mL^{-1} (OTA) 0.09 ng mL^{-1} (PAT)	4.3-8.5 (OTA) 4.5–7.8 (PAT)	0.10–50 ng L^{-1} (OTA and PAT)	[146]
24.	AFB1, FB1, OTA, ZEN	three infant foods	chemiluminescence optical fiber/aptasensor	0.032 pg mL^{-1} 0.015 pg mL^{-1} 0.432 pg mL^{-1} and 0.275 pg mL^{-1}, respectively	<7.2	0.3–2 × 10^4 pg mL^{-1} 0.3–3.2 × 10^4 pg mL^{-1} 2.5–6 × 10^4 pg mL^{-1} 2.0–3.5 × 10^4 pg mL^{-1} respectively	[87]
25.	OTA	wine, beer	electrochemiluminescence/aptamer	0.012 nM	2.25–8.16	0.05–5 nM	[147]
26.	OTA		electrochemiluminescence aptasensor	0.03 ng mL^{-1}		0.1–320 ng mL-^{1}	[148]
27.	OTA, STG, ZEN, DON	aqueous solutions	bioluminescence/Photobacte rium phosphoreum cells immobilized in poly(vinyl alcohol) cryogel			0.017–56 mg L^{-1}, 0.010–33 mg mL^{-1}, 0.009–14 mg L^{-1}, 0.026–177 mg L^{-1}, respectively	[149]

Table 2. *Cont.*

No.	Mycotoxin	Matrix	Detection/Bioelement	LOD	RSD%	Linearity	Ref.
28.	ZEN	corn flour extract	nanoscale affinity double layer evanescent wave optical-fiber/aptasensor	2.31 fM		1 fM–100 pM	[121]
29.	OTA	coffee samples	surface plasmon resonance/monoclonal ochratoxin A antibodies	5.7 ng mL^{-1} for chitosan and 3.8 ng mL^{-1} for carboxymethyl chitosan as nanomatrix substrates	coefficient of variance in coffee 16%	0–50 ng mL^{-1}	[150]
30.	AFB1, OTA, ZEN, DON	corn and wheat	surface plasmon resonance/mycotoxin antigens	0.59 ng mL^{-1}, 1.27 ng mL^{-1}, 7.07 ng mL^{-1} and 3.26 ng mL^{-1} respectively	2.52 to 9.8	0.99–21.92 ng mL^{-1} 1.98–28.22 ng mL^{-1} 10.37–103.31 ng mL^{-1} 5.31–99.37 ng mL^{-1} respectively	[151]
31.	AFB1	milk and groundnut samples	photo-electrochemical/aptasensor	1 pg mL^{-1}	4.5 inter-assay	0.005–50 ng mL^{-1}	[152]
32	OTA	red wine samples	electrochemical-graphene field-effect transistors/aptasensor	1.4 pM		6 pM–100 pM	[60]
33	AFB1		amperometry at MWCNTs-modified Pt transducers/enzyme sensor	0.5 ng mL^{-1}	6.1%	1–225 ng mL^{-1}	[62]
34.	AFM1	spiked milk samples	chronoamperometry at SWCNTs-modified silver transducers/immunosensor	0.0259 µg L^{-1}		0.01–1 µg L^{-1}	[153]
35.	OTA	paddy rice-spiked samples	current-voltage measurements at electrospun cellulose acetate-doped 3D-graphene nanofibre transducers/aptasensor	156 fg mL^{-1}		1 fg mL^{-1}–1 ng mL^{-1}	[154]
36.	AFB1	rice milk	cyclic voltammetry at functionalized gold screen-printed transducers/imunosensor (anti-AFB1 antibodies)	50 fg mL^{-1}		50 fg mL^{-1}–5 ng mL^{-1}	[155]
37.	OTA	wheat	alternating current voltammetry at modified gold transducers/aptasensor	3.3 pg mL^{-1}	3.9–5.2	0.01–10 ng mL^{-1}	[156]
38.	AFB1, OTA	corn and wheat	alternating current voltammetry at modified gold transducers/aptasensor	4.3 pg mL^{-1} 13.3 pg mL^{-1} for AFB1 and OTA	3.2 (hairpin DNA-based aptasensor) and 6.5 (single stranded DNA-based aptasensor)	10–3000 pg mL^{-1} 30–10,000 pg mL^{-1} for AFB1 and OTA	[157]
39.	AFB1	maize flour samples	differential pulse voltammetry at poly(aniline-anthranilic acid) modified graphite screen-printed transducers/aptamer	0.086 ng mL^{-1}	5–10	0.1–10 ng mL^{-1}	[158]
40.	AFB1	human blood plasma pasteurized cow milk	differential pulse voltammetry at graphene oxide nanosheets modified glassy carbon transducers/aptasensor	0.07 nM	2.9	0.5 nM–4 µM	[159]
41.	PAT	patulin solution	differential pulse voltammetry at graphene oxide-gold nanocomposite transducer s/immunosensor	5 µg L^{-1}		10–200 µg L^{-1}	[160]
42.	AFB1, FuB1	spiked corn samples	differential pulse voltammetry at indium tin oxide transducers/molecularly imprinted polymer	0.313 and 0.322 pg mL^{-1} for AFB1 and FuB1	2.73	1 pg mL^{-1}–500 ng mL^{-1}	[161]
43.	AFB1, OTA	spiked wine samples	differential pulse voltammetry at phosphorene-gold nanocomposite transducers/aptasensor	0.023 (AFB1), 0.039 ng mL^{-1} (OTA)	6.9	0.05–10 ng mL^{-1}	[162]
44.	ZEN	corn powder samples	differential pulse voltammetry at glassy carbon transducers/aptasensor	3.1×10^{-12} mol L^{-1}		10^{-11}–10^{-6} mol L^{-1}	[163]
45.	DON	maize flour samples	differential pulse voltammetry at polyaniline-gold nanoparticles-graphite screen-printed transducers/aptasensor	3.2 ng mL^{-1}	5	5.0–30.0 ng mL^{-1}	[164]
46.	ZEN	*semen coicis* real samples	differential pulse voltammetry at polyethyleneimine-functionalized multi-walled carbon nanotubes nanocomposite transducers/aptasensor	1.0×10^{-5} ng mL^{-1}	1.37–1.61%	5.0×10^{-5} to 50.0 ng mL^{-1}	[165]
47.	AFB1	wine and soy sauce	pulse voltammetry at gold thin-film transducers/aptasensor	0.016 pg mL^{-1}	<3	0.1–10 pg mL^{-1}	[120]
48.	AFB1	beer, withe grape wine	square wave voltammetry at gold transducers/aptasensor	2 nM	<4	2 nM–4 µM	[122]
49.	ZEN	extract of maize grain	square wave voltammetry at gold transducers/aptasensor	0.017 ng mL^{-1}		0.01–1000 ng mL^{-1}	[166]
50.	OTA	red wine	square wave voltammetry at $NiCo_2S_4$ nanoparticle-dispersed MoS_2 nanosheets transducers/aptasensor	0.42 pg mL^{-1}		0.5 pg mL^{-1}–1 ng mL^{-1}	[167]
51.	FB1, AFB1, ZEN, OTA	spiked corn flour samples	impedance spectroscopy at gold nanoparticles—indium tin oxide transducers/aptasensor	2.47, 3.19, 5.38, 4.87 ng mL^{-1} for FB1, AFB1, ZEN, OTA, respectively	7.5, 8.2, 6.6 and 7.2 for FB1, AFB1, ZEN, OTA, respectively	5–1000, 10–250, 10–1250, 10–1500 ng mL^{-1} for FB1, AFB1, ZEN, OTA, respectively	[123]
52.	OTA	wine (red and withe), grape juices	impedance spectroscopy at gold nanoparticles-cysteamine-gold transducers/aptasensor	0.030 ng mL^{-1}	1.30–8.20	0.1–10 ng mL^{-1}	[168]
53.	OTA	spiked beer samples	electrochemical impedance spectroscopy at pencil graphite transducers/impedimetric aptasensor	0.1 ng mL^{-1}	3.49–4.95	0.1–2.0 ng mL^{-1}	[169]
54.	OTA		electrochemical impedance spectroscopy at 4-carboxyphenyl monolayer-gold transducers/immunosensor	0.5 ng mL^{-1}	5.8	1–20 ng mL^{-1}	[68]
55.	AFB1		conductometric at interdigitated thin film transducers fabricated by gold vapor deposition /enzyme sensor based on acetylcholinesterase	0.05 µg mL^{-1}	7	0.25–1 mM	[73]
56.	T2-toxin, ZEN, FB1 semiquanti tative detection	saliva	mass sensitive/immunosensor	6.1 ng mL^{-1}, 3.6 ng mL^{-1}, 2.4 ng mL^{-1} for T2, FB1 and ZEN (sensitivities reported as IC50 values in the multiplex analysis with the portable microfluidic device)	for each toxin coefficients of variation are all below 18	0.1–10 ng mL^{-1}	[49]
57.	AFB1	contaminated samples (peanut, pistachio, rice, and wheat)	quartz crystal microbalance sensor	2.8 pg mL^{-1}	3.67	0.05–75 ng mL^{-1}	[170]

6. Comparative Overview and Future Perspective

The conventional analysis methods (chromatography, ELISA, and immunoassay techniques) have been largely applied to mycotoxin detection in food but suffer from a series of limitations, such as laborious steps concerning sample preparation (that may imply grinding, mixing, and homogenization), extraction, and clean up procedures. The use of solvents, the requirement for skilled personnel, the high analysis cost, and the difficulty of collecting representative samples given the heterogenous character represent other drawbacks [171]. The inconsistency linked to food analysis by these methods could be reduced by increasing sample size, the degree of crushing, and the number of aliquots analyzed [172]. Moreover, the use of organic solvents might lead to antibody denaturation in the case of ELISA and immunoaffinity analysis [173].

Hence, biosensors are classed among the novel approaches to minimize the aforementioned drawbacks of the traditional analysis. One important advantage of biosensors over other rapid screening strip tests is their recycling use. Even if their application has been reported as straightforward when compared to laborious conventional techniques, the use of biosensors as analytical tools may still involve sample cleanup [171].

Biosensors, in general, have proven to be useful analytical tools through the performances they achieve, depending on the nature of the bioreceptor, the nature of immobilization support, the transducer, the matrix, etc.

Optical detection based on optical fibers, fluorescence, optical waveguides, or colorimetry has experienced a special development due to the progress made in the field of optical measurements [82,86,87,174]. Fluorescence detection has been used for both immunosensors and aptamers [175]. Immunosensors with optical detection can guarantee good sensitivity and specificity. Thus, Wu et al. [176] analyzed FB1, ZEN, OTA, and AFB1 with an immunochromatographic nanosensor based on gold nanospheres, characterized by accurate, fast, and sensitive visual detection, obtaining LOD values of 3.27, 0.70, 0.10, and 0.06 ng mL^{-1}, respectively. Fluorescence imparts a viable optical detection for mycotoxins [176,177] by using organic dyes (e.g., fluorescein, rhodamine, etc.) and other fluorescence sensing compounds, such as silica nanoparticles, organic polymers nanoparticles, Au, or Ag nanoparticles, etc. When determining AFB1 from peanut, corn, soy sauce, vegetable oil, or mouse feed with a fluorescence-based immunosensor, an LOD between 0.06 and 0.12 μg kg^{-1} was obtained [178], and when determining ZEN from beer and wine with an aptasensor, a LOD of 0.5 ng mL^{-1} was obtained [179].

The analytical signal can also be measured colorimetrically. If the recognition bioelement is an enzyme, the measurement is based on the enzymatic transformation of the chromogenic substrate into colored products, followed by optical analysis (naked eye, spectrophotometric, or colorimetric) [180]. The most used enzymes are horseradish peroxidase, acetylcholinesterase, G-quadruplex sequences, or deoxyribozymes. When determining AFB1 from peanut samples using G-quadruplex as a signal reporter, a very good sensitivity was obtained, namely an LOD of 1 pM. The mentioned advantages are low-cost, facility of detection (e.g., naked-eye detection), good selectivity, simple operation, wash-free, label-free format, and applicability to samples with complex matrices. The long incubation time, about 40 min, is mentioned as a disadvantage, which increases the analysis time [180,181]. Another disadvantage is the need for mycotoxin extraction from complex samples, with the possibility of interference with proteins, lipids, sugars, and salts [180]. For the simultaneous detection of AFB1, OTA, and ZEN, ELISA-based methods demonstrated high sensitivity and selectivity [182,183].

Gold nanoparticles used in colorimetric biosensors impart stability, sensitivity, accuracy, and repeatability. They can be employed as markers by coupling with antibodies or ligands through electrostatic adsorption and chemical bonds [125].

The shortcomings of optical sensors have been discussed, along with the possibilities of counteracting them. Colorimetry is considered as a non-expensive, portable, and useful technique. Nevertheless, it is limited to the assay of colored samples. Interferent species or matrix components imparting the same color can lead to erroneous results. Moreover, the technique is not highly sensitive, accurate wavelength bandwidth selection is necessary, and changes in source light intensity may lead to errors [184].

Fluorescent dyes suffer from limitations such as hydrophobicity and photobleaching, and the analytical response is highly pH-sensitive. Nanomaterials, such as quantum dots and carbon-based dots, served as a viable alternative to fluorescent dyes, exhibiting high quantum yield, very good photochemical stability, and adaptive photoluminescence [185–187]. Fluorescent lateral flow immunochromatographic assay technology integrates the convenient optical properties of fluorescent magnetic quantum beads and the inexpensive, portable, rapid, and versatile lateral flow immunochromatographic detection [187].

Hence, by integrating nanomaterials, fluorescence-based biosensors could hamper the drawbacks of diminished stability, increased background interference, and photobleaching, optimizing assay time and sensitivity. However, some shortcomings that may be encountered are interference from the environment and sample autofluorescence [125].

Also, elevated costs, laborious synthesis, and high heavy metals toxicity (Cd and Se) are some shortcomings that cannot be overlooked when working with quantum dots-based transducers. In recent years, carbonaceous quantum dots (carbon dots, graphene quantum dots, and graphene oxide quantum dots) proved biocompatible, inexpensive, and benefited from easy synthesis and low toxicity [187,188].

Chemiluminescent detection proved low detection limit and low background signal interference factors and employs a combination of biomolecules (recognition elements) to analyze target compounds by recording the analytical signal coming from the chemical probes; no external light source is required, and the technique benefits from sensitivity and broad calibration range. Biorecognition elements such as antibodies or aptamers can function as tracers in chemiluminescent biosensors [125]. Some drawbacks are limited antigen detection, a limited panel of tested toxins, low reagent stability, and elevated costs, and the assay is restricted to closed analytical systems.

Labeled surface-enhanced Raman spectroscopy is an indirect assay technology employed to detect and characterize biotoxins using organic molecules such as dyes endowed with high Raman activity in contact with the metallic surface instead of targeted analytes. Nevertheless, regarding high-quality surface-enhanced Raman spectroscopy, an active substrate is necessary, which should possess a large area of high-density hotspots, very good uniformity and signal reproducibility, and an elevated high enhancement factor [125].

Improvement of optical biosensors' performances encompasses the following: the use of efficient enrichment and separation techniques applied to complex trace samples; the introduction of novel nano-materials with large specific area, enhanced conductivity, and magnetic separation capacity, enabling the use of multiple recognition elements, accelerating the electron transfer or facilitating separation steps; the use of novel recognition elements with remarkable affinity, molecular stability, long life, repeatable use, resulting in selectivity and versatility of the analytical tool; the quest for modern nanomaterials with enhanced activity, diminished cost and outstanding stability to enable signal amplification, to replace expensive and unstable natural enzymes; developing biosensing arrays for simultaneous microbial toxin detection; the integration of microelectronics and microfluidics technology for obtaining high-throughput, portable, miniaturized optical biosensors for real time detection; coupling biosensors with other detection techniques such as spectrographic or chromatographic approaches, to ensure accuracy; also, including wireless communication, using smartphone, "cloud" computing and data storage systems, to be integrated into optical biosensors, enables the achievement of high-frequency online analysis for long periods [187]. Smartphones may be embedded with an optical chemical or biosensing base, and different filters, lenses, diffraction gratings, and alternative light sources may be accommodated to enhance signal detection in colorimetric, fluorescent assays, chemi- or bioluminescence, as well as scattering-based techniques [184].

By considering the above-mentioned aspects, using modalities of development that promote the advantages and overcome the limitations, it has been concluded that optical biosensors can constitute a viable alternative for food control, pharmaceutical analysis, and environmental monitoring [187].

Various novel developments in optical biosensors have been reviewed by Singh et al. Surface plasmon resonance-based biosensors were considered as the most broadly used, versatile, and prone to a wide range of applications: food analysis, pharmacy, medical diagnosis, or military defense [77]. They can be applied with the facility; nevertheless, they require initial training and are prone to automation and portability, with biochips being regenerated. Results are provided in real time, with no washing steps and no incubation periods. Nevertheless, biosensors of this type are expensive and can require labeling or elevated antibody concentrations to enhance sensitivity [49].

The progress in nanotechnologies and novel materials is presently leading to miniaturization and portability [77].

In novel studies, biotin-labeled aptamers were bound to the surface of streptavidin-coated magnetic nanoparticles. The use of hybrid nanomaterials led to the reduction of sample preparation and treatment, improved performances, and, eventually, circumvented false positive and negative analytical responses [128].

When determining mycotoxins with the help of electrochemical biosensors, Farré et al. [189] note the following advantages: low cost, simplicity, sensitivity and selectivity, miniaturization, and portability.

Among the electrochemical biosensors, some authors consider amperometric biosensors as the most broadly used, characterizing them as more competitive than conductometric or potentiometric ones, being more sensitive, cheaper, and more available [54]. Graphene-coated electrodes represent effective electrochemical transducers. Chronoamperometry allows fast assay, and it is considered as appropriate for assessing the repeatability and stability of electrochemical biosensors [190]. Majer-Baranyi and collaborators [191] also emphasize that electrochemical biosensors are the most broadly used due to the selectivity and sensitivity of the determinations and the advantages imparted by low cost, miniaturization, simplicity, and portability. The introduction of screen-printed electrodes brings great advantages in that they can be developed starting from different materials: Au, Ag, magnetic nanoparticles, graphene, or other carbon-based nanotubes [192–194]. Electrochemical biosensors allow analysis in colored, turbid, or viscous media using small amounts of sample [193]. Carbon-based nanomaterials, especially graphene, have good conductivity, large surface area (which allows the fixation of biomolecules), good chemical stability, and low price [194]. SWCNTs achieved the increase in the surface area of the working electrodes (like Ag paste printed electrodes), enabling the attachment of more bioelements such as antibodies and promoting the electrode's sensitivity [153].

Hence, nanomaterials are considered as appropriate carriers for biomolecules, such as enzymes, antibodies, aptamers, cells, and tissues. They have a high specific area and electroconductivity and are prone to easy modification, enabling the increase in the number and variety of immobilized biorecognition elements, leading to the simultaneous detection of multiple analytes. Nanomaterials can preserve the activity of biomolecules and enhance their physiological stability [195]. Gong et al. [195] discussed comparatively the performances of different types of nanomaterials. Gold nanoparticles have proved to be excellent transducers for developing electrochemical biosensors. Nevertheless, noble metals are expensive, and there is a request to improve nano-biosensor stability. Graphene-based sensors using various biorecognition elements (antibodies or aptamers) had a stable response over a storage period of 60-90 days. Sensors based on carbon nanomaterials (carbon nanotubes, graphene, or their derivatives) showed a reproducible analytical response. To develop sensitive, versatile transducers, functionalized carbonaceous materials (MWCNTs, SWCNTs) were used in combination with metal (Au, Pd, Pt) or metal oxide-based nanoparticles (magnetite, indium tin oxide), integrating polymeric materials (polypyrrole, polyethylene imine or polyaniline) to promote electrochemical performance. The incorporation of materials to be used as modifiers should consider aspects such as the degree of toxicity or biocompatibility [195].

The analytical performances of biosensors in which the recognition bioelements are antibodies, antibody fragments, and antigens were analyzed comparatively. Such biosensors are called immunosensors and are characterized by very good analytical performances, LOD having values of 0.05 ng mL^{-1} (electrochemical impedance spectroscopy, AFB1), 0.5 pg mL^{-1} (differential pulse voltammetry, ZEN), 8.6 ppb (differential pulse voltammetry, DON) [193].

Aptasensors represent a category of biosensors that use DNA or RNA molecules as biological recognition elements [196]. Aptamers contain, in length, up to 80 nucleotides capable of recognizing different analytes [117]. The aptamers impart very good results in the determination of mycotoxins. Beheshti-Marnani et al. [159] obtained an LOD of 0.07 nM for the electrochemical determination of AFB1. Guo et al. [197] discussed comparatively the performances of immunosensors with those of aptamers in the detection of mycotoxins, showing that aptamers are more efficient. Although immunosensors are highly specific, the elevated costs and storage stability of antibodies hinder their applications, so aptasensors benefit from a broader range of target compounds. Aptamers used in biorecognition represent single-stranded DNA or RNA oligonucleotides that induce aptamer/target complex formation with excellent affinity and specificity through conformational change. Among the qualities of aptamers, the authors mention better stability (temperature-induced denaturation is reversible), they can be stored/transported at room temperature, and they can detect a wide range of target substances with lowered production costs and in a short time. Qian et al. [123] demonstrated that aptamers resulted in excellent selectivity, repeatability, long-term stability, great simplicity and portability, easy operation, and multiple mycotoxins recognition. By exploiting the stable 2D structure of hairpin DNA to provide binding sites for the aptamers, a highly specific, sensitive, and reliable electrochemical aptasensor was developed based on dual-ratiometric simultaneous detection of AFB1 and OTA. An anthraquinone-2-carboxylic acid-labeled complementary DNA, a ferrocene-labeled AFB1 aptamer, and a methylene blue-labeled OTA aptamer were used to develop the sensing interface. The oxidation current of anthraquinone gave the reference signal, whereas ferrocene and methylene blue resulted in simultaneous response signals. In the presence of AFB1 and OTA, the recognition step resulted in the dissociation of both ferrocene-labeled and methylene blue-labeled aptamers from the electrode, resulting in the diminution of the signals proper to ferrocene and methylene blue, while the oxidation current of anthraquinone remained unchanged. The ratios between the current intensities, ferrocene to anthraquinone and methylene blue to anthraquinone, were then exploited for quantification of AFB1 and OTA, respectively [157].

Biosensors based on electrochemical impedance spectroscopy as transduction mode [66], are appreciated for their sensitivity, selectivity, and portability [66,67,198]. Thus, Kesici and Erdem [198] achieved a detection limit for FUM of 3.69 ng mL^{-1} with an impedimetric biosensor. Modification of the electrode surface at which biorecognition takes place, increased sensitivity and electrocatalytic activities, and the analyte can diffuse more rapidly on the surface of the electrode: the graphite electrode modified with nanofibers developed by electrospinning technique was used for the determination of T2 toxin, by voltammetry and electrochemical impedance spectroscopy, minimizing interferences in complex polluted matrixes [199]. Apart from the advantages of impedimetric detection, such as low detection limit, high stability and response reproducibility, versatility, broad linear range, reduced power requirement, portability, and high resolution, some authors also mention several disadvantages, such as short shelf life, sensitivity toward the changes occurring in the environmental conditions (temperature), high susceptibility to cross-sensitivity [200].

The comparative assessment of the largely used voltammetric detection methods is revealed in differential pulse voltammetry; the difference between the two current intensities (before the application of the pulse and at the end of each pulse) is quantified, and this procedure leads to minimization of the capacitive current in favor of the Faradaic current. The background current is significantly reduced, and the low capacitive current improves sensitivity. The small potential step sizes give narrower peaks than in cyclic voltammetry, favoring discrimination of analytes possessing similar or very close oxidation potentials.

As in the case of other potential step techniques, one shortcoming is the duration of the experiment, which is reported as being longer than in amperometry or ramping techniques such as cyclic voltammetry [201]. Given the low detection limits imparted and excellent sensitivity, the square-wave voltammetric technique is reported as prone to simultaneous multiple analyte biosensing [190]. Nevertheless, some authors consider that electrochemical sensors, mostly those using aptamers as bioelements, though simple, sensitive, fast, and cost-effective, still require signal amplification protocols for sensitivity increase. In a novel electrochemical assay, sensitivities of the order of pM were obtained using exonuclease I and branched hybridization chain reaction of the biorecognition element, promoting signal amplification for zearalenone differential pulse voltammetric detection [163].

Mass-sensitive microarray biosensors were characterized as very simple to use and prone to regeneration and reuse; by clearing the surface of the previous coating analyte, they allow multiple analyses. They necessitate small reagent and sample volumes, are relatively inexpensive, sensitive, and label-free, with results available in real time, and require no long incubation periods and no washing steps. Nevertheless, automated biosensors are costly (particularly in the case of non-portable devices), and in portable technology, one sample can be analyzed at a time [49].

The mentioned trends [123,125,191,202–204] for the improvement of detection with biosensors are related to the efficiency of biomolecules, the improvement of their fixation on the transducer, modifications brought to the surfaces or to the pH, the use of nanomaterials, the improvement of detection signals, the possibility of multi-analyte detection, miniaturization, portability. Aptamers, regardless of the detection modality, are considered extremely efficient and described as being superior to ELISA antibody technology, although the affinity of aptamers is considered, in general, weaker compared to that of antibodies [197]. ELISA [205] is considered by some authors like Matson [206] to be a biosensor. In some biosensors, this type of enzyme immuno-assay is integrated for key signaling [206].

The detection of mycotoxins based on a single analytical signal has proven, in some cases, due to matrix effects, to be false negative or false positive. For this reason, multimodal biosensors have appeared, which can generate different analytical signals, resulting in linearity increase and accuracy [125]. OTA was determined with a dual-readout electrochemical/visual (paper-based) aptasensor. The linearity ranges were 0.1–200 ng mL^{-1} (colorimetry) and 0.0001–200 ng mL^{-1} (electrochemistry) [207]. AFB1 was determined with a dual biosensor based on electrostatically mediated fluorescence resonance energy transfer and being exploited as a signal enhancement approach. In the presence of the analyte, the aptamer selectively binds to AFB1, leading to the aggregation of bare gold nanoparticles, promoted by the presence of sodium chloride. This eventually leads to a color change of gold nanoparticle solution from wine-red to purple, exploited in a colorimetric assay. Measured analytical signals were of colorimetric or fluorescent nature, obtaining linearity domains of 10–320 ng mL^{-1} and 3–320 ng mL^{-1}, respectively [131]. The AFB1 photothermal detection based on Cu2-xSe-Au nanoparticles enhanced the linear range and sensitivity (LOD of 0.00842 μg/L) when compared to the simple visual analysis methods [208].

Very good selectivity and elevated sensitivity were obtained by integrating the features of photoelectrochemical transducers (semiconductors and semiconductor-based nanoheterostructures incorporating graphene oxide, metal or metal oxide-based nanoparticles) and the high-affinity recognition elements such as molecularly imprinted polymers. Sensitivities below 1 pg mL^{-1} were obtained in the case of aflatoxin B1 and ochratoxin. Analytical protocols based on ratiometric detection were used to minimize unstability factors that may originate from the light source [209].

Recently, a highly sensitive and selective electrochemiluminescent aptasensor relying on a self-enhanced luminophore enabled the detection of ochratoxin A. Polyethyleneimine functionalized multi-walled carbon nanotubes decorated with gold nanoparticles served as electrochemical transducers to promote electronic transfer and represented an adequate microenvironment for self-enhanced luminophore loading and electrochemiluminescent analytical signal enhancement. The electron transfer distance was significantly shortened, as black phosphorus quantum dots and oxidized tris (2,2′-bipyridyl) ruthenium(II) were bound within one nanoparticle, hence optimizing electrochemiluminescent efficiency to reach the "switch-on" state. Then, the luminophore was quenched using ferrocenes, which corresponded to the "switch-off" state of the sensor. Excellent analytical parameters were achieved, such as sensitivity (0.03 ppb detection limit), stability, and reproducibility [148].

A novel automated reaction equipment and nanozyme-amplified immunosorbent assay were developed for accurate and sensitive determination of AFB1. Highly effective signal probes were coupled with the automated immunoassay equipment. Polystyrene nanoparticles served as signal carriers for loading a robust in situ-synthesized platinum/palladium nanozyme. The horseradish peroxidase-labeled goat anti-mouse antibody present on the surface of the nanozyme led to the generation of a bimetallic nanozyme-bioenzyme hybrid material with analytical signal enhancement. The reported analytical parameters showed a broad linear range of 10–10^4 pg mL^{-1} and sensitivity, with a low detection limit of 5.52 pg mL^{-1}, 65-fold lower than that obtained by ELISA [210].

Recently, wearable biosensors using various biorecognition elements have attracted increasing attention, employing accurate electrochemical and optical detection [211]. Considering the analytical performances of the biosensors, the simplicity, the possibilities of miniaturization and use of nanomaterials, of the in situ application, of increasing the stability, we think that these have become essential tools in the analysis of mycotoxins, alternatives to other much more expensive methods (e.g., HPLC-MS). Future trends imply quantifying more than one analytical parameter (using multimodal detection), employing nanomaterials whose optical and electrochemical features can be exploited with great facility, achieving sensitivity and fast response, applying automation, integrating hybrid materials, and applying signal amplification protocols for analytical response enhancement. Electrode materials with high surface area and incorporated modifiers should be environmentally friendly and are expected to achieve versatility by accommodating multiple bioelements for recognition.

Thus, a market of commercial biosensors has been developed, including for the determination of mycotoxins. The commercial products grow steadily. The market developed from 7.3 billion in 2013 to 18.6 billion in 2018, then to 26.8 billion in 2022, with an estimated worth of 34.3 billion in 2025 and 36.7 billion USD in 2026 [212–215].

Author Contributions: A.M.P.: Conceptualization, Validation, Writing—original draft, Writing—review and editing, Supervision. F.I.: Conceptualization, Validation, Writing—original draft. L.S.: Conceptualization, Supervision, Writing—original draft. E.M.: Supervision, Validation, Writing—review and editing. L.B.S.: Supervision, Visualization, Writing—review and editing. O.I.G.: Supervision, Visualization, Writing—review and editing. L.B.: Validation, Supervision, Writing—review and editing. A.I.S.: Conceptualization, Validation, Writing—original draft. All authors have read and agreed to the published version of the manuscript.

Funding: This research received no external funding.

Institutional Review Board Statement: Not applicable.

Informed Consent Statement: Not applicable.

Data Availability Statement: Not applicable.

Conflicts of Interest: The authors declare no conflicts of interest.

References

1. Bennett, J.W.; Klich, M. Mycotoxins. *Clin. Microbiol. Rev.* **2003**, *16*, 497–516. [CrossRef]
2. Dohlman, E. Mycotoxin hazards and regulations-impacts on food and animal feed crop trade. In *International Trade and Food Safety Economic Theory and Case Studies*; Buzby, J.C., Ed.; Agricultural Economic Report No. 828; United States Department of Agriculture: Washington, DC, USA, 2003; Chapter 6; pp. 97–108. Available online: https://www.ers.usda.gov/webdocs/publications/41603/15644_aer828_1_.pdf?v=0 (accessed on 4 February 2024).

3. Ostry, V.; Malir, F.; Toman, J.; Grosse, Y. Mycotoxins as human carcinogens-the IARC Monographs classification. *Mycotoxin Res.* **2017**, *33*, 65–73. [CrossRef]
4. Alshannaq, A.; Yu, J.-H. Occurrence, toxicity, and analysis of major mycotoxins in food. *Int. J. Environ. Res. Public Health* **2017**, *14*, 632. [CrossRef]
5. Awuchi, C.G.; Ondari, E.N.; Ogbonna, C.U.; Upadhyay, A.K.; Baran, K.; Okpala, C.O.R.; Korzeniowska, M.; Guiné, R.P.F. Mycotoxins affecting animals, foods, humans, and plants: Types, occurrence, toxicities, action mechanisms, prevention, and detoxification strategies—A revisit. *Foods* **2021**, *10*, 1279. [CrossRef]
6. da Silva, J.V.B.; de Oliveira, C.A.F.; Ramalho, L.N.Z. An overview of mycotoxins, their pathogenic effects, foods where they are found and their diagnostic biomarkers. *Food Sci. Technol.* **2022**, *42*, e48520. [CrossRef]
7. FAO; WHO. Codex Alimentarius-Codex General Standard for Contaminants and Toxins in Food and Feed (Codex Stan 193-1995). Available online: https://www.fao.org/fileadmin/user_upload/livestockgov/documents/1_CXS_193e.pdf (accessed on 8 March 2024).
8. Commission Regulation (EU). 2023/915 of 25 April 2023 on Maximum Levels for Certain Contaminants in Food and Repealing Regulation (EC) No 1881/2006 (Text with EEA Relevance). *Off. J. Eur. Union* **2023**, *L119*, 103–157. Available online: https://eur-lex.europa.eu/legal-content/EN/TXT/PDF/?uri=CELEX:32023R0915 (accessed on 20 December 2023).
9. US FDA—Chemical Contaminants, Metals, Natural Toxins & Pesticides Guidance Documents & Regulations, 2000–2010. Available online: https://www.fda.gov/Food/GuidanceRegulation/GuidanceDocumentsRegulatoryInformation/ChemicalContaminantsMetalsNaturalToxinsPesticides/default.htm (accessed on 15 December 2023).
10. Ministry of Health and Family Welfare (Food Safety and Standards Authority of India). Notification, New Delhi, the 7th August, 2020. In *The Gazette of India: Extraordinary, Part. III, Sec 4*; Ministry of Health and Family Welfare: New Delhi, India, 2020; pp. 18–30. Available online: https://www.fssai.gov.in/upload/notifications/2020/08/5f3d09f97b78aGazette_Notification_Limit_Metal_19_08_2020.pdf (accessed on 29 November 2023).
11. Stein, R.A.; Bulboacă, A.E. Mycotoxins. In *Foodborne Diseases*, 3rd ed.; Dodd, C.E.R., Aldsworth, T., Stein, R.A., Cliver, D.O., Riemann, H.P., Eds.; Elsevier: Amsterdam, The Netherlands, 2017; pp. 407–446. [CrossRef]
12. Ráduly, Z.; Szabó, L.; Madar, A.; Pócsi, I.; Csernoch, L. Toxicological and medical aspects of *Aspergillus*-derived mycotoxins entering the feed and food chain. *Front. Microbiol.* **2020**, *10*, 2908. [CrossRef]
13. European Commission, Health & Consumer Protection Directorate-General, Scientific Commitee on Food, the 119th Pleanry Meeting, Opinion on Fusarium Toxins. 1999. Available online: https://food.ec.europa.eu/document/download/62e47971-e232-4e39-a9d7-2e3429eb5957_en?filename=cs_contaminants_catalogue_fusarium_out44_en.pdf (accessed on 14 May 2024).
14. Puel, O.; Galtier, P.; Oswald, I.P. Biosynthesis and Toxicological Effects of Patulin. *Toxins* **2010**, *2*, 613–631. [CrossRef]
15. International Agency for Research on Cancer. Mycotoxins and human health. In *Improving Public Health through Mycotoxin Control*; Pitt, J.I., Wild, C.P., Baan, R.A., Gelderblom, W.C.A., Miller, J.D., Riley, R.T., Wu, F., Eds.; IARC Scientific Publication No. 158, E, 2012, Chapter 6; International Agency for Research on Cancer: Lyon, France, 2012; pp. 87–104. Available online: https://publications.iarc.fr/Book-And-Report-Series/Iarc-Scientific-Publications/Improving-Public-Health-Through-Mycotoxin-Control-2012 (accessed on 16 May 2024).
16. Ahmed Adam, M.A.; Tabana, Y.M.; Musa, K.B.; Sandai, D.A. Effects of different mycotoxins on humans, cell genome and their involvement in cancer (Review). *Oncol. Rep.* **2017**, *37*, 1321–1336. [CrossRef]
17. EFSA (European Food Safety Authority). *Outcome of a Public Consultation on the Draft Risk Assessment of Aflatoxins in Food*; EFSA Supporting Publication: Parma, Italy, 2020; p. EN-1798. 53p. [CrossRef]
18. Mohebbi, A.; Nemati, M.; Mogaddam, M.R.A.; Farajzadeh, M.A.; Lotfipour, F. Dispersive micro-solid-phase extraction of aflatoxins from commercial soy milk samples using a green vitamin-based metal-organic framework as an efficient sorbent followed by high performance liquid chromatography-tandem mass spectrometry determination. *J. Chromatogr. A* **2022**, *1673*, 463099. [CrossRef]
19. Shuib, N.S.; Saad, B. In-syringe dispersive micro-solid phase extraction method for the HPLC-fluorescence determination of aflatoxins in milk. *Food Control* **2022**, *132*, 108510. [CrossRef]
20. Romero-Sánchez, I.; Ramírez-García, L.; Gracia-Lor, E.; Madrid-Albarrán, Y. Simultaneous determination of aflatoxins B1, B2, G1 and G2 in commercial rices using immunoaffinity column clean-up and HPLC-MS/MS. *Food Chem.* **2022**, *395*, 133611. [CrossRef]
21. Maneeboon, T.; Chuaysrinule, C.; Mahakarnchanakul, W. Optimization and validation of dispersive liquid-liquid microextraction for simultaneous determination of aflatoxins B1, B2, G1, and G2 in Senna leaves and pods using HPLC-FLD with pre-column derivatization. *Toxins* **2023**, *15*, 277. [CrossRef]
22. Wang, Y.Z.; Hou, C.; Dai, Y.Q.; Chu, L.L.; Geng, S.W.; Zheng, S.L.; Kang, X.J. Determination of aflatoxin B1 by novel nanofiber-packed solid-phase extraction coupled with a high performance liquid chromatography-fluorescence detector. *Anal. Methods* **2023**, *15*, 472–481. [CrossRef]
23. Noori, H.; Feizi, J.; Eshaghi, Z. Development of a nanoparticle-assisted fabric phase sorptive extraction technique coupled with high-performance liquid chromatography for sensitive determination of aflatoxins in food samples. *Anal. Bioanal. Chem. Res.* **2023**, *10*, 121–134. [CrossRef]
24. Sartori, A.V.; de Moraes, M.H.P.; dos Santos, R.P.; Souza, Y.P.; Candido, F.S.; da Nobrega, A.W. Determination of aflatoxins M1, M2, B1, B2, G1, G2 and ochratoxin A in infant formulas from Brazil using a modified QuEChERS method and UHPLC-MS/MS. *Food Anal. Methods* **2023**, *16*, 841–849. [CrossRef]
25. Medina, M.L.J.; Lafarga, T.; Frenich, A.G.; Romero-Gonzalez, R. Natural occurrence, legislation, and determination of aflatoxins using chromatographic methods in food: A review (from 2010 to 2019). *Food Rev. Int.* **2021**, *37*, 244–275. [CrossRef]

26. Schincaglia, A.; Aspromonte, J.; Franchina, F.A.; Chenet, T.; Pasti, L.; Cavazzini, A.; Purcaro, G.; Beccaria, M. Current developments of analytical methodologies for Aflatoxins' determination in food during the last decade (2013–2022), with a particular focus on nuts and nut products. *Foods* **2023**, *12*, 527. [CrossRef]
27. Pisoschi, A.M.; Iordache, F.; Stanca, L.; Ionescu Petcu, A.; Purdoiu, L.; Geicu, O.I.; Bilteanu, L.; Serban, A.I. Comprehensive overview and critical perspective on the analytical techniques applied to aflatoxin determination—A review paper. *Microchem. J.* **2023**, *191*, 108770. [CrossRef]
28. Anfossi, L.; Giovannoli, C.; Baggiani, C. Mycotoxin detection. *Curr. Opin. Biotechnol.* **2016**, *37*, 120–126. [CrossRef]
29. Pisoschi, A.M.; Negulescu, G.P.; Pisoschi, A. Ascorbic acid determination by an amperometric ascorbate oxidase-based biosensor. *Rev. Chim.* **2010**, *61*, 339–344.
30. Pisoschi, A.M.; Pop, A.; Serban, A.I.; Negulescu, G.P. Ethanol determination by an amperometric bienzyme sensor based on a Clark-type transducer. *J. Electroanal. Chem.* **2012**, *671*, 85–91. [CrossRef]
31. Pisoschi, A.M. Biosensors as bio-based materials in chemical analysis: A Review. *J. Biobased Mater. Bioenergy* **2013**, *7*, 19–38. [CrossRef]
32. Ge, L.; Liu, Q.; Hao, N.; Kun, W. Recent developments of photoelectrochemical biosensors for food analysis. *J. Mater. Chem. B* **2019**, *7*, 7283–7300. [CrossRef]
33. Kurbanoglu, S.; Erkmen, C.; Uslu, B. Frontiers in electrochemical enzyme based biosensors for food and drug analysis. *TRAC Trends Anal. Chem.* **2020**, *124*, 115809. [CrossRef]
34. Wang, Y.; Zhai, H.; Yin, J.; Guo, Q.; Zhang, Y.; Sun, X.; Guo, Y.; Yang, Q.; Zhang, Y.; Li, F.; et al. Recent advances and future prospects of aptamer-based biosensors in food safety analysis. *Int. J. Electrochem. Sci.* **2022**, *17*, 22019. [CrossRef]
35. Kuswandi, B.; Hidayat, M.A.; Noviana, E. Paper-based electrochemical biosensors for food safety analysis. *Biosensors* **2022**, *12*, 1088. [CrossRef]
36. Li, W.; Xiao, F.; Bai, X.; Xu, H. Magnetic nanoparticles for food hazard factors sensing: Synthesis, modification and application. *J. Chem. Eng.* **2023**, *465*, 142816. [CrossRef]
37. Sadanandan, S.; Meenakshi, V.S.; Ramkumar, K.; Pillai, N.P.; Anuvinda, P.; Sreelekshmi, P.J.; Devika, V.; Ramanunni, K.; Sankar, R.J.; Sreejaya, M.M. Biorecognition elements appended gold nanoparticle biosensors for the detection of food-borne pathogens-A review. *Food Control* **2023**, *148*, 109510. [CrossRef]
38. Tetyana, P.; Morgan Shumbula, P.; Njengele-Tetyana, Z. Biosensors: Design, development and applications. In *Nanopores*; Ameen, S., Akhtar, M.S., Shin, H.-S., Eds.; IntechOpen: Rijeka, Croatia, 2021. [CrossRef]
39. Morales, M.A.; Halpern, J.M. Guide to selecting a biorecognition element for biosensors. *Bioconjug. Chem.* **2018**, *29*, 3231–3239. [CrossRef]
40. Takeda, K.; Nakamura, N. Biosensors: Enzyme Sensors. In *Encyclopedia of Sensors and Biosensors*; Ikebukuro, K., Ed.; Elsevier: Amsterdam, The Netherlands, 2023; Volume 1, pp. 297–381. [CrossRef]
41. Sharma, S.; Byrne, H.; O'Kennedy, R.J. Antibodies and antibody-derived analytical biosensors. *Essays Biochem.* **2016**, *60*, 9–18. [CrossRef] [PubMed]
42. Hua, Y.; Ma, J.; Li, D.; Wang, R. DNA-based biosensors for the biochemical analysis: A review. *Biosensors* **2022**, *12*, 183. [CrossRef] [PubMed]
43. Yoshimatsu, K. Biosensors: Biomimetic sensors. In *Encyclopedia of Sensors and Biosensors*; Ikebukuro, K., Ed.; Elsevier: Amsterdam, The Netherlands, 2023; Volume 1, pp. 393–404. [CrossRef]
44. Cieplak, M.; Kutner, W. Artificial biosensors: How can molecular imprinting mimic biorecognition? *Trends Biotechnol.* **2016**, *34*, 922–941. [CrossRef]
45. Naresh, V.; Lee, N. A review on biosensors and recent development of nanostructured materials-enabled biosensors. *Sensors* **2021**, *21*, 1109. [CrossRef] [PubMed]
46. Sumitha, M.S.; Xavier, T.S. Recent advances in electrochemical biosensors—A brief review. *Hybrid Adv.* **2023**, *2*, 100023. [CrossRef]
47. Meira, D.I.; Barbosa, A.I.; Borges, J.; Reis, R.L.; Correlo, V.M.; Vaz, F. Recent advances in nanomaterial-based optical biosensors for food safety applications: Ochratoxin-A detection, as case study. *Crit. Rev. Food Sci. Nutr.* **2023**, 1–43. [CrossRef] [PubMed]
48. Khorshid, M.; Sichani, S.B.; Cornelis, P.; Wackers, G.; Wagner, P. The hot-wire concept: Towards a one-element thermal biosensor platform. *Biosens. Bioelectron.* **2021**, *179*, 113043. [CrossRef] [PubMed]
49. Nolan, P.; Auer, S.; Spehar, A.; Oplatowska-Stachowiak, M.; Campbell, K. Evaluation of mass sensitive micro-array biosensors for their feasibility in multiplex detection of low molecular weight toxins using mycotoxins as model compounds. *Talanta* **2021**, *222*, 121521. [CrossRef] [PubMed]
50. Nair, M.P.; Teo, A.J.T.; Li, K.H.H. Acoustic biosensors and microfluidic devices in the decennium: Principles and applications. *Micromachines* **2021**, *13*, 24. [CrossRef]
51. Ramesh, M.; Janani, R.; Deepa, C.; Rajeshkumar, L. Nanotechnology-enabled biosensors: A review of fundamentals, design principles, materials, and applications. *Biosensors* **2023**, *13*, 40. [CrossRef]
52. Thevenot, D.; Toth, K.; Durst, R.; Wilson, G. Electrochemical biosensors: Recommended definitions and classification. *Biosens. Bioelectron.* **2001**, *16*, 121–131. [CrossRef] [PubMed]
53. Grieshaber, D.; MacKenzie, R.; Voeroes, J.; Reimhult, E. Electrochemical biosensors-sensor principles and architectures. *Sensors* **2008**, *8*, 1400–1458. [CrossRef] [PubMed]

54. Mehrvar, M.; Abdi, M. Recent developments, characteristics, and potential applications of electrochemical biosensors. *Anal. Sci.* **2004**, *20*, 1113–1126. [CrossRef] [PubMed]
55. Rameil, S.; Schubert, P.; Grundmann, P.; Dietrich, R.; Märtlbauer, E. Use of 3-(4-hydroxyphenyl)propionic acid as electron donating compound in a potentiometric aflatoxin M1-immunosensor. *Anal. Chim. Acta* **2010**, *661*, 122–127. [CrossRef] [PubMed]
56. Stepurska, K.V.; Soldatkin, O.O.; Arkhypova, V.M.; Lagarde, F.; Jaffrezic-Renault, N.; Dzyadevych, S.V. Development of novel enzyme potentiometric biosensor based on pH-sensitive field effect transistors for aflatoxin B1 analysis in real samples. *Talanta* **2015**, *144*, 1079–1084. [CrossRef] [PubMed]
57. Wadhera, T.; Kakkar, D.; Wadhwa, G.; Raj, B. Recent advances and progress in development of the field effect transistor biosensor: A review. *J. Electron. Mater.* **2019**, *48*, 7635–7646. [CrossRef]
58. Sadighbayan, D.; Hasanzadeh, M.; Ghafar-Zadeh, E. Biosensing based on field-effect transistors (FET): Recent progress and challenges. *TrAC Trends Anal. Chem.* **2020**, *133*, 116067. [CrossRef] [PubMed]
59. Hao, R.; Liu, L.; Yuan, J.; Wu, L.; Lei, S. Recent advances in field effect transistor biosensors: Designing strategies and applications for sensitive assay. *Biosensors* **2023**, *13*, 426. [CrossRef] [PubMed]
60. Nekrasov, N.; Jaric, S.; Kireev, D.; Emelianov, A.V.; Orlov, A.V.; Gadjanski, I.; Nikitin, P.I.; Akinwande, D.; Bobrinetskiy, I. Real-time detection of ochratoxin A in wine through insight of aptamer conformation in conjunction with graphene field-effect transistor. *Biosens. Bioelectron.* **2022**, *200*, 113890. [CrossRef]
61. Nguyen, H.H.; Lee, S.H.; Lee, U.J.; Fermin, C.D.; Kim, M. Immobilized enzymes in biosensor applications. *Materials* **2019**, *12*, 121. [CrossRef]
62. Li, S.C.; Chen, J.H.; Cao, H.; Yao, D.S.; Liu, D.L. Amperometric biosensor for aflatoxin B1 based on aflatoxin-oxidase immobilized on multiwalled carbon nanotubes. *Food Control* **2011**, *22*, 43–49. [CrossRef]
63. Vidal, J.C.; Bonel, L.; Ezquerra, A.; Hernández, S.; Bertolín, J.R.; Cubel, C.; Castillo, J.R. Electrochemical affinity biosensors for detection of mycotoxins: A review. *Biosens. Bioelectron.* **2013**, *49*, 146–158. [CrossRef] [PubMed]
64. Tria, S.A.; Lopez-Ferber, D.; Gonzalez, C.; Bazin, I.; Guiseppi-Elie, A. Microfabricated biosensor for the simultaneous amperometric and luminescence detection and monitoring of Ochratoxin A. *Biosens. Bioelectron.* **2016**, *79*, 835–842. [CrossRef] [PubMed]
65. Bahadir, E.B.; Sezgintürk, M.K. A review on impedimetric biosensors. *Artif. Cells Nanomed. Biotechnol.* **2016**, *44*, 248–262. [CrossRef] [PubMed]
66. Magar, H.S.; Hassan, R.Y.A.; Mulchandani, A. Electrochemical impedance spectroscopy (EIS): Principles, construction, and biosensing applications. *Sensors* **2021**, *21*, 6578. [CrossRef] [PubMed]
67. Lazanas, A.C.; Prodomidis, M.I. Electrochemical impedance spectroscopy—A tutorial. *ACS Meas. Sci. Au* **2023**, *3*, 162–193. [CrossRef]
68. Radi, A.E.; Muñoz-Berbel, X.; Lates, V.; Marty, J.L. Label-free impedimetric immunosensor for sensitive detection of ochratoxin A. *Biosens. Bioelectron.* **2009**, *24*, 1888–1892. [CrossRef] [PubMed]
69. Malvano, F.; Albanese, D.; Crescitelli, A.; Pilloton, R.; Esposito, E. Impedimetric label-free immunosensor on disposable modified screen-printed electrodes for Ochratoxin A. *Biosensors* **2016**, *6*, 33. [CrossRef]
70. Dzyadevych, S.; Jaffrezic-Renault, N. Conductometric biosensors. In *Biological Identification*; Paul Schaudies, R., Ed.; Elsevier: Amsterdam, The Netherlands, 2014; pp. 153–193. [CrossRef]
71. Adley, C.C.; Ryan, M.P. Conductometric biosensors for high throughput screening of pathogens in food. In *High Throughput Screening for Food Safety Assessment Biosensor Technologies, Hyperspectral Imaging and Practical Applications*; Bhunia, A.K., Kim Moon, S., Taitt, C.R.T., Eds.; Elsevier: Amsterdam, The Netherlands, 2015; pp. 315–326. [CrossRef]
72. Bahadır, E.B.; Sezgintürk, M.K. Electrochemical biosensors for hormone analyses. *Biosens. Bioelectron.* **2015**, *68*, 62–71. [CrossRef]
73. Soldatkin, O.O.; Burdak, O.S.; Sergeyeva, T.A.; Arkhypova, V.M.; Dzyadevycha, S.V.; Soldatkin, A.P. Acetylcholinesterase-based conductometric biosensor for determination of aflatoxin B1. *Sens. Actuators B Chem.* **2013**, *188*, 999–1003. [CrossRef]
74. Soldatkin, O.O.; Stepurska, K.V.; Arkhypova, V.M.; Soldatkin, A.P.; El'skaya, A.V.; Lagarde, F.; Dzyadevych, S.V. Conductometric enzyme biosensor for patulin determination. *Sens. Actuators B Chem.* **2017**, *239*, 1010–1015. [CrossRef]
75. Damborský, P.; Švitel, J.; Katrlík, J. Optical biosensors. *Essays Biochem.* **2016**, *60*, 91–100. [CrossRef] [PubMed]
76. Samuel, V.R.; Jagajjanani Rao, K. A review on label free biosensors. *Biosens. Bioelectron. X* **2022**, *11*, 100216. [CrossRef]
77. Singh, A.K.; Mittal, S.; Das, M.; Saharia, A.; Tiwari, M. Optical biosensors: A decade in review. *Alex. Eng. J.* **2023**, *67*, 673–691. [CrossRef]
78. Sun, Y.; Fan, X. Optical ring resonators for biochemical and chemical sensing. *Anal. Bioanal. Chem.* **2011**, *399*, 205–211. [CrossRef] [PubMed]
79. Sarkaleh, A.K.; Lahijani, B.V.; Saberkari, H.; Esmaeeli, A. Optical ring resonators: A platform for biological sensing applications. *J. Med. Signals Sens.* **2017**, *7*, 185–191. [CrossRef] [PubMed]
80. Xu, Y.; Xiong, M.; Yan, H. A portable optical fiber biosensor for the detection of zearalenone based on the localized surface plasmon resonance. *Sens. Actuators B Chem.* **2021**, *336*, 129752. [CrossRef]
81. Campell, D.P. Interferometric biosensors. In *Principles of Bacterial Detection: Biosensors, Recognition Receptors and Microsystems*; Zourob, M., Elwary, S., Turner, A., Eds.; Springer: New York, NY, USA, 2008; pp. 169–211. [CrossRef]
82. Nabok, A.; Al-Rubaye, A.G.; Al-Jawdah, A.M.; Tsargorodska, A.; Marty, J.-L.; Catanante, G.; Szekacs, A.; Takacs, E. Novel optical biosensing technologies for detection of mycotoxins. *Opt. Laser Technol.* **2019**, *109*, 212–221. [CrossRef]

83. Kozma, P.; Kehl, F.; Ehrentreich-Förster, E.; Stamm, C.; Bier, F.F. Integrated planar optical waveguide interferometer biosensors: A comparative review. *Biosens. Bioelectron.* **2014**, *58*, 287–307. [CrossRef]
84. Lin, Y.C.; Chen, L.Y. Subtle application of electrical field-induced lossy mode resonance to enhance performance of optical planar waveguide biosensor. *Biosensors* **2021**, *11*, 86. [CrossRef]
85. Nabok, A.; Al-Jawdah, A.M.; Gémes, B.; Takács, E.; Székács, A. An optical planar waveguide-based immunosensors for determination of fusarium mycotoxin zearalenone. *Toxins* **2021**, *13*, 89. [CrossRef]
86. Al-Jawdah, A.; Nabok, A.; Jarrah, R.; Holloway, A.; Tsargorodska, A.; Takacs, E.; Szekacs, A. Mycotoxin biosensor based on optical planar waveguide. *Toxins* **2018**, *10*, 272. [CrossRef] [PubMed]
87. Jia, Y.; Zhao, S.; Li, D.; Yang, J.; Yang, L. Portable chemiluminescence optical fiber aptamer-based biosensors for analysis of multiple mycotoxins. *Food Control* **2023**, *144*, 109361. [CrossRef]
88. Li, S.; Zhong, X.; Xu, Y.; Zheng, Y.; Shi, X.; Li, F.; Guo, S.; Yang, J. Smartphone-based reading system integrated with phycocyanin-enhanced latex nanospheres immunoassay for on-site determination of aflatoxin b1 in foodstuffs. *Food Chem.* **2021**, *360*, 130019. [CrossRef] [PubMed]
89. Kłos-Witkowska, A. Enzyme-based fluorescent biosensors and their environmental, clinical and industrial applications. *Pol. J. Environ. Stud.* **2015**, *24*, 19–25. [CrossRef]
90. Selvin, P.R. The renaissance of fluorescence resonance energy transfer. *Nat. Struct. Mol. Biol.* **2000**, *7*, 730–734. [CrossRef]
91. Das, A.P.; Kumar, P.S.; Swain, S. Recent advances in biosensor based endotoxin detection. *Biosens. Bioelectron.* **2014**, *51*, 62. [CrossRef]
92. Nawrot, W.; Drzozga, K.; Baluta, S.; Cabaj, J.; Malecha, K. A Fluorescent Biosensors for Detection Vital Body Fluids' Agents. *Sensors* **2018**, *18*, 2357. [CrossRef]
93. Tan, H.; Ma, L.; Guo, T.; Zhou, H.; Chen, L.; Zhang, Y.; Dai, H.; Yu, Y. A novel fluorescence aptasensor based on mesoporous silica nanoparticles for selective and sensitive detection of aflatoxin B1. *Anal. Chim. Acta* **2019**, *1068*, 87–95. [CrossRef]
94. Ebanks, F.; Nasrallah, H.; Garant, T.M.; McConnell, E.M.; DeRosa, M.C. Colorimetric detection of aflatoxins B1 and M1 using aptamers and gold and silver nanoparticles. *Adv. Agrochem.* **2023**, *2*, 221–230. [CrossRef]
95. Dies, H.; Siampani, M.; Escobedo, C.; Docoslis, A. Direct detection of toxic contaminants in minimally processed food products using dendritic surface-enhanced Raman scattering substrates. *Sensors* **2018**, *18*, 2726. [CrossRef]
96. Petersen, M.; Yu, Z.; Lu, X. Application of Raman spectroscopic methods in food safety: A review. *Biosensors* **2021**, *11*, 187. [CrossRef]
97. Mehrotra, P. Biosensors and their applications—A review. *J. Oral Biol. Craniofac. Res.* **2016**, *6*, 153–159. [CrossRef]
98. Monošík, R.; Streďanský, M.; Šturdík, E. Biosensors—Classification, characterization and new trends. *Acta Chim. Slovaca* **2012**, *5*, 109–120. [CrossRef]
99. Pohanka, M. Overview of piezoelectric biosensors, immunosensors and DNA sensors and their applications. *Materials* **2018**, *11*, 448. [CrossRef] [PubMed]
100. Fogel, R.; Limson, J.; Seshia, A.A. Acoustic biosensors. *Essays Biochem.* **2016**, *60*, 101–110. [CrossRef] [PubMed]
101. Juodeikiene, G.; Basinskiene, L.; Vidmantiene, D.; Bartkiene, E.; Kunigelis, V.; de Koe, W.J. Rapid acoustic screening of deoxynivalenol (DON) in grain. *World Mycotoxin J.* **2008**, *1*, 267–274. [CrossRef]
102. Ramanathan, K.; Danielsson, B. Principles and applications of thermal biosensors. *Biosens. Bioelectron.* **2001**, *16*, 417–423. [CrossRef]
103. Vasuki, S.; Varsha, V.; Mithra, R.; Dharshni, R.A.; Abinaya, S.; Dharshini, R.D.; Sivarajasekar, N. Thermal biosensors and their applications. *Am. Int. J. Res. Sci. Technol. Eng. Math.* **2019**, *1*, 262–264. Available online: http://iasir.net/AIJRSTEMpapers/IBCFT-2019.pdf (accessed on 12 January 2024).
104. Bhardwaj, T. Review on immobilization techniques of biosensors. *Int. J. Eng. Res. Technol.* **2014**, *3*, 294–298.
105. Liébana, S.; Drago, G.A. Bioconjugation and stabilisation of biomolecules in biosensors. *Essays Biochem.* **2016**, *60*, 59–68. [CrossRef]
106. Homaei, A.A.; Sariri, R.; Vianello, F.; Stevanato, R. Enzyme immobilization: An update. *J. Chem. Biol.* **2013**, *6*, 185–205. [CrossRef] [PubMed]
107. Martinkova, P.; Kostelnik, A.; Valek, T.; Pohanka, M. Main streams in the construction of biosensors and their applications. *Int. J. Electrochem. Sci.* **2017**, *12*, 7386–7403. [CrossRef]
108. Frutiger, A.; Tanno, A.; Hwu, S.; Tiefenauer, R.F.; Vörös, J.; Nakatsuka, N. Nonspecific binding fundamental concepts and consequences for biosensing applications. *Chem. Rev.* **2021**, *121*, 8095–8160. [CrossRef] [PubMed]
109. Asal, M.; Özen, Ö.; Sahinler, M.; Baysal, H.T.; Polatoglu, I. An overview of biomolecules, immobilization methods and support materials of biosensors. *Sens. Rev.* **2019**, *39*, 377–386. [CrossRef]
110. Rivero, P.J.; Goicoechea, J.; Arregui, F.J. Layer-by-layer nano-assembly: A powerful tool for optical fiber sensing applications. *Sensors* **2019**, *19*, 683. [CrossRef] [PubMed]
111. Campbell, J.; Vikulina, A.S. Layer-by-layer assemblies of biopolymers: Build-up, mechanical stability and molecular dynamics. *Polymers* **2020**, *12*, 1949. [CrossRef] [PubMed]
112. Iost, R.M.; Crespilho, F.N. Layer-by-layer self-assembly and electrochemistry: Applications in biosensing and bioelectronics. *Biosens. Bioelectron.* **2012**, *31*, 1–10. [CrossRef]
113. Gibbson, T.D. Biosensors: The stability problem. *Analusis* **1999**, *27*, 630–638. [CrossRef]
114. Bhalla, N.; Jolly, P.; Formisano, N.; Estrela, P. Introduction to biosensors. *Essays Biochem.* **2016**, *60*, 1–8. [CrossRef]

115. Panjan, P.; Ohtonen, E.; Tervo, P.; Virtanen, V.; Sesay, A.M. Shelf life of enzymatic electrochemical sensors. *Proc. Technol.* **2017**, *27*, 306–308. [CrossRef]
116. Puggioni, G.; Calia, G.; Arrigo, P.; Bacciu, A.; Bazzu, G.; Migheli, R.; Fancello, S.; Serra, P.A.; Rocchitta, G. Low-temperature storage improves the over-time stability of implantable glucose and lactate biosensors. *Sensors* **2019**, *19*, 422. [CrossRef] [PubMed]
117. Alhamoud, Y.; Yang, D.; Kenston, S.S.F.; Liu, G.; Liu, L.; Zhou, H.; Ahmed, F.; Zhao, J. Advances in biosensors for the detection of ochratoxin A: Bio-receptors, nanomaterials, and their applications. *Biosens. Bioelectron.* **2019**, *141*, 111418. [CrossRef] [PubMed]
118. Zhai, W.; Wei, D.; Cao, M.; Wang, Z.; Wang, M. Biosensors based on core–shell nanoparticles for detecting mycotoxins in food: A review. *Food Chem.* **2023**, *429*, 136944. [CrossRef] [PubMed]
119. Chen, L.C.; Wang, E.; Tai, C.S.; Chiu, Y.C.; Li, C.W.; Lin, Y.R.; Lee, T.H.; Huang, C.W.; Chen, J.C.; Chen, W.L. Improving the reproducibility, accuracy, and stability of an electrochemical biosensor platform for point-of-care use. *Biosens. Bioelectron.* **2020**, *155*, 112111. [CrossRef] [PubMed]
120. Zhang, Y.; Lin, T.; Shen, Y.; Li, H. A high-performance self-supporting electrochemical biosensor to detect Aflatoxin B1. *Biosensors* **2022**, *12*, 897. [CrossRef] [PubMed]
121. Zhao, H.; Ren, S.; Wei, Z.; Lou, X. Evanescent wave optical-fiber aptasensor for rapid detection of zearalenone in corn with unprecedented sensitivity. *Biosensors* **2022**, *12*, 438. [CrossRef] [PubMed]
122. Wang, C.; Li, Y.P.; Zhao, Q. A signal-on electrochemical aptasensor for rapid detection of aflatoxin B1 based on competition with complementary DNA. *Biosens. Bioelectron.* **2019**, *144*, 111641. [CrossRef]
123. Qian, J.; Liu, Y.; Cui, H.; Yang, H.; Hussain, M.; Wang, K.; Wei, J.; Long, L.; Ding, L.; Wang, C. Fabrication of a disposable aptasensing chip for simultaneous label-free detection of four common coexisting mycotoxins. *Anal. Chim. Acta* **2023**, *1282*, 341921. [CrossRef]
124. Song, M.; Lin, X.; Peng, Z.; Xu, S.; Jin, L.; Zheng, X.; Luo, H. Materials and methods of biosensor interfaces with stability. *Front. Mater.* **2021**, *7*, 583739. [CrossRef]
125. Tang, X.; Zuo, J.; Yang, C.; Jiang, J.; Zhang, Q.; Ping, J.; Li, P. Current trends in biosensors for biotoxins (mycotoxins, marine toxins, and bacterial food toxins): Principles, application, and perspective. *TRAC Trends Anal. Chem.* **2023**, *165*, 117144. [CrossRef]
126. Kasoju, A.; Shrikrishna, N.S.; Shahdeo, D.; Khan, A.A.; Alanazi, A.M.; Gandhi, S. Microfluidic paper device for rapid detection of aflatoxin B1 using an aptamer based colorimetric assay. *RSC Adv.* **2020**, *10*, 11843–11850. [CrossRef] [PubMed]
127. Zhu, W.; Li, L.; Zhou, Z.; Yang, X.; Hao, N.; Guo, Y.; Wang, K. A colorimetric biosensor for simultaneous ochratoxin A and aflatoxins B1 detection in agricultural products. *Food Chem.* **2020**, *319*, 126544. [CrossRef] [PubMed]
128. Rafati, A.; Dorosti, N.; Gil, P. Smartphone-based technology for nanomolecular detection of aflatoxin B1 by aptamer-conjugated magnetic nanoparticles. *World Mycotoxin J.* **2022**, *15*, 159–169. [CrossRef]
129. Contreras-Trigo, B.; Diaz-Garcia, V.; Oyarzun, P. A novel preanalytical strategy enabling application of a colorimetric nanoaptasensor for on-site detection of AFB1 in cattle feed. *Sensors* **2022**, *22*, 9280. [CrossRef] [PubMed]
130. Mousivand, M.; Javan-Nikkhah, M.; Anfossi, L.; Di Nardo, F.; Salina, M.; Bagherzadeh, K. High performance aptasensing platform development through in silico aptamer engineering for aflatoxin B1 monitoring. *Food Control* **2023**, *145*, 109418. [CrossRef]
131. Xiong, J.; He, S.; Qin, L.; Zhang, S.; Shan, W.; Jiang, H. Aptasensor-based assay for dual-readout determination of aflatoxin B1 in corn and wheat via an electrostatic force-mediated FRET strategy. *Microchim. Acta* **2023**, *190*, 80. [CrossRef] [PubMed]
132. Anastasiadis, V.; Koukouvinos, G.; Petrou, P.S.; Economou, A.; Dekker, J.; Harjanne, M.; Heimala, P.; Goustouridis, D.; Raptis, I.; Kakabakos, S.E. Multiplexed mycotoxins determination employing white light reflectance spectroscopy and silicon chips with silicon oxide areas of different thickness. *Biosens. Bioelectron.* **2020**, *153*, 112035. [CrossRef]
133. Al-Jawdah, A.; Nabok, A.; Abu-Ali, H.; Catanante, G.; Marty, J.-L.; Szekacs, A. Highly sensitive label-free in vitro detection of aflatoxin B1 in an aptamer assay using optical planar waveguide operating as a polarization interferometer. *Anal. Bioanal. Chem.* **2019**, *411*, 7717–7724. [CrossRef]
134. Wang, C.; Tan, R.; Li, J. Exonuclease I-assisted fluorescent method for ochratoxin A detection using iron-doped porous carbon, nitrogen-doped graphene quantum dots, and double magnetic separation. *Anal. Bioanal. Chem.* **2019**, *411*, 2405–2414. [CrossRef]
135. Ye, H.; Lu, Q.; Duan, N.; Wang, Z. GO-amplified fluorescence polarization assay for high-sensitivity detection of aflatoxin B1 with low dosage aptamer probe. *Anal. Bioanal. Chem.* **2019**, *411*, 1107–1115. [CrossRef] [PubMed]
136. Guo, X.; Wen, F.; Qiao, Q.; Zheng, N.; Saive, M.; Fauconnier, M.-L.; Wang, J. A novel graphene oxide-based aptasensor for amplified fluorescent detection of Aflatoxin M1 in milk powder. *Sensors* **2019**, *19*, 3840. [CrossRef] [PubMed]
137. Niazi, S.; Khan, I.M.; Yan, L.; Khan, M.I.; Mohsin, A.; Duan, N.; Wu, S.; Wang, Z. Simultaneous detection of fumonisin B1 and ochratoxin a using dual-color, time-resolved luminescent nanoparticles ($NaYF_4$: Ce, Tb and NH_2-Eu/DPA@SiO_2) as labels. *Anal. Bioanal. Chem.* **2019**, *411*, 1453–1465. [CrossRef] [PubMed]
138. Sergeyeva, T.; Yarynka, D.; Dubey, L.; Dubey, I.; Piletska, E.; Linnik, R.; Antonyuk, M.; Ternovska, T.; Brovko, O.; Piletsky, S.; et al. Sensor based on molecularly imprinted polymer membranes and smartphone for detection of Fusarium contamination in cereals. *Sensors* **2020**, *20*, 4304. [CrossRef] [PubMed]
139. Peltomaa, R.; Farka, Z.; Mickert, M.J.; Brandmeier, J.C.; Pastucha, M.; Hlaváček, A.; Martínez-Orts, M.; Canales, Á.; Skládal, P.; Benito-Peña, E.; et al. Competitive upconversion-linked immunoassay using peptide mimetics for the detection of the mycotoxin zearalenone. *Biosens. Bioelectron.* **2020**, *170*, 112683. [CrossRef] [PubMed]

140. Li, Y.; Xu, L.; Fu, X.; Liu, H.; Ding, G.B.; Li, L.S.; Zhu, J.; Guo, Y. A competitive immunoassay based on engineered magnetic/fluorescent nanoparticles and biolayer interferometry-based assay for T-2 toxin determination. *Microchim. Acta* **2020**, *187*, 514. [CrossRef] [PubMed]
141. Song, X.; Wang, D.; Kim, M. Immunoliposome-based fluorometric patulin assay by using immunomagnetic nanoparticles. *Microchim. Acta* **2019**, *186*, 834. [CrossRef]
142. Song, X.L.; Ding, Q.; Pu, Y.P.; Zhang, J.; Sun, R.L.; Yin, L.H.; Wei, W.; Liu, S.Q. Application of the dimeric G-quadruplex and toehold-mediated strand displacement reaction for fluorescence biosensing of ochratoxin A. *Biosens. Bioelectron.* **2021**, *192*, 113537. [CrossRef] [PubMed]
143. Wang, C.; Yu, H.; Zhao, Q. A simple structure-switch aptasensor using label-free aptamer for fluorescence detection of aflatoxin B1. *Molecules* **2022**, *27*, 4257. [CrossRef]
144. Wang, Y.; Yu, L.; Zhang, H.; Zhu, R.; Meng, Z. Competitive ELISA based on pH-responsive persistent luminescence nanoparticles for autofluorescence-free biosensor determination of ochratoxin A in cereals. *Anal. Bioanal. Chem.* **2023**, *415*, 1877–1887. [CrossRef]
145. Ge, G.; Wang, T.; Liu, Z.; Liu, X.; Li, T.; Chen, Y.; Fan, J.; Bukye, E.; Huang, X.; Song, L. A self-assembled DNA double-crossover-based fluorescent aptasensor for highly sensitivity and selectivity in the simultaneous detection of aflatoxin M1 and aflatoxin B1. *Talanta* **2023**, *265*, 124908. [CrossRef] [PubMed]
146. Ma, P.; Guo, H.; Li, K.; Zhang, Y.; Guo, H.; Wang, Z. Simultaneous detection of patulin and ochratoxin A based on enhanced dual-color AuNCs modified aptamers in apple juice. *Talanta* **2024**, *266*, 124949. [CrossRef] [PubMed]
147. Wei, M.; Wang, C.; Xu, E.; Chen, J.; Xu, X.; Wei, W.; Liu, S. A simple and sensitive electrochemiluminescence aptasensor for determination of ochratoxin A based on a nicking endonuclease-powered DNA walking machine. *Food Chem.* **2019**, *282*, 141–146. [CrossRef] [PubMed]
148. Sang, M.; Meng, X.; Zhang, Y.; Li, Z.; Zhou, Q.; Jing, X.; Sun, X.; Zhao, W. An "on-off-on" electrochemiluminescence aptasensor based on a self-enhanced luminophore for ochratoxin A detection. *Anal. Bioanal. Chem.* **2023**, *415*, 5833–5844. [CrossRef] [PubMed]
149. Senko, O.; Stepanov, N.; Maslova, O.; Akhundov, R.; Ismailov, A.; Efremenko, E. Immobilized luminescent bacteria for the detection of mycotoxins under discrete and flow-through conditions. *Biosensors* **2019**, *9*, 63. [CrossRef] [PubMed]
150. Rehmat, Z.; Mohammed, W.S.; Sadiq, M.B.; Somarapalli, M.; Kumar Anal, A. Ochratoxin A detection in coffee by competitive inhibition assay using chitosan-based surface plasmon resonance compact system. *Colloids Surf. B Biointerfaces* **2019**, *174*, 569–574. [CrossRef]
151. Wei, T.; Ren, P.P.; Huang, L.L.; Ouyang, Z.C.; Wang, Z.Y.; Kong, X.F.; Li, T.J.; Yin, Y.L.; Wu, Y.N.; He, Q.H. Simultaneous detection of aflatoxin B1, ochratoxin A, zearalenone and deoxynivalenol in corn and wheat using surface plasmon resonance. *Food Chem.* **2019**, *300*, 125176. [CrossRef]
152. Asl, G.B.; Arvand, M.; Habibi, M.F. High affinity aptamers for ultra-sensitive detection of aflatoxin B1 in milk and groundnut samples with label-free photo-electrochemical aptasensor. *Food Chem.* **2022**, *397*, 133829. [CrossRef] [PubMed]
153. Abera, B.D.; Falco, A.; Ibba, P.; Cantarella, G.; Petti, L.; Lugli, P. Development of flexible dispense-printed electrochemical immunosensor for Aflatoxin M1 detection in milk. *Sensors* **2019**, *19*, 3912. [CrossRef]
154. Al-Dhahebi, A.M.; Gopinath, S.C.B.; Saheed, M.S.M.; Mustapha, M. Electrospun cellulose acetate-doped 3D-graphene nanofibre for enhanced transduction of ochratoxin A determination. *Bull. Mater. Sci.* **2022**, *45*, 166. [CrossRef]
155. Ben Abdallah, Z.; Grauby-Heywang, C.; Beven, L.; Cassagnere, S.; Moroté, F.; Maillard, E.; Sghaier, H.; Bouhacina, T.C. Development of an ultrasensitive label-free immunosensor for fungal aflatoxin B1 detection. *Biochem. Eng. J.* **2019**, *150*, 107262. [CrossRef]
156. Zhu, C.; Liu, D.; Li, Y.; Shen, X.; Ma, S.; Liu, Y.; You, T. Ratiometric electrochemical aptasensor for ultrasensitive detection of Ochratoxin A based on a dual signal amplification strategy: Engineering the binding of methylene blue to DNA. *Biosens. Bioelectron.* **2020**, *150*, 111814. [CrossRef]
157. Zhu, C.; Liu, D.; Li, Y.; Ma, S.; Wang, M.; You, T. Hairpin DNA assisted dual-ratiometric electrochemical aptasensor with high reliability and anti-interference ability for simultaneous detection of aflatoxin B1 and ochratoxin A. *Biosens. Bioelectron.* **2021**, *174*, 112654. [CrossRef]
158. Selvolini, G.; Lettieri, M.; Tassoni, L.; Gastaldello, S.; Grillo, M.; Maran, C.; Marrazza, G. Electrochemical enzyme-linked oligonucleotide array for aflatoxin B1 detection. *Talanta* **2019**, *203*, 49–57. [CrossRef] [PubMed]
159. Beheshti-Marnani, A.; Hatefi-Mehrjardi, A.; Es'haghi, Z. A sensitive biosensing method for detecting of ultra-trace amounts of AFB1 based on "Aptamer/reduced graphene oxide" nano-bio interaction. *Colloids Surf. B* **2019**, *175*, 98–105. [CrossRef]
160. Song, X.; Wang, D.; Kimb, M. Development of an immuno-electrochemical glass carbon electrode sensor based on graphene oxide/gold nanocomposite and antibody for the detection of patulin. *Food Chem.* **2021**, *342*, 128257. [CrossRef] [PubMed]
161. Singh, A.K.; Lakshmi, G.B.V.S.; Fernandes, M.; Sarkar, T.; Gulati, P.; Singh, R.P.; Solanki, P.R. A simple detection platform based on molecularly imprinted polymer for AFB1 and FuB1 mycotoxins. *Microchem. J.* **2021**, *171*, 106730. [CrossRef]
162. Jiang, H.; Guo, Q.; Liu, Y.; Qin, M.; Bikila, T.L.; Weng, X. A simple paper-based dual-analyte electrochemical nanobiosensor for mycotoxins using phosphorene-gold nanocomposites. *IEEE Sens. J.* **2022**, *22*, 19144–19151. [CrossRef]
163. Liao, Z.; Guo, W.; Ning, G.; Wu, Y.; Wang, Y.; Ning, G. A sensitive electrochemical aptasensor for zearalenone detection based on target-triggered branched hybridization chain reaction and exonuclease I-assisted recycling. *Anal. Bioanal. Chem.* **2023**, *415*, 4911–4921. [CrossRef]

164. Subak, H.; Selvolini, G.; Macchiagodena, M.; Ozkan-Ariksoysal, D.; Pagliai, M.; Procacci, P.; Marrazza, G. Mycotoxins aptasensing: From molecular docking to electrochemical detection of deoxynivalenol. *Bioelectrochemistry* **2020**, *138*, 107691. [CrossRef]
165. Lai, H.; Ming, P.; Wu, M.; Wang, S.; Sun, D.; Zhai, H. An electrochemical aptasensor based on P-Ce-MOF@MWCNTs as signal amplification strategy for highly sensitive detection of zearalenone. *Food Chem.* **2023**, *423*, 136331. [CrossRef] [PubMed]
166. Azri, F.A.; Eissa, S.; Zourob, M.; Chinnappan, R.; Sukor, R.; Yusof, N.A.; Raston, N.H.A.; Alhoshani, A.; Jinap, S. Electrochemical determination of zearalenone using a label-free competitive aptasensor. *Microchim. Acta* **2020**, *187*, 266. [CrossRef] [PubMed]
167. Gao, H.; Yao, J.; Jiang, B.; Yuan, R.; Xiang, Y. $NiCo_2S_4$ nanoparticle-dispersed MoS_2 nanosheets for catalytic and sensitive electrochemical aptamer sensing of ochratoxin A via cascaded amplifications. *Sens. Actuators B Chem.* **2022**, *371*, 132530. [CrossRef]
168. Nan, M.; Bi, Y.; Xue, H.; Xue, S.; Long, H.; Pu, L.; Fu, G. Rapid determination of Ochratoxin A in grape and its commodities based on a label-free impedimetric aptasensor constructed by layer-by-layer self-assembly. *Toxins* **2019**, *11*, 71. [CrossRef] [PubMed]
169. Gökçe, G.; Ben Aissa, S.; Nemčeková, K.; Catanante, G.; Raouafi, N.; Marty, J.L. Aptamer-modified pencil graphite electrodes for the impedimetric determination of ochratoxin A. *Food Control* **2020**, *115*, 107271. [CrossRef]
170. Gu, Y.; Wang, Y.; Wu, X.; Pan, M.; Hu, N.; Wang, J.; Wang, S. Quartz crystal microbalance sensor based on covalent organic framework composite and molecularly imprinted polymer of poly(o-aminothiophenol) with gold nanoparticles for the determination of aflatoxin B1. *Sens. Actuators B Chem.* **2019**, *291*, 293–297. [CrossRef]
171. Boshra, M.H.; El-Housseiny, G.S.; Farag, M.M.S.; Aboshanab, K.M. Innovative approaches for mycotoxin detection in various food categories. *AMB Express* **2024**, *14*, 7. [CrossRef] [PubMed]
172. Whitaker, T.B. Detecting mycotoxins in agricultural commodities. *Mol. Biotechnol.* **2003**, *23*, 61–71. [CrossRef]
173. Liu, X.; Liu, X.; Huang, P.; Wei, F.; Ying, G.; Lu, J.; Zhou, L.; Kong, W. Regeneration and reuse of immunoafnity column for highly efficient clean-up and economic detection of ochratoxin A in malt and ginger. *Toxins* **2018**, *10*, 462. [CrossRef]
174. Li, R.; Wen, Y.; Wang, F.; He, P. Recent advances in immunoassays and biosensors for mycotoxins detection in feedstuffs and foods. *J. Anim. Sci. Biotechnol.* **2021**, *12*, 108. [CrossRef]
175. Sharma, A.; Khan, R.; Catanante, G.; Sherazi, T.A.; Bhand, S.; Hayat, A.; Marty, J.L. Designed strategies for fluorescence-based biosensors for the detection of mycotoxins. *Toxins* **2018**, *10*, 197. [CrossRef] [PubMed]
176. Wu, Y.; Zhou, Y.; Huang, H.; Chen, X.; Leng, Y.; Lai, W.; Hang, X.; Xiong, Y. Engineered gold nanoparticles as multicolor labels for simultaneous multi-mycotoxin detection on the immunochromatographic test strip nanosensor. *Sens. Actuators B Chem.* **2020**, *316*, 128107. [CrossRef]
177. Altunbas, O.; Ozdas, A.; Yilmaz, M.D. Luminescent detection of Ochratoxin a using terbium chelated mesoporous silica nanoparticles. *J. Hazard. Mater.* **2020**, *382*, 121049. [CrossRef]
178. Zhang, Z.; Tang, X.; Wang, D.; Zhang, Q.; Li, P.; Ding, X. Rapid on-site sensing aflatoxin B1 in food and feed via a chromatographic time-resolved fluoroimmunoassay. *PLoS ONE* **2015**, *10*, e0123266. [CrossRef]
179. Yugender Goud, K.; Hayat, A.; Satyanarayana, M.; Sunil Kumar, V.; Catanante, G.; Vengatajalabathy Gobi, K.; Marty, J.L. Aptamer-based zearalenone assay based on the use of a fluorescein label and a functional graphene oxide as a quencher. *Microchim. Acta* **2017**, *184*, 4401–4408. [CrossRef]
180. Majdinasab, M.; Ben Aissa, S.; Marty, J.L. Advances in colorimetric strategies for mycotoxins detection: Toward rapid industrial monitoring. *Toxins* **2020**, *13*, 13. [CrossRef] [PubMed]
181. Wu, J.; Zeng, L.; Li, N.; Liu, C.; Chen, J. A wash-free and label-free colorimetric biosensor for naked-eye detection of aflatoxin B1 using G-quadruplex as the signal reporter. *Food Chem.* **2019**, *298*, 125034. [CrossRef] [PubMed]
182. Urusov, A.; Zherdev, A.; Petrakova, A.; Sadykhov, E.; Koroleva, O.; Dzantiev, B. Rapid multiple immunoenzyme assay of mycotoxins. *Toxins* **2015**, *7*, 238–254. [CrossRef]
183. Sheini, A. Colorimetric aggregation assay based on array of gold and silver nanoparticles for simultaneous analysis of aflatoxins, ochratoxin and zearalenone by using chemometric analysis and paper based analytical devices. *Microchim. Acta* **2020**, *187*, 167. [CrossRef]
184. Kumari Shrestha, Y.; Krishna Shrestha, S. Fundamentals of colorimetry. In *Advances in Colorimetry*; Samanta, A.K., Ed.; IntechOpen: Rijeka, Croatia, 2023. [CrossRef]
185. Rene, W.; Lenoble, V.; Chioukh, M.; Branger, C. A turn-on fluorescent ion-imprinted polymer for selective and reliable optosensing of lead in real water samples. *Sens. Actuators B Chem.* **2020**, *319*, 128252. [CrossRef]
186. Jo, E.-J.; Byun, J.-Y.; Mun, H.; Bang, D.; Son, J.H.; Lee, J.Y.; Lee, L.P.; Kim, M.-G. Single-step LRET aptasensor for rapid mycotoxin detection. *Anal. Chem.* **2018**, *90*, 716–722. [CrossRef] [PubMed]
187. Yi, Z.; Ren, Y.; Li, Y.; Li, Y.; Long, F.; Zhu, A. Optical biosensors for microbial toxin detection: Recent advances and future trends. *Microchem. J.* **2023**, *191*, 108894. [CrossRef]
188. Li, Y.; Liu, W.; Sun, C.; Zheng, M.; Zhang, J.; Liu, B.; Wang, Y.; Xie, Z.; Xu, N. Hybrids of carbon dots with subunit B of ricin toxin for enhanced immunomodulatory activity. *J. Colloid Interface Sci.* **2018**, *523*, 226–233. [CrossRef]
189. Farré, M.; Kantiani, L.; Pérez, S.; Barceló, D. Sensors and biosensors in support of EU Directives. *TRAC Trends Anal. Chem.* **2009**, *28*, 170–185. [CrossRef]
190. Kaur, M.; Gaba, J.; Singh, K.; Bhatia, Y.; Singh, A.; Singh, N. Recent advances in recognition receptors for electrochemical biosensing of mycotoxins—A review. *Biosensors* **2023**, *13*, 391. [CrossRef]

191. Majer-Baranyi, K.; Adányi, N.; Székács, A. Biosensors for Deoxynivalenol and Zearalenone determination in feed quality control. *Toxins* **2021**, *13*, 499. [CrossRef] [PubMed]
192. Rhouati, A.; Bulbul, G.; Latif, U.; Hayat, A.; Li, Z.-H.; Marty, J.L. Nano-aptasensing in mycotoxin analysis: Recent updates and progress. *Toxins* **2017**, *9*, 349. [CrossRef] [PubMed]
193. Evtugyn, G.; Hianik, T. Electrochemical immuno-and aptasensors for mycotoxin determination. *Chemosensors* **2019**, *7*, 10. [CrossRef]
194. Le, V.T.; Vasseghian, Y.; Dragoi, E.-N.; Moradi, M.; Khaneghah, A.M. A review on graphene-based electrochemical sensor for mycotoxins detection. *Food Chem. Toxicol.* **2021**, *148*, 111931. [CrossRef]
195. Gong, Z.; Huang, Y.; Hu, X.; Zhang, J.; Chen, Q.; Chen, H. Recent progress in electrochemical nano-biosensors for detection of pesticides and mycotoxins in foods. *Biosensors* **2023**, *13*, 140. [CrossRef]
196. Abd-Ellatief, R.; Abd-Ellatief, M.R. Electrochemical aptasensors: Current status and future perspectives. *Diagnostics* **2021**, *11*, 104. [CrossRef]
197. Guo, X.D.; Wen, F.; Zheng, N.; Saive, M.; Fauconnier, M.L.; Wang, J.Q. Aptamer-based biosensor for detection of mycotoxins. *Front. Chem.* **2020**, *8*, 195. [CrossRef] [PubMed]
198. Kesici, E.; Erdem, A. Impedimetric detection of Fumonisin B1 and its biointeraction with fsDNA. *Int. J. Biol Macromol.* **2019**, *139*, 1117–1122. [CrossRef] [PubMed]
199. Moradi, M.; Azizi-Lalabadi, M.; Motamedi, P.; Sadeghi, E. Electrochemical determination of T2 toxin by graphite/polyacrylonitrile nanofiber electrode. *Food Sci. Nutr.* **2021**, *9*, 1171–1179. [CrossRef]
200. He, S.; Yuan, Y.; Nag, A.; Feng, S.; Afsarimanesh, N.; Han, T.; Mukhopadhyay, S.C.; Organ, D.R. A review on the use of impedimetric sensors for the inspection of food quality. *Int. J. Environ. Res. Public Health* **2020**, *17*, 5220. [CrossRef]
201. Venton, B.J.; DiScenza, D.J. Voltammetry. In *Electrochemistry for Bioanalysis*, 1st ed.; Elsevier: Amsterdam, The Netherlands, 2021; pp. 27–50. [CrossRef]
202. Meliana, C.; Liu, J.; Show, P.L.; Low, S.S. Biosensor in smart food traceability system for food safety and security. *Bioengineered* **2024**, *15*, 2310908. [CrossRef]
203. Zhang, M.; Guo, X.; Wang, J. Advanced biosensors for mycotoxin detection incorporating miniaturized meters. *Biosens. Bioelectron.* **2023**, *224*, 115077. [CrossRef]
204. Gupta, R.; Raza, N.; Bhardwaj, S.K.; Vikrant, K.; Kim, K.-H.; Bhardwaj, N. Advances in nanomaterial-based electrochemical biosensors for the detection of microbial toxins, pathogenic bacteria in food matrices. *J. Hazard. Mater.* **2021**, *401*, 123379. [CrossRef] [PubMed]
205. Geicu, O.I.; Bilteanu, L.; Stanca, L.; Ionescu Petcu, A.; Iordache, F.; Pisoschi, A.M.; Serban, A.I. Composition-based risk estimation of mycotoxins in dry dog foods. *Foods* **2023**, *12*, 110. [CrossRef]
206. Matson, R.S. ELISA-based biosensors. *Methods Mol. Biol.* **2023**, *2612*, 225–238. [CrossRef]
207. Zhang, X.; Zhi, H.; Zhu, M.; Wang, F.; Meng, H.; Feng, L. Electrochemical/visual dual-readout aptasensor for ochratoxin a detection integrated into a miniaturized paper-based analytical device. *Biosens. Bioelectron.* **2021**, *180*, 113146. [CrossRef] [PubMed]
208. Wang, Q.; Li, S.; Zhang, Y.; Wang, S.; Guo, J.; Wang, J. A highly sensitive photothermal immunochromatographic sensor for detection of aflatoxin B1 based on Cu_2-xSe-Au nanoparticles. *Food Chem.* **2024**, *401*, 134065. [CrossRef]
209. Zhou, Q.; Tang, D. Recent advances in photoelectrochemical biosensors for analysis of mycotoxins in food. *TrAC Trends Anal. Chem.* **2020**, *124*, 115814. [CrossRef]
210. Zhao, Y.; Wang, X.; Pan, S.; Hong, F.; Lu, P.; Hu, X.; Jiang, F.; Wu, L.; Chen, Y. Bimetallic nanozyme-bioenzyme hybrid material-mediated ultrasensitive and automatic immunoassay for the detection of aflatoxin B1 in food. *Biosens. Bioelectron.* **2024**, *248*, 115992. [CrossRef] [PubMed]
211. Lahcen, A.A.; Amine, A. Biorecognition elements (Chapter 3). In *Wearable Physical, Chemical and Biological Sensors*; Morales-Narvaez, E., Dincer, C., Eds.; Elsevier: Amsterdam, The Netherlands, 2022; pp. 41–70. [CrossRef]
212. Oliveira, I.S.; da Silva Junior, A.G.; de Andrade, C.A.S.; Oliveira, M.D.L. Biosensors for early detection of fungi spoilage and toxigenic and mycotoxins in food. *Curr. Opin. Food Sci.* **2019**, *29*, 64–79. [CrossRef]
213. Sivasubramanian, S.P.; Vhanbatte, S.; Rajagopalan, S. Biosensor global market potential. *Asian Tex. J.* **2020**, *29*, 43–45.
214. Bhide, A.; Ganguly, A.; Parupudi, T.; Ramasamy, M.; Muthukumar, S.; Prasad, S. Next-generation continuous metabolite sensing toward emerging sensor needs. *ACS Omega* **2021**, *6*, 6031–6040. [CrossRef]
215. Herrera-Domínguez, M.; Morales-Luna, G.; Mahlknecht, J.; Cheng, Q.; Aguilar-Hernández, I.; Ornelas-Soto, N. Optical biosensors and their applications for the detection of water pollutants. *Biosensors* **2023**, *13*, 370. [CrossRef]

chemosensors

MDPI

Review

Humidity Sensing Using Polymers: A Critical Review of Current Technologies and Emerging Trends

Jintian Qian [1], Ruiqin Tan [1,*], Mingxia Feng [1], Wenfeng Shen [2,3], Dawu Lv [2,3] and Weijie Song [2,3,*]

1 Faculty of Electrical Engineering and Computer Science, Ningbo University, Ningbo 315211, China
2 Ningbo Institution of Materials Technology and Engineering, Chinese Academy of Sciences, Ningbo 315201, China; wenfengshen@nimte.ac.cn (W.S.); lvdawu@nimte.ac.cn (D.L.)
3 University of Chinese Academy of Sciences, Beijing 100049, China
* Correspondence: tanruiqin@nbu.edu.cn (R.T.); weijiesong@nimte.ac.cn (W.S.)

Abstract: In the post-pandemic era, human demand for a healthy lifestyle and a smart society has surged, leading to vibrant growth in the field of flexible electronic sensor technology for health monitoring. Flexible polymer humidity sensors are not only capable of the real-time monitoring of human respiration and skin moisture information but also serve as a non-contact human–machine interaction method. In addition, the development of moist-electric generation technology is expected to break free from the traditional reliance of flexible electronic devices on power equipment, which is of significant importance for the miniaturization, reliability, and environmentally friendly development of flexible devices. Currently, flexible polymer humidity sensors are playing a significant role in the field of wearable electronic devices and thus have attracted considerable attention. This review begins by introducing the structural types and working principles of various humidity sensors, including the types of capacitive, impedance/resistive, frequency-based, fiber optic, and voltage-based sensors. It mainly focuses on the latest research advancements in flexible polymer humidity sensors, particularly in the modification of humidity-sensitive materials, sensor fabrication, and hygrosensitivity mechanisms. Studies on material composites including different types of polymers, polymers combined with porous nanostructured materials, polymers combined with metal oxides, and two-dimensional materials are reviewed, along with a comparative summary of the fabrication and performance mechanisms of related devices. This paper concludes with a discussion on the current challenges and opportunities faced by flexible polymer humidity sensors, providing new research perspectives for their future development.

Keywords: humidity sensors; polymer sensors; human health monitoring; contactless human-machine interaction; moisture power generation

1. Introduction

In the post-pandemic era, the demand for healthy lifestyles and a smart society has grown significantly, driving the rapid development of flexible, wearable electronic sensing devices [1–3]. Among these, flexible humidity sensors play a crucial role. They can not only be used to monitor human respiratory status and skin moisture but also help prevent contact with germs through non-contact human–computer interaction. Humidity refers to the amount of water vapor present in air or other gases. It can be expressed in several ways, including absolute humidity, relative humidity, and dew point temperature, with relative humidity being the most commonly used measure. Absolute humidity, or vapor density, is defined as the ratio of the mass of water vapor in the air to the volume of the air, and is typically measured in grams per cubic meter or grains per cubic foot. Relative humidity (RH) is the ratio of the actual moisture content of the air to the maximum moisture level it can hold at a given temperature and pressure. Humidity sensors measure an environment's humidity by utilizing the physical or chemical interaction of hygroscopic materials with water molecules. Typically, humidity sensors need to meet several key criteria such as repeatability, high sensitivity, linearity, having low hysteresis, rapid response and recovery speeds, stability, being low cost, and ease of integration with control units. The development of devices that meet these criteria has long been a focal point in scientific research [4].

Flexible humidity sensors are generally composed of three main components: a flexible substrate, hygroscopic materials, and peripheral interface circuits. Of these, the development of and research on hygroscopic materials are undoubtedly the core of sensor technology. The early research on hygroscopic materials primarily focused on electrolytes, ceramics, porous metal oxides, and semiconductors. However, due to the existing processing techniques and inherent material limitations, these materials have not seen widespread practical application. In contrast, organic polymer materials, with their advantages of ease of processing and being low cost, have gained great popularity, particularly due to the rapid development of wearable flexible devices. The ability of polymers to integrate with various substrates has drawn increasing attention to their potential in humidity sensor development [5–7].

This article will focus on polymer-based sensitive material humidity sensors, covering their working principles, their types, and the research progress related to them in different fields, aiming to provide a reference and inspiration for researchers and engineering technicians in this field.

2. The Working Principle and Structure of Polymer Humidity Sensors

With the continuous advancement of science and technology, alongside the growing demand for applications in diverse environments, various polymer-based humidity sensors have been developed. These sensors can be classified based on their output signal types, which primarily include impedance-based, capacitive, optical, acoustic frequency, and voltage-based humidity sensors.

2.1. *Capacitive Humidity Sensors*

Capacitive humidity sensors consist of a substrate, a hygroscopic sensitive material layer, and electrode components. Based on their electrode configuration, these sensors can be classified into two structural types: parallel plate and interdigital electrodes, as illustrated in Figure 1a(i,ii) [8,9]. Each of these two structures offers distinct advantages. The sensitivity of parallel plate capacitive sensors is generally superior to that of sensors based on interdigital electrodes, while the interdigital electrode structure is easier to fabricate. It is important to note that structural parameters such as the width, length, and spacing of the interdigital electrodes, as well as the thickness of the sensitive film coating, directly impact the sensor's performance.

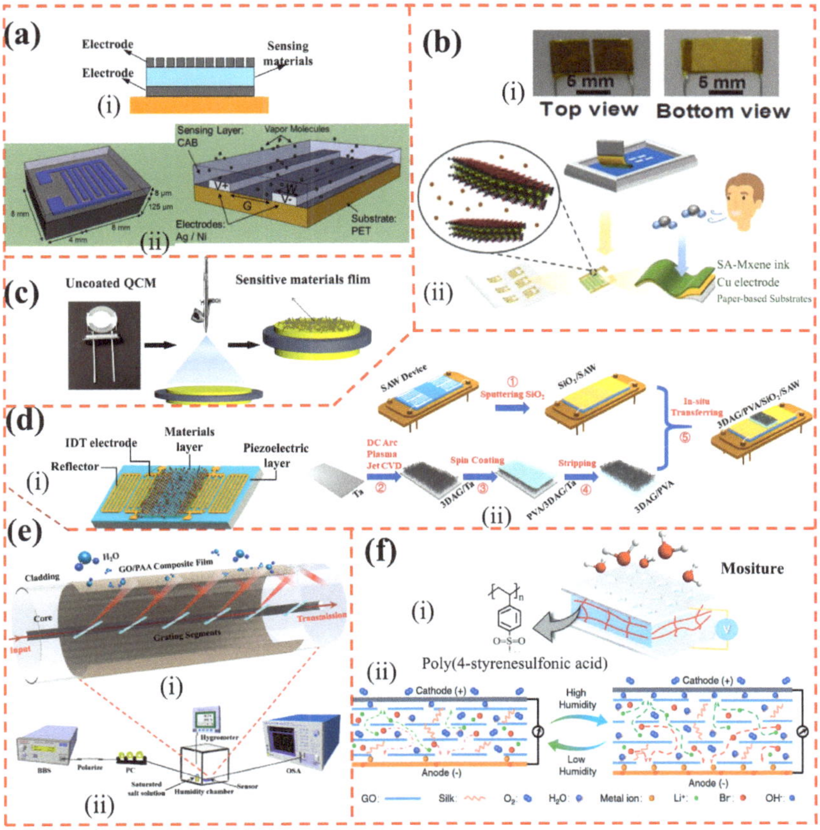

Figure 1. (**a**) (**i**) Schematic diagram of parallel plate capacitor structure [8]; (**ii**) schematic diagram of interdigital electrode structure [9]; (**b**) (**i**) schematic diagram of resistive/impedance structure [10]; (**ii**) schematic diagram of the fabrication process for flexible resistive/impedance humidity sensors [11]; (**c**) flowchart of the fabrication of a QCM (quartz crystal microbalance) humidity sensor [12]; (**d**) (**i**) schematic diagram of SAW (surface acoustic wave) structure [13]; (**ii**) schematic diagram of the fabrication process for SAW humidity sensors [14]; (**e**) (**i,ii**) schematic and humidity measurement setup for fiber optic humidity sensors [15]; (**f**) (**i**) schematic diagram of a self-powered humidity sensor generating potential difference through proton concentration gradient [16]; (**ii**) schematic diagram of the working principle of an electrochemical humidity sensor [17].

The working principle of capacitive humidity sensors is as follows: the polymer layer, acting as the humidity-sensitive material, continuously adsorbs water molecules from the environment. As the number of adsorbed water molecules, which have a high dielectric constant, increases, the capacitance of the sensor rises exponentially [18].

2.2. Resistive/Impedence Humidity Sensors

Resistive/impedance humidity sensors have a similar structure to that of interdigital capacitive sensors. However, because resistive/impedance types of sensors do not need to account for parasitic capacitance or the electric field distribution of the device structure to the same extent, they offer greater flexibility and diversity compared to capacitive sensors with interdigital electrodes. This flexibility is particularly evident when they are used on flexible substrates, as shown in Figure 1b(i) [10], where the electrodes can simply consist of two conductive tapes symmetrically attached to the hygroscopic material.

Resistive/impedance humidity sensors offer the advantages of a simple structure and an easy fabrication process. Figure 1b(ii) [11] illustrates a typical three-step method for the preparation of resistive/impedance humidity sensors: the first step involves preparing the sensitive material ink, the second step is the deposition of a stable interdigital electrode pattern on the flexible substrate, and the final step involves screen-printing the ink onto the electrode layer to complete the device.

Resistive/impedance-based humidity-sensing mechanisms, which use polymers as the sensitive layer material, are generally divided into two categories. The first category involves the use of polyelectrolytes with ionic group structures as the sensor′s sensitive layer. In these cases, electrolytes in the polymer ionize in the presence of water molecules, leading to an increase in the electrical conductivity of the sensitive material. The second category uses hydrophilic polymers, the principle of which can be explained by the Grotthuss mechanism [19]. In this process, the migration of H_3O^+ ions between the multiple layers of physically adsorbed water molecules on the surface of the polymer film significantly reduces the impedance, facilitating the adsorption of water molecules.

2.3. *Frequency-Based Humidity Sensors*

Frequency-based humidity sensors include the surface acoustic wave (SAW) and bulk acoustic wave (BAW) types. Their working principle is based on the absorption or desorption of water molecules by the sensitive film, which induces changes in the wave velocity and frequency of the device. The primary distinction is that BAW sensors transmit sound waves through the bulk of a quartz crystal or other piezoelectric material, and these propagate within the crystal itself. In contrast, SAW devices generate sound waves that propagate along the surface of the piezoelectric crystal, with the waves traveling parallel to the surface.

The quartz crystal microbalance (QCM) type is a representative of the BAW type. QCM sensors are mass-sensitive sensors that detects shifts in the resonant frequency of the piezoelectric material and oscillation circuit that are caused by mass changes as water molecules are absorbed by the sensitive material in response to humidity.

2.3.1. QCM Humidity Sensors

The mass sensitivity principle of QCM sensors is based on the well-known Sauerbrey equation [20]:

$$\Delta f = -\frac{2{f_0}^2}{A\sqrt{\rho_q \mu_q}}\Delta m$$

where Δf is the resonant frequency shift of the QCM, f_0 is the base resonant frequency, Δm is the mass change, A is the electrode surface area, and ρ_q and μ_q are the density and shear modulus of the quartz crystal, respectively. This relation is only valid with the following conditions: (i) the $\Delta f << f_0$, (ii) the added mass is rigid, and (iii) the mass is evenly distributed over the sensing area.

Zhang et al. [12] reported a typical preparation process for a quartz crystal microbalance (QCM) humidity sensor. As illustrated in Figure 1c, the sensitive material solution is evenly sprayed onto the piezoelectric quartz crystal at the center of the device, followed by a simple thermal treatment to fabricate the QCM humidity-sensitive device.

2.3.2. SAW Humidity Sensors

The structure and fabrication process of a SAW-type humidity sensor are shown in Figure 1d(i,ii) [13,14]. The working principle is that, when the sensitive material adsorbs water molecules, the propagation speed or frequency of its surface acoustic wave will change, thereby reflecting the information on humidity changes. The mutual conversion between the ultrasonic waves and electrical signals is accomplished by preparing interdigital transducers (IDT) on the surface of the piezoelectric substrate.

2.4. Fiber Optic Humidity Sensors

Optical sensing technology, a relatively new and emerging field, has recently found applications in humidity sensing. Its working principle typically involves utilizing the optical properties—such as the reflection coefficient, frequency, or phase of light propagation—of sensitive materials that change in response to variations in environmental relative humidity [21,22].

Xia et al. [15] reported an excessively tilted fiber grating (ex-TFG) humidity sensor. Figure 1e(i) presents a three-dimensional schematic diagram of the proposed fiber optic humidity sensor, while (ii) shows a schematic diagram of the sensor testing device. This type of grating combines the advantages of fiber Bragg gratings and long-period fiber gratings, with a functional composite hygroscopic film coated on the ex-TFG that enhances the modulation effect of external humidity changes on the optical signal.

Compared with traditional capacitive and impedance humidity sensors, optical flexible humidity sensors offer obvious advantages such as resistance to electromagnetic interference, having a small size, and the ability to transmit signals over long distances and can be applied in some specific scenarios. However, due to the high production cost and limited accuracy of optical flexible humidity sensors, their widespread adoption across various environments remains challenging.

2.5. Voltage Humidity Sensors

The traditional humidity sensors discussed above are all passive sensors, requiring an external power supply to generate electrical signals in practical applications. Voltage-type humidity sensors, however, can convert environmental humidity directly into a voltage output, offering the potential for self-powered development. Currently, two primary mechanisms for humidity-driven power generation in voltage-output sensors have been explored: (1) the ionization of water molecules along a gradient, and (2) reliance on redox reactions.

2.5.1. Voltage Humidity Sensors Based on Ion Diffusion

The concept of power generation using moisture was first proposed by Qu et al. [23] in 2015. They discovered that graphene oxide films with a gradient variation in the concentration of oxygen-containing groups can generate an open-circuit voltage of 20–30 mV under specific humidity conditions. The structure of this type of moisture-powered humidity sensor is illustrated in Figure 1f(i) [16]. In this design, hydrophobic polystyrene sulfonate is prepared asymmetrically, and its polar functional groups react with water molecules, with OH^- binding to the functional groups via hydrogen bonds, thereby releasing protons. The proton concentration gradient leads to ion drift and current generation, creating a potential difference between the electrodes. The formation of this proton concentration gradient is crucial for the sensor's performance.

Increasing the ion concentration gradient is key to enhancing the ion migration and producing a greater potential difference. With thoughtful material design by establishing an asymmetric distribution of functional groups or a water content gradient within the material, the ion concentration difference can be amplified, thus boosting the potential difference.

2.5.2. Voltage Humidity Sensors Based on Redox Reactions

Electrochemical humidity power generation sensors are inspired by the structure and working principle of metal–air batteries. The commonly used hygroscopic electrolyte consists of humidity-sensitive materials and electrolyte substances [24,25]. The humidity-sensitive material promotes the adsorption of water molecules, while the electrolyte facilitates ion conduction. When the material absorbs moisture, an anion diffusion channel is formed, triggering oxidation-reduction reactions at the electrodes, which in turn causes the metal electrode to lose electrons and generate a current.

Li et al. [17] employed an aSF/GO/LiBr composite film as the solid electrolyte, as shown in Figure 1f(ii). By connecting electrodes to both sides of the film, ion transfer channels are established within the material layer as water is absorbed, and oxidation-reduction reactions occur at the positive and negative electrodes. The reaction equations at the respective electrodes are as follows (Equations (1) and (2)):

$$O_2 + 4e^- + 2H_2O \rightarrow 4OH^- \quad (1)$$

$$M \rightarrow M^{n+} + ne^- \quad (2)$$

where M refers to the active metal at the anode, and electrons are transferred to the cathode through the external circuit.

It is noteworthy that, although the two aforementioned types of humidity sensors have the potential for self-powered operation and do not require external power consumption, their active power output remains relatively low, and they are prone to interference. Additionally, challenges persist in extending their service life and maintaining their operational stability. Enhancing the output power while ensuring stable and sustained operation remains a persistent challenge.

3. Research Progress in Polymer Humidity Sensors

To date, a variety of materials such as ceramics [26], organic polymers, metal oxides [27,28], and two-dimensional materials [29–31] have been studied for use in humidity sensors. With the rapid development of flexible and wearable electronic technology, the application fields of humidity sensors have expanded, imposing more stringent requirements for their functionality and performance. Therefore, the development of humidity sensors that are fast-responding, are linear, exhibit low hysteresis, have high sensitivity, have low power consumption, and are economically and environmentally friendly has become a research focus for scholars in the field.

Due to their lightweight, simple preparation methods, low-cost large-scale production, and structural flexibility, polymers have gained significant attention in recent decades as humidity materials for flexible devices. There are many organic polymers used as hygroscopic materials, including conductive polymers such as polyaniline (PANI) and polypyrrole (PPy) [6,32,33], long-chain polymer electrolytes with ionizable groups, such as quaternary ammonium salts and sulfonate salts [34,35], and lipids like polyimide (PI) [36–38], polymethyl methacrylate (PMMA), and polyethylene terephthalate (PET) [39,40], as well as hydrophobic polymers like polydimethylsiloxane (PDMS) [41]. Biopolymers with a large number of hydrophilic groups, such as chitosan (CS) [42–44], cellulose [45], sodium alginate [46], and silk fibroin (SF) [17], are increasingly being used in humidity sensors due to their good biodegradability and non-toxicity to humans and nature.

Overall, polymer humidity sensors still have the following limitations.

(1) Hydrophilic polymers experience significant chain/segment dissolution/migration/relaxation at high humidity levels, greatly restricting their application range.
(2) When polymers are used as resistive/impedance humidity sensors, their conductivity is too low at low humidity levels, making detection difficult.
(3) Individual polymer humidity sensors often suffer from low sensitivity or long response/recovery times, which is unfavorable for applications of flexible devices that require rapid and sensitive human health monitoring.

Single types of hygroscopic material are increasingly unable to address these challenges, making the combination of different materials a key direction for future development. The following is a summary of typical composite material approaches based on polymers: composites of polymers with differing properties, polymers with nanoporous structures, polymers combined with metal oxides, and polymers integrated with novel two-dimensional materials. These composite materials are effectively combined in various experimental designs, creative sensor structures, and configurations that harness these materials' complementary properties.

3.1. Polymer-Polymer Humidity Sensors

Leveraging the advantages of different polymers, composite materials can achieve an enhanced overall performance. Moreover, optimizing the ratios and processing techniques of these polymers can further improve the performance of humidity sensors, enabling high sensitivity, rapid responses, and extended operational lifespans.

Hydrophilic polymers such as polyethyleneimine (PEI), sodium alginate, and chitosan exhibit excellent moisture-sensing responses due to their high affinity for water molecules. However, their long-term stability in high-humidity environments is limited, constraining their functional ranges [47–49]. In contrast, some polymers such as polyacrylonitrile (PAN), cellulose, PPy etc. [50–52], which demonstrate superior water resistance and mechanical stability, can effectively improve the long-term stability of humidity sensors. PAN, in particular, is an excellent supporting membrane with high mechanical stability. Aditya et al. [47] and Tang et al. [48] reported the fabrication of QCM humidity sensors by grafting hydrophilic polymers such as PEI and sodium alginate onto electrospun PAN nanofibers, which resulted in sensors with both high sensitivity and excellent mechanical stability. Cellulose, which is insoluble in water and possesses remarkable mechanical strength, can further enhance the structural stability of sensor films [49,50]. Liu et al. [52] fabricated CS/PPy QCM humidity sensors by combining chitosan, which has abundant amino and hydroxyl groups and excellent film-forming properties, with PPy, a polymer that is easy to synthesize and environmentally stable. These sensors exhibited a total frequency shift of 5132.12 Hz over a humidity range of 0–97% RH, along with good repeatability and stability, highlighting that combining polymers with superior flexibility and film-forming capabilities with highly conductive polymers can not only improve the response sensitivity of sensors but also enhance their durability and environmental stability.

In addition to combining mechanically stable polymers, other strategies are also commonly employed to address the poor water resistance of hydrophilic polymers. Researchers have chemically modified polymer-sensitive materials through grafting [53], copolymerization [54], crosslinking reactions [55–58], and the development of interpenetrating network structures to achieve an optimal balance between hydrophobicity and hydrophilicity [58–60]. He et al. [58] effectively addressed the issue of polyethyleneimine (PEI) becoming easily deliquescent under high humidity conditions by employing a Michael addition reaction between PEI and tannic acid (TA) in an aqueous solution (Figure 2a). As illustrated in Figure 2b, compared to PEI that is not crosslinked or inadequately crosslinked, the PEI−TA material retains structural stability even after 24 h of water immersion.

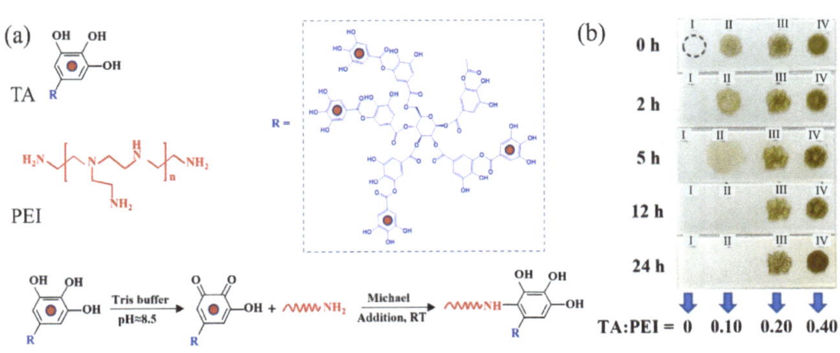

Figure 2. (**a**) The mechanism of crosslinking reaction between TA and PEI through Michael addition, and (**b**) the water resistance test of PEI with different proportions of TA [58].

When hydrophilic polymers are employed in impedance-based humidity sensors, it is important to note that, in addition to the issue of polymer hydrolysis under high humidity conditions, there is often a challenge of excessively high sensor impedance at lower humidity levels due to insufficient water molecule adsorption, which impedes the formation of ionic channels. Incorporating conductive polymers can be an effective composite solution to address this challenge.

Yang et al. [61] successfully prepared quaternized and crosslinked poly (4-vinylpyridine) (QC-PVP) with an interpenetrating network structure using materials such as poly (4-vinylpyridine) and poly (glycerol methacrylate). The researchers then coated polypyrrole onto the QC-PVP using vapor-phase polymerization technology, forming a QC-PVP/PPy composite hygroscopic membrane. This innovative design reduced the sensor's impedance in low humidity, improving its practicality in low-humidity environments. The researchers also investigated a double-layer composite structure combining QC-PVP with polyaniline (PANI) [62], similarly reducing the device's resistance in response to humidity. Suresha K. et al. [63] developed a cellulose/PPy nanocomposite using a polymerization-induced adsorption method, opening new avenues for the application of cellulose in humidity sensing technologies. Additionally, this composite can enhance the electrical properties of sensors by chemical modification or through the use of incorporated conductive materials, such as electrolytes (KOH, $CaCl_2$, sodium carboxylate (COONa), etc. [64–66]) and highly conductively noble metal particles (Au, Ag, Pt, etc. [67–69]). It is worth noting that the effect of noble metal nanoparticles such as Au, promoting the adsorption of hydrogen atoms, can enhance the detection performance of sensors for water molecules [70].

A wide variety of polymers are utilized in humidity sensors, and Table 1 summarizes several typical composite humidity sensors based on polymer combinations. Each polymer possesses distinct characteristics, along with specific limitations. In practical applications, it is essential to leverage the strengths of various polymer materials while mitigating their weaknesses. Achieving optimal sensor performance requires carefully selecting and combining materials, as well as employing appropriate fabrication techniques.

Table 1. Comparison of several typical polymer–polymer composite humidity sensors.

Sensing Materials	Sensor Type	Range (% RH)	Sensitivity /Response	Response/ Recovery Times (s)	Hysteresis (%)	Reference
PAN/PEI	QCM	30–75	164 Hz/% RH	13/7	-	[47]
SA-PAN	QCM	0–97	63.33 Hz/% RH	14.5/2.5	1.6	[48]
GG/EC-PVP	QCM	0–97	55.72 Hz/% RH	26/2	2.8	[50]
CA/KGM	QCM	0–97	-	12.3/0.1	0.64	[49]
PPy/CS	QCM	0–97	-	13/2	1.68	
NaSPF/PDEB	SAW	20–85	~0.4 kHz/% RH	-	-	[51]
QC-PVP/PPy	Impedance	33–97	-	33/110	5	[61]
QC-PVP/PANI	Impedance	1–98	10,000	24/35	3	[62]
PEI/TA	Impedance	35–90	29,900	28/12	2	[58]
Cellulose/PPy	Capacitance	27.8–92.4	0.0852 pF/% RH	<416	-	[63]

3.2. Nano- and Porous- Structured Polymer Humidity Sensors

Traditional organic polymer films, due to their semi-closed characteristics and relatively small specific surface area, have a limited adsorption capacity for water molecules. The incorporation of nano-porous structures can significantly increase the specific surface area available for humidity sensing in polymers, thereby enhancing their sensitivity to moisture. Nano-porous structures, such as mesoporous SiO_2, Cu-ZnS, and halloysite nanotubes (HNTs), not only exhibit high stability but also possess large specific surface areas, providing numerous active sites for sensitive groups. These features make them ideal frameworks for constructing polymer-based hygroscopic materials.

In recent years, Fei et al. [71] developed an MCM-41/PPy humidity sensor by employing self-polymerizing pyrrole vapor within MCM-41, a type of hexagonal mesoporous silica. Compared with sensors made solely from MCM-41 or PPy, this composite sensor demonstrated a superior capacitive humidity sensing performance. In 2022, the same team [72] further developed MCM-41/PEDOT nano-flower structures (Figure 3a), which reduced the response time of PEDOT-based humidity sensors by approximately 5 min and expanded their humidity sensing range.

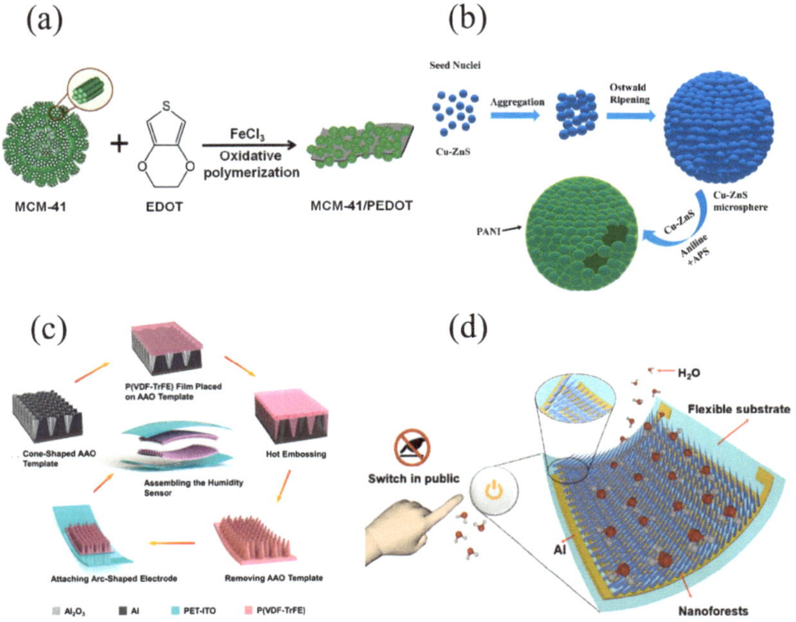

Figure 3. (**a**) Schematic diagram of the synthesis of MCM-41/PEDOT [72]; (**b**) schematic diagram of the synthesis of PANI/Cu-ZnS [73]; (**c**) schematic diagram of the fabrication process of the nanocone P(VDF-TrFE) arc-shaped hollow structure [74]; (**d**) schematic diagram of the PI nanoforest structure [75];.

Hemalatha et al. [73] synthesized PANI-coated Cu-ZnS using hydrothermal and in situ polymerization methods. As shown in Figure 3b, the zinc acetate, copper acetate, and thiourea formed seed nuclei, which subsequently produced ZnS solid porous microspheres under the appropriate hydrothermal conditions. The microspheres were then dispersed in an acidic aniline solution, where π–π^* stacking interactions between aniline functional groups and aniline monomers facilitated the coating of PANI on the Cu-ZnS microspheres after polymerization. The resultant PANI/Cu-ZnS composite exhibited a significantly improved response and recovery performance, with low humidity hysteresis (~1.2% RH) and excellent stability.

As shown in Figure 3c, Niu et al. [74] developed nano-cone arrays of poly(vinylidene fluoride-trifluoroethylene) (P(VDF-TrFE)) with arc-shaped hollow structures by using a combination of hot pressing and anodic aluminum oxide (AAO) template-transfer methods. These arrays were assembled into a high-performance, flexible capacitive humidity sensor. Unlike traditional capacitive structures where the electrode and dielectric layers are closely attached, the arc-shaped hollow structure enabled water molecules to be adsorbed over a large area of the sensitive material. The three-dimensional conical design significantly reduced the adsorption and desorption times to just a few seconds.

In a 2023 study, Mu et al. [38] modified halloysite nanotubes (HNTs) using silane coupling agents to facilitate the integration of HNTs with polyimide, forming an efficient humidity-sensing sensing layer. Combined with advanced MEMS technology, this sensor achieved an outstanding sensitivity of 0.87 pF/% RH in the 10–90% RH humidity range, which was 1.81 times greater than that of a pure PI humidity sensor. In addition to using nanoporous materials as templates to fabricate various nanostructured patterns, some specialized fabrication methods can also be employed to construct nanostructures. Chen et al. [76] developed a polyimide humidity sensor based on a nanoforest structure embedded on silicon substrate by using O_2 plasma reaction etching. The unique nanoforest morphology on the PI layer exhibited an especially large surface area and thus provided numerous active sites for adsorbing molecules. This innovative design resulted in a humidity sensor that was 15 times more sensitive than traditional polyimide sensors in the 10–90% RH range. Zhao et al. [75] used the same method to fabricate a nanoforest-structured PI on a flexible substrate (Figure 3d). Due to its ultra-high sensitivity, it can detect the humidity levels on fingertips.

It is worth noting that, in addition to forming nano-porous characteristics by compounding with these special structural materials, also it is also possible to utilize nano-film preparation techniques on polymers to achieve the same effect. The commonly used polymer nano-film techniques include electrospinning [77–80], electrostatic self-assembly [81–84], inkjet printing [85–87], etc. Nanotechnology has greatly enhanced the effectiveness of humidity sensors, due to allowing for a high specific surface area and porosity related to water molecule adsorption. Table 2 summarizes polymer-based humidity sensors fabricated using nano-porous structure templates or nanotechnology.

Table 2. Comparison of several typical nanostructured polymer humidity sensors.

Sensing Materials	Sensor Type	Range (% RH)	Sensitivity /Response	Response/ Recovery Times (s)	Hsteresis (%)	Reference
MCM-41/PPy	Capacitance	11–95	119 pF/% RH	915/100	-	[71]
MCM-41/PEDOT	Capacitance	11–95	10,000	165/115	6	[72]
Cu-ZnS /PANI	Capacitance	30–90	12 pF/% RH	42/24	1.2	[73]
HNTs/PI	Capacitance	10–90	0.87 pF/% RH	12/8	2.18	[38]
P(VDF-TrFE)	Capacitance	50–90	-	3.693/3.43	9.1	[74]
PI-Nanoforest	Capacitance	10–90	-	8/5	-	[76]
PANI/PVB-Nanofiber	SAW	20–90	75 kHz/% RH	1/2	-	[77]
PMMA-nanofiber	Optical fiber	35–85	0.28	16/126	-	[78]
PVA/PEDOT:PSS-nanofiber	Optical fiber	20–80	−0.990 nm/% RH	-	-	[79]

3.3. Polymer-Metal Oxide Humidity Sensors

Metal oxides possess active adsorption sites that readily interact with water molecules through the chemical adsorption of hydroxyl groups [88,89]. Therefore, incorporating metal oxides into organic polymer materials significantly enhances their physical adsorption capacity for water molecules. This leads to the formation of a water layer within the composite material, increasing the number of ion transport channels and stabilizing the impedance rate of change [90].

SnO_2 is a typical metal oxide semiconduction material and has a wide band gap, suitable electrochemical stability, and abundant oxygen vacancies, which is not only beneficial for absorbing water but also allows forming biocomposites more easily with polymer [91–93]. As shown in Figure 4a, Shukla et al. [94] synthesized a nano-sized SnO_2/PANI nanocomposite. Under the synergistic effects of SnO_2 and PANI [95,96], the nanocomposite exhibited a 10% improvement in humidity sensitivity compared to pure PANI. Feng et al. [92] wrapped SnO_2/PVA nanofibers onto excessively tilted fiber grating (Ex-TFG), which exhibited an ultrafast response of ~67 ms.

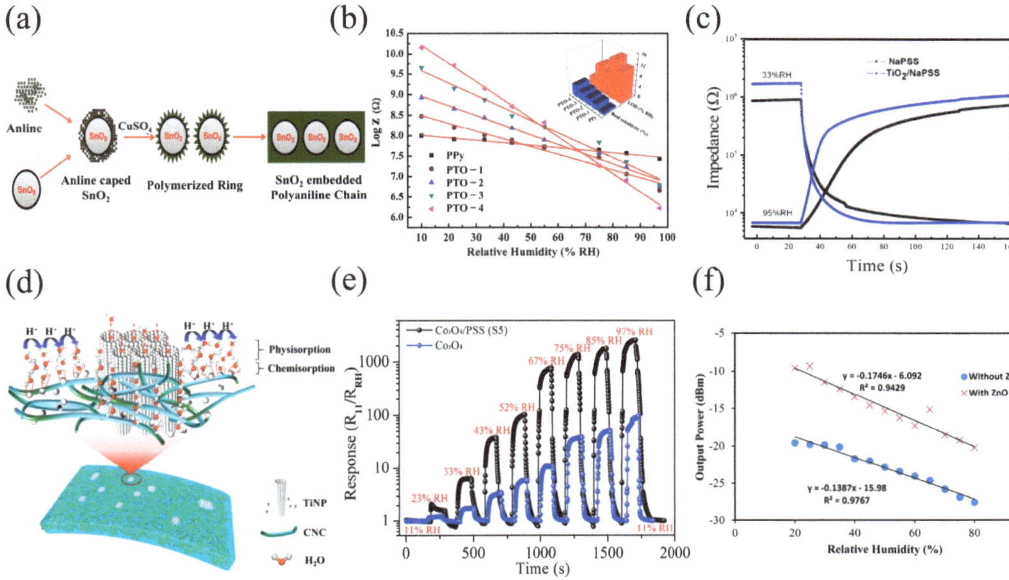

Figure 4. (**a**) Schematic diagram of the synthetic route for nano SnO_2/PANI [94]; (**b**) humidity sensing performance graph of PPy-Ta_2O_5 [97]; (**c**) comparison chart of adsorption/desorption time for NaPSS and TiO_2/NaPSS [98]; (**d**) explanation diagram of the humidity sensing mechanism for ZnO/CNC [99]; (**e**) comparison chart of humidity responsiveness for Co_3O_4 and Co_3O_4/PSS [82]; (**f**) PMMA/ZnO humidity sensors [100].

Other metal oxides also possess similar properties, and there have been many reports on the characteristics of their composites with polymers. B. Chethana [70] investigated the humidity sensing properties of a core-shell structured polypyrrole/tantalum pentoxide (Ta_2O_5) composite (Figure 4b). They mechanically blended polypyrrole with Ta_2O_5, and the resultant PPy-Ta_2O_5 composite displayed a significant increase in porosity, water absorption, and material expansion when compared to pure PPy. The sensor achieved response and recovery times of 6 s and 7 s, respectively, and demonstrated stable performance over two months. Su et al. [98] utilized 1 μm polystyrene microspheres as a substrate to synthesize microstructured porous TiO_2 films. These were subsequently immersed in a sodium polystyrene sulfonate (NaPSS) solution, resulting in an inorganic/polymer composite film. The ordered arrangement of TiO_2 within the composite film yielded an exceptionally fast response time in the 33–90% RH range (Figure 4c). After 2 years, the team [101] further optimized the process, discovering that microspheres with a 100 nm diameter produced the best results. In 2022, Tong et al. [99] transformed spherical TiO_2 into a tubular structure and embedded it in hydrophilic cellulose with a porous structure. As depicted in Figure 4d, the tubular channels not only enhanced the water adsorption capacity of the material but also facilitated water molecule migration from regions of high to low relative humidity. This advancement, alongside the synergistic properties of cellulose and semiconductors, significantly improved the sensor's humidity sensitivity.

Zhang et al. [82] developed a composite humidity-sensitive film using Co_3O_4 and PSS through layer-by-layer self-assembly technology. Benefiting from the strong adsorption capacity of Co_3O_4 and the layered nanostructure of PSS, the film displayed a superior response performance across a broad relative humidity range of 11–97% RH (Figure 4f). The sensor does not require a heating device and operates effectively at room temperature, demonstrating excellent repeatability and long-term stability.

N. Irawati et al. [100] demonstrated that adding a nanostructured ZnO coating to the surface of a microfiber loop resonator fabricated from PMMA fibers markedly improved the sensitivity of sensors (Figure 4f). Sahoo et al. [76] also explored the role of ZnO in low-relative humidity environments, revealing that an electrostatic field generated by water adsorption at oxygen-deficient sites on ZnO surfaces promotes water molecule dissociation, enhancing their sensor's performance.

Table 3 summarizes several classic polymer-metal oxide composite humidity sensors. While the introduction of metal oxides enhances the performance of humidity sensors, it is worth noting that certain mechanisms remain unclear. Metal oxides may exhibit sensitivity to other gas molecules besides water, which poses a challenge for impedance-based signal output humidity sensors. Improving the selectivity of metal oxide/polymer humidity sensors selectivity a significant challenge that must be addressed to enable their broader application.

Table 3. Comparison of several polymer/metal oxide humidity sensors.

Sensing Materials	Sensor Type	Range (% RH)	Sensitivity /Response	Response/ Recovery Times (s)	Hsteresis (%)	Reference
SnO_2/PANI	Impedance	5–95	0.22 kΩ/% RH	26/30	-	[94]
SnO_2/PVA	Optical fiber	35–75	0.43 dB/% RH	0.067/0.087	-	[92]
Ta_2O_5/PPy	Impedance	11–97	0.044 kΩ/% RH	6/7	2	[97]
TiO_2/NaPSS	Impedance	11–95	100,000	2/20	-	[98]
Co_3O_4/PSS	Impedance	11–98	~1.5 MΩ/% RH	37/23	-	[82]
TiO_2/CNC	Resistance	11–97	~190	34/18	-	[99]
PMMA/ZnO_2	Optical fiber	20–89	0.1746 dBm/% RH	-	-	[100]

3.4. Polymer-Two-Dimensional Material Humidity Sensor

Two-dimensional materials, including graphene oxide (GO), carbon nanotubes (CNTs), transition metal carbides or nitrides (MXenes), and metal-organic frameworks (MOFs), have demonstrated immense potential across various fields due to their exceptional properties. These materials feature high specific surface areas and hydrophilic groups, along with surface vacancies that facilitate the adsorption of water molecules through hydrogen bonding. Given these advantages, the development of composite structures that integrate polymers and two-dimensional materials for humidity sensors has garnered significant attention from researchers.

GO is particularly notable for its unique layered structure, high specific surface area, and rich oxygen-containing functional groups, which confer excellent hydrophilicity. In 2023, Han et al. [102] modified the PI aerogel with GO. The researchers used laser direct writing technology to reduce the GO on both the upper and lower surface layers of the aerogel into reduced graphene oxide (rGO), forming planar electrodes (Figure 5a). The resultant device was a self-supporting, flexible, parallel plate capacitive humidity sensor. In addition to its high sensitivity, this sensor has the potential to detect moisture in common solvents, presenting new possibilities for humidity detection applications. The chemical reduction of GO removes many oxygen-containing groups and restores aromatic carbon double bonds, facilitating electron mobility and improving conductivity in the resulting film [103,104]. The reduction process often leaves behind some oxygen-containing functional groups, making the rGO conductive and chemically active due to the resulting existence of defect sites [103]. Ravikiran et al. [104] showed that PPy/rGO composites prepared using a similar method exhibited superior sensitivity, a lower detection limit, and reduced hysteresis compared to both PPy and PPy/GO (Figure 5b).

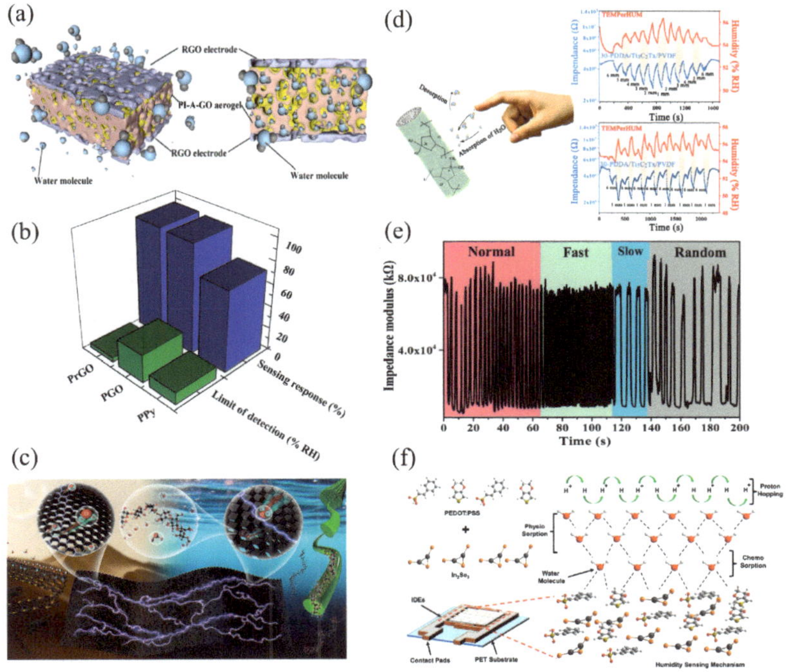

Figure 5. (**a**) Schematic diagram of the PI/GO aerogel humidity sensor structure [102]; (**b**) performance comparison of PPy, PPy/GO, and PPy/rGO humidity sensors [104]; (**c**) schematic diagram of the CNFs/MWCNTs sensor mechanism [105]; (**d**) schematic diagram of the gap between fingertip and PDDA/Ti_3C_2Tx/PVDF sensor [35]; (**e**) schematic diagram of the MOF/polyelectrolyte sensor monitoring human breathing [106]; (**f**) schematic diagram of the PEDOT:PSS/In_2Se_3 hygroscopic mechanism [107].

Polymer-CNT composite materials have garnered significant attention in the field of flexible humidity sensing, largely due to their high sensitivity, rapid response, and excellent stability [108]. As shown in Figure 5c, Jin et al. [105] advanced the traditional "ice-casting" method, successfully fabricating CNFs/CNT (cellulose nanofibers/CNT) aerogel thin films with an oriented porous structure. The honeycomb structure not only enhances the structure's air permeability but also accelerates moisture exchange between the gas and material, significantly improving the sensor's response speed in practical applications. This innovative structural design represents a new direction in the development of high-performance flexible humidity sensors.

Yang et al. [11] introduced sodium ascorbate (SA) to modify multi-layer MXene, followed by a simple screen-printing of SA-MXene ink onto paper substrate to fabricate a highly sensitive humidity sensor. The enediol groups in SA form a charge transfer complex with surface and edge Ti atoms in the MXene, preventing MXene's oxidation in humid environments and improving the sensor's long-term stability. Zhao et al. [35] similarly demonstrated the outstanding performance of PDDA-modified MXene sensors, which are capable of detecting minute movements, such as finger motions as small as 1 mm (Figure 5d).

MOFs, with their high specific surface area, precisely controllable structure, persistent porosity, and tunable properties, are an ideal platform for constructing porous electrolytes and chemically processing sensitive films. Through an in situ thiolene click crosslinking reaction, Zhang et al. [106] developed a humidity sensor based on a polyelectrolyte film derived from UIO-66. The inherent pore size of UIO-66 and structural defects introduced by sulfonic acid enabled the rapid adsorption and desorption of water molecules, effectively allowing the sensor to recognize various states of human breathing (Figure 5e).

Indium selenide (In_2Se_3), a hydrophilic two-dimensional material with a large specific surface area, high dielectric constant, and excellent semiconductor characteristics, has emerged as a promising material for high-performance humidity sensors. Ali Khan et al. [107] reported a composite humidity sensor comprising In_2Se_3 and PEDOT:PSS. As illustrated in Figure 5f, water molecules interact with the hydrophilic sulfonic acid groups and selenium atoms, resulting in chemical adsorption in low humidity and physical adsorption at higher humidity levels. These interactions form multiple layers of water molecules, amplifying the capacitance changes due to hygroscopicity. The addition of In_2Se_3, with its high dielectric constant, significantly enhances the sensor's sensitivity over a broader humidity range. Both In_2Se_3 and PEDOT:PSS exhibit inherent hygroscopic properties, and their combination in appropriate proportions results in an enhanced overall humidity sensitivity. Through a synergistic combination of chemical and physical adsorption processes, the sensor effectively covers a wide range of humidity levels with increased sensitivity.

Table 4 summarizes these typical two-dimensional material and polymer composite humidity sensors. The large specific surface area and abundant adsorption sites of two-dimensional materials significantly enhance the performance of humidity sensors. However, given the relatively short history of two-dimensional material research, the long-term stability of the polymer composites which incorporate these materials requires further exploration and verification.

Table 4. Summary of the hygroscopic performance of several typical polymer/two-dimensional material composites.

Sensing Materials	Sensor Type	Range (% RH)	Sensitivity /Response	Response/ Recovery Times (s)	Hsteresis (%)	Reference
PI/GO	Capacitance	11–98	1000	39/37	-	[102]
rGO/PPy	Resistance	11–97	0.042 Ω/% RH	2/4	4	[104]
CNFs/CNT	Resistance	0–75	71.5%	18/47	-	[105]
PVA/Mxene	Resistance	11–97	40	0.9/6.3	-	[2]
SA/Mxene	Capacitance	11–97	131.4%	9.38/12.94	-	[11]
UIO-66-S3-NH-AA	Impedance	33–95	1000	3.1/1.5	-	[106]
PEDOT:PSS/In_2Se_3	Capacitance	5–95	0.177 μF/% RH	1.2/1.9	-	[107]

4. Application of Polymer Humidity Sensors

With the rapid advancement of internet of things (IoT) technology and the growth of flexible wearable electronic devices, as well as the increasing demand for an enhanced quality of life, humidity sensors have gained significant attention. Beyond these sensors' traditional roles in monitoring environmental humidity in fields such as industry and agriculture, these sensors are being developed for emerging applications, expanding their utility and value. This review focuses primarily on three key areas of application: human health, contactless switches, and moisture-based power generation.

4.1. Application in Human Healthcare Detection

The human respiratory system is regulated by the respiratory center in the brain, controlling the levels of oxygen and carbon dioxide in the arterial blood. Respiratory patterns can provide critical insights into a person's health, as well as their physical and mental activity [1,109].The human body releases significant amounts of water vapor during respiration, making flexible humidity sensors an appealing non-contact method for monitoring breathing patterns. This innovative detection approach has garnered the attention of numerous researchers. Additionally, other aspects of human health, such as skin moisture detection and the monitoring of baby diapers [110,111] can be effectively addressed by integrating flexible humidity sensors into external devices.

Park et al. [112] developed a flexible substrate that allows a sensor to be attached under the nose, as shown in Figure 6a. The sensor is connected to a signal processing and communication module worn on the arm, enabling real-time data recording and analysis via a computer. The displayed capacitive response on the screen can effectively distinguish between two respiratory states: walking and running. As illustrated in Figure 6b(i), Zheng et al. [113] embedded a humidity sensor into a mask. A program was designed to automatically calculate the duration of data stability shown in the red box in Figure 6b(ii). Periods of no fluctuation are classified into six risk alert levels; upon reaching the sixth level, the sensor automatically sends an SOS alarm to a monitoring terminal, helping to prevent accidents.

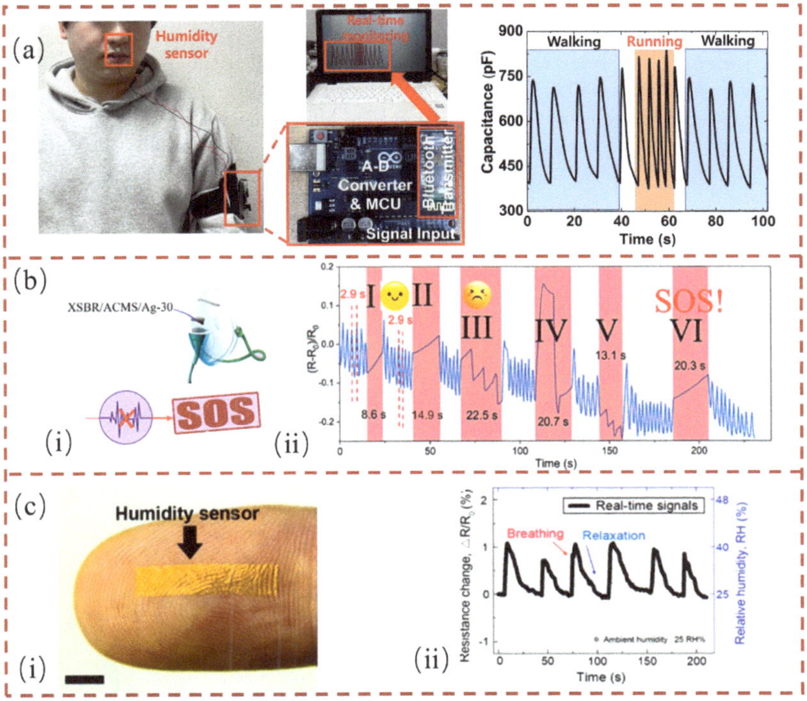

Figure 6. (**a**) Physical image of the flexible humidity sensor for breath detection [112]; (**b**) (**i**) schematic diagram of the breath detection device; (**ii**) real-time monitoring of dangerous and healthy breathing [113]; (**c**) (**i**) schematic diagram of the flexible hygroscopic membrane on the finger (length = 4 mm); (**ii**) standardized real-time response graph of the sensor to sweat on the skin surface [111].

Jeong et al. [111] developed a breathable nano-net humidity sensor designed for long-term skin moisture monitoring (Figure 6c(i)). Its ultrathin, flexible structure enables easy attachment to the skin, allowing for the continuous recording of moisture levels on the user's skin surface. Figure 6c(ii) demonstrates how the sensor's resistance changes in response to sweat production after the user finishes exercising.

4.2. Application of Humidity Sensors in Noncontact Human-Machine Interaction Methods

Human–machine interaction (HMI) has significantly transformed how humans interact with their environment. However, traditional contact-based interaction methods pose a risk of bacterial or viral infections, a concern that has become increasingly prominent, particularly following the outbreak of the novel coronavirus disease in 2019. To mitigate the risk of infectious disease transmission, the development of non-contact human–machine interaction methods has gained critical importance. Humidity sensors, which can sensitively detect humidity fields generated by breathing, sweat, and skin hydration, offer a flexible, low-cost, and adaptable solution for a variety of applications.

Li et al. [59] developed a highly sensitive flexible humidity sensor. As shown in Figure 7a(i), the sensor demonstrates a significant change in its impedance response as a finger approaches or moves away from it. The sensor exhibits good repeatability, and can estimate the distance between the finger and the sensor based on the magnitude of the impedance response. Building on this capability, the team created a 3 × 3 sensor array that effectively tracks the position of an operator's fingertip and simulates keyboard button functions (Figure 7a(ii)). Yang et al. [88] enhanced this sensor array by analyzing and processing the signals from the 3 × 3 humidity sensing array using a microcontroller, enabling the accurate display of numbers on a computer screen (with each sensor corresponds to a specific number). As illustrated in Figure 7b(i), the screen displays the three positions in the array where the user has pressed. The array can not only detect finger positions near the sensor but also recognize non-contact gestures. As shown in Figure 7b(ii), the array captures movements tracing the letters "J", "L", and "U". The more sensors that are incorporated into the array, the more information that can be gathered based on humidity.

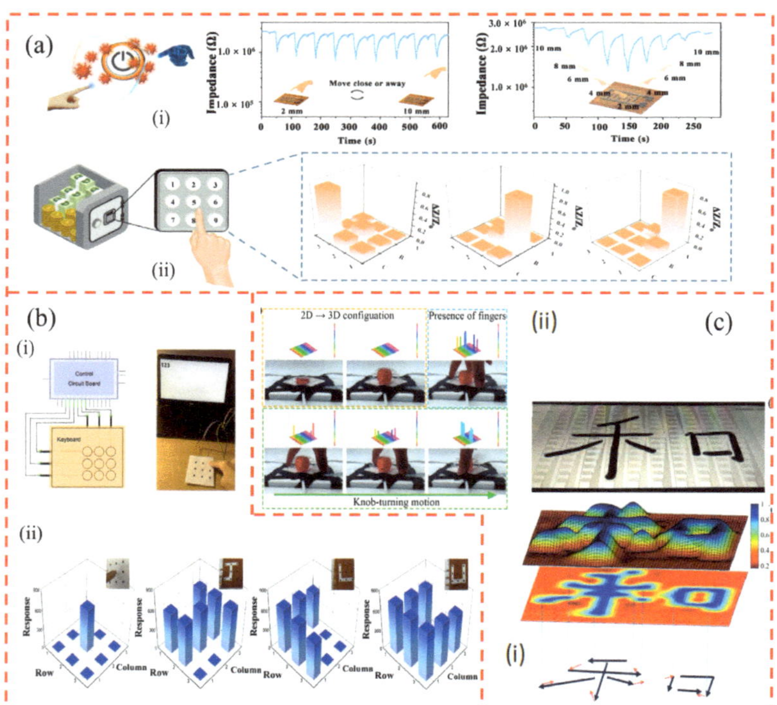

Figure 7. (**a**) (**i**) Real-time impedance response of the sensor to changes in distance from the fingertip; (**ii**) sensor response when the finger approaches a specific point in the sensor array, which in the box diagram, the numbers "1", "2", "3" and the letters "A", "B", "C" are used for coordinate positioning to simulate a keyboard [59]; (**b**) (**i**) schematic diagram of the humidity sensing array simulating part of the keyboard circuit; (**ii**) record of the direction of movement as the finger moves on the array [114]; (**c**) (**i**) humidity level reconstruction map recorded by the sensor array when the finger writes the Chinese character "He" in the air above the humidity sensing array; (**ii**) response of the sensor array to three-dimensional shapes, the presence of multiple fingers, and non-contact rotary knob motion of the finger [87].

Li et al. [87] furthered this concept by fabricating a 15 × 10 humidity sensor array on a PET substrate using inkjet printing technology. An analyzer was connected to monitor the capacitive response of each sensor, and the team mounted the sensor matrix on a display screen. When a user traced the Chinese character "He" in the air above the screen, the sensor accurately recorded the finger's trajectory and height changes. As shown in Figure 7c(i), after the finger movement is completed, a humidity reconstruction map is generated based on the capacitive signals from the array's sensors, demonstrating that non-contact interfaces based on humidity sensors can accurately capture users' writing. To further expand its application in 3D space, the sensor array can be fabricated into a spherical structure. As shown in Figure 7c(ii), the 3D sensor array can detect both the number and direction of fingers surrounding it.

4.3. Appliacation of Humidity Sensor in Technology of Moist-Electric Generation

As fossil fuel resources dwindle and environmental pollution worsens, the search for safe, reliable, and clean energy alternatives has become a central focus in global energy research [16,115,116]. Water, as an abundant and recyclable resource, is not only essential for life but also serves as Earth's largest energy carrier [117,118]. Moist-electric generation (MEG) technology, which converts the chemical energy of ambient humidity into electrical energy, is gaining increasing attention [119]. By integrating MEG with humidity sensors, self-powered humidity sensors can be developed, eliminating the need for external power supplies. This makes the devices lighter, more energy-efficient, and well-suited for large-scale applications.

As depicted in Figure 8a, Li et al. [120] demonstrated that, in a cellulose/MXene/PSSA composite film, water molecules induce the release of free protons from sulfonic and hydroxyl groups. The protons diffuse along a concentration gradient, causing charge accumulation on the opposite side of the film, which generates an electric field. The strength of this electric field is approximately linearly correlated with the surrounding humidity; the maximum output voltage can reach 300 mV. However, for humidity-based power generation to be practically viable, it is essential not only to achieve output voltages that meet the device activation thresholds but also to provide stable and continuous power for self-powered devices. Zhong et al. [121] reported a quaternized cellulose aerogel self-powered humidity sensor that, thanks to the aerogel's porous structure, enhances the moisture capture and facilitates rapid ion transfer. The device generates electrical signals over a broad humidity range (30–90% RH) and produces varying electrical potentials based on the humidity field around a nearby finger (Figure 8b(i)). The aerogel system has demonstrated highly stable power generation for over 4000 min (Figure 8b(ii)).

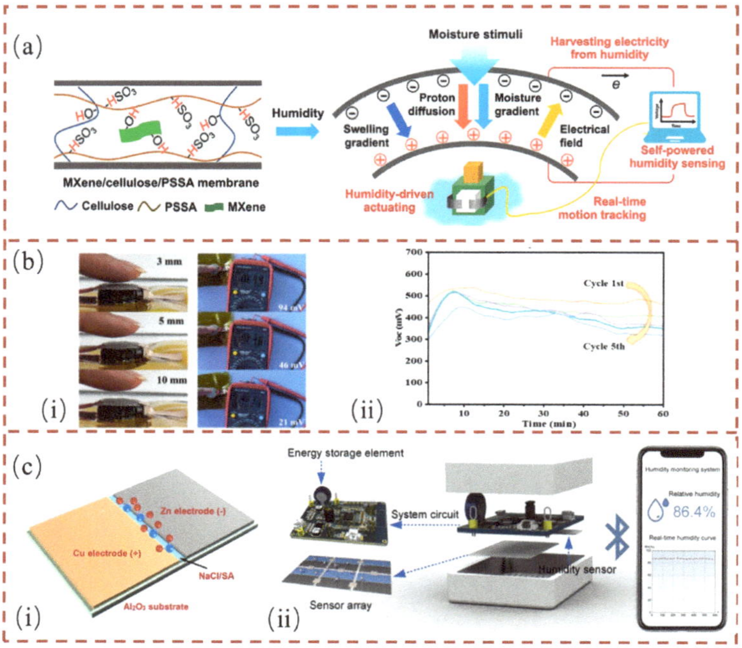

Figure 8. (**a**) Schematic of the working principle of the gradient water molecule ionization type MEG [120]; (**b**) (**i**) generation of electromotive force through non-contact interaction between the finger and the sensor; (**ii**) stability test of the sensor's voltage output over five cycles [121]; (**c**) (**i**) structural diagram of the NaCl/sodium electrochmecial humidity sensor; (**ii**) physical image of the self-powered wireless humidity monitoring system [122].

In addition to ion diffusion-based humidity power generation designs, electrochmecial humidity devices based on redox reaction have also attracted significant interest [123–125]. Electrochemical reactions rely on electrode potential and ion conduction, and ion conduction is influenced by the ion concentration and adsorbed water molecules [123]. Therefore, to achieve a stronger voltage output performance, alkali metal salts (such as LiBr [17], NaCl [126], and LiCl [124]) are used either individually or in combination with some hydrophilic materials to form the sensitive layer of electrochemical humidity sensors. Tai Huiling's research group [123] reported a high-performance power generation humidity sensor based on a NaCl/sodium alginate (SA) humidity sensing electrolyte and Cu/Zn electrodes. As illustrated in Figure 8c(i), the device has a high response voltage (~0.7 V), a large short circuit current (~24 μA), and a large loading power (~2.63 μW) at 91.5% RH. Zhang et al. [122] used NaCl and hydroxylated multi-walled carbon nanotubes (OH-MWCNTs) as a humidity-sensing electrolyte. The team developed a self-powered wireless humidity monitoring system (Figure 8c(ii)) for which the system power module is composed of an array formed by connecting several sensors in series and parallel with a supercapacitor. By generating voltage in the array under humidity, the capacitor is charged to power the peripheral low-power circuit modules. The system was capable of automatically detecting humidity changes and transmitting real-time data to a mobile phone app, offering users a convenient and continuous humidity-monitoring solution without an external power source.

5. Conclusions and Outlook

This article presents a comprehensive review of the latest research progress in polymer-based humidity sensors. It reviews the various principles and structures of humidity sensors and different types of composite constructions, such as compounding with other polymers, nano-porous structural materials, metal oxides, and two-dimensional materials. The review also highlights recent applications of high-sensitivity flexible humidity sensors for human health monitoring, non-contact human-machine interaction, and self-powered devices utilizing moisture-based power generation. It also outlines various fabrication methods and compares the performance of different humidity sensitive materials.

The application prospects for polymer humidity sensors in the future are exceedingly promising. However, researchers inevitably confront a range of challenges during their development.

(1) Although composite materials can provide excellent humidity sensitivity performance, the research history of these materials is relatively short, and the stability of the complex structural characteristics during long-term operation needs further investigation;
(2) Currently, humidity sensors face high demands for their sensitivity and response speed when dealing with new applications such as contactless switches. Furthermore, there is a lack of research on the relevant circuit design and signal processing in this area;
(3) Electrochemical and ionic diffusion-based humidity sensors, which derive power from environmental moisture, currently encounter limitations in terms of power generation and operational duration, necessitating further advancements for practical deployment.

Author Contributions: R.T., M.F., D.L. and J.Q. conceived and designed the study; J.Q., M.F., D.L., R.T. and W.S. (Wenfeng Shen) analyzed and summarized the relevant articles; J.Q., M.F., R.T. and W.S. (Weijie Song) wrote the manuscript; and R.T. revised the manuscript. All authors have read and agreed to the published version of the manuscript.

Funding: This work is supported by the Ningbo Key Scientific and Technological Project (NBSTI 2023Z021).

Institutional Review Board Statement: Not applicable.

Informed Consent Statement: Not applicable.

Data Availability Statement: Not applicable.

Conflicts of Interest: The authors declare no conflicts of interest.

References

1. Khan, Y.; Ostfeld, A.E.; Lochner, C.M.; Pierre, A.; Arias, A.C. Monitoring of Vital Signs with Flexible and Wearable Medical Devices. *Adv. Mater.* **2016**, *28*, 4373–4395. [CrossRef] [PubMed]
2. Wang, D.; Zhang, D.; Li, P.; Yang, Z.; Mi, Q.; Yu, L. Electrospinning of Flexible Poly(Vinyl Alcohol)/MXene Nanofiber-Based Humidity Sensor Self-Powered by Monolayer Molybdenum Diselenide Piezoelectric Nanogenerator. *Nano-Micro Lett.* **2021**, *13*, 57. [CrossRef]
3. Luo, Y.; Abidian, M.R.; Ahn, J.-H.; Akinwande, D.; Andrews, A.M.; Antonietti, M.; Bao, Z.; Berggren, M.; Berkey, C.A.; Bettinger, C.J.; et al. Technology Roadmap for Flexible Sensors. *ACS Nano* **2023**, *17*, 5211–5295. [CrossRef] [PubMed]
4. Delipinar, T.; Shafique, A.; Gohar, M.S.; Yapici, M.K. Fabrication and Materials Integration of Flexible Humidity Sensors for Emerging Applications. *ACS Omega* **2021**, *6*, 8744–8753. [CrossRef] [PubMed]
5. Choi, J.; Chen, Y.; Abbel, R.; Visagie, I.; Parker, K. Flexible Humidity Sensors for Wireless Monitoring Based on Electrospun Sulfonated Polyether Ether Ketone (SPEEK) Nanofibres. *Sens. Actuators B Chem.* **2020**, *324*, 128704. [CrossRef]
6. Ragazzini, I.; Gualandi, I.; D'Altri, G.; Di Matteo, V.; Yeasmin, L.; Cassani, M.C.; Scavetta, E.; Bernardi, E.; Ballarin, B. Polyaniline/Poly (2-Acrylamido-2-Methyl-1-Propanesulfonic Acid) Modified Cellulose as Promising Material for Sensors Design. *Carbohydr. Polym.* **2023**, *316*, 121079. [CrossRef]
7. Yang, T.; Xu, C.; Liu, C.; Ye, Y.; Sun, Z.; Wang, B.; Luo, Z. Conductive Polymer Hydrogels Crosslinked by Electrostatic Interaction with PEDOT:PSS Dopant for Bioelectronics Application. *Chem. Eng. J.* **2022**, *429*, 132430. [CrossRef]
8. Zampetti, E.; Pantalei, S.; Pecora, A.; Valletta, A.; Maiolo, L.; Minotti, A.; Macagnano, A.; Fortunato, G.; Bearzotti, A. Design and Optimization of an Ultra Thin Flexible Capacitive Humidity Sensor. *Sens. Actuators B Chem.* **2009**, *143*, 302–307. [CrossRef]
9. Molina-Lopez, F.; Briand, D.; de Rooij, N.F. All Additive Inkjet Printed Humidity Sensors on Plastic Substrate. *Sens. Actuators B Chem.* **2012**, *166–167*, 212–222. [CrossRef]

10. Duan, Z.; Jiang, Y.; Yan, M.; Wang, S.; Yuan, Z.; Zhao, Q.; Sun, P.; Xie, G.; Du, X.; Tai, H. Facile, Flexible, Cost-Saving, and Environment-Friendly Paper-Based Humidity Sensor for Multifunctional Applications. *ACS Appl. Mater. Interfaces* **2019**, *11*, 21840–21849. [CrossRef]
11. Yang, M.; Huang, M.; Li, Y.; Feng, Z.; Huang, Y.; Chen, H.; Xu, Z.; Liu, H.; Wang, Y. Printing Assembly of Flexible Devices with Oxidation Stable MXene for High Performance Humidity Sensing Applications. *Sens. Actuators B Chem.* **2022**, *364*, 131867. [CrossRef]
12. Zhang, D.; Wang, D.; Zong, X.; Dong, G.; Zhang, Y. High-Performance QCM Humidity Sensor Based on Graphene Oxide/Tin Oxide/Polyaniline Ternary Nanocomposite Prepared by in-Situ Oxidative Polymerization Method. *Sens. Actuators B Chem.* **2018**, *262*, 531–541. [CrossRef]
13. Le, X.; Liu, Y.; Peng, L.; Pang, J.; Xu, Z.; Gao, C.; Xie, J. Surface Acoustic Wave Humidity Sensors Based on Uniform and Thickness Controllable Graphene Oxide Thin Films Formed by Surface Tension. *Microsyst. Nanoeng.* **2019**, *5*, 1–10. [CrossRef] [PubMed]
14. Su, Y.; Li, C.; Li, M.; Li, H.; Xu, S.; Qian, L.; Yang, B. Surface Acoustic Wave Humidity Sensor Based on Three-Dimensional Architecture Graphene/PVA/SiO_2 and Its Application for Respiration Monitoring. *Sens. Actuators B Chem.* **2020**, *308*, 127693. [CrossRef]
15. Xia, B.; Liu, B.; Wang, N.; Liao, C.; Long, G.; Zhao, C.; Liao, Z.; Lyu, D. Polyelectrolyte/Graphene Oxide Nano-Film Integrated Fiber-Optic Sensors for High-Sensitive and Rapid-Response Humidity Measurement. *ACS Appl. Mater. Interfaces* **2022**, *14*, 41379–41388. [CrossRef]
16. Xu, T.; Ding, X.; Huang, Y.; Shao, C.; Song, L.; Gao, X.; Zhang, Z.; Qu, L. An Efficient Polymer Moist-Electric Generator. *Energy Environ. Sci.* **2019**, *12*, 972–978. [CrossRef]
17. Li, S.; Zhang, Y.; Liang, X.; Wang, H.; Lu, H.; Zhu, M.; Wang, H.; Zhang, M.; Qiu, X.; Song, Y.; et al. Humidity-Sensitive Chemoelectric Flexible Sensors Based on Metal-Air Redox Reaction for Health Management. *Nat. Commun.* **2022**, *13*, 5416. [CrossRef] [PubMed]
18. Ullah, A.; Zulfiqar, M.H.; Khan, M.A.; Zubair, M.; Mehmood, M.Q.; Massoud, Y. Fast Response Facile Fabricated IDE-Based Ultra-Sensitive Humidity Sensor for Medical Applications. *ACS Omega* **2023**, *8*, 16842–16850. [CrossRef]
19. Agmon, N. The Grotthuss Mechanism. *Chem. Phys. Lett.* **1995**, *244*, 456–462. [CrossRef]
20. Yuan, Z.; Tai, H.; Ye, Z.; Liu, C.; Xie, G.; Du, X.; Jiang, Y. Novel Highly Sensitive QCM Humidity Sensor with Low Hysteresis Based on Graphene Oxide (GO)/Poly(Ethyleneimine) Layered Film. *Sens. Actuators B Chem.* **2016**, *234*, 145–154. [CrossRef]
21. Traversa, E. Ceramic Sensors for Humidity Detection: The State-of-the-Art and Future Developments. *Sens. Actuators B Chem.* **1995**, *23*, 135–156. [CrossRef]
22. Rittersma, Z.M. Recent Achievements in Miniaturised Humidity Sensors—a Review of Transduction Techniques. *Sens. Actuators Phys.* **2002**, *96*, 196–210. [CrossRef]
23. Zhao, F.; Cheng, H.; Zhang, Z.; Jiang, L.; Qu, L. Direct Power Generation from a Graphene Oxide Film under Moisture. *Adv. Mater.* **2015**, *27*, 4351–4357. [CrossRef] [PubMed]
24. Jiang, Y.; Duan, Z.; Fan, Z.; Yao, P.; Yuan, Z.; Jiang, Y.; Cao, Y.; Tai, H. Power Generation Humidity Sensor Based on NaCl/Halloysite Nanotubes for Respiratory Patterns Monitoring. *Sens. Actuators B Chem.* **2023**, *380*, 133396. [CrossRef]
25. Guo, Y.; Xi, H.; Gu, Z.; Li, M.; Li, X.; Gao, D. A Self-Powered PVA-Based Flexible Humidity Sensor with Humidity-Related Voltage Output for Multifunctional Applications. *Colloids Surf. Physicochem. Eng. Asp.* **2023**, *658*, 130700. [CrossRef]
26. Angadi, V.J.; Chethan, B.; Pattar, V.; Shigihalli, N.B.; Patil, S.A.; Ubaidullah, M.; Sehgal, S.S.; Prakash, C.; Manjuantha, S.O.; Manjunatha, K. Graphene-Cobalt Chromate Ceramics Composite for Humidity Sensor Applications. *J. Alloys Compd.* **2023**, *947*, 169438. [CrossRef]
27. Zhang, Y.; Wu, Y.; Duan, Z.; Liu, B.; Zhao, Q.; Yuan, Z.; Li, S.; Liang, J.; Jiang, Y.; Tai, H. High Performance Humidity Sensor Based on 3D Mesoporous Co_3O_4 Hollow Polyhedron for Multifunctional Applications. *Appl. Surf. Sci.* **2022**, *585*, 152698. [CrossRef]
28. Guo, P.; Tian, B.; Liang, J.; Yang, X.; Tang, G.; Li, Q.; Liu, Q.; Zheng, K.; Chen, X.; Wu, W. All-Printed, Fast Response Flexible Humidity Sensor Based on Hexagonal-WO_3 Nanowires for Multifunctional Applications. *Adv. Mater.* **2023**, *35*, 2304420. [CrossRef]
29. Lei, D.; Zhang, Q.; Liu, N.; Su, T.; Wang, L.; Ren, Z.; Zhang, Z.; Su, J.; Gao, Y. Self-Powered Graphene Oxide Humidity Sensor Based on Potentiometric Humidity Transduction Mechanism. *Adv. Funct. Mater.* **2022**, *32*, 2107330. [CrossRef]
30. Janica, I.; Montes-García, V.; Urban, F.; Hashemi, P.; Nia, A.S.; Feng, X.; Samorì, P.; Ciesielski, A. Covalently Functionalized MXenes for Highly Sensitive Humidity Sensors. *Small Methods* **2023**, *7*, 2201651. [CrossRef]
31. Zeng, S.; Pan, Q.; Huang, Z.; Gu, C.; Wang, T.; Xu, J.; Yan, Z.; Zhao, F.; Li, P.; Tu, Y.; et al. Ultrafast Response of Self-Powered Humidity Sensor of Flexible Graphene Oxide Film. *Mater. Des.* **2023**, *226*, 111683. [CrossRef]
32. Zhao, H.; Wang, Z.; Li, Y.; Yang, M. Single-Sided and Integrated Polyaniline/Poly(Vinylidene Fluoride) Flexible Membrane with Micro/Nanostructures as Breathable, Nontoxic and Fast Response Wearable Humidity Sensor. *J. Colloid Interface Sci.* **2022**, *607*, 367–377. [CrossRef] [PubMed]
33. Heredia-Rivera, U.; Kasi, V.; Krishnakumar, A.; Kadian, S.; Barui, A.K.; He, Z.; Wang, H.; Stanciu, L.; Rahimi, R. Cold Atmospheric Plasma-Assisted Direct Deposition of Polypyrrole-Ag Nanocomposites for Flexible Electronic Sensors. *ACS Appl. Mater. Interfaces* **2023**, *15*, 17078–17090. [CrossRef]
34. Shen, L.; Feng, W.; Yu, D.; Wang, W. High Sensitive Humidity Sensor Based on PEDOT:PSS/CMC-Na Coated Polyester Fabric with Directional Moisture Transport Performance. *Colloids Surf. Physicochem. Eng. Asp.* **2024**, *682*, 132880. [CrossRef]

35. Zhao, H.; Chen, H.; Yang, M.; Li, Y. Facile Fabrication of Poly (Diallyldimethyl Ammonium Chloride)/$Ti_3C_2T_x$/Poly (Vinylidene Fluoride) 3D Hollow Fiber Membrane Flexible Humidity Sensor and Its Application in the Monitoring of Health-Related Physiological Activity. *Sens. Actuators B Chem.* **2023**, *374*, 132773. [CrossRef]
36. Wang, N.; Tong, J.; Wang, J.; Wang, Q.; Chen, S.; Sheng, B. Polyimide-Sputtered and Polymerized Films with Ultrahigh Moisture Sensitivity for Respiratory Monitoring and Contactless Sensing. *ACS Appl. Mater. Interfaces* **2022**, *14*, 11842–11853. [CrossRef]
37. Jiang, X.; Chen, K.; Long, Y.; Liu, S.; Chi, Z.; Xu, J.; Zhang, Y. Design and Synthesis of Vertical Gradient of Expansion Structure Based on Polyimide Humidity Sensing Layer with Ultra-Fast Response, High Sensitivity, and Large Deformation Driven by Humidity. *Chem. Eng. J.* **2023**, *468*, 143805. [CrossRef]
38. Mu, Y.; Jin, P.; Zheng, L.; Wang, C.; Hou, Y.; Liu, W.; Si, L.; Liu, Z. An Enhanced MEMS-Based Polyimide Capacitive-Type Relative-Humidity Sensor with Halloysite Nanotube as a Modifier. *Microchem. J.* **2023**, *191*, 108934. [CrossRef]
39. Roman, C.; Bodea, O.; Prodan, N.; Levi, A.; Cordos, E.; Manoviciu, I. A Capacitive-Type Humidity Sensor Using Crosslinked Poly(Methyl Methacrylate-Co-(2 Hydroxypropyl)-Methacrylate). Sens. *Actuators B Chem.* **1995**, *25*, 710–713. [CrossRef]
40. Meanna Pérez, J.M.; Freyre, C. A Poly(Ethyleneterephthalate)-Based Humidity Sensor. *Sens. Actuators B Chem.* **1997**, *42*, 27–30. [CrossRef]
41. Xu, D.; Liu, B.; Wang, N.; Zhou, J.; Tang, L.; Zhang, D.; Sheng, B. Ultrasensitive and Flexible Humidity Sensors Fabricated by Ion Beam Sputtering and Deposition from Polydimethylsiloxane. *Vacuum* **2023**, *213*, 112125. [CrossRef]
42. Liu, B.-H.; Xie, G.-Z.; Li, C.-Z.; Wang, S.; Yuan, Z.; Duan, Z.-H.; Jiang, Y.-D.; Tai, H.-L. A Chitosan/Amido-Graphene Oxide-Based Self-Powered Humidity Sensor Enabled by Triboelectric Effect. *Rare Met.* **2021**, *40*, 1995–2003. [CrossRef]
43. Kumari, P.; Kumar, A.; Yadav, A.; Gupta, G.; Gupta, G.; Shivagan, D.D.; Bapna, K. Chitosan-Based Highly Sensitive Viable Humidity Sensor for Human Health Monitoring. *ACS Omega* **2023**, *8*, 39511–39522. [CrossRef] [PubMed]
44. Nasution, T.I.; Nainggolan, I.; Dalimunthe, D.; Balyan, M.; Cuana, R.; Khanifah, S. Humidity Detection Using Chitosan Film Based Sensor. *IOP Conf. Ser. Mater. Sci. Eng.* **2018**, *309*, 012080. [CrossRef]
45. Huang, L.; Tang, Y.; Liu, W.; Hu, Q.; Wei, X. Cellulose Paper-Based Humidity Power Generator with High Open Circuit Voltage Based on Zinc-Air Battery Structure. *Carbohydr. Polym.* **2024**, *326*, 121649. [CrossRef]
46. Zhao, Q.; Jiang, Y.; Duan, Z.; Yuan, Z.; Zha, J.; Wu, Z.; Huang, Q.; Zhou, Z.; Li, H.; He, F.; et al. A Nb2CTx/Sodium Alginate-Based Composite Film with Neuron-like Network for Self-Powered Humidity Sensing. *Chem. Eng. J.* **2022**, *438*, 135588. [CrossRef]
47. Rianjanu, A.; Julian, T.; Hidayat, S.N.; Yulianto, N.; Majid, N.; Syamsu, I.; Wasisto, H.S.; Triyana, K. Quartz Crystal Microbalance Humidity Sensors Integrated with Hydrophilic Polyethyleneimine-Grafted Polyacrylonitrile Nanofibers. *Sens. Actuators B Chem.* **2020**, *319*, 128286. [CrossRef]
48. Tang, M.; Liu, X.; Zhang, D.; Zhang, H.; Xi, G. Ultra-Sensitive Humidity QCM Sensor Based on Sodium Alginate/Polyacrylonitrile Composite Film for Contactless Morse Code Communication. *Sens. Actuators B Chem.* **2024**, *407*, 135429. [CrossRef]
49. Zhang, Y.; Zhang, D.; Liu, X.; Yao, Y.; Tang, M.; Zhang, H.; Xi, G. Ultralow-Hysteresis Quartz Crystal Microbalance Humidity Sensor Based on Electrospinned Cellulose Acetate/Konjac Glucomannan Network-like Film. *Sens. Actuators B Chem.* **2024**, *410*, 135643. [CrossRef]
50. Yan, W.; Zhang, D.; Liu, X.; Chen, X.; Yang, C.; Kang, Z. Guar Gum/Ethyl Cellulose-Polyvinyl Pyrrolidone Composite-Based Quartz Crystal Microbalance Humidity Sensor for Human Respiration Monitoring. *ACS Appl. Mater. Interfaces* **2022**, *14*, 31343–31353. [CrossRef]
51. Li, Y.; Yang, M.; Ling, M.; Zhu, Y. Surface Acoustic Wave Humidity Sensors Based on Poly(p-Diethynylbenzene) and Sodium Polysulfonesulfonate. *Sens. Actuators B Chem.* **2007**, *122*, 560–563. [CrossRef]
52. Liu, X.; Zhang, D.; Wang, D.; Li, T.; Song, X.; Kang, Z. A Humidity Sensing and Respiratory Monitoring System Constructed from Quartz Crystal Microbalance Sensors Based on a Chitosan/Polypyrrole Composite Film. *J. Mater. Chem. A* **2021**, *9*, 14524–14533. [CrossRef]
53. Sakai, Y.; Sadaoka, Y.; Matsuguchi, M.; Rao, V.L.; Kamigaki, M. A Humidity Sensor Using Graft Copolymer with Polyelectrolyte Branches. *Polymer* **1989**, *30*, 1068–1071. [CrossRef]
54. Li, Y.; Zhang, L.; Yang, M.; He, W. Improving Humidity Sensing Properties of Copolymer-Based Polyelectrolytes by Modifying the Chemical Structure and Content of the Comonomers. *Sens. Actuators B Chem.* **2019**, *301*, 127061. [CrossRef]
55. Liu, L.; Xu, X.; Zhu, M.; Cui, X.; Feng, J.; Rad, Z.F.; Wang, H.; Song, P. Bioinspired Strong, Tough, and Biodegradable Poly(Vinyl Alcohol) and Its Applications as Substrates for Humidity Sensors. *Adv. Mater. Technol.* **2023**, *8*, 2201414. [CrossRef]
56. Guan, X.; Yu, Y.; Hou, Z.; Wu, K.; Zhao, H.; Liu, S.; Fei, T.; Zhang, T. A Flexible Humidity Sensor Based on Self-Supported Polymer Film. *Sens. Actuators B Chem.* **2022**, *358*, 131438. [CrossRef]
57. Zhao, H.; Lin, X.; Qi, R.; Dai, J.; Liu, S.; Fei, T.; Zhang, T. A Composite Structure of In Situ Cross-Linked Poly(Ionic Liquid)s and Paper for Humidity-Monitoring Applications. *IEEE Sens. J.* **2019**, *19*, 833–837. [CrossRef]
58. He, H.; Yao, Y.; Liu, T. Flexible Humidity Sensor Based on Crosslinked Polyethyleneimine/Tannic Acid and Porous Carbonaceous Interdigitated Electrode. *Sens. Actuators B Chem.* **2023**, *393*, 134194. [CrossRef]
59. Chen, H.; Han, K.; Li, Y. Laser-Direct-Writing Assisted Preparation of Flexible Humidity Sensors Based on Semi-Interpenetrating Polymer Network for Applications in Non-Contact Human-Machine Interaction. *Sens. Actuators B Chem.* **2023**, *394*, 134486. [CrossRef]
60. Lin, W.-D.; Chang, H.-M.; Wu, R.-J. Applied Novel Sensing Material Graphene/Polypyrrole for Humidity Sensor. *Sens. Actuators B Chem.* **2013**, *181*, 326–331. [CrossRef]

61. Li, Y.; Hong, L.; Yang, M. Crosslinked and Quaternized Poly(4-Vinylpyridine)/Polypyrrole Composite as a Potential Candidate for the Detection of Low Humidity. *Talanta* **2008**, *75*, 412–417. [CrossRef]
62. Li, Y.; Fan, K.; Ban, H.; Yang, M. Bilayer-Structured Composite Sensor Based on Polyaniline and Polyelectrolyte for Sensitive Detection of Low Humidity. *Synth. Met.* **2015**, *199*, 51–57. [CrossRef]
63. Mahadeva, S.K.; Yun, S.; Kim, J. Flexible Humidity and Temperature Sensor Based on Cellulose–Polypyrrole Nanocomposite. *Sens. Actuators Phys.* **2011**, *165*, 194–199. [CrossRef]
64. Wang, Y.; Zhang, L.; Zhou, J.; Lu, A. Flexible and Transparent Cellulose-Based Ionic Film as a Humidity Sensor. *ACS Appl. Mater. Interfaces* **2020**, *12*, 7631–7638. [CrossRef] [PubMed]
65. Yu, J.; Feng, Y.; Sun, D.; Ren, W.; Shao, C.; Sun, R. Highly Conductive and Mechanically Robust Cellulose Nanocomposite Hydrogels with Antifreezing and Antidehydration Performances for Flexible Humidity Sensors. *ACS Appl. Mater. Interfaces* **2022**, *14*, 10886–10897. [CrossRef]
66. Zhu, L.; Li, X.; Kasuga, T.; Uetani, K.; Nogi, M.; Koga, H. All-Cellulose-Derived Humidity Sensor Prepared via Direct Laser Writing of Conductive and Moisture-Stable Electrodes on TEMPO-Oxidized Cellulose Paper. *J. Mater. Chem. C* **2022**, *10*, 3712–3719. [CrossRef]
67. Su, P.-G.; Hsu, C.-C. Flexible Humidity Sensor Based on Au Nanoparticles/Organosilica-Containing Polyelectrolyte Composite. *Chemosensors* **2023**, *11*, 291. [CrossRef]
68. He, J.; Zheng, X.; Zheng, Z.; Kong, D.; Ding, K.; Chen, N.; Zhang, H.; Yang, W. Pair Directed Silver Nano-Lines by Single-Particle Assembly in Nanofibers for Non-Contact Humidity Sensors. *Nano Energy* **2022**, *92*, 106748. [CrossRef]
69. Tsai, M.-S.; Su, P.-G.; Lu, C.-J. Fabrication of a Highly Sensitive Flexible Humidity Sensor Based on Pt/Polythiophene/Reduced Graphene Oxide Ternary Nanocomposite Films Using a Simple One-Pot Method. *Sens. Actuators B Chem.* **2020**, *324*, 128728. [CrossRef]
70. Ma, Z.; Yu, Y.; Wu, K.; Song, Y.; Liu, S.; Yang, X.; Fei, T.; Zhang, T. Au Loaded Mesoporous SiO_2/Gelatin Hydrogel: Detecting Low Humidity and NH_3. Chem. *Eng. J.* **2023**, *471*, 144788. [CrossRef]
71. Qi, R.; Lin, X.; Dai, J.; Zhao, H.; Liu, S.; Fei, T.; Zhang, T. Humidity Sensors Based on MCM-41/Polypyrrole Hybrid Film via in-Situ Polymerization. *Sens. Actuators B Chem.* **2018**, *277*, 584–590. [CrossRef]
72. Qi, R.; Zhang, T.; Guan, X.; Dai, J.; Liu, S.; Zhao, H.; Fei, T. Capacitive Humidity Sensors Based on Mesoporous Silica and Poly(3,4-Ethylenedioxythiophene) Composites. *J. Colloid Interface Sci.* **2020**, *565*, 592–600. [CrossRef] [PubMed]
73. Parangusan, H. Capacitive Type Humidity Sensor Based on PANI Decorated Cu–ZnS Porous Microspheres. *Talanta* **2020**, *219*, 121361. [CrossRef] [PubMed]
74. Niu, H.; Yue, W.; Li, Y.; Yin, F.; Gao, S.; Zhang, C.; Kan, H.; Yao, Z.; Jiang, C.; Wang, C. Ultrafast-Response/Recovery Capacitive Humidity Sensor Based on Arc-Shaped Hollow Structure with Nanocone Arrays for Human Physiological Signals Monitoring. *Sens. Actuators B Chem.* **2021**, *334*, 129637. [CrossRef]
75. Zhao, Y.; Chen, G.; Zhao, Y.; Li, M.; Zhang, N.; Wen, J.; Zhou, N.; Li, S.; Mao, H.; Huang, C. Wafer-Level, High-Performance, Flexible Sensors Based on Organic Nanoforests for Human–Machine Interactions. ACS Appl. *Mater. Interfaces* **2023**, *15*, 30793–30803. [CrossRef] [PubMed]
76. Chen, G.; Liu, Y.; Shi, M.; Zhou, N.; Dai, X.; Mao, H.; Chen, D. Performance Enhanced Humidity Sensor by In-Situ Integration of Nanoforests. *IEEE Electron Device Lett.* **2021**, *42*, 585–588. [CrossRef]
77. Lin, Q.; Li, Y.; Yang, M. Highly Sensitive and Ultrafast Response Surface Acoustic Wave Humidity Sensor Based on Electrospun Polyaniline/Poly(Vinyl Butyral) Nanofibers. *Anal. Chim. Acta* **2012**, *748*, 73–80. [CrossRef]
78. Yuan, T.; Qi, X.; Liu, Z.; Yang, J.; Guan, C.; Long, Q.; Cao, J.; Luo, M.; Yang, X.; Yuan, L. Humidity Sensor Based on Micro Optical Fiber Array Fabricated by Electrospinning. *Opt. Commun.* **2018**, *427*, 517–521. [CrossRef]
79. Wen, H.-Y.; Liu, Y.-C.; Chiang, C.-C. The Use of Doped Conductive Bionic Muscle Nanofibers in a Tennis Racket–Shaped Optical Fiber Humidity Sensor. *Sens. Actuators B Chem.* **2020**, *320*, 128340. [CrossRef]
80. Zu, Y.; Duan, Z.; Yuan, Z.; Jiang, Y.; Tai, H. Electrospun Nanofiber-Based Humidity Sensors: Materials, Devices, and Emerging Applications. *J. Mater. Chem. A* **2024**, *12*, 27157–27179. [CrossRef]
81. Squillaci, M.A.; Cipriani, A.; Melucci, M.; Zambianchi, M.; Caminati, G.; Samorì, P. Self-Assembly of Functionalized Oligothiophene into Hygroscopic Fibers: Fabrication of Highly Sensitive and Fast Humidity Sensors. *Adv. Electron. Mater.* **2018**, *4*, 1700382. [CrossRef]
82. Zhang, D.; Jiang, C.; Sun, Y.; Zhou, Q. Layer-by-Layer Self-Assembly of Tricobalt Tetroxide-Polymer Nanocomposite toward High-Performance Humidity-Sensing. *J. Alloys Compd.* **2017**, *711*, 652–658. [CrossRef]
83. Liu, W.; Qu, H.; Hu, J.; Pang, W.; Zhang, H.; Duan, X. A Highly Sensitive Humidity Sensor Based on Ultrahigh-Frequency Microelectromechanical Resonator Coated with Nano-Assembled Polyelectrolyte Thin Films. *Micromachines* **2017**, *8*, 116. [CrossRef]
84. Nohria, R.; Khillan, R.K.; Su, Y.; Dikshit, R.; Lvov, Y.; Varahramyan, K. Humidity Sensor Based on Ultrathin Polyaniline Film Deposited Using Layer-by-Layer Nano-Assembly. *Sens. Actuators B Chem.* **2006**, *114*, 218–222. [CrossRef]
85. Yuan, Y.; Peng, B.; Chi, H.; Li, C.; Liu, R.; Liu, X. Layer-by-Layer Inkjet Printing SPS:PEDOT NP/RGO Composite Film for Flexible Humidity Sensors. *RSC Adv.* **2016**, *6*, 113298–113306. [CrossRef]
86. Yuan, Y.; Zhang, Y.; Liu, R.; Liu, J.; Li, Z.; Liu, X. Humidity Sensor Fabricated by Inkjet-Printing Photosensitive Conductive Inks PEDOT:PVMA on a Paper Substrate. *RSC Adv.* **2016**, *6*, 47498–47508. [CrossRef]

87. Li, N.; Jiang, Y.; Xiao, Y.; Meng, B.; Xing, C.; Zhang, H.; Peng, Z. A Fully Inkjet-Printed Transparent Humidity Sensor Based on a Ti3C2/Ag Hybrid for Touchless Sensing of Finger Motion. *Nanoscale* **2019**, *11*, 21522–21531. [CrossRef]
88. Hertl, W.; Hair, M.L. Hydrogen Bonding between Adsorbed Gases and Surface Hydroxyl Groups on Silica. *J. Phys. Chem.* **1968**, *72*, 4676–4682. [CrossRef]
89. Henderson, M.A. The Interaction of Water with Solid Surfaces: Fundamental Aspects Revisited. *Surf. Sci. Rep.* **2002**, *46*, 1–308. [CrossRef]
90. Dai, J.; Zhao, H.; Lin, X.; Liu, S.; Liu, Y.; Liu, X.; Fei, T.; Zhang, T. Ultrafast Response Polyelectrolyte Humidity Sensor for Respiration Monitoring. *ACS Appl. Mater. Interfaces* **2019**, *11*, 6483–6490. [CrossRef]
91. Gupta, L.K.; Kumar, K.; Yadav, B.C.; Yadav, T.P.; Dzhardimalieva, G.I.; Uflyand, I.E. Shripal Comparative Study on Humidity Sensing Abilities of Synthesized Mono and Poly Rhodium Acryl Amide Tin Oxide (RhAAm/SnO_2) Nanocomposites. *Sens. Actuators Phys.* **2021**, *330*, 112839. [CrossRef]
92. Feng, D.; Zheng, H.; Sun, H.; Li, J.; Xi, J.; Deng, L.; Guo, Y.; Jiang, B.; Zhao, J. SnO2/Polyvinyl Alcohol Nanofibers Wrapped Tilted Fiber Grating for High-Sensitive Humidity Sensing and Fast Human Breath Monitoring. *Sens. Actuators B Chem.* **2023**, *388*, 133807. [CrossRef]
93. Wang, S.; Yan, H.; Zheng, H.; He, Y.; Guo, X.; Li, S.; Yang, C. Fast Response Humidity Sensor Based on Chitosan/Graphene Oxide/Tin Dioxide Composite. *Sens. Actuators B Chem.* **2023**, *392*, 134070. [CrossRef]
94. Shukla, S.K.; Shukla, S.K.; Govender, P.P.; Agorku, E.S. A Resistive Type Humidity Sensor Based on Crystalline Tin Oxide Nanoparticles Encapsulated in Polyaniline Matrix. *Microchim. Acta* **2016**, *183*, 573–580. [CrossRef]
95. Su, P.-G.; Huang, L.-N. Humidity Sensors Based on TiO_2 Nanoparticles/Polypyrrole Composite Thin Films. *Sens. Actuators B Chem.* **2007**, *123*, 501–507. [CrossRef]
96. Shukla, S.K. Synthesis and Characterization of Polypyrrole Grafted Cellulose for Humidity Sensing. *Int. J. Biol. Macromol.* **2013**, *62*, 531–536. [CrossRef]
97. Chethan, B.; Prakash, H.G.R.; Ravikiran, Y.T.; Vijayakumari, S.C.; Thomas, S. Polypyyrole Based Core-Shell Structured Composite Based Humidity Sensor Operable at Room Temperature. *Sens. Actuators B Chem.* **2019**, *296*, 126639. [CrossRef]
98. Sun, A.; Huang, L.; Li, Y. Study on Humidity Sensing Property Based on TiO_2 Porous Film and Polystyrene Sulfonic Sodium. *Sens. Actuators B Chem.* **2009**, *139*, 543–547. [CrossRef]
99. Tong, X.; Wang, H.; Ding, H.; Li, J.; Zhao, H.; Lin, Z.; Xi, H.; Zhang, X. Flexible Humidity Sensors Based on Multidimensional Titanium Dioxide/Cellulose Nanocrystals Composite Film. *Nanomaterials* **2022**, *12*, 1970. [CrossRef]
100. Irawati, N.; Abdullah, T.N.R.; Rahman, H.A.; Ahmad, H.; Harun, S.W. PMMA Microfiber Loop Resonator for Humidity Sensor. *Sens. Actuators Phys.* **2017**, *260*, 112–116. [CrossRef]
101. Sun, A.; Huang, H.; Chu, C.; Li, Y. Effect of the Pore Size of TiO_2 Porous Film on Humidity Sensitive Properties of TiO_2/NaPSS Composite Films. *Sens. Actuators B Chem.* **2011**, *160*, 1335–1339. [CrossRef]
102. Han, K.; Li, Y. Flexible Parallel-Type Capacitive Humidity Sensors Based on the Composite of Polyimide Aerogel and Graphene Oxide with Capability of Detecting Water Content Both in Air and Liquid. *Sens. Actuators B Chem.* **2024**, *401*, 135050. [CrossRef]
103. Guo, L.; Jiang, H.-B.; Shao, R.-Q.; Zhang, Y.-L.; Xie, S.-Y.; Wang, J.-N.; Li, X.-B.; Jiang, F.; Chen, Q.-D.; Zhang, T.; et al. Two-Beam-Laser Interference Mediated Reduction, Patterning and Nanostructuring of Graphene Oxide for the Production of a Flexible Humidity Sensing Device. *Carbon* **2012**, *50*, 1667–1673. [CrossRef]
104. Ravikiran, Y.T.; Chethan, B.; Prasad, V.; Raj Prakash, H.G.; Prashantkumar, M.; Tiwari, S.K.; Thomas, S. Polypyrrole/Reduced Graphene Oxide Composite as a Low-Cost Novel Sensing Material for Fast-Response Humidity Sensor. *Mater. Chem. Phys.* **2023**, *303*, 127800. [CrossRef]
105. Jin, G.; Sun, M.; Gao, Y.; Zhou, X.; Wei, C.; Lyu, L. A CNFs/MWCNTs Aerogel Film-Based Humidity Sensor with Directionally Aligned Porous Structure for Substantially Enhancing Both Sensitivity and Response Speed. *Chem. Eng. J.* **2023**, *473*, 145304. [CrossRef]
106. Wu, K.; Guan, X.; Hou, Z.; Liu, L.; Zhao, H.; Liu, S.; Fei, T.; Zhang, T. Humidity Sensors Based on Metal Organic Frameworks Derived Polyelectrolyte Films. *J. Colloid Interface Sci.* **2021**, *602*, 646–653. [CrossRef]
107. Khan, S.A.; Saqib, M.; Khan, M.; Rehman, M.M.; Rahman, S.A.; Kim, W.Y. Wide-Range, Fast-Responsive Humidity Sensor Based on In2Se3/PEDOT:PSS Nanocomposite. ACS Appl. *Electron. Mater.* **2023**, *5*, 4473–4484. [CrossRef]
108. Huang, L.; Yang, Y.; Ti, P.; Su, G.; Yuan, Q. Graphene Oxide Quantum Dots Attached on Wood-Derived Nanocellulose to Fabricate a Highly Sensitive Humidity Sensor. *Carbohydr. Polym.* **2022**, *288*, 119312. [CrossRef]
109. Duan, Z.; Jiang, Y.; Tai, H. Recent Advances in Humidity Sensors for Human Body Related Humidity Detection. *J. Mater. Chem. C* **2021**, *9*, 14963–14980. [CrossRef]
110. Su, L.; Vélez, P.; Casacuberta, P.; Muñoz-Enano, J.; Martín, F. Microwave Humidity Sensor for Early Detection of Sweat and Urine Leakage. *Electronics* **2023**, *12*, 2276. [CrossRef]
111. Jeong, W.; Song, J.; Bae, J.; Nandanapalli, K.R.; Lee, S. Breathable Nanomesh Humidity Sensor for Real-Time Skin Humidity Monitoring. *ACS Appl. Mater. Interfaces* **2019**, *11*, 44758–44763. [CrossRef]
112. Park, S.-J.; Kim, M.-H.; Ha, T.-J. All-Printed Wearable Humidity Sensor with Hydrophilic Polyvinylpyrrolidone Film for Mobile Respiration Monitoring. *Sens. Actuators B Chem.* **2023**, *394*, 134395. [CrossRef]

113. Zheng, Z.; Yang, L.; Yang, Y.; Li, L.; Lin, B.; Fu, L.; Xu, C. Flexible, Sensitive and Rapid Humidity-Responsive Sensor Based on Rubber/Aldehyde-Modified Sodium Carboxymethyl Starch for Human Respiratory Detection. *Carbohydr. Polym.* **2023**, *306*, 120625. [CrossRef] [PubMed]
114. Yang, Y.; Wang, J.; Lou, J.; Yao, H.; Zhao, C. Fast Response Humidity Sensor Based on Hyperbranched Zwitterionic Polymer for Respiratory Monitoring and Non-Contact Human Machine Interface. *Chem. Eng. J.* **2023**, *471*, 144582. [CrossRef]
115. Feron, S.; Cordero, R.R.; Damiani, A.; Jackson, R.B. Climate Change Extremes and Photovoltaic Power Output. *Nat. Sustain.* **2021**, *4*, 270–276. [CrossRef]
116. Veers, P.; Sethuraman, L.; Keller, J. Wind-Power Generator Technology Research Aims to Meet Global-Wind Power Ambitions. *Joule* **2020**, *4*, 1861–1863. [CrossRef]
117. Rodell, M.; Famiglietti, J.S.; Wiese, D.N.; Reager, J.T.; Beaudoing, H.K.; Landerer, F.W.; Lo, M.-H. Emerging Trends in Global Freshwater Availability. *Nature* **2018**, *557*, 651–659. [CrossRef]
118. Cooley, S.W.; Ryan, J.C.; Smith, L.C. Human Alteration of Global Surface Water Storage Variability. *Nature* **2021**, *591*, 78–81. [CrossRef]
119. Liu, X.; Gao, H.; Ward, J.E.; Liu, X.; Yin, B.; Fu, T.; Chen, J.; Lovley, D.R.; Yao, J. Power Generation from Ambient Humidity Using Protein Nanowires. *Nature* **2020**, *578*, 550–554. [CrossRef]
120. Li, P.; Su, N.; Wang, Z.; Qiu, J. A Ti_3C_2Tx MXene-Based Energy-Harvesting Soft Actuator with Self-Powered Humidity Sensing and Real-Time Motion Tracking Capability. *ACS Nano* **2021**, *15*, 16811–16818. [CrossRef]
121. Zhong, H.; Wang, S.; Wang, Z.; Jiang, J. Asymmetric Self-Powered Cellulose-Based Aerogel for Moisture-Electricity Generation and Humidity Sensing. *Chem. Eng. J.* **2024**, *486*, 150203. [CrossRef]
122. Zhang, M.; Duan, Z.; Zhang, B.; Yuan, Z.; Zhao, Q.; Jiang, Y.; Tai, H. Electrochemical Humidity Sensor Enabled Self-Powered Wireless Humidity Detection System. *Nano Energy* **2023**, *115*, 108745. [CrossRef]
123. Duan, Z.; Zhang, B.; Zhang, M.; Yuan, Z.; Jiang, Y.; Tai, H. High-Performance Electrochemical Power Generation Humidity Sensor Based on NaCl/Sodium Alginate Humidity Sensing Electrolyte and Cu/Zn Electrodes for Visual Humidity Indication and Respiratory Patterns Detection. *Sens. Actuators B Chem.* **2024**, *409*, 135585. [CrossRef]
124. Facile Primary Battery-Based Humidity Sensor for Multifunctional Application. *Sens. Actuators B Chem.* **2022**, *370*, 132369. [CrossRef]
125. Zu, Y.; Hu, J.; Yang, M.; Duan, Z.; Zhang, M.; Yuan, Z.; Jiang, Y.; Tai, H. Electrochemical Power Generation Humidity Sensor Based on WS2 Nanoflakes. *Sens. Actuators B Chem.* **2024**, *405*, 135325. [CrossRef]
126. Duan, Z.; Yuan, Z.; Jiang, Y.; Zhao, Q.; Huang, Q.; Zhang, Y.; Liu, B.; Tai, H. Power Generation Humidity Sensor Based on Primary Battery Structure. *Chem. Eng. J.* **2022**, *446*, 136910. [CrossRef]

chemosensors

MDPI

Review

Nanomaterial-Based Electrochemical Sensors for the Detection of Pharmaceutical Drugs

Shweta J. Malode [1], Mohammed Ali Alshehri [2] and Nagaraj P. Shetti [1,*]

[1] Center for Energy and Environment, School of Advanced Sciences, KLE Technological University, Vidyanagar, Hubballi 580031, Karnataka, India; shweta.malode@kletech.ac.in

[2] Department of Biology, University of Tabuk, Tabuk 71491, Saudi Arabia; ma.alshehri@ut.edu.sa

* Correspondence: dr.npshetti@gmail.com

Abstract: The rapidly increasing human population has led to new biological and environmental challenges. These challenges, in turn, have contributed to the rapid growth of the pharmaceutical sector. Quality control in pharmaceutical manufacturing and drug delivery necessitates portable, sensitive, precise, and cost-effective devices to monitor patient dosing and assess pharmaceutical hazards. This study highlights the attributes and applications of the current nanomaterial-based sensors for drug detection, emphasizing the potential of these devices to advance the detection of bioactive molecules, thereby promoting human health and environmental protection on a large scale. Electrochemical sensors, in particular, have become invaluable in bioimaging, electrochemical analysis, and drug delivery due to their high specificity, selectivity, and stability across cycles. This review focuses on recent advancements in electrochemical devices for healthcare applications, detailing their production, analytical performance, and clinical uses.

Keywords: pharmaceutical drug; electrochemistry; nanomaterial-based sensors; electrochemical methods

1. Introduction

There is increasing interest in the utilization of electrochemical sensors and drug delivery platforms in personalized healthcare and point-of-care (POC) diagnostics [1,2]. These devices demonstrate versatility, non-invasive application, safety, implantability/wearability, a lightweight structure, and cost-effectiveness. The development of integrated platforms capable of operating in direct conjunction with biological systems—whether remotely, on epithelial surfaces, or within soft tissue—is paramount in achieving precise and reliable real-time assessments of physiological parameters or biomarker concentrations [3]. Such parameters encompass the pH, temperature, heart rate, neurophysiological signals, and blood pressure. These electrochemical sensors are characterized by their non-toxic nature and exhibit a minimal immunogenic response upon integration into biological matrices, thereby ensuring biocompatibility [4] and ease of fabrication [5–7].

The development of flexible (bio)sensors often eschews the incorporation of complex substrates, in contrast to conventionally fabricated rigid sensing devices, in response to end-user demands for portable or self-screening solutions [8,9]. The analytical efficacy of these proposed sensors is markedly enhanced through the utilization of advanced transducer materials in the primary sensing element [10,11]. Due to their mechanical properties and material characteristics, paper-based and fabric-integrated detection devices are particularly attractive, as they can be readily modified with nanomaterials and biomolecules [12,13]. Autonomous micro- and nanoscale machines are increasingly integrated into biomedical instrumentation for targeted drug delivery and diagnostics [14]. Biorecognition components are pivotal in ensuring the analytical performance of biosensors, supplemented by novel interface materials such as engineered nanoobjects—especially nanoparticles—employed as immobilization and detection platforms, alongside contemporary carbon-based nanomaterials like graphene and its analogs. Newly synthesized polymers and copolymers are proposed as effective matrices for the immobilization of active components and the enhancement of sensor signal transduction [15,16].

The comprehensive market for pharmacological enterprises was appraised at approximately USD 1.25 trillion in 2019, with projections indicating a surge to USD 1.64 trillion by 2025, driven by the escalating human population. A contextual analysis reveals that pharmaceutical transactions increased by 358.5% from 2005 to 2024 [16]. The pervasive misapplication and abuse of pharmaceuticals have culminated in two critical dilemmas: (i) the imperative need for cost-effective, portable, and precise sensors applicable to diverse practical contexts and (ii) the necessity to monitor and mitigate pharmaceutical contamination in aquatic environments to safeguard both human and ecological health. The demand for affordable, portable, and accurate sensors in clinical contexts is underscored by the rapid advancement of precise diagnostic modalities for infectious diseases, which have markedly influenced global health paradigms. Recent innovations in miniaturized biosensor technologies tailored to point-of-care (POC) testing have yielded significantly enhanced sensitivity, reliability, rapidity, and cost-effectiveness in detection methodologies, obviating the requirement for elaborate instrumentation. These advancements have facilitated the development of user-ready devices that are now available on the market. Moreover, wearable sensors for kinematic tracking have emerged as promising instruments in rehabilitative medicine, enabling the systematic quantification of motor behavior across diverse patient demographics. These devices enhance remote monitoring and telerehabilitation, augmenting care for individuals with neurological or musculoskeletal disorders. The confluence of big data sourced from these applications propels the transition towards personalized and precision medicine. In sweat analysis, flexible, wearable sweat sensors facilitate the continuous, real-time, non-invasive monitoring of sweat analytes, yielding insights into human physiological states. Electrochemical sensors are particularly suitable for these applications due to their superior performance, cost-effectiveness, and extensive applicability. Collectively, advancements in biosensor technology enhance the diagnostic capabilities and optimize the efficiency and efficacy of clinical practices, establishing them as indispensable instruments in contemporary healthcare [11].

The laxity in the regulatory frameworks governing prescription pharmaceuticals and the enforcement of corresponding laws has precipitated a critical epidemic of drug overdoses across numerous nations. For instance, data from the National Center for Health Statistics indicated that, from February 2018 to February 2019, there were 69,029 reported fatalities attributable to overdoses of non-steroidal anti-inflammatory drugs (NSAIDs), representing a 5.5% increase from the previous year [17]. Furthermore, in 2017, over 5000 deaths were documented due to antidepressant overdoses, in contrast to 3889 in 2010, with the US National Center for Health Statistics reporting a consistent annual increment of approximately 6% in mortality associated with antidepressant overdoses from 2005 to 2018. A report from the German Service for the Climate revealed the presence of 203 pharmaceuticals, encompassing significant concentrations, within the aquatic ecosystems of 71 distinct nations. The majority consisted of analgesics, antibiotics, and anti-inflammatory and antifungal agents. Notably, the concentrations of antibiotics in 37 rivers subjected to analysis by Japanese health authorities reached levels as high as 626 ng/L [18]. However, traditional detection methodologies remain constrained due to their high costs and limited mobility. Consequently, electrochemical detection techniques have emerged as promising alternatives to conventional methods [3]. The integration of nanomaterials has significantly enhanced the development of electrochemical sensors; these nanomaterials can be engineered with tunable morphologies, dimensions, surface charges, and physical and chemical properties. This versatility allows for the tailored adjustment of specific nanomaterials to optimize their efficacy in detecting diverse analytes. To fully exploit the capabilities of contemporary electrochemical sensors, a comprehensive understanding of the physicochemical and electrostatic interactions at the interfaces between nanomaterial-based electrodes and target analytes is essential. This knowledge is crucial in detecting vital pharmaceutical compounds, including analgesics, stimulants, antibacterials, antivirals, antifungals, and anticancer agents.

Biosensing technology has undergone significant advancement since the inception of the first biosensor utilizing glucose oxidase in the 20th century [19,20]. It has evolved into a multidisciplinary field that integrates aspects of human physiology with environmental science [21–24]. Biosensors find utility across various interdisciplinary domains, including medicine, materials science, and biological research [25,26]. Despite notable progress aimed at enhancing biosensors' efficacy, these devices remain susceptible to background interference within reaction samples, which can introduce measurement bias and uncertainty. Consequently, it is imperative to develop alternative analytical methodologies to overcome the limitations inherent in conventional biosensors [27]. Electrochemical sensing has emerged as a promising analytical technique, extensively employed in clinical, biological, and pharmacological investigations. Electrochemical sensors offer several advantages over alternative methods, notably their ease of miniaturization, operational simplicity, and cost-effectiveness in detection [28–30].

Furthermore, designs incorporating integrated electrochemical transducers are often characterized by portability, disposability, and user accessibility [31–33]. The advent of simultaneous physiological monitoring through electrochemical biosensors has facilitated the detection of specific biomarkers within human biological fluids [34,35], enabling their identification via wireless data acquisition systems [36–38]. High-performance electrochemical biosensors enhance the electronic conductivity, accelerating advancements in diagnostic assays, environmental surveillance, and pharmaceutical applications [39,40]. An extensive body of literature has emerged that evaluates electrochemical sensors from diverse perspectives, particularly with novel materials and specialized fabrication methodologies [41]. We have synthesized a comprehensive overview of the analytical performance metrics and electrochemical device fabrication techniques employed to achieve targeted enhancements in sensitivity and selectivity [42]. The applications of these electrochemical sensors were then systematically analyzed, emphasizing their innovative roles in human healthcare, including wearable sensor technology, disease diagnostics, and pharmacological screening. Lastly, a concise discourse is presented regarding the prospective developments and challenges associated with electrochemical technologies (Figure 1).

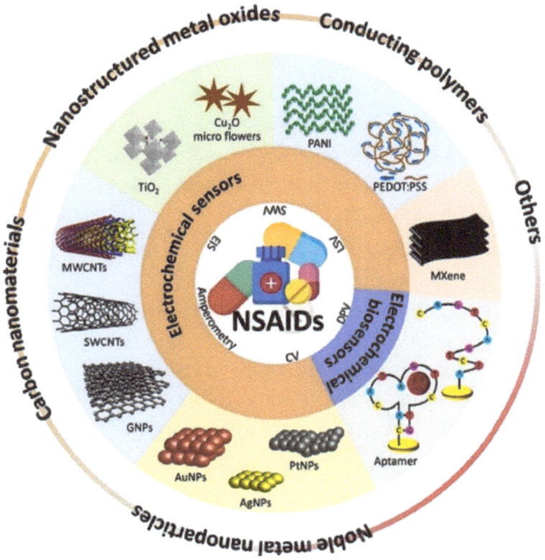

Figure 1. Electrochemical sensors and biosensors based on various nanostructured materials. Reproduced with permission from [42].

1.1. Electrochemical Methods

Various electroanalytical techniques can be used for the electrochemical detection of drugs. Specific methods might be more appropriate for distinguishing drug accumulation in light of explicit electrochemical connection points between the nanomaterials utilized, the analytes of interest, and the typical application. Examples of popular electrochemical systems include voltammetry, electrochemical impedance spectroscopy (EIS), potentiometry, and amperometry. The cyclic voltammetry (CV) technique measures the current by varying the applied potential of the working electrode during forward and reverse scans. CV can be used to calculate the response current, considering the stoichiometry, number of electrons transferred, and reversibility [43]. The dissemination coefficient, charge move coefficient, and initiation boundary may also be determined using this approach, which helps to clarify the framework's response energy. For electrochemical research, beat methods, including square wave voltammetry (SWV), differential pulse voltammetry (DPV), and normal pulse voltammetry (NPV), are more frequently utilized because of their rapid response compared to CV. The Faradaic reply under mobility and linear distribution circumstances is displayed just after the root of the capacitance current by the Cottrell condition, intending for the Faradaic current to be substituted proportionally to the time [44]. DPV is typically suitable to obtain location cutoff points of 10^{-8} M or lower. NPV and DPV both utilize a series of potential pulses; however, DPV differs in that it applies a fixed pulse amplitude superimposed onto a gradually increasing potential range, instead of progressively increasing the pulse amplitude, as in NPV. The current is estimated not long before the utilization of each pulse and towards the end of each pulse. The boundaries, especially the beat width and number, are essential for these pulse methods to enhance the sign reaction [45]. The material used significantly impacts how the beat width and number are enhanced. The number may need to be lowered to remove a sizeable capacitive current from a detecting substrate with high capacitance. Conversely, the beat width may need to be increased for more delicate detection. Even if there are more oxidation/decrease actions occurring at the surface, for sensing phases with large surfaces in particular, the capacitive current may overcome any Faradaic current as it slowly decomposes. This issue could be resolved by using a lower pulse amplitude; however, this may decrease the Faradaic response. One more dominant electrochemical method for detection applications is SWV. This method, as its name implies, utilizes a square wave superimposed on a staircase-like potential, similar to differential pulse voltammetry (DPV). The square wave features both forward and reverse pulses. The difference between the resulting forward and reverse currents is then plotted against the staircase potential to generate the final measurement [46]. The benefit of SWV, as opposed to DPV, is the elimination of capacitive limitations while removing the forward beat from the opposite beat, bringing about more refined identification limits. SWV is likewise helpful in clarifying the terminal energy for some responses by utilizing a fast output rate (~1 V/s) and a quick information assortment speed combined with PC handling. This strategy has a few limits because of its swift sweep rate; SWV is more suitable for examining reversible and fast terminal cycles and those combined with quick substance responses, rather than for semi-reversible responses with low cathode energy. A higher capacitive current in a material can cause more significant peaks in the Faradaic reaction. Amperometric sensors depend on ongoing estimation at an applied cathode potential; they display a few main benefits—for example, a low location breaking point and high selectivity, contrasting with voltammetry-based electrochemical sensors [47]. Due to their excellent responsiveness and selectivity, protein-based amperometric sensors have received much attention [48]. Safety is a major concern in enzymatic electrochemical monitoring, as factors such as protein denaturation, sample array clogging, and interference from microorganisms can impact the reliability.

CV and DPV are widely used in drug detection due to their ability to identify and quantify drugs at low concentrations, particularly when integrated with nanomaterial-based sensors. One study focused on the electrochemical determination of novel psychoactive substances, specifically examining the electroanalytical behavior of compounds such as 25B-NBOMe, benzylpiperazine, 1-(3-chlorophenyl)piperazine, and N,N-dimethyltryptamine. Utilizing DPV on boron-doped diamond electrodes, the researchers achieved high sensitivity in their measurements. The detection limits for these compounds ranged from 0.15 μg/mL to 1.8 μg/mL, indicating the method's effectiveness. Additionally, the technique was used to successfully analyze spiked oral fluid samples, with impressive recovery rates ranging between 98% and 103% [32].

A recent study explored the simultaneous electrochemical determination of non-steroidal anti-inflammatory drugs using innovative electrode materials. Specifically, the researchers employed a combination of fullerene–carbon nanofiber and graphene–carbon nanotube paste electrodes to detect three common medications: diclofenac, naproxen, and ibuprofen. Utilizing the DPV technique, they achieved impressive detection limits—0.230 nM for diclofenac, 0.310 nM for naproxen, and 0.180 nM for ibuprofen. The results indicated robust reproducibility and stability when tested with real surface water samples, showcasing the efficacy of these electrodes in environmental monitoring [34]. A square wave cathodic adsorptive stripping voltammetric method was developed to detect nitrofurantoin. This method demonstrated a well-defined reduction peak, attributed to the reduction of the -NO_2 group present in the compound. Notably, it showcased a linear concentration range of 2×10^{-5} to 1×10^{-7} mol L^{-1}, highlighting its sensitivity. With a limit of detection of just 0.06 ng/mL, the method proved to be highly effective in identifying this toxic drug [36].

A novel biosensor was developed to detect acetaminophen in human blood, utilizing a combination of ruthenium-doped vanadium carbide and a polymeric nanohybrid. Through the application of CV and DPV, this biosensor demonstrated impressive performance, achieving a detection limit of 0.024 μM. Furthermore, it operated effectively within a linear range of 0.1 to 382.72 μM. Notably, the biosensor showed reasonable recovery rates in human blood samples, underscoring its potential for practical application in clinical settings [38]. A dual-functional sensor was developed to detect and degrade tetracycline, which utilized silver-doped zinc ferrite embedded in chitosan-functionalized carbon nanofibers. Electrochemical tests demonstrated the sensor's impressive capabilities, showing a low detection limit of 1 nM and a wide linear range of 0.2 to 53.2 μM. Furthermore, it exhibited high recovery values in real environmental and food samples, underscoring its effectiveness in monitoring this antibiotic [39].

Atenolol was determined in pharmaceutical formulations using a gold nanoparticle-modified indium tin oxide electrode. This innovative method utilized DPV, which had been shown to produce a linear calibration curve within the range of 0.5 μM to 1.0 mM. Notably, the detection limit was established at an impressive 0.13 μM. Additionally, the recovery rates for this technique fell between 95.7% and 105.2%, indicating its reliability for quantitative analysis in both drug formulations and urine samples [41]. The voltammetric methods, combined with nanomaterial-modified electrodes, provide the specificity, sensitivity, and low detection limits needed for practical drug detection across pharmaceuticals, environmental safety, and clinical diagnostics.

1.2. Electrochemical Sensors

A major subgroup of substance sensors is represented by electrochemical sensors. A substance sensor is a tool that uses systems-based data on the chemical qualities of the area. A compound delivers specific reactivity that is directly relevant to the concentration of a particular chemical in various species. The sensor element is the central point of a sensor. In an unusual scenario, the sensor identifies and links to the species as it interfaces with an identifier. A quantifiable result signal is constituted by the identifiers using a substance signal transmitted by the sensor component for the targeted species [49]. The cathode serves as the critical indicator component in electrochemical sensors. An electrocoagulation sensor consists of a counter electrode and receiving cathode isolated by a thin electrolyte layer [50]. Electrochemical sensors usually operate by using the cathode surface species' redox reaction to generate an electrical signal, analogous to gathering the analyte species. The reference electrode is placed inside the electrolyte setup, in close proximity to the working electrode, in a sensor that needs an additional voltage to function and maintain the working electrode's performance. In an ideal situation, no specific current flows between the reference terminal and the functional cathode. Generally speaking, a suitable sensor should have the following characteristics [51]: (1) the signal result must be adequate for the species and size of the target group; (2) it must identify the species; (3) it must set high standards and be extremely selective; (4) it must be highly precise and repeatable; (5) it must have a quick response time for a brief period; (6) it must exhibit a lack of response to ecological factors such as the temperature and ionic strength. Such sensors have reached the commercial stage. Currently, they stand out among the sensors that are in use. For instance, glucose meters with electrochemical sensors can measure the blood glucose levels in diabetics. The idea behind these devices is an enzymatic reaction that is used to calculate blood glucose. According to [52,53], electrochemical sensors may be divided into the following five classes: conductometric sensors, amperometric sensors, impedimetric sensors, voltammetric sensors, and potentiometric sensors. Electrochemical sensors are classified as coulometric and electrochemiluminescence sensors in some cases.

2. Novel Materials for Sensors

2.1. Significance of Nanomaterials in Electrochemical Sensing

The product that completes the identification step requires an excellent and reliable electrochemical sensor. As a result, nanomaterials have several advantages in sensor development that support the electrochemical stage. Given the characteristics of the nanoscale, sensors have several advantages over other types of devices, including their tiny size, high awareness, and selectivity. Different nanomaterials have unique features, such as a large surface area, conductivity, and strong chemical properties, enabling them to interact synergistically with analytes, playing a critical role in enhancing drug detection.

i. Large Surface Area: Nanomaterials have an exceptionally large surface-to-volume ratio, providing more active sites for the adsorption of analyte molecules. This increased interaction area maximizes the binding of drug molecules, improving the sensor's sensitivity. An enhanced surface area also means that more analyte molecules can be captured simultaneously, enabling detection even at low concentrations. This is crucial for the monitoring of trace levels of pharmaceutical compounds.

ii. Enhanced Conductivity: Many nanomaterials, such as carbon nanotubes, graphene, and metal nanoparticles, exhibit excellent electrical conductivity, essential for electrochemical sensors. High conductivity facilitates the rapid transfer of electrons between the nanomaterial and the analyte, which can lead to quick and precise current responses in electrochemical sensors. This rapid electron transfer enhances the detection limit, enabling fast response times and high sensitivity to the presence of drugs in a sample.

iii. Chemical Functionalization and Selectivity: Nanomaterials can be chemically modified to have specific functional groups that selectively interact with particular drug molecules on their surfaces. For instance, surface modifications with functional groups like carboxyl, amino, or thiol can create more robust, selective bonds with target drugs. This selective affinity improves the detection specificity, allowing sensors to distinguish between similar molecules, reducing false positives, and improving the accuracy.

These properties, in combination, make nanomaterial-based sensors highly effective in drug detection by maximizing the sensitivity, selectivity, and response speed, which is crucial for healthcare and environmental monitoring applications. The following can be used as examples of noteworthy nanosensor qualities: • More modest and less expensive; • Increased surface region of the terminal; • Increased pace of mass exchange; • Quick electron movement, in contrast with cathodes, in light of mass materials; • Further developed selectivity; • Greater awareness; • Increased reaction to excessive proportions—as the molecule size decreases, the surface region increases.

The surface energy is significantly influenced by the expansion of a particle's surface area. Modifications in the interparticle spacing or the separation between their constituent atoms are necessary. Incorporating nanoparticles enhances the surface adhesion and influences the voltammetric conductivity when deposited onto electrode surfaces. This results in an increased dynamic surface area, improved selectivity, the enhanced mass transport of reactants, and a better signal-to-noise ratio, among other enhancements. Due to their unique physicochemical properties, nanomaterials are particularly advantageous for electrochemical applications. Advances have been made in integrating mass transport mechanisms with nano-anodes to facilitate the investigation of electrochemical cycles. Previously unavailable at macroscopic scales, glass-like materials are now accessible at the nanoscale, leading to improved interactions and catalytic processes [54]. Additionally, nanosensor materials should exhibit durability and possess excellent dielectric strength. While nanosensors are inherently more delicate and diminutive, they may present a more cost-effective solution than conventional sensor types. Incorporating nanoparticles into a terminal results in two effects: (1) diminished detection probabilities and (2) enhanced reactivity, attributable to the increased surface area of nanostructured entities, thereby leading to a more extensive redox scale. Consequently, this results in augmented peak intensities. It is essential to emphasize that increased reactivity does not necessarily correlate with lower detection thresholds. In certain instances, the baseline noise levels may increase by an equivalent magnitude or even exceed the signal amplitude. This phenomenon is occasionally observed in modified carbon nanotube films. Meanwhile, (3) in situations where the signal amplification surpasses the noise levels, the detection limit can be improved; (4) they exhibit increased stability. These qualities allow for better reproducibility [54].

2.2. Advanced Materials for Electrodes

The configuration of universal or typical electrode materials, including graphite, smooth carbon, carbon filaments, deeply oriented pyrolytic graphite, and boron-doped diamond, has been augmented through the exploration of innovative carbonaceous substances [55–59]. Pencil graphite cathodes have emerged as substitutes for conventional anode materials owing to their advantageous electrical properties, economic viability, and potential for disposable applications [60]. Carbon-based interconnects, such as carbon particulates aggregated in a folio and carbon nanostructures utilizing surface engineering, remain subjects of investigation. These materials are frequently enhanced via the incorporation of electrocatalysts, redox mediators, or biorecognition elements, as biosensors facilitate improved detection capabilities. Recently, boron-doped diamond (BDD) has established an important position within materials science and engineering as a substrate with advanced performance. Fojta and his collaborators [61] gathered the latest advancements in BBD cathode applications, focusing on electrochemical processes involving biomolecules. The primary objective is to synthesize advanced films exhibiting superior BDD characteristics. This involves the modification of the BDD interfaces through the integration of diverse materials, including the incorporation of metallic particulates, the establishment of covalent linkages, and the assembly of metallic or metal oxide nanoparticles and nanorods at designated junctions. Techniques such as chemisorption and the formation of self-assembled monolayers (SAMs) are being investigated to engineer a robust biorecognition layer that mitigates contamination risks. Various methodologies are being explored to leverage nanostructured materials and judiciously select (bio)chemical agents to develop a specialized functional surface. This tailored surface may be employed for a multitude of applications. Sometimes, it is necessary to accept the costs associated with specific advantages, such as smaller windows, increased noise, lower resistance to passivation, and a shorter lifespan [62]. Immobilizing biorecognition elements on terminal surfaces is critical in advancing biosensor technology. Integrating relevant materials at these interfaces enhances the surface-to-volume ratio, significantly augmenting the analytical performance of the sensors. The research conducted by Trnkova has proposed various modification techniques, elucidating the advantageous characteristics of engineered layers composed of diverse terminal materials, tailored to amplified electrochemical DNA-based biosensors [63]. The capability to evaluate a broad spectrum of proteins across extensive concentration ranges holds considerable promise for multiplex disease diagnostics. An electrochemical ultrasensitive immunosensing platform was developed, utilizing human immunoglobulin G (HIgG) as the target analyte, featuring an oligonucleotide self-assembled monolayer that mediated the detection interface on a gold cathode. This design mitigates nonspecific adsorption and cross-reactivity while enabling the efficient modulation of the electrochemical signal [64–66]. Electrochemical nucleic acid biosensors are particularly significant in diagnostic applications, especially for the detection of specific DNA or RNA sequences associated with pathogens and viruses [67,68]. Thus, investigating the hybridization dynamics between an immobilized capture probe on the catalytic interface and the target nucleic acid within biological samples is essential. The electrochemical steric hindrance hybridization strategy demonstrates a low nanomolar detection limit, permitting the quantitative localization of larger biomolecules, such as antibodies, within 10 min.

Furthermore, printable electrodes represent a versatile material, commonly employed in fabricating point-of-care (POC) devices [69]. Screen-printing techniques continue to facilitate the cost-effective production of carbon paste, gold, and other screen-printed electrodes (SPEs) that exhibit heightened sensitivity and selectivity. The inherent simplicity of their integration with various devices paves the way for the development of disposable and user-friendly electrochemical platforms for health monitoring and continuous self-assessment [70]. The versatility of SPEs lies in their potential for chemical modification akin to traditional electrodes or even during the screen-printing process itself. Consequently, SPEs are promising candidates for the rapid screening of pharmaceuticals and biomolecules within complex matrices [71,72]. For instance, the work by Yamanaka et al. [73] has elucidated the fabrication and surface modification strategies of SPEs for the detection of specific DNA sequences, incorporating reverse transcription polymerase chain reactions (RT-PCR) for analytical applications.

2.3. Sensing Systems That Are Integrated into Both Paper and Textiles

Paper has consistently served as a substrate in fabricating paper-based analytical systems, enabling diverse methodologies for current detection and facilitating the differentiation of target biomolecules. This material is attractive and versatile and possesses a semi-normal structural composition, enhancing its utility in various scientific applications. The advancement of paper-based nanobiosensors has facilitated the early detection of immunological reactions and DNA/RNA hybridization events. Specific proteins can function as biotin–avidin or antigen–neutralizer conjugates, establishing a connection between the DNA/RNA molecules and the paper substrate. This interaction has been documented through various synthesis methods, design protocols, and applications [74–80]. The employment of inkjet [81], wax, and screen-printing technologies [82,83] has enabled the production of wearable biosensors suitable for in situ testing. These biosensors exhibit remarkable thermal stability across various temperatures and durations.

Innovative materials, such as Carnage TEX and other smart materials, including nylon, fleece, and cotton, have garnered significant attention due to their incorporation potential in devices for the monitoring of human fluids and tissue compositions. However, electrochemical biosensors often encounter challenges related to the non-conductivity of the materials. Therefore, integrating an additional conductive medium, a cathode, is essential in enhancing the material's electrode surface. The ideal materials and filaments should not interfere with analyte signaling and exhibit biocompatibility for efficient sensor integration. A relatively limited number of publications have highlighted the applications of fiber-based electrochemical biosensors [84]. Due to its hydrophobic characteristics, test absorption resistance, high print fidelity, and ability to maintain electroactivity under strain, GORE-TEX has emerged as an excellent candidate for incorporation into electrochemical sensing devices [85]. The convergence of electrochemical sensors and nanomaterials is increasingly manifesting in clinical applications, progressing from laboratory-based research to practical deployment in clinical trials and pharmaceutical research and development. This evolution is driven by the significant demand for rapid, sensitive, and precise diagnostic methodologies. Nanotechnology-enhanced biosensors demonstrate significant potential across various medical fields, particularly in monitoring health statuses and disease diagnostics. For example, the amalgamation of electrochemical techniques and nanomaterials significantly enhances biosensors' performance, facilitating the detection of specific biomarkers associated with diseases such as cancer and diabetes [3]. Early and accurate diagnosis is pivotal for effective therapeutic interventions and improved clinical outcomes.

Pharmaceutical enterprises, such as Abbott and Medtronic, have pioneered biosensors embodying this transformative trend. Abbott's continuous glucose monitoring systems utilize electrochemical sensors to deliver real-time glucose measurements, which is critical for diabetes management. These sensors have undergone stringent validation protocols within clinical environments to ensure their reliability and precision, rendering them appropriate for patient utilization [11]. Likewise, Medtronic has developed implantable sensors capable of monitoring various physiological parameters. These devices exploit nanomaterials to enhance their sensitivity and biocompatibility, effectively addressing the challenges associated with prolonged implantation periods. The validation of these technologies in clinical settings demands extensive trials to substantiate their efficacy and safety, ultimately culminating in regulatory approvals for broad-based applications. The integration of electrochemical sensors and nanomaterials into clinical frameworks represents a noteworthy advancement in medical technology [21]. Continuous collaboration between researchers and pharmaceutical entities is pivotal in refining these innovations and ensuring their successful transition from laboratory settings to clinical utilization.

2.4. Self-Propelled Micro- and Nanomachines

Miniature and nanomotors (MNMs) have achieved considerable prominence as remarkably sophisticated mechanistic devices and vehicles in the last decade [86–90]. They find application in numerous high-stakes scientific domains. Exhibiting an extensive array of exceptional mechanical properties, MNMs facilitate a range of dynamic functionalities, including rotation, rolling, transportation, delivery, contraction, and collective motion, rendering them highly adaptable for intricate detection systems. The construction of MNMs typically involves foundational materials, which are often fabricated from silicon-based substrates [91], polymers [92–94], or noble and various metals [95]. The self-propulsion phenomenon driven by gradients from adjacent electrochemical reactions is an intriguing mechanism for independent movement [96]. Utilizing specific responsive materials is paramount for the efficacy of the determination system. These materials facilitate the transmutation of the compound energy generated by forces, particularly hydrogen peroxide, into kinetic energy, propelling molecular nanomachines forward. This propulsion is essential in achieving the particular material's synthesis of the MNM surface, including various synergistic materials employed [97]. Merkoçi's consortium [98] has elucidated advancements in micro-/nanomotor science and technology, concentrating on elucidating the motion dynamics, exploring novel energy sources, and developing such motors with bioactive molecules as surface modifiers, predominantly tailored to analytical applications. For prospective biotechnological implementations, the organization of self-propelling nano- and micromotors leveraging Janus architectures is particularly compelling [99]. Notably, these nanomotors show promise in the delivery of chemotherapeutic agents, such as Tamoxifen [100]. Self-propelled micro-nanoscale machines present numerous benefits due to being ecologically benign, mainly through their remarkably efficient conversion of chemical energy into mechanical energy. This transformation employs non-toxic energy sources and external stimuli, such as photonic inputs, as an abundant, controllable, and zero-waste propulsion medium. Consolidating such properties with valuable materials and promoting their practical application would lead to an increase in the use of long-lifetime (bio)sensing frameworks.

2.5. Self-Powered Biofuel Cells

Biofuel cells (BFCs) have recently emerged as a novel analytical platform, harnessing naturally dynamic biomolecules, primarily proteins [101]. BFCs provide a distinctive and autonomous biosensing mechanism, diverging from the conventional methodologies employed in the fabrication of electrochemical biosensors. This innovative system proficiently transduces the stored chemical energy inherent in biomolecules into electrochemical energy, facilitating advanced biosensing applications. This aspect enhances their functionality in fabricating wearable and adaptable sensing devices for the self-monitoring of health parameters, as many developed biosenors are contingent upon an energy source. Thus, either an electromagnetic field or a non-recyclable lithium battery is needed [102]. Modified electrodes have been proposed for the detection of lactate [103], oxygen, and glucose [104,105], as well as the initial phase of malignant growth [106] in human physiological liquids [107]. These electrical frameworks offer remarkable potential for future research and biomedical applications because of their unique biological nature, which makes them appealing for in vivo testing [108].

2.6. Regulatory Standards and Current Challenges

For FDA approval, medical sensors must undergo extensive clinical testing to ensure their accuracy, reliability, reproducibility, and safety. Electrochemical sensors for drug detection face challenges due to the need for high precision at low analyte concentrations. The FDA typically requires multiple phases of clinical trials, including robust double-blind studies, to assess effectiveness compared to established methods. These sensors must also demonstrate stability, biocompatibility, and repeatability, which can be complex due to the variability in nanomaterials. While these sensors show promise, achieving consistent reproducibility and accuracy across diverse patient populations remains difficult. Factors like enzyme degradation and interference from biological matrices can affect readings. Additionally, clinical trials require large sample sizes and lengthy testing, increasing the development costs. Companies like Abbott and Medtronic, known for their successful glucose monitoring biosensors, have navigated these regulatory demands through rigorous testing. For instance, Abbott's FreeStyle Libre and Medtronic's glucose sensors met the FDA standards by demonstrating sustained accuracy in extensive clinical trials, followed by ongoing post-market surveillance [87]. The future of electrochemical sensors in drug detection may involve advancements in nanomaterial stability and integration with digital health systems. Regulatory bodies are increasingly open to innovative technologies, such as the FDA's Breakthrough Devices Program, which could expedite the approval of promising sensor technologies that demonstrate significant clinical benefits.

3. Nanomaterials for Electrochemical Sensing

The integration of nanomaterials has allowed novel and viable detection platforms to be created. This section covers a few significant nanomaterials and nanocomposites, generally utilized to plan the advanced execution of electrochemical sensors and biosensors to distinguish drug compounds (Figure 2).

3.1. Carbon-Based Nanomaterials

In contrast to many other nanomaterials, carbon-based materials have a few unique advantages. They exhibit large surface-to-volume ratios, increased mechanical strength, strong electrical conductivity, and long-range material solidity [109]. Due to these qualities, carbon-based nanomaterials can have greater awareness and lower recognition limits. They are frequently also suitable as supports for surface chemistry with aptamers, pharmaceuticals, and other nanomaterials.

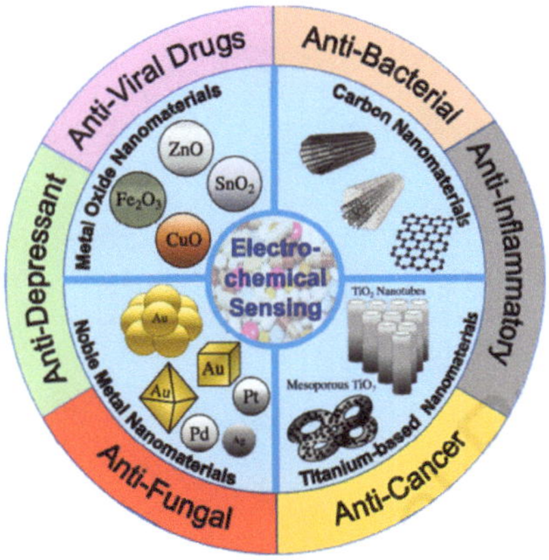

Figure 2. Electrocatalysts used for drug detection. Reproduced with permission from [109].

3.1.1. Carbon Nanotubes

Due to their superior conductivity and outstanding processability, carbon nanotubes (CNTs) are increasingly preferred for electrochemical devices. Contingent upon the particular atomic design and synthetic creation of drugs, CNTs might be utilized to advance electron movement in numerous responses and work with the adsorption of natural particles. Additionally, CNTs can serve as platforms for new device fabrication [110–118]. Their strong conductivity and large surface-to-volume ratio can increase the surface-level presentation of driving factors. Moreover, CNTs might deliver synergetic outcomes that advance detection. SWCNTs, or single-walled carbon nanotubes, are cylindrical tubes with a single graphene sheet and a wall thickness ranging from 0.4 to 2.5 nm. The tiny size and three-dimensionality of nanoparticles can enhance the energy of electron transport in many ways, in addition to their high electrical conductivity.

Their enormous surface-to-volume ratios may have a considerable impact on the overall signal-to-noise percentages. The fact that the nanotubes' constituent parts can be adjusted to enhance the desired response is crucial. For instance, Bandyopadhyay et al. described how they could successfully intercalate or trap harmful insect sprays by changing the SWCNTs' spans, enhancing the particles' electrochemical oxidation [119]. With varying widths of up to 100 nm, MWCNTs are incorporated into various settling graphene sheet layers. MWCNTs have large surface-to-volume ratios, excellent conductivity, and profound tunability, much like SWCNTs. Nevertheless, while constructing electrochemical sensors, significant distinctions between SWCNTs and MWCNTs must also be considered [120]. MWCNTs are relatively rigid, but SWCNTs are typically more flexible. Likewise, the development of SWCNTs requires more resources and is often more costly.

3.1.2. Graphene and Graphene Oxide

Graphene is a hexagonal sheet of sp^2-hybridized carbon, known for its exceptional electrical and structural properties. It is valuable for phase determination and electrochemical detection [121]. While the beneficial oxygen groups in graphene oxide (GO) can enhance the detection of specific analytes, their presence often reduces the surface conductivity [122]. Interestingly, these oxygen functional groups can be intentionally reduced through electrochemical or thermal methods, potentially leading to defects like monovacancies, which can significantly accelerate the catalysis of various atoms. Additionally, doping graphene with heteroatoms can activate surface charges, creating synergistic sites for different particles and aiding in electrostatic interactions [123–128].

Like carbon nanotubes (CNTs), graphene-based nanostructures can serve as frameworks for further derivatization. Preserved nanoparticles (NPs) can be balanced with graphene and GO materials, preventing aggregation and enhancing the performance [129].

The large specific surface area, carrier mobility, and electrical conductivity of graphene allow for the development of low-cost electrode materials that boost the sensitivity and selectivity of electrochemical sensors. The rapid electron transfer facilitated by graphene lowers the activation energy for reactions, improving the overall kinetics of detection [130].

Furthermore, the unique properties of graphene enable the formation of various nanocomposites, optimizing sensors' performance through enhanced electrochemical responses [122]. Functionalization with oxygenated groups increases the hydrophilicity, promoting better interaction with analytes. This is essential in achieving lower detection limits and faster response times. Overall, integrating graphene into sensor technology improves the electrochemical detection process and contributes to the creation of highly efficient biosensing platforms for diverse applications [128,129].

3.2. Noble Metal Nanomaterials

Because of their excellent reactant capacities, large reactant sizes, and diverse forms, MNs are frequently applied for the detection of pharmacological analytes. Through the careful planning of their surfaces and application circumstances, utilizing coating materials and supramolecular interactions, which play a crucial role in the production of nanoparticles, it is possible to manage the nanoparticles' sizes, forms, and characteristics [131]. The size, adsorption power, orientation, and substantial components of the molecules all play a role in identifying nanoparticles for a given analyte. To improve reactant detection, bi- or trimetallic NPs can be used for synergistic effects. Examples include the edge locations of cucurbituril groups or the interiors or exteriors of cyclodextrin rings [132]. As detection platforms, various three-dimensional (3D) nanomaterials, such as those containing nanopores, blank forms, and circles, might be used [133]. Since the compounds may have synergistic effects, bi- and trimetallic composites occasionally enhance the detection power. The alteration of intermediates, improvements in analyte adsorption, proton movement, and reduction in the energizing barrier of the interactions between the analytes and the composite may be attributed to the synergetic effects of different metals [134].

3.3. Metal–Carbon Nanocomposites

Metal–carbon matrix composites have primarily been studied for detection because of their high conductance, huge surface areas, and affordable prices. Nanoparticles can adhere to the vast surface areas of carbon nanomaterials, increasing the population in sensitive regions. Combining materials based on graphene commonly results in blended metal oxides and metal nanoparticles. In particular, GO can decrease particle agglomeration and resolve it, thanks to graphene/GO–metal nanoparticle nanocomposites.

3.4. TiO_2-Supported Nanomaterials

Due to their substance persistence and low cytotoxicity, TiO_2-supported nanostructures are frequently utilized in electrochemical detection. They have outstanding photosynergetic capabilities and adaptability. When TiO_2 nanorods or nanotubes are ornamented with metal nanoparticles, for example, the well-known features of numerous materials might be utilized. To reduce the possibility of coupling among electron transporters and side reactions, the conductivity and charge movement are enhanced by the nanoparticles' dynamic nature, rather than by the TiO_2 support material. Ti also has the advantage of being a biocompatible substance, making it particularly suitable for biomedical applications. Ti is often plentiful, reducing the production costs compared to products with noble metals. TiO_2 can also be considered in more severe circumstances when the electrochemical sensor and nanomaterial are joined and active [135–139].

3.5. Conductive Polymers

Conducive polymers have been included in composites for detection applications over the past ten years. Because of their intriguing behavior when exposed to the electroactive properties of the applied electric field, especially their conductance, conductive polymers are promising [140]. Most of the atoms in these polymers originate from nature. Conductive polymers can improve the discrimination and susceptibility of sensors for specific analytes. Due to their ability to strengthen the particular series of connections between the detection point and the analyte, atomically engraved polymer (MIP) composites have recently attracted attention. These composites are particularly helpful in identifying analytes in complex organic lattices, where selectivity and fouling are significant problems [141]. Furthermore, because MIPs are typically much less expensive than natural transducers, they offer superior practicality and reusability compared to organic receptors. By restricting target atoms, MIPs may also operate as signal transducers that alter the mass, absorption coefficient, absorptivity, conductivity, electric potential, and movement. The development of MIPs is typically supported by computational screening approaches, explaining how possible MIP–analyte interactions work. Additionally, adding MIPs to carbon or metal materials may make the resulting electrochemical sensors more sensitive.

4. Drug Detection Using Electrochemical Sensors and Biosensors

Sensors have been developed for the recognition of numerous types of essential medications. However, due to the underlying medical structures, these sensors frequently require explicit connection points to exploit their tremendous potential for recognition. New electrochemical sensors are being continuously developed to improve their awareness and power and address identification limits. Based on their traits, they can be divided into six distinct groups of clinical applications and properties. These categories include calming, energizing, antibacterial, parasitic, viral, and malignant growth.

4.1. Anti-Inflammatory Drugs

Inflammation is treated with nonsteroidal anti-inflammatory drugs (NSAIDs), which also lessen discomfort, itching, and heat. NSAIDs and painkillers can be used to treat various ailments, making them important medical treatments. When they were identified in the middle of the 19th century, which made it possible to synthesize these substances, this led to the creation of the acetylsalicylic acid or aspirin. NSAIDs, the majority of which are organic acids, were also created due to the chemical discoveries of the 19th and 20th centuries. Following World War II, NSAIDs were first discovered during the pre-prostaglandin era, prior to the 1970s; then, during the later half of the 20th century, the drug discovery process included testing for their impacts on production. Among their physiological functions are those related to the gastrointestinal system, the kidneys, the vascular system, and various other organs. Prostaglandins (PGs) and thromboxane (TxA2) are prostanoids. Two cyclo-oxygenases (COX) control prostanoid production: COX-1 produces PGs and TxA2, which regulates inflammation, pain, and fever, and COX-2 produces prostanoids. COX-2-specific medications were developed in the 1990s to limit COX-2 and spare COX-1; these play a significant role in physiological functioning and are thought to play an essential role in the emergence of adverse reactions, especially those involving the gastrointestinal (GI) tract. Despite the introduction of two new COX-2 inhibitors, which were promoted as having low GI side effects, there was a tremendous amount of commercial development at the turn of the century. In addition to arthritis and pain, COX isoforms have been implicated in several non-arthritic and non-pain-related diseases with inflammation within their etiology, such as cancer, Alzheimer's disease, and other neurodegenerative conditions. The utilization of novel drug delivery technologies for NSAIDs and, to a lesser extent, safer applications of corticosteroids are more recent technological advancements, occurring in the twenty-first century. Moreover, the drowsiness caused by medications like acetaminophen is not very strong. NSAIDs are generally available without a prescription; thus, they are possibly the most poorly handled pharmaceuticals. Consumers' widespread use of NSAIDs has resulted in severe issues with water pollution [142]. Because cyclooxygenase (COX-1 or COX-2) helps to produce prostaglandins, it is implicated in the aggravation and flagging cycle, and all NSAIDs operate by blocking their movement [143].

4.1.1. Naproxen

Ibuprofen and naproxen, two of the most well-known NSAIDs, are propanoic acid subordinates that independently have one and two benzene rings in their synthetic compositions. Both isoniazid and naproxen undergo electrochemical oxidation; typically, a one-electron move causes fast oxidation after the decarboxylation event to create a liquid subsidiary to the material [144]. Shokri et al. examined the impact of fluorescence probe for detection of naproxen in pharmaceutical formulations and water samples using MPA-capped CdTe/ZnS core-shell nanocrystal-neutral red [145]. The increase in fluorescence intensity displayed a direct correlation with the concentration of naproxen, adhering to a linear pattern within the concentration range of 2.00×10^{-1} to 27.3 μmol/L, with detection limits established at 7.0×10^{-2} μmol/L. A disposable electrochemical sensor (AgNPs@GO-Cd) was developed, composed of a computerized circular chip holding gold and altered by silver nanoparticles [146]. The produced terminals demonstrated their value and potential for numerous applications by recognizing naproxen pills and naproxen in human urine tests. Enzymatic electrochemical sensors are usually used to identify biological species, since they are precise, and their practical applications are supported by real-world evidence. Specific proteins of interest are combined with nanoparticles to settle the chemicals and enhance sensors' responses. A cytochrome-P450-based electrochemical sensor was used by Rossi et al. to develop an amperometric biosensor that could detect naproxen by dropping microsomal P4501A2 (msCYP1A2) and MWCNTs onto a screen-printed electrode for graphite (SPE) [147]. A tiny commercial osmotic siphon was used to examine drug transport, and this electrochemical sensor was shown to have a slightly better LOD than other approaches.

Alagumalai et al. [148] studied naproxen electrooxidation using a noble metal efficiently doped on oxidized SWCNTs with GO on its surface. Using the ultrasound-assisted sonication technique, a hybrid nanocomposite, Au@f-CNT/GO, was created and used to accurately quantify the medication NPZ. The proposed sensor also exhibited excellent selectivity, stability, reproducibility, and repeatability. Further evidence that the recommended sensor may be helpful in accurately detecting NPZ in various water and biological samples was derived from an accurate sample analysis.

Díaz et al. [149] investigated the degradation of naproxen using CV and three different MWCNT working electrodes (MWCNT, MWCNT-COOH, and MWCNT-NH_2). The process of electrochemical oxidation results in two peaks that align with the oxidation of deprotonated NPX, which is followed by decarboxylation and additional electron transfer oxidation. The highest removal efficiency, which was 82.5%, was achieved at a constant potential of +1.5 V after a duration of 20 hours at 500 rpm.

Kanagasabapathy et al. [150] used peroxide to aid the electrochemical oxidation process of nano-spinel zinc ferrite films (ZFO). The films' shapes, textures, and electrochemical properties, as well as their lattice structures, were investigated. It was determined that the anodic oxidation and oxyhydroxide deposition electrochemical kinetics were quasi-reversible. Through electropolymerization, Hung et al. [151] produced a poly(L-serine)-modified glassy carbon electrode (PLS/GCE) to investigate naproxen detection. A calibration curve for linear sweep voltammetry was created in the concentration range of 4.3–65 μM, corresponding to a detection limit and standard retrieval of 0.69 μM and $104 \pm 2.5\%$, respectively (Figure 3).

A CPE modified with carbon nanofibers (CNFs), gold nanoparticles (Au), and polyaniline was used by Afzali et al. [152] to conduct a voltammetric analysis of naproxen. The ionic compound Bmim[PF_6], which has a butyl-3-methylimidazolium and hexafluorophosphate anion, could be used as an electrode modifier.

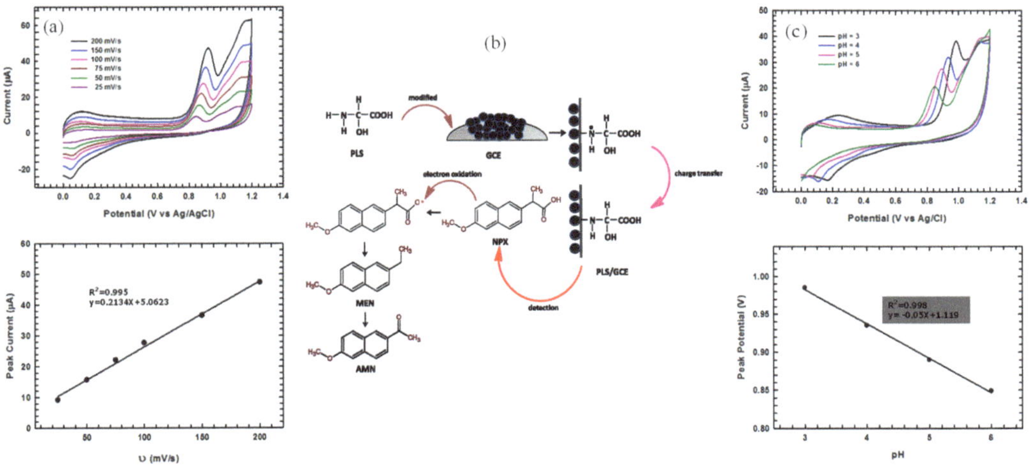

Figure 3. (**a**) Effects of the scan rate on the NPX CV curves produced for the PLS/GCE in PBS. (**b**) Effect of the pH on the NPX CV curves for the PLS/GCE in PBS. (**c**) The schematic of naproxen. Reproduced with permission from [151].

4.1.2. Ibuprofen

To create the ultrasensitive electrochemical sensor described by Roushani et al. for the discovery of ibuprofen, a covalent bond between an aptamer and gold nanoparticles was formed on a polished carbon terminal (GCE) surface. Ibuprofen's oxidation was aided by adding AuNPs, which enhanced the active surface area. The aptamer improved the analyte reaction's signal-to-noise ratio and the sensor's selectivity and awareness. In this system, a static self-assembled monolayer (SAM) was created using cysteamine, and terephthalate was used as the connecting agent to covalently bond an ibuprofen-explicit aptamer (ssDNA2) to the AuNP/GCE surface [153]. Stable SAMs were created by functionalizing AuNPs stored on the GCE with cysteine. The addition of terephthalate and a 3′-amine-ended catch test came next (ssDNA1). Because the ibuprofen compound covered the terminal's surface and impeded the electron's mobility with the redox species, the current decreased as the analyte's centralization increased. Nair et al. also created an AgNP-modified, acid-functionalized GO electrochemical sensor for naproxen that was wrapped in a polymer. Compared to a GO-only sensor, this sensor demonstrated enhanced responsiveness and a lower detection limit [154]. Electrochemical sensors have shown significant promise in detecting and quantifying ibuprofen in pharmaceutical formulations, clinical samples, and environmental monitoring. They can reliably quantify ibuprofen, which is crucial for real-time patient monitoring and quality control, achieving excellent recovery rates above 95%. These sensors also addressed concerns about pharmaceutical contamination in water systems by detecting ibuprofen at concentrations as low as several parts per billion (ppb). Their high sensitivity and selectivity make them valuable for the monitoring of pharmaceutical contamination and in ensuring safety and efficacy across various applications.

Mutharani et al. [155] created an electrochemical sensor for the detection of the anti-inflammatory medication ibuprofen (IBU) in human body fluids, which was studied. It was verified through the facile wet-chemical synthesis of 3D copper tellurate (Cu_3TeO_6), a powerful electrocatalyst. Different methods were used to characterize the synthesized Cu_3TeO_6. The dynamic detection range for the electrochemical determination of IBU was 0.02–5 M and 9–246 M, respectively (Figure 4). Because of its properties, ibuprofen is a frequently recommended medication. In sensor and medication delivery systems, fullerenes and carbon nanotubes were studied as innovative components by Parlak et al. [156]. It was discovered that SiC59 strongly interacted with IBU and had higher electrical sensitivity than the Si@SWCNT system.

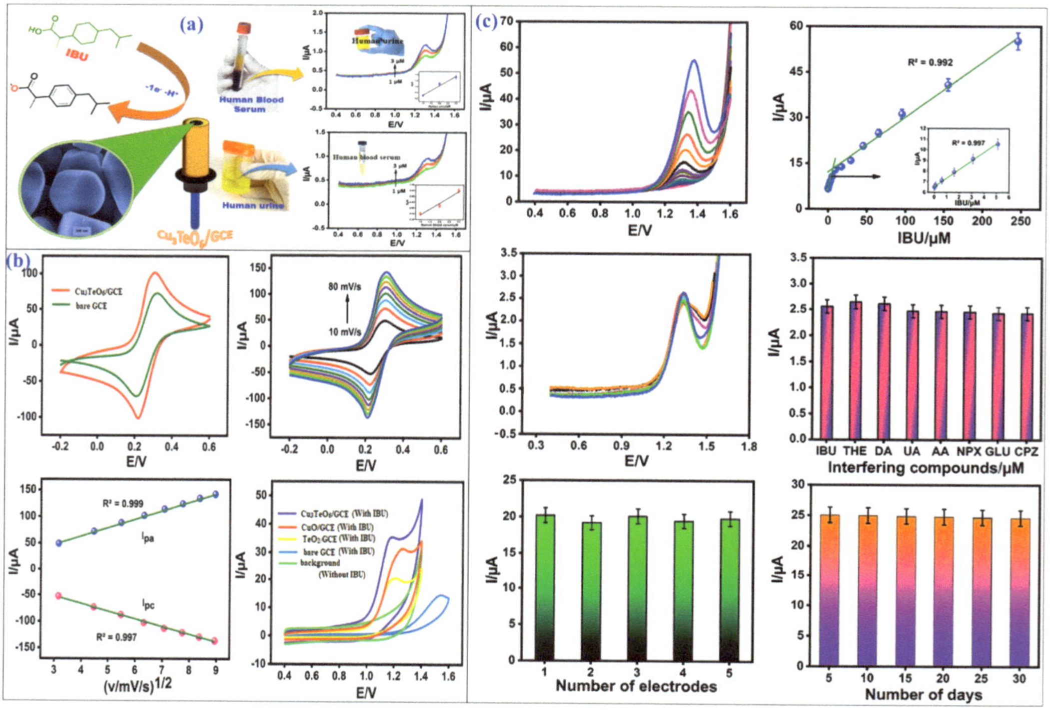

Figure 4. (a) DPVs obtained for ibuprofen−spiked blood and urine samples. **(b)** CVs for IBU at Cu_3TeO_6−modified GCE (red) versus bare GCE (green). CVs of IBU at various scan rates ranging from 10 mV/s to 80 mV/s. The plot of current (I/µA) vs. square root of scan rate $(\upsilon/mV/s)^{1/2}$. The CVs of IBU at CuO/GCE (red), TeO_2/GCE (yellow), Cu_3TeO_6/GCE (purple), and bare GCE (green). **(c)** Analysis of the Cu_3TeO_6−modified GCE for escalating IBU concentrations. DPVs generated for a 15 µM IBU solution in the presence of various interfering substances (THE, DA, UA, AA, NPX, GLU, CPZ). A bar graph illustrated I/µA for the interfering compounds, while a final bar graphs presented the stability of the electrode in terms of current over time and with respect to the number of storage days. Reproduced with permission from [155].

4.1.3. Aspirin

Painkillers are acetylated salicylates with benzene rings and carboxylic groups, which are analogous to propionic acids. Ibuprofen is hydrolyzed into salicylic acid during the oxidation of headache medications. Salicylic acid is exposed to a one-electron deficit to form a free radical. The radical is converted to 2,5-dihydroxybenzoic acid through the combination of another radical and the loss of an electron [157]. Poly-4-vinylpyridine (P4VP) was found to be folded over MWCNTs and drop-projected onto a GCE surface, according to Ghadimi et al. According to the research in [158], joining conductive polymers affects the compound's conductivity, electron transport energy, and electrocatalytic action. Diouf et al. published a paper on an electrochemical sensor composed of self-collecting chitosan wrapped in AuNPs on a screen-printed carbon cathode (SPCE). The chitosan was electrically protective, while showing excellent synergistic movement for anti-inflammatory drugs. To overcome this, AuNPs were combined, increasing the conductivity and promoting catalytic activity. Because of their significant synergistic properties, large surface-to-volume ratio, and high conductivity, AuNPs are frequently used to detect analytes. Through DPV, this fabricated sensor achieved an LOD of 0.03 ng/L [159].

The interest in creating pharmacological diagnostics techniques has recently increased due to the rise in inflammatory illnesses. When taken in therapeutic doses, acetylsalicylic acid (ASA or aspirin) can be used to treat several diseases. However, ASA overdoses can cause adverse side effects, such as ulcers and gastrointestinal damage. This makes it perfect for the development of sensitive, rapid, and portable ASA detection techniques. Diouf et al. [159] used an electrochemical sensor and an electronic voltammeter to analyze aspirin levels in urine, saliva, and a medication tablet. The electrochemical sensor was self-assembled on a screen-printed carbon electrode (SPCE) with chitosan-coated gold nanoparticles. From the data for both devices, prediction models were created using the partial least squares (PLS) method, which produced a regression correlation coefficient R^2 = 0.99. As shown in Figure 5, both the VE-Tongue and the SPCE/(Cs + AuNPs) electrochemical sensors may offer practical tools for the examination of the biological effects of drugs.

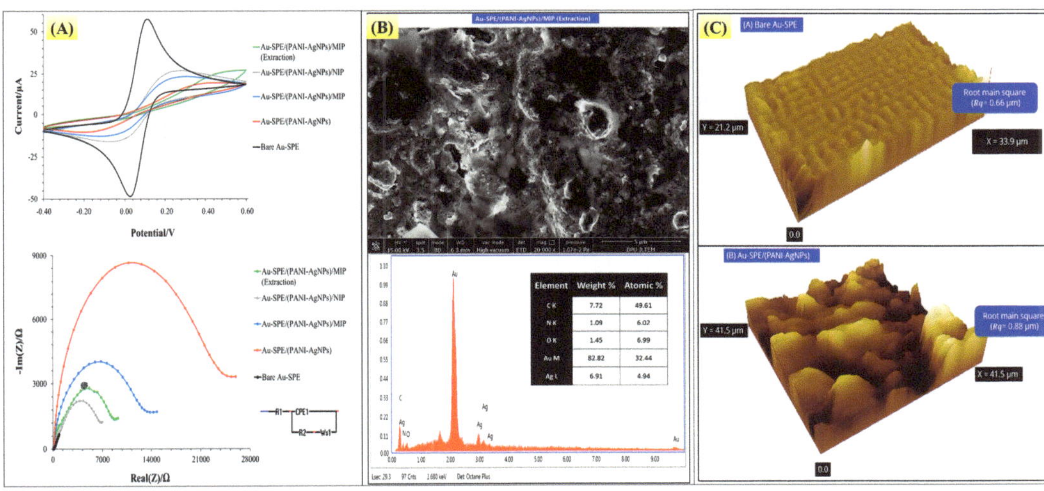

Figure 5. The cyclic voltammograms and Nyquist plots in (**A**) correlate to the undeveloped Au−SPE and the various MIP sensor development stages. (**B**) The table demonstrates that the percentages of O and C drop to 1.45% and 7.72% following the TRA extraction stage. (**C**) The electrodes' AFM pictures. Reproduced with permission from [159].

Xia et al. created a new indium (In)-doped PbO_2 electrode for the electrochemical degradation of refractory organic contaminants using the electrodeposition process [160]. After doping, there were energy savings of up to 30.56%. This finding matched the surface characterization data of PbO_2 electrodes quite well.

4.1.4. Diclofenac and Celecoxib

Diclofenac is a non-steroidal anti-inflammatory medicine that is widely used worldwide to treat various illnesses, including osteoarthritis, ankylosing spondylitis, and ailments that cause severe muscle pain. Diclofenac has no side effects when taken in the recommended amounts, but an overdose can negatively affect the body [161]. Additionally, even trace amounts of diclofenac in ecosystems harm the health of living things. As a result, it is necessary to create analytical methods for diclofenac monitoring. Biosensing and electrochemical sensing techniques have been widely described in this field.

Diclofenac and indomethacin play a role in gathering NSAID residues, although they are less common than ibuprofen, headache medicines, and naproxen. Sataraddi et al. effectively utilized an MWCNT-modified GCE for the electrochemical detection of indomethacin, which was used to verify the precision of commercial drug tests and identify diclofenac in complex human liquids [162]. The diclofenac particle is divided through the nitrogen molecule during electrochemical oxidation. The one-electron irreversible oxidation process is part of the electrochemical oxidation process. Celecoxib, a less popular NSAID, lessens discomfort by inhibiting COX-2, the enzyme that starts inflammatory responses. Arkan et al. [163] illustrated a graphene–gold nanocomposite carbon ionic fluid cathode to select celecoxib. The graphene and gold nanoparticles demonstrated superior interactions compared to the electrochemical sensor.

Shalauddin et al. [164] presented the electrochemical detection of acetaminophen and diclofenac sodium using a nanocomposite composed of nanocellulose (NC), functionalized multiwalled carbon nanotubes (fMWCNTs), and biosynthesized copper nanoparticles (CuN) (NC-fMWCNT-CuN/GCE). Green tea leaf extract was used as a reducing and stabilizing agent in the biosynthesized CuN process for the first time. The SWV approach was used to perform the simultaneous determination. The substantial recoveries and low RSDs show the sensor's potential for use in accurate sample detection. It offers a potential sensing platform for the detection of pharmaceutical formulations in human blood and serum.

Honakeri et al. [165] developed a novel core–shell nanostructure-modified sensor based on carbon electrodes, demonstrating improved sensitivity towards diclofenac. A discrete voltammetric technique was used to determine diclofenac's electrochemical behavior and applications (DCF). According to the proposed modified electrode, DCF was electrooxidized and electrocatalyzed strongly compared to the bare electrode, with a higher peak shift. In addition to being fast, consistent, repeatable, and reproducible, the modified electrode possessed other unique qualities. The authors considered how different performance parameters affected the peak improvement. The limit of quantification (LOQ) was determined at 11.3×10^{-8} M, and the limit of detection (LOD) was 3.41×10^{-8} M. The relevance of the proposed scheme was assessed by analyzing DCF in drug products and human samples. The DCF recovery in the tablet reached 97.5%, with an RSD of 0.7%.

4.2. *Antidepressants*

Antidepressants may currently rank among the most abused and widely prescribed drugs. Most antidepressants disrupt sleep—namely, the physiological patterns of the several stages of sleep, which can be monitored overnight using EEG and other physiological markers. The most effective antidepressants for rapid eye movement (REM) sleep are those that improve serotonin activity by slowing metabolism or preventing reuptake. Early in treatment, the reduction in REM sleep seems to be the greatest. However, after the use of monoamine oxidase drugs, when REM sleep is frequently absent for several months, it steadily decreases after long-term medication use. Antidepressants can impact sleep onset and maintenance, but the effects vary considerably among medications. Early in treatment, some antidepressants—including clomipramine and SSRIs, particularly fluoxetine—are sleep-disturbing, whereas others, including amitriptyline and the more recent serotonin 5-HT2-receptor antagonists, promote sleep. After a few weeks of treatment, these effects are comparatively fleeting, and there are not many noticeable distinctions among such medicines. In general, within the first 3–4 weeks of the use of some effective antidepressant treatments, depressed patients' objectively measured sleep and subjective sleep quality was improved. When insomnia is bothersome, or to ensure compliance, improving sleep early in therapy may be an essential clinical aim for some patients. In these patients, it is advised to choose an antidepressant that is well tolerated and effective and enhances short-term sleep. Before selecting a course of treatment, it is essential to rule out other sleep problems in patients, such as REM sleep behavior disorders and restless leg syndrome, which some antidepressants can exacerbate. On the other hand, there is proof that some antidepressants may help with sleep disturbances, including anxiety attacks.

Dopamine, norepinephrine, and serotonin—the three types of monoamines—serve as synapses at which signals are sent to the cerebrum's nerve receptors. For individuals who experience depression or other mental health issues, antidepressants work by enhancing the effects of these synapses. There are five different classes of antidepressants, but selective serotonin reuptake inhibitors (SSRIs), which prevent serotonin reuptake, are the most well-known class. The three most well-known types, paroxetine (Paxil), fluoxetine (Prozac), and sertraline (Zoloft), are typically larger, making their electrochemical oxidation more challenging. Because of this, contrary to NSAIDs and medications from all other classes, these medicines are manufactured with fewer electrochemical sensors.

4.2.1. Fluoxetine

MIP NPs with fluoxetine (combined by precipitation polymerization) were recently included in a CPE [166]. The coordinated terminal's graphene significantly increased the awareness. A fluoxetine-engraved polymer was created using methacrylic acid and vinyl benzene (VB). The former provides hydrogen-bonding interactions with fluoxetine using its alternative amine and fluorine groups. By analyzing different strategies, the inclusion of graphene to increase the conductivity was considered. Two techniques for the consolidation of graphene were used with nano-MIP-modified carbon glue anodes. The subsequent method (nano-MIP/G2-CP) combined graphene with an orchestrated polymer, instead of the original method's combination of graphene, graphite, and MIP powder. The nano-MIP/G2-CP produced the best results. The cathode demonstrated excellent responsiveness while revealing an LOD of 2.8 nM. Ardelean et al. developed a carbon nanofiber–epoxy composite cathode for fluoxetine, and antibiotics were detected electrochemically in water simultaneously [167].

The demand for healthy products that aid in weight loss is rising due to the global obesity pandemic. However, unstated adulterants are frequently added to improve their performance, and the creation of quick procedures for the identification of these substances is crucial. Ramos et al. [168] showed that the doping agent fluoxetine could be quickly detected and quantified in samples with boron-doped diamond as the working electrode. After simple sample dilution in a supportive electrolyte solution, quick fluoxetine screening is feasible. These findings imply that the technique has much potential as a quick and easy screening test to detect FLU in natural items used in obesity treatment.

4.2.2. Paroxetine

Another SSRI that is widely used to treat severe anxiety problems is paroxetine, marketed under the trade name Paxil and comparable to other SSRIs [169]. Oghli et al. demonstrated a polyoxometalate/diminished graphene oxide (rGO)-modified pencil graphite sensor after subsequently identifying paroxetine [170]. Pencil graphite anodes (PGEs) offer an advantage over other carbon-based cathodes because of their inexpensive costs, excellent mechanical dependability, low foundation currents, and wide anticipated window. A small portion of the graphite cathode surface had to be removed to eliminate memory effects and the adsorbed species that caused terminal fouling. The rGO was combined with the proton-moving phosphotungstic acid, which was then used to modify the PGE. The electrochemical sensor performed flawlessly to break down paroxetine in serum and urine.

4.2.3. Sertraline

Another well-known SSRI is sertraline, which is marketed as Zoloft. Khosrokhavar et al. [171] created a graphene nanosheet for sertraline that consolidated an MIP as an SPCE. The electrocatalyst for the identification of sertraline was a Ni–levodopa film bound to AuNPs, and, in the modified GCE, AuNPs and MWCNTs cooperated in providing a substantial surface area that could electropolymerize more Ni(II)-LD, leading to the increased electrochemical oxidation of sertraline. In a study by Shoja et al. [172], the use of Ni(II)-Ni(III) redox couples along with levodopa was proven to have a strong synergist effect for the oxidation of natural components like amines, carboxylic groups, and alcohols.

Based on estimations of this system's reliability, sertraline could undergo electrochemical oxidation consisting of two electrons and two protons.

4.2.4. Venlafaxine

SNRIs, or serotonin and norepinephrine reuptake inhibitors, are a unique class of antidepressants. SNRIs are more effective than SSRIs in alleviating more severe anxiety [173]. Iron oxide (Fe_3O_4) has become a sought-after electrocatalyst for the oxidation of natural particles and detection of organic molecules [174]. To differentiate between venlafaxine and venlafaxine, Khalilzadeh et al. created an electrochemical sensor with iron oxide nanoparticles stored on a cellulose nanocrystal–copper nanocomposite (Fe_3O_4@CNC/Cu) [175]. Petasites hybridus leaf was used to develop electrocatalysts and served as a copper settler. This cycle could continue spontaneously [175]. The creators of the proposed electrical detector used DPV to analyze venlafaxine quantitatively in samples; Figure 4c shows the DPV bending. The electrochemical sensor showed acceptable responsiveness and a wide range, with a lower detection limit than in other literature reports.

4.2.5. TCAs

Tricyclic antidepressants (TCAs), among the first antidepressants that were widely recommended in the 1950s, continue to be a popular option [176]. A nitrogen molecule is consolidated in their design's focal ring, consisting of three freely measured connected rings. Additionally, TCAs can prevent neuroreceptors from reabsorbing serotonin, norepinephrine, and acetylcholine. To detect imipramine, Jankowska-Sliwinska et al. developed a DNA-based electrochemical sensor. Using oligonucleotide successions and their integral strands that had been thiol-marked, electrochemical sensors for gold glue were tuned. Unexpectedly, the DNA-adjusted sensor outperformed an exposed gold adhesive and DNA terminals [177]. A simple one-pot sonochemical synthesis method was used to create a bismuth oxide nano-tile-enhanced peeling graphite terminal, which demonstrated a respectable detection range (0.02–82.3 μM) and a feasible detection limit (6 nM) for imipramine [178]. While SPEs and fine carbon in natural grids demonstrated great results in experiments with desipramine [179], an improved electrochemical sensor, composed of palladium nanoparticle-brightened rGO, showed promise in assessing the amount of imipramine in human urine [180]. According to adsorptive stripping voltammetry, Sanghavi and Srivastava [181] simultaneously identified imipramine, trimipramine, and desipramine, when adopting titanium dioxide with an Amberlite XAD-2-modified CPE.

4.3. Antibacterial Medications

Antibacterial drugs (antitoxins) are generally utilized to treat bacterial infections in humans, animals, and plants. These medications are broadly used given the diverse distribution of microbes through different systems. Their activity follows four distinct pathways, including the inhibition of chemicals in cell wall amalgamation, nucleic acid digestion, protein combination, and cell film disturbance. Bacteria are targeted by antibiotics, which belong to the class of antimicrobial agents. Due to the effectiveness of antibiotics in treating and preventing bacterial infections, they are frequently used in this field. The growth of bacteria can be suppressed or terminated. Only a small number of antibiotics also have antiprotozoal qualities. In contrast to antibiotics, which are ineffective against viruses like the flu or the common cold, antiviral drugs or antivirals are pharmaceuticals that prevent the growth of viruses. The word "antibiotic", which means "opposing life", is derived from the Greek words "anti", which means "against", and "bios", which means "life", and is used to refer to any medication intended to target bacteria. However, in standard medical practice, only naturally occurring antibiotics (like penicillin) are used (by one microorganism fighting another). Sulfonamides and antiseptics are examples of non-antibiotic antibacterials that are entirely manufactured. However, both types are included in antimicrobial chemotherapy and have the same goal of destroying or limiting bacterial growth. In contrast to antibiotics, a substantial number of antibacterials are utilized in medicine and, on occasion, in animal feed. "Antibacterials" include antiseptic drugs, antibacterial soaps, and chemical disinfectants. Antibiotics have been used since the beginning of time. The therapeutic value of moldy bread has been mentioned in Ancient Egypt, Nubia, China, Serbia, Greece, and Rome, among other cultures. The earliest formal record of the use of mold to treat ailments was created by John Parkinson (1567–1650). In the 20th century, antibiotics changed medicine. Modern penicillin was discovered in 1928 by Alexander Fleming (1881–1955), and its widespread use was beneficial throughout the war. However, because antibiotics are so powerful and accessible, certain bacteria have developed resistance to them due to abuse.

As anti-infection agents have gained increased interest as a solution for an expansive range of illnesses, from rankles to tuberculosis, the development of anti-infection agents and their misuse have increased. Because of the unreasonable use of antimicrobials for various conditions, microorganisms have developed resistance to these medications. These resistant bacterial strains increase the spread of viral diseases, which necessitates frequent monitoring among patients. Excess consumption can trigger numerous detrimental side effects, like sensitivities, bone marrow damage, cancer, nephropathy, immunopathological effects, hepatoxicity, and regenerative problems. To achieve the close monitoring of these medications to limit the adverse consequences for the climate and general human well-being, further developments should be made in light of new advancements and materials. These medications can be ordered by their structures and chiefly include sulfonamide (sulfamethizole), macrolides (erythromycin), antibiotic medications (oxytetracycline), fluoroquinolones (ciprofloxacin), and β-lactam (penicillin). The electrochemical identification of some of these basic antimicrobials is examined below.

4.3.1. Penicillin

The antitoxin penicillin is most frequently used to treat staphylococcal and streptococcal infections. The catalysts trapped on crossover Pt-nanowire/Au-NP clusters displayed high responsiveness for the identification of penicillin and antibiotic medications, according to an electrochemical detection platform designed for the oxidation of penicillin to penicillin acid, with the arrival of carbon dioxide within sight of the penicillinase catalyst, as shown in Figure 6 [182]. Most electrochemical identification techniques focus on a few distinct types of penicillin [183]. Feier and colleagues investigated the electrochemical behaviors of each of the five penicillin types with a boron-doped precious stone terminal (BDDE). This demonstrated that this group of drug particles can likely be highly oxidized [184]. With a detection limit of 57 ng/L when recognizing penicillin, a GCE modified with graphene, poly(3,4-ethylenedioxythiophene (PEDOT), and AuNPs displayed excellent responsiveness [185]. The interaction of Printex 6L Carbon (P6LC) and CdTe quantum dots (QDs) inside a PEDOT, namely poly(3,4-ethylenedioxythiophene)-poly(styrene sulfonate) (PSS) film, enabled the creation of another electrochemical sensor for the detection of amoxicillin (AMX) [186]. A gold sign transducer was used to demonstrate the electrochemical detection of penicillin G in milk, which revealed a detection limit of 2 μM [187]. This research focused on distinguishing penicillin G from other types of penicillin and antimicrobials by a factor of about 10. Li et al. developed gold-based immunosensors with a bilayer lipid screen that was hostile to penicillin G to detect trace amounts penicillin G at the value specified by the European Association (4 μg/L) [183]. The intended sensor might also be used as a fast penicillin G screening detection tool. This sensor proved to be more effective and beneficial than standard HPLC.

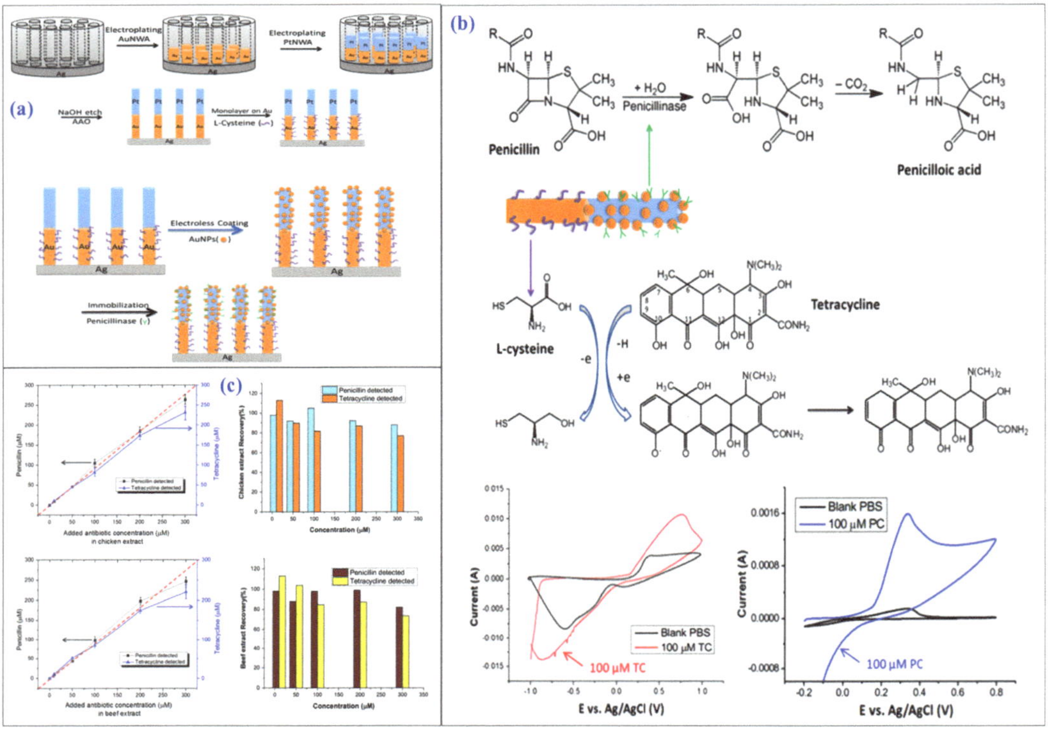

Figure 6. (**a**) Schematic representation of Au−Pt multisegment nanowire array fabrication with immobilization of L−cysteine on Au segment and electroless plating of Au nanoparticles on Pt segment, followed by localization of penicillinase enzyme. (**b**) Penicillinase and penicillin sensing mechanisms; L−cysteine and tetracycline sensing mechanisms. CV scans of Au (L−cysteine) nanowire arrays sensing 100 μM tetracycline and Pt (penicillinase) nanowire arrays monitoring penicillin were conducted. (**c**) Evaluation of penicillin and tetracycline in samples employing multiple extracts. Reproduced with permission from [182].

4.3.2. Tetracycline

Antibiotic medicines (TET) have numerous applications in targeting Gram-positive and Gram-negative bacteria and pathogens. They are also often used as food additives in farming areas. Tang et al. designed a sensor to detect TET. When used as a cover for a GCE and AuNPs, MoS_2 and TiO_2 provided a large surface area due to their circular design [188]. A roundabout electrochemical identification approach for TET was used to complete the suggested sensor. In a different investigation, CV and EIS were used to investigate the ability of stepwise-produced Fe_3O_4/AuNPs with chitosan to detect TET. This platform was used to test food, and the results revealed a 95.9% recovery rate with a 1.86% standard deviation. Using impedance antimicrobials, the particularity and security of the sensors were investigated [189]. An MIP was also used to create a TET sensor using MWCNTs and AuNPs. As a result, the cathode was projected to have the most detection locations and a higher electron transport rate. The cathode's improved electrocatalytic performance with AuNPs led to a low LOD of 90 nM for TET when using CV. When the sensor's selectivity was tested under prevalent disruptions (such as those caused by oxytetracycline, chloramphenicol, and nafcillin), it was discovered that oxytetracycline had a more significant impact than the other two compounds [190].

4.3.3. Kanamycin

As substrates for biosensing, Qin et al. improved a progressive thionine-functionalized graphene and nanoporous (HNP) Pt-Cu composite (GR-TH). When using an HNP-PtCu/GR-TH/GCE, the aptamer designated for kanamycin was arranged using strong interactions among the aptamer and the PtNPs' amine groups. For kanamycin, the sensor generated a lower LOD of 0.86 pM and a total direct response within the range of 0.001 to 100 nM [191,192]. The sensor also demonstrated good sensitivity for kanamycin in the presence of other competing species, proving its potential for analytical techniques. In addition, the sensor exhibited great functional use and good solidness in milk tests.

4.3.4. Chloramphenicol

A specialist medication in fighting both Gram-negative and -positive bacterial microorganisms is chloramphenicol (CAP). An electrochemical sensor was developed using rGO and palladium nanoparticles [193] to degrade CAP. It involved a transmission electron magnifying lens in its construction. The electrochemical experiment was achieved by utilizing a sensor that was examined by CV and DPV as an easy-to-understand procedure for the recognition of actual samples, such as honey and tap water. The creators inspected the impacts of different boundaries. They found upgraded dependability, selectivity, and a broad range for the detection of CAP utilizing the electrochemical sensor. CAP's nitroso subordinates were considered, and the response component was presented as a two-electron and two-proton movement mechanism. Chen et al. used a molybdenum sulfide/polyaniline nanocomposite (MoS2/PANI) to construct an electrochemical sensor that demonstrated a broad range over three significant degrees and additional notable electrochemical benefits. Under a neutral pH, its actual capability for CAP detection was confirmed [194]. Recently, the electrocatalyst europium oxide (Eu_2O_3) has come into focus as a possible CAP detection catalyst. The Eu_2O_3/rGO nanocomposite showed increased repeatability and awareness for the detection of CAP in honey and milk and had excellent electric conductivity, dependability, and adaptability and a large, electrochemically accessible surface area [195].

4.4. Antifungal Drugs

The progress in creating drugs to combat fungal infections has not kept pace with the advancements in the development of drugs to fight bacterial infections. This is not surprising given the cellular characteristics of the species involved in such interactions. Bacteria, being prokaryotic organisms, present various structural and metabolic aspects that are different from those found in the human host. In contrast, because fungi are eukaryotes, most poisonous substances harm the organisms that they infect. Additionally, the measurement of fungi is more complex than that of bacteria due to their frequent adoption of multicellular forms and slow growth rates. This problem complicates the process of conducting trials to evaluate the potential antifungal properties of a substance, whether in the laboratory or in living organisms. Despite these drawbacks, there have been significant advancements in the discovery of novel antifungal drugs and our knowledge of those already in use.

Parasitic medications (antimycotics) are utilized to combat infectious diseases by destroying or preventing the spread of low-risk growths within an organism. The activity of such drugs can occur in the interior or exterior, where their performance depends on their communication with the host's immune system. For instance, organisms that affect the feet exhibit strong odors but are not unsafe; meanwhile, contagious diseases of the blood and tissue can be deadly. This section explains how fungicides like polyenes, azoles, and allylamine may be used in various electrochemical biosensing and detection applications.

4.4.1. Natamycin

Natamycin is the sole approved polyene-type drug for the treatment of infectious keratitis. One group studied the electrochemical properties of natamycin by employing a carbon paste electrode (CPE) and conducting differential pulse voltammetry (DPV) within feasible packaging conditions [196]. SWCNTs were immobilized on the poly(L-serine)/GCE surface, leading to another approach to identifying natamycin. The current was significantly increased and made as low as feasible by altering the open circuit potential [197]. A robust, high-strength, and high-selectivity integrated graphene oxide/MWCNT sensor was developed for the detection of natamycin [198]. Authors have also explored the electrochemical detection of natamycin by modifying an SPCE using nanocomposites of MWCNTs with platinum-doped cadmium sulfide [199]. A homogenized yogurt beverage spiked with a known type of natamycin was used to evaluate the suggested Pt-compact disc/MWCNT/SPCE sensor, proving the practicality of this method for the specific determination of natamycin in the food industry.

4.4.2. Fluconazole

The fluorine-joined bis-triazole called fluconazole (influenza) is an anti-contagious drug for the treatment of vaginitis caused by vaginal yeast and recurrent Candida infections. Additionally, it serves as a preventative and healing medication for people who have undergone bone marrow transplants. The electrochemical analysis of this drug at the surface of a Pt electrode and GCE exhibited a pH-dependent oxidation mechanism that enhanced the current at pH 8, and it revealed anodic potential of ~0.85 V. This process involved passing a triazolic ring electron, producing an extreme charge, and then performing additional dimerization steps to create a bis-compound object. Utilizing an electrochemical approach, the ability of the drug to securely adsorb to the cathode surface was examined, raising questions regarding its scientific limitations, including its awareness, linearity, and reproducibility. An innovative Fe_3O_4@PA-Ni@Pd/chitosan nanocomposite-modified carbon ionic fluid terminal, as shown in Figure 7, was prepared for the sensitive detection of influenza to solve this problem [200]. Several relapse examinations were used to optimize the trial conditions. This figure illustrates how the collection duration and nanoparticle fixation affect the 3D response surface of the electrochemical current. The CV responses of the developed sensor to influenza were recorded at various output rates ranging between 10 and 500 mV/s. The proposed sensor was approved by quantifying influenza in plasma and urine samples, demonstrating excellent selectivity. With an LOD of 3.5 nM, it also displayed a broad detection range of 0.01 to 400 μM [200].

Nagatani et al. described a semi-real-time electrochemical monitoring approach for influenza virus RNA based on reverse transcription loop-mediated isothermal amplification (RT-LAMP) in [201]. The peak height of the current was determined by the amount of input RNA and the degree of DNA amplification used.

4.4.3. Ketoconazole

This drug is utilized as an oral medication because of its low toxicity and flexible application throughout the circulation system, urine, saliva, and other liquids. Peng and associates used CV and a GCE to investigate ketoconazole's electrochemical and adsorptive characteristics. On the other hand, DPV demonstrated good awareness and selectivity when used for electrochemical identification in the presence of potential contaminant particles. In another study, ciclopirox olamine, a pyridine antagonist to certain compounds used in beauty products, was identified using a BDDE and the electrochemical analysis of ketoconazole. Ketoconazole and ciclopirox olamine's optimum electrochemical oxidation were examined using SWV, and the results showed that ketoconazole had a dependence ratio of 0.29 to 3.13 μM. In comparison, that of ciclopirox olamine ranged from 25.3 to 419 μM. The qualitative and quantitative electrochemical tests using ketoconazole succeeded with a straightforward setup. For the evaluation of ciclopirox olamine, however, a neutral pH seemed preferable [202].

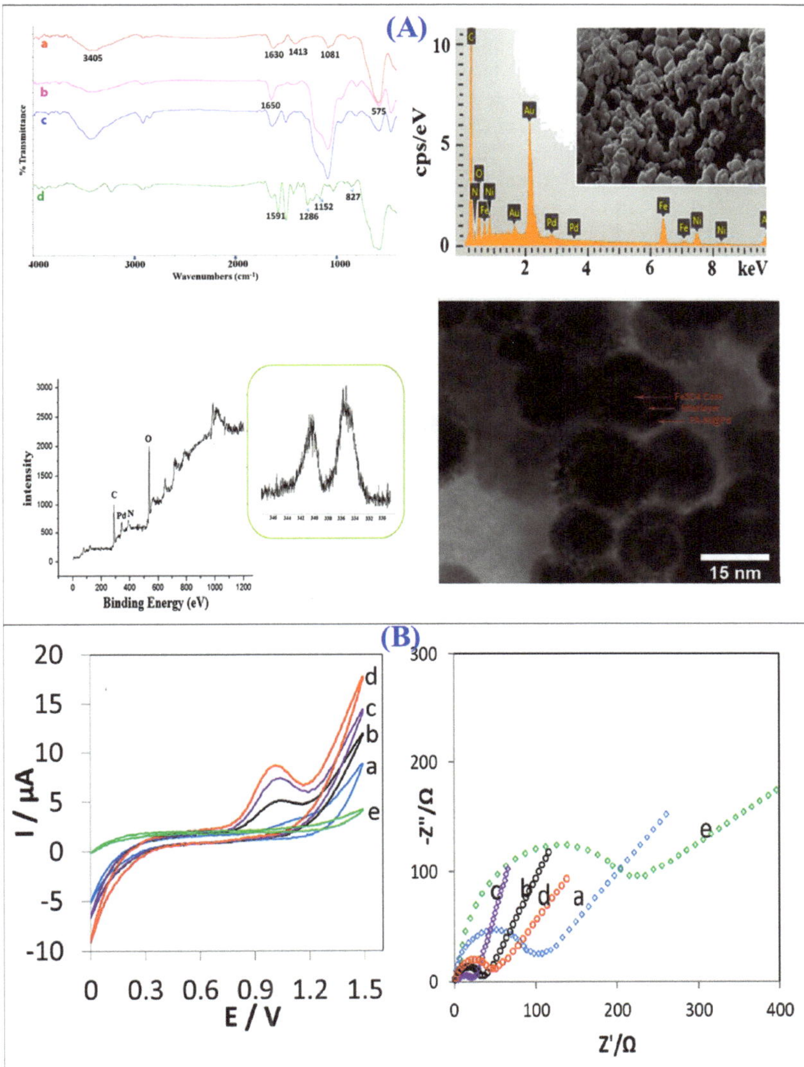

Figure 7. (**A**) FT−IR spectra of Fe_3O_4, $Fe_3O_4@SiO_2$, $Fe_3O_4@SiO_2@PA$, and yolk−shell $Fe_3O_4@PA$. EDS, SEM, XPS, and TEM images of yolk−shell $Fe_3O_4@PA{-}Ni@Pd$. (**B**) CVs 10μmolL^{-1} FLU and EIS in the presence of 10.0 mmolL^{-1} $[Fe(CN)_6]^{3-/4-}$ and 0.1 molL^{-1} KCl solution. Reproduced with permission from [200].

4.4.4. Tolnaftate

An antifungal medication called tolnaftate (TNF) has been used for a long time to target various microbes and other types of microspores, which can cause several infectious disorders. For the electroanalysis of TNF, disposable SPEs were used, providing a sensitive and repeatable electrochemical platform for the differentiation of TNF and its dynamic hydrolysis products. When the pH ranged from 2 to 10, reasonable irreversible oxidation was seen at 1.20 V with a direct range of 0.24 to 3.76 μM. It was shown that the electrooxidation was a dispersion-controlled process that involved a single electron moving in response to the entrance of a water particle [203].

4.4.5. Clioquinol

A skin medication called clioquinol (CQL) is used to treat subacute myeloid-optic neuropathies and gastrointestinal infections. Tin molybdate (SnMoO4)2 nanoplates demonstrated improved responsiveness, remarkable stability, and good selectivity when used for the electrochemical detection of CQL. With only a few common metal particles in its field of view, this sensor displayed an LOD of 14 nM. Three-layered blossom-like cerium vanadate ($CeVO_4$) was used to continuously examine CQL in organic samples. CV and DPV evaluated the $CeVO_4$-modified SPCE's electrocatalytic performance for the electrochemical detection of CQL [204]. The developed platform's progressive application to the examination of the spiking of CQL (a known focus) in human urine tests yielded a recovery range of 97.5 to 105% for various durations, illuminating the potential uses of the developed sensor in various electrochemical detection applications [205].

4.5. Antiviral Medicines

The antiviral medications currently available consist of over 40 substances that have been officially certified for clinical consumption. At least half of the licensed drugs are used to treat human immunodeficiency virus (HIV) infections, most of which are recent discoveries from the past five years. The other antivirals currently on the market are mainly used to treat infections caused by the virus. Antiviral medications include a number of compounds used to treat various common illnesses, from seasonal infections to human immunodeficiency virus. Most popular drugs are controlled intravenously as opposed to orally. The excessive consumption of antiviral medicines can render the body incapable of fighting other viral diseases; hence, quantitative and subjective investigation is essential.

4.5.1. Acyclovir

Acyclovir (ACV) is an oral and intravenous drug that is used to treat viral illnesses such as varicella zoster, hepatitis B, and herpes simplex. The improved direct electrochemical identification of ACV in a broad range was made possible by the collective energy between MWCNTs and dihexadecyl hydrogen phosphate (DHP). Due to its highly electrochemically dynamic surface region, the empty nanostructured film anode improved the electrochemical identification of ACV. The suggested detection platform was used to study an economically viable ACV pill, demonstrating potential and practical use. Wang et al. modified a CPE using polyvinylpyrrolidone (PVP) and a macromolecule surfactant [206]. The PVP-modified CPE terminal significantly boosted the oxidation signal with an LOD of 2.5 nM, with two-electron and two-proton oxidation components involved in the electrochemical oxidation. For the electrochemical identification of ACV, a few parameters, including the pH, collection time, collection potential, and PVP focus, were enhanced. The method used for the electrochemical investigation was compared to HPLC, demonstrating excellent results and validating its accuracy. Radical hydroxy-guanine and oxo-guanine were produced because the ACV was electrochemically oxidized on the PGE, which was found to be an extensive and irreversible oxidation process [207].

There has been much interest in manufacturing chemically synthesized electrodes for sensor applications. For the minute detection of compounds, CPEs coated with one or more nanoparticles have provided impressive results in the search for novel materials. In the work of Shetti et al. [208], γ-Fe_2O_3 nanoparticles and bentonite clay particles were used as modifiers in a CPE to measure the antiviral drug ACV. The outcomes also demonstrated the sensor's sensitive pharmacokinetic performance.

4.5.2. Ganciclovir (GCV)

For the treatment of Epstein–Barr virus, herpes, and cytomegalovirus, GCV has received clinical approval. It has been confirmed that electrochemical oxidation in a GCE is a simple, quick, and delicate approach for the identification of GCV in serum and drug testing [209]. The crucial process that caused the current to increase was the oxidation of the guanine component using electrochemistry. However, regarding the degree of GCV oxidation, the analyte particles were not oxidized concurrently. A boron-doped nanocrystal jewel (BDND) cathode performed well in a different investigation when used with GCV at pH 2.5; when employing DPV, the peak current at 1.2 V rose directly with the increase in focus. The BDND sensor also showed significantly better security than a GCE, thanks to the decreased oxygen groups created following electrooxidation, which reduced the extent of the infection [210]. The CV of 100 μM GCV with different electrodes revealed that the electrochemical oxidation of GCV was more active with AuNPs/MIP/MWCNTs/GCE [211].

4.5.3. Zanamivir (ZAV)

ZAV is another medication utilized against influenza A H5N1 and H1N1 infections. Although ZAV is a fascinating compound, its electrochemical examination has yet to be considered because it is not among the most popular medications. Skrzypek used square wave adsorptive stripping voltammetry on a mercury-doped cathode to investigate the electrochemical oxidation of ZAV. They discovered that the solution's pH had no significant effect on the process, with the greatest current obtained at pH 2.2 [212]. Focusing on the electrochemical oxidation of ZAV, an Au-based sensor was proposed by Wahyuni et al. to identify the exosialidase protein neuraminidase (NA), which is involved in several diseases. This is because, although NA is not directly electrochemically oxidized, its connection to ZAV shifts the maximum potential for ZAV decomposition while considering the unique position of NA [213].

4.5.4. Valacyclovir (VCV) and Acetaminophen

The use of numerous medications is a standard clinical procedure to treat infections and their side effects. Antiviral and antipyretic drugs can offer resources in the fight against many diseases. However, the observation of these groups of medications is required in this context. In this way, the synchronous detection of VCV and acetaminophen was proposed using rGO. The CV of acetaminophen and VCV obtained using a GCE and rGO/GCE demonstrated the potential for simultaneous acetaminophen and VCV detection utilizing rGO/GCEs [214]. To create 8-oxovalacyclovir, two electrons and two protons are used in an electrooxidation interaction. They are not entirely predetermined to be diffusion-controlled and irreversible.

4.6. Anticancer Medication

In the context of disease, drugs show usefulness in eliminating malignant cells, combating cancer, preventing the disease from metastasizing and spreading, and alleviating different side effects. These medications' creation and standard clinical utilization require ready-to-use, subjective, and quantitative examination tools. This section features a few recent improvements in the electrochemical detection of anticancer drugs.

4.6.1. Taxol

Taxol is obtained from a standard mixture of the Pacific yew tree's stem bark. It is a powerful medication to target cancerous growth in the breast, ovarian cancer, and non-small-cell lung cancer. An insightful technique was created to detect Taxol by utilizing cathodic stripping SWV. Taxol was discovered under a soluble base using a mercury drop electrode with an interfacial contact area of 0.0278 cm^2 [215]. The primary basis of efforts to produce and develop Taxol detectors has been DPV using PGEs, which is hindered by its interaction with twofold abandoned DNA (ds-DNA). In a study, this interaction lowered the strength of the guanine and adenine oxidation signals in the predicted range of 0.5 to 1.3 V, allowing the electroanalysis of Taxol to be completed with a detection range of 0.2 to 10.0 μM [216]. The favorable electron motion characteristics and the highly dynamic regions increased the voltammetric oxidation of Taxol. The designed nanocomposite electrode offers a sensitive, robust, and specific detection platform [217].

4.6.2. Doxorubicin

Doxorubicin, an anthracycline drug produced by the bacterium Streptomyces peucetius var. caesius, is applied to treat many leukemias and lung and breast cancers. Using a working electrode composed of carbon, doxorubicin was swiftly and thoroughly examined. The pseudo-reversible reaction involved an acetic acid derivative, which was suggested as the driving force behind the electrochemical catalysis. This was supported by a unique change that occurred when the pH value was increased, potentially leading to undesirable results [218]. The final uses for these sensors lie in medicine and the environment. Nicole and colleagues developed a drug discovery technique using single nucleic acids that could attach to target particles (aptasensor). The experiment continued with an extensive detection range of 4 to 1000 nM, with the immersion of the aptamer–gold cathode occurring at 125 nM [219]. In contrast, distinguishing between two drugs increases a particular detection platform's cost, viability, and effectiveness. It could be possible to devise an approach to identify doxorubicin and another anti-disease agent (methotrexate) for the evaluation of pharmaceutical, healthcare, and natural products. An integrated cyclodextrin–graphene nanocomposite on a GCE (Cd GN/GCE) was used to distribute doxorubicin and methotrexate concurrently. Doxorubicin and methotrexate's peak flows on the disc, compared to the data displayed on an exposed GCE, rose by 26.5 and 23.7 times, respectively [220]. Another oligonucleotide metal (DNA/silver)-dependent detector for the identification of doxorubicin was designed using steady-state voltammetry. The TEM images of the silver nanoparticles following synthesis with the introduction of doxorubicin confirmed that the Ag nanoparticles were successful. When doxorubicin stacking with AgNPs amounting to ~17 (red line) and ~1 (dark line) was used in the proposed system, the correlation of the voltammetric data calculated using 0.3 M of KCl showed that the responsiveness dropped as the level of doxorubicin stacking increased because of the drug's complex binding.

4.6.3. Imatinib and Flutamide

Malignant growth inhibitors for gastrointestinal and stromal tumors and leukemia, such as imatinib (IMA), are effective in the treatment of these diseases (essences). This type of medicine should be monitored in bodily fluids such as plasma, urine, cerebral fluid, and blood. A dendrimer-layered empty fiber graphene oxide sensor was developed to micro-extract and electrochemically identify biochemical samples, including IMA [221]. Three cancer-preventative drugs with excellent selectivity for IMA and an identity threshold of 7.39 nM were used in obstruction research. SPCEs were used to disseminate sensor information, enabling inexpensive, quick-acting, and simple sensors to quantitatively identify numerous drugs [222]. For instance, the voltammetric detection of IMA was accomplished utilizing SPCEs (CNT). It exhibited the piperazine ring oxidative conductivity of IMA at a peak potential of 0.75 V. Despite any additional decrease due to the massive increase in current from 0.71 V, this electrode showed outstanding results under a synergistic and irreversible cycle and it was found to be an adsorption-controlled process.

Additionally, the suitability of the SPCEs for the projected area was compared with that of platinum- and gold-functionalized electrocatalysts, where the two anodes were successful. Several drugs are given to immunocompromised individuals directly, orally, forcibly, or chronically. In this case, one medication may restrict the activity of another, which could bring about serious side effects, or changes to their doses might be required. To avoid these problems, synchronous medication detection is attractive. With the aid of a metal oxide/carbon-based electrode (NiO-ZnO/MWCNT-COOH/GCE), the simultaneous recognition of a drug (IMA) and an antifungal (Itraconazole) was investigated. Itraconazole's maximum oxidation current increased in DPV with an LOD of 4.1 nM and 2.64 $\mu A/\mu M/cm^2$, indicating excellent responsiveness. IMA had responsiveness of 9.64 $\mu A/\mu M/cm^2$, an LOD of 2.4 nM, and a linear range of 0.015 to 2.0 μM [223]. Moreover, Tseng et al. described a nanocatalyst for the electrochemical detection of flutamide, a non-steroidal antiandrogen used in the medical field to treat leukemia and prostate conditions, consisting of graphene oxide sheets and calcium titanium oxide (GOS/$CaTiO_3$). Based on the XRD, TEM, and EDX results, Figure 8 shows the proposed nanocatalyst's shape, design, and structure. This figure demonstrates a broad range (0.015 to 1184 μM), a low LOD (5.7 nM), and high responsiveness (1.073 μA/μM/cm^2). Human blood and urine tests were used to evaluate the sensor, demonstrating its potential for use in malignant growth and drug localization [224]. Table 1 shows various electrochemical sensors for the detection of pharmaceutical drugs.

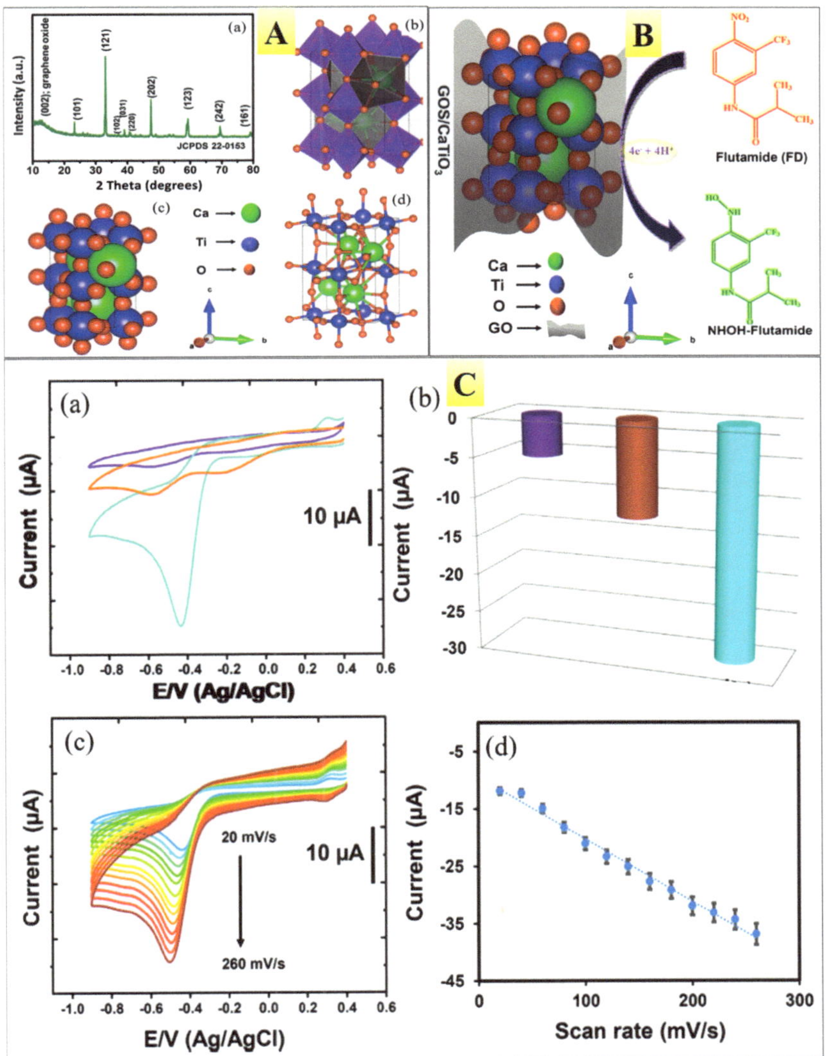

Figure 8. (**A**) (**a**) XRD study of GOS/CaTiO$_3$ nanocomposite. (**b**) The polyhedral model's orthorhombic CaTiO$_3$ crystal structure, (**c**) the space−filling model, and (**d**) the ball−and−stick model. (**B**) Flutamide electrochemical reduction mechanism. (**C**) (**a**) CV of flutamide−containing GOS/GCE, GOS/CaTiO$_3$ NC/GCE, and bare GCE. (**b**) Calibration plot. (**c**) Flutamide at GOS/CaTiO$_3$ NC/GCE with a varying scan rates. (**d**) Relationship between scan rate against the cathodic peak current. Reproduced with permission from [224].

Table 1. Various electrochemical sensors for the detection of pharmaceutical drugs. Reproduced with permission from [42].

Electrode	Analyte	LOD (µmol/L)	Linear Range (µmol/L)	Ref.
SPCE/(CSþAuNPs)	Aspirin	0.03 pg/mL	1 pg/mL–1 µg/mL	[225]
CuNCs/CuE	Mefenamic acid	1 nM	4 nM–10 mM	[226]
CS-CuNCs/CuE	Indomethacin	1 nM	1 nM–10 mM	[226]
AuNPs/MWCNTs/GCE	Diclofenac sodium	0.02 µM	0.03–200 µM	[227]
PtNFs/RGO/SPE	Diclofenac	40 nM	0.1–100 µM	[228]
G-DVD/GO/AgNPs@b-CD	Naproxen	0.023 µM	0.4–80 µM	[146]
GO-COOH/GCE	Diclofenac	0.09 µM	1.2–400 µM	[229]
GO/GCE	Naproxen	1.94 µM	10 µM–1 µM	[230]
GO/CPE	Flufenamic acid	5.0 nM	0.001–0.09 µM	[231]
Graphite rod	Diclofenac	0.76 µM	2.56–9.5 µM	[232]
PDDA-GR/GCE	Diclofenac	0.609 µM	10–100 µM	[233]
Nano-sepiolite/MWCNTs/PGE	Paracetamol	0.018 µM	0.059–60 µM	[234]
SD-MWCNTs/GCE	Ibuprofen	1.9 µM	10–1000 µM	[235]
FMWCNTs/b-CD/CPE	Piroxicam	0.7 µM	10^{-6}–10^{-2} M	[236]
Pt-N-RGO-SWCNTs/GCE	Piroxicam	5.0 ng/mL	0.02–20 µg/mL	[237]
GNP-CNF/GCE	Nepafenac	63 nM	4.0–15 µM	[238]
NDCNDs/CoTAPhPcNPs/GCE	Aspirin	9.66 nM	-	[239]
CuO/GCE	ASA	0.037 µM	0.1–714 µM	[240]
TiO_2 NPs/GCE	Nimesulide	3.37 nM	0.1–40 µM	[241]
N-CQD/Cu_2O/GCE	Aspirin	0.002 µM	1–907 µM	[242]
GNS/PANI/Bi2O3/GCE	Etodolac	10.03 ngmL^{-1}	20–100 ngmL^{-1}	[243]
f-CNF/$LaCoO_3$/GCE	4-AAP	1.0 nM	0.001–1374 µM	[244]
Iron oxide NPs/CPE	Diclofenac	2.45 nM	0.01–100 µM	[245]
Pt-NiO/MWCNTs/GCE	Piroxicam, Amlodipine	0.061 µM	0.6–320.0 mM	[246]
XAD/CPE	Flufenamic acid	3.6 nM	0.05–8.0 µM	[247]
Ag-TiO_2/XAD/CPE	Flufenamic acid	1.2 nM	0.05–8.0 µM	[247]
Ru-TiO_2/MWCNTs/CPE	Flufenamic acid	0.68 nM	0.01–0.9 µM	[248]
Ru-TiO_2/MWCNTs/CPE	Mefenamic acid	0.45 nM	0.01–0.9 µM	[248]
Oxygen plasma-treated ZnO/SPE	Dopamine, Diclofenac	0.28 µM	0.1–300 µM	[249]
$Cu_5V_2O_{10}$/CPE	Mefenamic acid	2.34 nM	0.01–470 µM	[250]
AgNPs-ChCl-GO/CPE	Celecoxib	2.51 nM	9.6 nM–0.74 µM	[251]
AuNPs-ChCl-GO/CPE	Meloxicam	1.008 nM	9.0 nM–0.85 µM	[252]
ER-GONRs/SPCE	Nimesulide	3.50 nM	0.01 µM–1.50 mM	[253]
NiNPs/ERGO/GCE	Diclofenac	0.09 µM	0.25–125.00 µM	[254]
f-MWCNTs/NC/GCE	Diclofenac	0.012 µM	0.05–250.0 µM	[255]
$BaNb_2O_6$NFs/CPE	Lornoxicam	0.639 nM	4.0 nM–0.25 mM	[256]
SWCNTs/GCE	Mefenamic acid	13.4 nM	0.1–35 µM	[257]
CP-BDDE	Pravastatin	0.204 µM	1.08–16.4 µM	[258]
MWCNTs/CPE	Diclofenac	0.74 µM	2.49–10 µM	[259]
Nano-smectite/MWCNTs/PGE	AA	0.096 µM	0.319–60.0 µM	[260]

Table 1. *Cont.*

Electrode	Analyte	LOD (μmol/L)	Linear Range (μmol/L)	Ref.
Fe_3O_4/Gluta/MWCNTs/CPE	Aspirin	11.8 nM	20–170 μM	[261]
AuNPs/Graphene/CILE	Celecoxib	0.2 μM	0.5–15 μM	[163]
AgNPs/SWCNTs/rGO/GCE	Piroxicam	0.5 μM	1.5–400 μM	[262]
Al_2O_3 microparticles/GCE	Naproxen	12 nM	50–500 nM	[263]
FTO/$BiVO_4$/CuO	Naproxen	5 nM	5–480 nM	[264]
MWCNTs-IL/CCE	Indomethacin	260 nM	1–50 μM	[265]
Polychitosan-CuNPs/CuE	Mefenamic acid	0.004 μM	0.004–10,000 μM	[266]
Carbon paper-based sensor	Ketoprofen	0.11 μM	0.088–1.96 μM	[267]
PANI-rGO-MIP/CPE	Diclofenac	1.1 mgL^{-1}	5–80 mgL^{-1}	[268]
PANI/MnO_2-Sb_2O_3/FTO	ASA	0.20 nM	1.2–228.68 nM	[269]
PEDOT/GCE	Diclofenac	9.06 nM	50.0–250 nM	[270]
RGO-PEDOT-PSS/GCE	Piroxicam, Nimesulide	0.1 μM	0.87–26 μM	[271]
TiO_2-PEDOT/GCE	AA	0.02 μM	6–46 μM	[272]
PEDOT/TiO_2/[BMIM]Cl/CPE	Diclofenac	11.7 nM	50–100 μM	[273]
Glucose/CPE	Mefenamic acid	1.01 nM	25 nM–500 μM	[274]
Nano-silica/CPE	Mefenamic acid	1.0 nM	0.2–5 μM	[275]
Fe(III)-SBMCP/CPE	Mefenamic acid	0.02 μM	0.05–150 μM	[276]
Carbon ionic liquid electrode	Piroxicam	40 μM	0.2–60 μM	[277]
Nanoclay/CPE	Nimesulide	1.01 nM	0.01–0.35 μM	[278]
HMDE	Tetrazine	27.8 nM	0.02–15.2 μM	[279]
MB/Cu/$Ti_3C_2T_x$/GCE	Piroxicam	0.05 μM	0.1–80 μM	[280]
MB/Apt/MWCNTs/IL/Chitosan/GCE	Ibuprofen	20 pM	70 pM–6 μM	[281]
Apt-Den-QDs/GCE	Ibuprofen	333 fM	0.001–12 nM	[282]
MWCNTs/msCYP1A2-SPE	Naproxen	16 μM	9–300 μM	[147]
Apt/MWCNTs/GO/Fe_3O_4/GCE	Diclofenac	33 pM	100–1300 pM	[283]
DCF-Probe/E-Probe/GCE	Diclofenac	0.1 pM	10^{-14} M–10^{-10} M	[284]
Apt/NiHCF/PtNPs/PEI/MWCNTs/Au	Diclofenac	2.7 nM	10–200 nM	[285]
GCE/AHA/DBA	Diclofenac	0.27 μM	0–5 μM	[286]
Apt/CdTeQD/GCE	Ibuprofen	16 pM	0.05–20,000 nM	[287]
Au/SAM/Hydrogel/Apt	Diclofenac	0.02 nM	30 pM^{-1} μM	[288]
Apt/AuNPs/GCE	Ibuprofen	0.5 pM	0.05–7 nM	[153]
Apt/AuNPs@N-GQDs/GCE	Ibuprofen	33.33 aM	10^{-7}–200 nM	[289]

5. Limitations

Nanomaterial-based electrochemical sensors hold great promise for drug detection and monitoring applications but face several potential drawbacks. Challenges include signal interference, durability under clinical conditions, and the scaling of these technologies for widespread use.

5.1. Signal Interference

Electrochemical sensors are commonly used in complex biological fluids like blood, serum, and urine but face performance challenges. A significant issue is fouling, where proteins and biomolecules adsorb onto the sensor surface, obstructing access to active sites and reducing the sensitivity. For example, substances like albumin can hinder the accurate detection of target analytes. Redox interference is another challenge, as biological samples often contain endogenous redox-active species that can mimic the target analyte, leading to false positives. Compounds like ascorbic acid may interfere with medications like ibuprofen. Additionally, matrix effects from variations in the biological fluid's composition—such as the pH, ionic strength, and temperature—can complicate signal interpretation, resulting in inconsistent readings.

i. Interference from complex biological fluids

Biological fluids, like blood and serum, present challenges for electrochemical sensors due to their complex composition. Fouling is vital, where proteins and biomolecules coat the sensor's surface, obstructing the interaction with target analytes such as ibuprofen, thereby reducing the sensitivity and specificity. Additionally, redox interference complicates detection, as endogenous redox-active species like ascorbic acid can produce overlapping signals with the analyte, resulting in false positives or negatives. Variability in the pH and ionic strength further affect sensors' performance. Fluctuations in these parameters can alter the charge and solubility of the target analyte, leading to inconsistent results and decreased reliability.

ii. Nanomaterial instability

Nanomaterials enhance sensors' sensitivity but face stability issues that affect their performance. A significant concern is oxidation, especially in carbon-based materials, which can result in decreased conductivity and reduced active surface areas, lowering the responsiveness. Agglomeration also poses a problem, as nanoparticles clump together, diminishing the surface area for essential electrochemical reactions and impacting the sensitivity. Additionally, the leaching of components, such as polymers or ions from gold nanoparticles, may alter the sensor characteristics and lead to inconsistent readings.

iii. Mitigation strategies

Researchers are tackling the challenges of developing electrochemical sensors through innovative strategies. One key approach is surface modification with biocompatible coatings, which reduce fouling and enhance the stability by minimizing nonspecific adsorption and protecting nanomaterials. Additionally, the combination of various nanomaterials, like carbon nanotubes with metal nanoparticles, creates effective nanocomposites that boost sensors' performance. Advanced signal processing algorithms and machine learning techniques also improve the accuracy by differentiating target signals from interferences in complex biological samples.

5.2. Durability Under Clinical Conditions

Nanomaterials often face stability challenges that affect the long-term performance of electrochemical sensors, particularly in clinical settings, where the conditions can vary. They are sensitive to the temperature, humidity, and reactive species, leading to issues like the oxidation or clumping of metal nanoparticles, which reduces their effectiveness. Mechanical durability is critical; sensors must withstand temperature shifts and physical stress. Fragile nanostructures may deteriorate over time, resulting in decreased performance or failure. Additionally, prolonged use can cause chemical degradation, leading to the loss of active sites that reduces the sensitivity and alters the selectivity—critical factors for reliable clinical performance.

5.3. Challenges in Scaling for Widespread Use

Transitioning from laboratory-scale development to the large-scale production of nanomaterial-based sensors presents significant challenges. Key hurdles include the complexity and cost of manufacturing high-quality nanomaterial coatings and the difficulty of standardizing the processes for mass production while maintaining performance. Quality control is also crucial, as uniformity in the properties of nanomaterials across production batches is essential. Even minor variations can lead to significant differences in sensor behavior, making quality assurance complex. Additionally, the navigation of regulatory challenges is necessary before electrochemical sensors can be approved for clinical use. The lengthy process of demonstrating safety and efficacy can delay the adoption of these technologies in healthcare.

6. Conclusions and Outlook

Advanced electrochemical sensors offer great potential for the detection of drug intensities, but it is crucial to understand the physical, chemical, and electrical interactions between the nanomaterials and target analytes. Investigating the subatomic structures of various pharmacological compounds and nanomaterials, as well as the electrochemical techniques and associated factors, would contribute to the current detector and biomarker research, particularly regarding their sensitivities and LODs. Combining metal nanoparticles, quantum dots, scalable organic groups, and nanocomposites in carbon-based nanostructures produces a synergistic effect to react with the analyte. Nanoparticle- or natural particle-functionalized cathodes have shown a low LOD and superior performance for small subatomic medicines such as headache medications, ibuprofen, and sertraline.

Electrochemical technology has advanced biomedical applications in disease prediction, real-time monitoring, and drug screening. However, there are still significant difficulties in acquiring target signals due to the method's dependency on wires, slow response times, and difficulties in verification. New technologies such as Bluetooth, wireless power transfer (WPT), and near-field communication (NFC) could make electrochemical data transmission quicker and better.

It is crucial to consider wireless platforms and the desired usability to adopt electrochemical biosensors, while the miniaturization of electrochemical instruments and advancements in the assembly of biosensors are expected. Electrochemical sensors and biosensors should have their costs and reliability carefully evaluated, along with their responsiveness and selectivity.

One of the emerging trends is the combination of mass spectrometry or fluid chromatography with electrochemical detection to identify therapeutic molecules effectively. In summary, developing advanced electrochemical sensors and biosensors to detect drug intensities requires a comprehensive understanding of nanomaterials and their interactions with target analytes.

The integration of quantum computing and AI with emerging technologies is poised to significantly enhance the capabilities in various fields, particularly electrochemical sensing and materials science. As quantum computing evolves, it could facilitate the development of advanced algorithms that optimize the electrospinning process for nanofiber production. This optimization could lead to nanofibers with tailored properties for specific applications, such as drug delivery and tissue engineering. Moreover, using AI with electrochemical sensors could improve real-time data processing and analysis, enabling the faster and more accurate detection of chemical compounds. This synergy could revolutionize personalized medicine by allowing for the rapid assessment of drug efficacy and patient-specific responses, thus paving the way for more effective treatment plans. In the context of materials science, combining quantum computing with hybrid chip technologies could enhance electronic systems' performance, addressing energy consumption and sustainability challenges. By leveraging the unique properties of 2D materials and their integration into IoT applications, researchers can develop more efficient sensors and communication systems, which are essential for the future of connected devices. The intersection of quantum computing, AI, and advanced materials technologies is promising to drive innovation in drug detection, personalized medicine, and sustainable electronic systems.

Author Contributions: Conceptualization, S.J.M. and N.P.S.; methodology, S.J.M.; software, S.J.M. and N.P.S.; validation, S.J.M. and N.P.S.; formal analysis, S.J.M., N.P.S. and M.A.A.; investigation, S.J.M.; resources, S.J.M.; data curation, S.J.M. and N.P.S.; writing—original draft preparation, S.J.M.; writing—review and editing, S.J.M. and N.P.S.; visualization, S.J.M., N.P.S. and M.A.A.; supervision, N.P.S. All authors have read and agreed to the published version of the manuscript.

Funding: This research received no external funding.

Conflicts of Interest: The authors state that they have no known financial conflicts of interest.

References

1. Ahmed, M.U.; Hossain, M.M.; Safavieh, M.; Wong, Y.L.; Rahman, I.A.A.; Zourob, M.; Tamiya, E. Toward the development of smart and low-cost point-of-care biosensors based on screen printed electrodes. *Crit. Rev. Biotechnol.* **2016**, *36*, 495–505. [CrossRef] [PubMed]
2. Yang, Y.; Gao, W. Wearable and flexible electronics for continuous molecular monitoring. *Chem. Soc. Rev.* **2019**, *48*, 1465–1491. [CrossRef] [PubMed]
3. Malode, S.J.; Pandiaraj, S.; Alodhayb, A.; Shetti, N.P. Carbon Nanomaterials for Biomedical Applications: Progress and Outlook. *ACS Appl. Bio Mater.* **2024**, *7*, 752–777. [CrossRef] [PubMed]
4. Rodrigues, D.; Barbosa, A.I.; Rebelo, R.; Kwon, I.K.; Reis, R.L.; Correlo, V.M. Skin-integrated wearable systems and implantable biosensors: A comprehensive review. *Biosensors* **2020**, *10*, 79. [CrossRef]
5. Joseph, J.I.; Eisler, G.; Diaz, D.; Khalf, A.; Loeum, C.; Torjman, M.C. Glucose sensing in the subcutaneous tissue: Attempting to correlate the immune response with continuous glucose monitoring accuracy. *Diabetes Technol. Ther.* **2018**, *20*, 321–324. [CrossRef]
6. Ruiz-Valdepeñas Montiel, V.; Sempionatto, J.R.; Campuzano, S.; Pingarrón, J.M.; Esteban Fernández de Ávila, B.; Wang, J. Direct electrochemical biosensing in gastrointestinal fluids. *Anal. Bioanal. Chem.* **2019**, *411*, 4597–4604. [CrossRef]
7. Yu, Y.; Nyein, H.Y.Y.; Gao, W.; Javey, A. Flexible electrochemical bioelectronics: The rise of in situ bioanalysis. *Adv. Mater.* **2020**, *32*, e1902083. [CrossRef]
8. Kassal, P.; Steinberg, M.D.; Steinberg, I.M. Wireless chemical sensors and biosensors: A review. *Sens. Actuators B* **2018**, *266*, 228–245. [CrossRef]
9. da Silva Neves, M.M.P.; González-García, M.B.; Hernández-Santos, D.; Fanjul-Bolado, P. Future trends in the market for electrochemical biosensing. *Curr. Opin. Electrochem.* **2018**, *10*, 107–111. [CrossRef]
10. Kannan, P.K.; Late, D.J.; Morgan, H.; Rout, C.S. Recent developments in 2D layered inorganic nanomaterials for sensing. *Nanoscale* **2015**, *7*, 13293–13312. [CrossRef]
11. Manasa, G.; Mascarenhas, R.J.; Shetti, N.P.; Malode, S.J.; Mishra, A.; Basu, S.; Aminabhavi, T.M. Skin Patchable Sensor Surveillance for Continuous Glucose Monitoring. *ACS Appl. Bio Mater.* **2022**, *5*, 945–970. [CrossRef] [PubMed]
12. Lee, V.B.C.; Mohd-Naim, N.F.; Tamiya, E.; Ahmed, M.U. Trends in paper-based electrochemical biosensors: From design to application. *Anal. Sci.* **2018**, *34*, 7–18. [CrossRef] [PubMed]
13. Economou, A.; Kokkinos, C.; Prodromidis, M. Flexible plastic, paper and textile lab-on-a chip platforms for electrochemical biosensing. *Lab Chip* **2018**, *18*, 1812–1830. [CrossRef]
14. Chałupniak, A.; Morales-Narváez, E.; Merkoçi, A. Micro and nanomotors in diagnostics. *Adv. Drug Deliv. Rev.* **2015**, *95*, 104–116. [CrossRef]
15. Evtugyn, G.; Hianik, T. Electrochemical DNA sensors and aptasensors based on electropolymerized materials and polyelectrolyte complexes. *TrAC Trends Anal. Chem.* **2016**, *79*, 168–178. [CrossRef]
16. Cole, M.A.; Seabrook, G.R. On the horizon—The value and promise of the global pipeline of Alzheimer's disease therapeutics. *Alzheimer's Dement. Transl. Res. Clin. Interv.* **2020**, *6*, e12009. [CrossRef]
17. National Center for Health Statistics. *With Chartbook on Long-Term Trends in Health*; Health Communications; Department of Health And Human Services: Washington, DC, USA, 2017.
18. Hall, A.J.; Logan, J.E.; Toblin, R.L.; Kaplan, J.A.; Kraner, J.C.; Bixler, D.; Crosby, A.E.; Paulozzi, L.J. Patterns of abuse among unintentional Pharmaceutical overdose fatalities. *JAMA* **2008**, *300*, 2613–2620. [CrossRef]
19. Kalambate, P.K.; Dhanjai; Sinha, A.; Li, Y.; Shen, Y.; Huang, Y. An electrochemical sensor for ifosfamide, acetaminophen, domperidone, and sumatriptan based on self-assembled MXene/MWCNT/chitosan nanocomposite thin film. *Mikrochim. Acta* **2020**, *187*, 402. [CrossRef] [PubMed]
20. Kalambate, P.K.; Gadhari, N.S.; Li, X.; Rao, Z.; Navale, S.T.; Shen, Y.; Patil, V.R.; Huang, Y. Recent advances in MXene–based electrochemical sensors and biosensors. *TrAC Trends Anal. Chem.* **2019**, *120*, 115643. [CrossRef]
21. Malode, S.J.; Bilagi, S.; Shetti, N.P. Synthesis of biowaste-derived nanostructured material for the nanomolar detection of glucose: Biological sample analysis. *J. Pharm. Biomed. Anal. Open* **2024**, *3*, 100026. [CrossRef]
22. Prabhu, K.; Malode, S.J.; Shetti, N.P.; Pandiaraj, S.; Alodhayb, A.; Muthuramamoorthy, M. Electro-sensing layer constructed of a WO_3/CuO nanocomposite, for the electrochemical determination of 2-phenylphenol fungicide. *Environ. Res.* **2023**, *236*, 116710. [CrossRef] [PubMed]
23. García-Guzmán, J.J.; Pérez-Ràfols, C.; Cuartero, M.; Crespo, G.A. Microneedle based electrochemical (Bio)Sensing: Towards decentralized and continuous health status monitoring. *TrAC Trends Anal. Chem.* **2021**, *135*, 116148. [CrossRef]

24. Malode, S.J.; Joshi, M.; Shetti, N.P.; Alshehri, M.A. Biowaste-derived carbon nanomaterial-based sensor for the electrochemical analysis of mefenamic acid in the presence of CTAB. *Mater. Today Commun.* **2024**, *39*, 108723. [CrossRef]
25. Ilager, D.; Malode, S.J.; Kulkarni, R.M.; Shetti, N.P. Electrochemical sensor based on Ca-doped ZnO nanostructured carbon matrix for algicide dichlone. *J. Hazard. Mater. Adv.* **2022**, *7*, 100132. [CrossRef]
26. Prabhu, K.; Malode, S.J.; Shetti, N.P.; Pandiaraj, S.; Alodhayb, A.; Muthuramamoorthy, M. Determination of fungicide at Ru-doped TiO_2/reduced graphene oxide decorated electrochemical sensor. *Microchem. J.* **2023**, *197*, 109722. [CrossRef]
27. Chung, T.H.; Dhar, B.R. Paper-based platforms for microbial electrochemical cell-based biosensors: A review. *Biosens. Bioelectron.* **2021**, *192*, 113485. [CrossRef]
28. Sreenivasulu, M.; Malode, S.J.; Alqarni, S.A.; Shetti, N.P. Graphitic carbon nitride (g–C3N4)-based electrochemical sensors for the determination of antiviral drug acyclovir. *Mater. Chem. Phys.* **2024**, *312*, 128650. [CrossRef]
29. Goud, K.Y.; Reddy, K.K.; Khorshed, A.; Kumar, V.S.; Mishra, R.K.; Oraby, M.; Ibrahim, A.H.; Kim, H.; Gobi, K.V. Electrochemical diagnostics of infectious viral diseases: Trends and challenges. *Biosens. Bioelectron.* **2021**, *180*, 113112. [CrossRef]
30. Wang, T.; Wang, H.; Kou, Z.; Liang, W.; Luo, X.; Verpoort, F.; Zeng, Y.J.; Zhang, H. Xenes as an emerging 2D monoelemental family: Fundamental electrochemistry and energy applications. *Adv. Funct. Mater.* **2020**, *30*, 2002885. [CrossRef]
31. Prabhu, K.; Malode, S.J.; Shetti, N.P.; Pandiaraj, S.; Alodhayb, A.N. Electro-sensing of biocide and its applications based on the Ru-doped TiO_2 and reduced GO nanocomposite fabricated electrode. *Mater. Chem. Phys.* **2024**, *317*, 129152. [CrossRef]
32. González-Hernández, J.; Alvarado-Gámez, A.L.; Arroyo-Mora, L.E.; Barquero-Quirós, M. Electrochemical determination of novel psychoactive substances by differential pulse voltammetry using a microcell for boron-doped diamond electrode and screen-printed electrodes based on carbon and platinum. *J. Electroanal. Chem.* **2021**, *882*, 114994. [CrossRef]
33. Vernekar, P.R.; Shetti, N.P.; Shanbhag, M.M.; Malode, S.J.; Malladi, R.S.; Reddy, K.R. Novel layered structured bentonite clay-based electrodes for electrochemical sensor applications. *Microchem. J.* **2020**, *159*, 105441. [CrossRef]
34. Motoc, S.; Manea, F.; Baciu, A.; Vasilie, S.; Pop, A. Highly sensitive and simultaneous electrochemical determinations of non-steroidal anti-inflammatory drugs in water using nanostructured carbon-based paste electrodes. *Sci. Total Environ.* **2022**, *846*, 157412. [CrossRef] [PubMed]
35. Xu, K.; Chen, Q.; Zhao, Y.; Ge, C.; Lin, S.; Liao, J. Cost-effective, wireless, and portable smartphone-based electrochemical system for on-site monitoring and spatial mapping of the nitrite contamination in water. *Sens. Actuators B* **2020**, *319*, 128221. [CrossRef]
36. Jain, R.; Dwivedi, A.; Mishra, R. Stripping voltammetric behaviour of toxic drug nitrofurantoin. *J. Hazard. Mater.* **2009**, *169*, 667–672. [CrossRef]
37. Malode, S.J.; Prabhu, K.; Pandiaraj, S.; Alodhayb, A.N.; Shetti, N.P. Development of a 1D-WO_3 and CuO nanocomposite modified electrode for enhanced detection of 2,4-dichlorophenol. *Surf. Interfaces* **2024**, *54*, 105219. [CrossRef]
38. Duraisamy, M.; Elancheziyan, M.; Eswaran, M.; Ganesan, S.; Ansari, A.A.; Rajamanickam, G.; Lee, S.L.; Tsai, P.-C.; Chen, Y.-H.; Ponnusamy, V.K. Novel ruthenium-doped vanadium carbide/polymeric nanohybrid sensor for acetaminophen drug detection in human blood. *Int. J. Biol. Macromol.* **2023**, *244*, 125329. [CrossRef]
39. Sebastian, N.; Yu, W.-C.; Balram, D.; Hong, G.-T.; Alharthi, S.S.; Al-Saidi, H.M. Ultrasensitive detection and photocatalytic degradation of polyketide drug tetracycline in environment and food samples using dual-functional Ag doped zinc ferrite embedded functionalized carbon nanofibers. *Chemosphere* **2023**, *348*, 140692. [CrossRef]
40. Prabhu, K.; Malode, S.J.; Veerapur, R.S.; Shetti, N.P. Clay-based carbon sensor for electro-oxidation of nimesulide. *Mater. Chem. Phys.* **2021**, *272*, 124992. [CrossRef]
41. Goyal, R.N.; Gupta, V.K.; Oyama, M.; Bachheti, N. Differential pulse voltammetric determination of atenolol in pharmaceutical formulations and urine using nanogold modified indium tin oxide electrode. *Electrochem. Commun.* **2005**, *8*, 65–70. [CrossRef]
42. Kalambate, P.K.; Noiphung, J.; Rodthongkum, N.; Larpant, N.; Thirabowonkitphithan, P.; Rojanarata, T.; Hasan, M.; Huang, Y.; Laiwattanapaisal, W. Nanomaterials-based electrochemical sensors and biosensors for the detection of non-steroidal anti-inflammatory drugs. *TrAC Trends Anal. Chem.* **2021**, *143*, 116403. [CrossRef]
43. Elgrishi, N.; Rountree, K.J.; McCarthy, B.D.; Rountree, E.S.; Eisenhart, T.T.; Dempsey, J.L. A Practical Beginner's Guide to Cyclic Voltammetry. *J. Chem. Educ.* **2018**, *95*, 197–206. [CrossRef]
44. Malode, S.J.; Keerthi, P.K.; Shetti, N.P.; Kulkarni, R.M. Electroanalysis of carbendazim using MWCNT/Ca-ZnO modified electrode. *Electroanalysis* **2020**, *32*, 1590–1599. [CrossRef]
45. Shetti, N.P.; Shanbhag, M.M.; Malode, S.J.; Srivastava, R.K.; Reddy, K.R. Amberlite XAD-4 modified electrodes for highly sensitive electrochemical determination of nimesulide in human urine. *Microchem. J.* **2020**, *153*, 104389. [CrossRef]
46. Malode, S.J.; Navada, N.; Shanbhag, M.M.; Shetti, N.P.; Alodhayb, A.N.; Alzahrani, K.E.; Albrithen, H.; Assaifan, A.K. Fe-doped WO_3-Modified sensor for the improved electrochemical detection of curcumin. *Microchem. J.* **2024**, 111655. [CrossRef]
47. Malode, S.J.; Ullagaddimath, P.V.; Shanbhag, M.S.; Alodhayb, A.N.; Alzahrani, K.E.; Albrithen, H.; Assaifan, A.K.; Shetti, N.P. Nickel-doped tungsten fabricated electrode for electrochemical sensing of amoxicillin. *Inorg. Chem. Commun.* **2024**, *169*, 112970. [CrossRef]
48. Rocchitta, G.; Spanu, A.; Babudieri, S.; Latte, G.; Madeddu, G.; Galleri, G.; Nuvoli, S.; Bagella, P.; Demartis, M.I.; Fiore, V.; et al. Enzyme Biosensors for Biomedical Applications: Strategies for Safeguarding Analytical Performances in Biological Fluids. *Sensors* **2016**, *16*, 780. [CrossRef] [PubMed]
49. Thévenot, D.R.; Toth, K.; Durst, R.A.; Wilson, G.S. Electrochemical biosensors: Recommended definitions and classification. *Biosens. Bioelectron.* **2001**, *16*, 121–131. [CrossRef] [PubMed]

50. Majder-Łopatka, M.; Węsierski, T.; Dmochowska, A.; Salamonowicz, Z.; Polanczyk, A. The influence of hydrogen on the indications of the electrochemical carbon monoxide sensors. *Sustainability* **2019**, *12*, 14. [CrossRef]
51. Bhalla, N.; Jolly, P.; Formisano, N.; Estrela, P. Introduction to biosensors. *Essays Biochem.* **2016**, *60*, 1–8.
52. McGrath, M.J.; Scanaill, C.N. Sensing and sensor fundamentals. In *Sensor Technologies: Healthcare, Wellness, and Environmental Applications*; Springer: Berlin/Heidelberg, Germany, 2013; pp. 15–50.
53. Aragay, G.; Merkoçi, A. Nanomaterials application in electrochemical detection of heavy metals. *Electrochim. Acta* **2012**, *84*, 49–61. [CrossRef]
54. Pumera, M.; Escarpa, A. Nanomaterials as electrochemical detectors in microfluidics and CE: Fundamentals, designs, and applications. *Electrophoresis* **2009**, *30*, 3315–3323. [CrossRef]
55. Yang, C.; Denno, M.E.; Pyakurel, P.; Venton, B.J. Recent trends in carbon nanomaterial-based electrochemical sensors for biomolecules: A review. *Anal. Chim. Acta* **2015**, *887*, 17–37. [CrossRef] [PubMed]
56. Zhang, W.; Zhu, S.; Luque, R.; Han, S.; Hu, L.; Xu, G. Recent development of carbon electrode materials and their bioanalytical and environmental applications. *Chem. Soc. Rev.* **2016**, *45*, 715–752. [CrossRef]
57. Eksin, E.; Zor, E.; Erdem, A.; Bingol, H. Electrochemical monitoring of biointeraction by graphene-based material modified pencil graphite electrode. *Biosens. Bioelectron.* **2017**, *92*, 207–214. [CrossRef]
58. Hasoň, S.; Daňhel, A.; Schwarzová-Pecková, K.; Fojta, M. Carbon electrodes in electrochemical analysis of biomolecules and bioactive substances: Roles of surface structures and chemical groups. In *Nanotechnology and Biosensors*; Elsevier: Amsterdam, The Netherlands, 2018; pp. 51–111.
59. Heydari-Bafrooei, E.; Ensafi, A.A. Typically used carbon-based nanomaterials in the fabrication of biosensors. In *Electrochemical Biosensors*; Elsevier: Amsterdam, The Netherlands, 2019; pp. 77–98.
60. Torrinha, Á.; Amorim, C.G.; Montenegro, M.C.B.S.M.; Araújo, A.N. Biosensing based on pencil graphite electrodes. *Talanta* **2018**, *190*, 235–247. [CrossRef] [PubMed]
61. Baluchová, S.; Daňhel, A.; Dejmková, H.; Ostatná, V.; Fojta, M.; Schwarzová-Pecková, K. Recent progress in the applications of boron doped diamond electrodes in electroanalysis of organic compounds and biomolecules—A review. *Anal. Chim. Acta* **2019**, *1077*, 30–66. [CrossRef]
62. Svítková, J.; Ignat, T.; Švorc, Ľ.; Labuda, J.; Barek, J. Chemical modification of boron-doped diamond electrodes for applications to biosensors and biosensing. *Crit. Rev. Anal. Chem.* **2016**, *46*, 248–256. [CrossRef]
63. Sharma, V.K.; Jelen, F.; Trnkova, L. Functionalized solid electrodes for electrochemical biosensing of purine nucleobases and their analogues: A review. *Sensors* **2015**, *15*, 1564–1600. [CrossRef]
64. Liu, D.; Luo, Q.; Deng, F.; Li, Z.; Li, B.; Shen, Z. Ultrasensitive electrochemical biosensor based on the oligonucleotide self-assembled monolayer-mediated immunosensing interface. *Anal. Chim. Acta* **2017**, *971*, 26–32. [CrossRef]
65. Levrie, K.; Jans, K.; Vos, R.; Ardakanian, N.; Verellen, N.; Van Hoof, C.; Lagae, L.; Stakenborg, T. Multiplexed site-specific electrode functionalization for multitarget biosensors. *Bioelectrochemistry* **2016**, *112*, 61–66. [CrossRef] [PubMed]
66. Yáñez-Sedeño, P.; Campuzano, S.; Pingarrón, J.M. Integrated affinity biosensing platforms on screen-printed electrodes electro-grafted with diazonium salts. *Sensors* **2018**, *18*, 675. [CrossRef]
67. Rashid, J.I.A.; Yusof, N.A. The strategies of DNA immobilization and hybridization detection mechanism in the construction of electrochemical DNA sensor: A review. *Sens. Bio Sens. Res.* **2017**, *16*, 19–31. [CrossRef]
68. Švorc, Ľ.; Jambrec, D.; Vojs, M.; Barwe, S.; Clausmeyer, J.; Michniak, P.; Marton, M.; Schuhmann, W. Doping level of boron-doped diamond electrodes controls the grafting density of functional groups for DNA assays. *ACS Appl. Mater. Interfaces* **2015**, *7*, 18949–18956. [CrossRef] [PubMed]
69. Mahshid, S.S.; Vallée-Bélisle, A.; Kelley, S.O. Biomolecular steric hindrance effects are enhanced on nanostructured microelectrodes. *Anal. Chem.* **2017**, *89*, 9751–9757. [CrossRef]
70. Mishra, R.K.; Nunes, G.S.; Souto, L.; Marty, J.L. Screen printed technology-an application towards biosensor development. In *Encyclopedia of Interfacial Chemistry: Surface Science and Electrochemistry*; Elsevier: Amsterdam, The Netherlands, 2018; pp. 487–498.
71. Couto, R.A.S.; Lima, J.L.F.C.; Quinaz, M.B. Recent developments, characteristics and potential applications of screen-printed electrodes in pharmaceutical and biological analysis. *Talanta* **2016**, *146*, 801–814. [CrossRef]
72. Yáñez-Sedeño, P.; Campuzano, S.; Pingarrón, J.M. Screen-printed electrodes: Promising paper and wearable transducers for (Bio)sensing. *Biosensors* **2020**, *10*, 76. [CrossRef] [PubMed]
73. Yamanaka, K.; Vestergaard, M.C.; Tamiya, E. Printable electrochemical biosensors: A focus on screen-printed electrodes and their application. *Sensors* **2016**, *16*, 1761. [CrossRef] [PubMed]
74. Alizadeh, A.; Burns, A.; Lenigk, R.; Gettings, R.; Ashe, J.; Porter, A.; McCaul, M.; Barrett, R.; Diamond, D.; White, P.; et al. A wearable patch for continuous monitoring of sweat electrolytes during exertion. *Lab Chip* **2018**, *18*, 2632–2641. [CrossRef]
75. Xia, Y.; Si, J.; Li, Z. Fabrication techniques for microfluidic paper-based analytical devices and their applications for biological testing: A review. *Biosens. Bioelectron.* **2016**, *77*, 774–789. [CrossRef]
76. Punjiya, M.; Moon, C.H.; Matharu, Z.; Nejad, H.R.; Sonkusale, S. A threedimensional electrochemical paper-based analytical device for low-cost diagnostics. *Analyst* **2018**, *143*, 1059–1064. [CrossRef] [PubMed]
77. Nery, E.W.; Kubota, L.T. Sensing approaches on paper-based devices: A review. *Anal. Bioanal. Chem.* **2013**, *405*, 7573–7595. [CrossRef]

78. Ratajczak, K.; Stobiecka, M. High-performance modified cellulose paper-based biosensors for medical diagnostics and early cancer screening: A concise review. *Carbohydr. Polym.* **2020**, *229*, 115463. [CrossRef]
79. Mettakoonpitak, J.; Boehle, K.; Nantaphol, S.; Teengam, P.; Adkins, J.A.; Srisa-art, M.; Henry, C.S. Electrochemistry on paper-based analytical devices: A review. *Electroanalysis* **2016**, *28*, 1420–1436. [CrossRef]
80. Brunauer, A.; Ates, H.C.; Dincer, C.; Früh, S.M. Integrated paper-based sensing devices for diagnostic applications. In *Comprehensive Analytical Chemistry*; Elsevier: Amsterdam, The Netherlands, 2020; pp. 397–450.
81. Sjöberg, P.; Määttänen, A.; Vanamo, U.; Novell, M.; Ihalainen, P.; Andrade, F.J.; Bobacka, J.; Peltonen, J. Paper-based potentiometric ion sensors constructed on ink-jet printed gold electrodes. *Sens. Actuators B* **2016**, *224*, 325–332. [CrossRef]
82. Lu, Y.; Shi, W.; Qin, J.; Lin, B. Fabrication and characterization of paper-based microfluidics prepared in nitrocellulose membrane by Wax printing. *Anal. Chem.* **2010**, *82*, 329–335. [CrossRef]
83. Lu, J.; Ge, S.; Ge, L.; Yan, M.; Yu, J. Electrochemical DNA sensor based on three-dimensional folding paper device for specific and sensitive point-of-care testing. *Electrochim. Acta* **2012**, *80*, 334–341. [CrossRef]
84. Windmiller, J.R.; Wang, J. Wearable electrochemical sensors and biosensors: A review. *Electroanalysis* **2013**, *25*, 29–46. [CrossRef]
85. Kim, J.; De Araujo, W.R.; Samek, I.A.; Bandodkar, A.J.; Jia, W.; Brunetti, B.; Paixão, T.R.L.C.; Wang, J. Wearable temporary tattoo sensor for real-time trace metal monitoring in human sweat. *Electrochem. Commun.* **2015**, *51*, 41–45. [CrossRef]
86. Wang, J.; Gao, W. Nano/Microscale motors: Biomedical opportunities and challenges. *ACS Nano* **2012**, *6*, 5745–5751. [CrossRef]
87. Yeung, A.W.K.; Torkamani, A.; Butte, A.J.; Glicksberg, B.S.; Schuller, B.; Rodriguez, B.; Ting, D.S.W.; Bates, D.; Schaden, E.; Peng, H.; et al. The promise of digital healthcare technologies. *Front. Public Health* **2023**, *11*, 1196596. [CrossRef] [PubMed]
88. Baylis, J.R.; Yeon, J.H.; Thomson, M.H.; Kazerooni, A.; Wang, X.; John, A.E.S.S.; Lim, E.B.; Chien, D.; Lee, A.; Zhang, J.Q.; et al. Self-propelled particles that transport cargo through flowing blood and halt hemorrhage. *Sci. Adv.* **2015**, *1*, e1500379. [CrossRef] [PubMed]
89. Tu, Y.; Peng, F.; Sui, X.; Men, Y.; White, P.B.; Van Hest, J.C.M.; Wilson, D.A. Selfpropelled supramolecular nanomotors with temperature-responsive speed regulation. *Nat. Chem.* **2017**, *9*, 480–486. [CrossRef] [PubMed]
90. Wei, X.; Beltrán-Gastélum, M.; Karshalev, E.; De Ávila, B.E.-F.; Zhou, J.; Ran, D.; Angsantikul, P.; Fang, R.H.; Wang, J.; Zhang, L. Biomimetic micromotor enables active delivery of antigens for oral vaccination. *Nano Lett.* **2019**, *19*, 1914–1921. [CrossRef]
91. Gibbs, J.G.; Zhao, Y.P. Design and characterization of rotational multicomponent catalytic nanomotors. *Small* **2009**, *5*, 2304–2308. [CrossRef]
92. Wu, Y.; Si, T.; Lin, X.; He, Q. Near infrared-modulated propulsion of catalytic Janus polymer multilayer capsule motors. *Chem. Commun.* **2015**, *51*, 511–514. [CrossRef]
93. Orozco, J.; Cortés, A.; Cheng, G.; Sattayasamitsathit, S.; Gao, W.; Feng, X.; Shen, Y.; Wang, J. Molecularly imprinted polymer-based catalytic micromotors for selective protein transport. *J. Am. Chem. Soc.* **2013**, *135*, 5336–5339. [CrossRef]
94. Gao, W.; Sattayasamitsathit, S.; Orozco, J.; Wang, J. Highly efficient catalytic microengines: Template electrosynthesis of polyaniline/platinum microtubes. *J. Am. Chem. Soc.* **2011**, *133*, 11862–11864. [CrossRef]
95. Gibbs, J.G.; Fragnito, N.A.; Zhao, Y. Asymmetric Pt/Au coated catalytic micromotors fabricated by dynamic shadowing growth. *Appl. Phys. Lett.* **2010**, *97*, 253107. [CrossRef]
96. Lee, T.C.; Alarcón-Correa, M.; Miksch, C.; Hahn, K.; Gibbs, J.G.; Fischer, P. Selfpropelling nanomotors in the presence of strong Brownian forces. *Nano Lett.* **2014**, *14*, 2407–2412. [CrossRef]
97. Safdar, M.; Khan, S.U.; Jänis, J. Progress toward catalytic micro- and nanomotors for biomedical and environmental applications. *Adv. Mater.* **2018**, *30*, e1703660. [CrossRef] [PubMed]
98. Guix, M.; Mayorga-Martinez, C.C.; Merkoçi, A. Nano/micromotors in (bio)chemical science applications. *Chem. Rev.* **2014**, *114*, 6285–6322. [CrossRef] [PubMed]
99. Ye, Y.; Luan, J.; Wang, M.; Chen, Y.; Wilson, D.A.; Peng, F.; Tu, Y. Fabrication of self-propelled micro- and nanomotors based on Janus structures. *Chemistry* **2019**, *25*, 8663–8680. [CrossRef]
100. Tejeda-Rodríguez, J.A.; Núñez, A.; Soto, F.; García-Gradilla, V.; Cadena-Nava, R.; Wang, J.; Vazquez-Duhalt, R. Virus-based nanomotors for cargo delivery. *ChemNanoMat* **2019**, *5*, 194–200. [CrossRef]
101. Kashyap, D.; Venkateswaran, P.S.; Dwivedi, P.K.; Kim, Y.H.; Kim, G.M.; Sharma, A.; Goel, S. Recent developments in enzymatic biofuel cell: Towards implantable integrated micro-devices. *Int. J. Nanoparticles* **2015**, *8*, 61–81. [CrossRef]
102. Gonzalez-Solino, C.; Di Lorenzo, M.D. Enzymatic fuel cells: Towards self-powered implantable and wearable diagnostics. *Biosensors* **2018**, *8*, 11. [CrossRef]
103. Garcia, S.O.; Ulyanova, Y.V.; Figueroa-Teran, R.; Bhatt, K.H.; Singhal, S.; Atanassov, P. Wearable sensor system powered by a biofuel cell for detection of lactate levels in sweat. *ECS J. Solid State Sci. Technol.* **2016**, *5*, M3075–M3081. [CrossRef]
104. Göbel, G.; Beltran, M.L.; Mundhenk, J.; Heinlein, T.; Schneider, J.; Lisdat, F. Operation of a carbon nanotube-based glucose/oxygen biofuel cell in human body liquids—Performance factors and characteristics. *Electrochim. Acta* **2016**, *218*, 278–284. [CrossRef]
105. Majdecka, D.; Draminska, S.; Janusek, D.; Krysinski, P.; Bilewicz, R. A self-powered biosensing device with an integrated hybrid biofuel cell for intermittent monitoring of analytes. *Biosens. Bioelectron.* **2018**, *102*, 383–388. [CrossRef]
106. Gai, P.; Song, R.; Zhu, C.; Ji, Y.; Wang, W.; Zhang, J.R.; Zhu, J.J. Ultrasensitive selfpowered cytosensors based on exogenous redox-free enzyme biofuel cells as point-ofcare tools for early cancer diagnosis. *Chem. Commun.* **2015**, *51*, 16763–16766. [CrossRef]

107. Wang, X.; Falk, M.; Ortiz, R.; Matsumura, H.; Bobacka, J.; Ludwig, R.; Bergelin, M.; Gorton, L.; Shleev, S. Mediatorless sugar/oxygen enzymatic fuel cells based on gold nanoparticle-modified electrodes. *Biosens. Bioelectron.* **2012**, *31*, 219–225. [CrossRef] [PubMed]
108. Di Trocchio, L.; Carucci, C.; Sindhu, K.R.; Morel, C.; Lachaud, J.L.; Bichon, S.; Gounel, S.; Mano, N.; Boiziau, C.; Dejous, C.; et al. Wireless in vivo biofuel cell monitoring. *IEEE J. Electromagn. RF Microw. Med. Biol.* **2020**, *5*, 25–34. [CrossRef]
109. Qian, L.; Durairaj, S.; Prins, S.; Chen, A. Nanomaterial-based electrochemical sensors and biosensors for the detection of pharmaceutical compounds. *Biosens. Bioelectron.* **2021**, *175*, 112836. [CrossRef] [PubMed]
110. Shetti, N.P.; Malode, S.J.; Nayak, D.S.; Reddy, C.V.; Reddy, K.R. Novel biosensor for efficient electrochemical detection of Methdilazine using carbon nanotubes-modified electrodes. *Mater. Res. Express* **2019**, *6*, 116308. [CrossRef]
111. Prabhu, K.; Malode, S.J.; Shetti, N.P.; Kulkarni, R.M. Analysis of herbicide and its applications through a sensitive electrochemical technique based on MWCNTs/ZnO/CPE fabricated sensor. *Chemosphere* **2022**, *287*, 132086. [CrossRef]
112. Patil, V.B.; Malode, S.J.; Tuwar, S.M.; Alshehri, M.A.; Shetti, N.P. Development of a glycine-MWCNT nanohybrid via electropolymerization for enhanced electrochemical detection of diclofenac. *J. Mol. Struct.* **2024**, *1319*, 139535. [CrossRef]
113. Malode, S.J.; Prabhu, K.K.K.; Shetti, N.P. Electrocatalytic behavior of a heterostructured nanocomposite sensor for aminotriazole. *New J. Chem.* **2020**, *44*, 19376–19384. [CrossRef]
114. Manasa, G.; Mascarenhas, R.J.; Shetti, N.P.; Malode, S.J.; Aminabhavi, T.M. Biomarkers for early diagnosis of ovarian carcinoma. *ACS Biomater. Sci. Eng.* **2022**, *8*, 2726–2746. [CrossRef]
115. Malode, S.J.; Shetti, N.P. New generation biomarkers for the detection of prostate cancer. *Biosens. Bioelectron.* **2022**, *12*, 100250. [CrossRef]
116. Prabhu, K.; Malode, S.J.; Shetti, N.P. Carbon-based electrochemical sensor for the detection and degradation of persistent toxic carbendazim in soil and water sample. *Electrocatalysis* **2022**, *14*, 88–97. [CrossRef]
117. Manasa, G.; Bhakta, A.K.; Bafna, J.; Mascarenhas, R.J.; Malode, S.J.; Shetti, N.P. An amperometric sensor composed of carbon hybrid-structure for the degradation of aminotriazole herbicide. *Environ. Res.* **2022**, *212*, 113541. [CrossRef] [PubMed]
118. Shetti, N.P.; Nayak, D.S.; Malode, S.J.; Kulkarni, R.M. Fabrication of MWCNTs and Ru doped TiO2 nanoparticles composite carbon sensor for biomedical application. *ECS J. Solid State Sci. Technol.* **2018**, *7*, Q3070–Q3078. [CrossRef]
119. Bandyopadhyay, A.; Ghosh, D.; Pati, S.K. Trapping and sensing of hazardous insecticides by chemically modified single walled carbon nanotubes. *Phys. Chem. Chem. Phys.* **2017**, *19*, 24059–24066. [CrossRef] [PubMed]
120. Duclaux, L. Review of the doping of carbon nanotubes (multiwalled and single-walled). *Carbon* **2002**, *40*, 1751–1764. [CrossRef]
121. Donarelli, M.; Ottaviano, L. 2D Materials for Gas Sensing Applications: A Review on Graphene Oxide, MoS_2, WS_2 and Phosphorene. *Sensors* **2018**, *18*, 3638–3683. [CrossRef]
122. Lu, C.; Huang, P.J.J.; Liu, B.; Ying, Y.; Liu, J. Comparison of Graphene Oxide and Reduced Graphene Oxide for DNA Adsorption and Sensing. *Langmuir* **2016**, *32*, 10776–10783. [CrossRef]
123. Killedar, L.S.; Shanbhag, M.M.; Manasa, G.; Malode, S.J.; Veerapur, R.S.; Shetti, N.P.; Mascarenhas, R.J.; Kakarla, R.R. An electrochemical sensor based on graphene oxide/cholesterol nanohybrids for the sensitive analysis of cetirizine. *J. Environ. Chem. Eng.* **2022**, *10*, 108894. [CrossRef]
124. Killedar, L.S.; Shanbhag, M.M.; Shetti, N.P.; Malode, S.J.; Veerapur, R.S.; Reddy, K.R. Novel graphene-nanoclay hybrid electrodes for electrochemical determination of theophylline. *Microchem. J.* **2021**, *165*, 106115. [CrossRef]
125. Shanbhag, M.M.; Shetti, N.P.; Malode, S.J.; Veerapur, R.S.; Reddy, K.R. Cholesterol intercalated 2D graphene oxide sheets fabricated sensor for voltammetric analysis of theophylline. *FlatChem* **2021**, *28*, 100255. [CrossRef]
126. Ilager, D.; Malode, S.J.; Shetti, N.P. Development of 2D graphene oxide sheets-based voltammetric sensor for electrochemical sensing of fungicide, carbendazim. *Chemosphere* **2022**, *303*, 134919. [CrossRef]
127. Malode, S.J.; Prabhu, K.; Pollet, B.G.; Kalanur, S.S.; Shetti, N.P. Preparation and performance of WO_3/rGO modified carbon sensor for enhanced electrochemical detection of triclosan. *Electrochim. Acta* **2022**, *429*, 141010. [CrossRef]
128. Manasa, G.; Mascarenhas, R.J.; Malode, S.J.; Shetti, N.P. Graphene-based electrochemical immunosensors for early detection of oncomarker carcinoembryonic antigen. *Biosens. Bioelectron.* **2022**, *11*, 100189. [CrossRef]
129. Kong, X.K.; Le Chen, C.L.; Chen, Q.W. Doped graphene for metal-free catalysis. *Chem. Soc. Rev.* **2014**, *43*, 2841–2857. [CrossRef] [PubMed]
130. Ravat, V.; Nongwe, I.; Coville, N.J. N-doped ordered mesoporous carbon supported PdCo nanoparticles for the catalytic oxidation of benzyl alcohol. *Micropor. Mesopor. Mater.* **2016**, *225*, 224–231. [CrossRef]
131. Verma, H.N.; Singh, P.; Chavan, R.M. Gold nanoparticle: Synthesis and characterization. *Vet. World* **2014**, *7*, 72–77. [CrossRef]
132. Dumestre, F.; Chaudret, B.; Amiens, C.; Renaud, P.; Fejes, P. Superlattices of iron nanocubes synthesized from $Fe[N(SiMe_3)_2]_2$. *Science* **2004**, *303*, 821–823. [CrossRef]
133. White, R.J.; Luque, R.; Budarin, V.L.; Clark, J.H.; Macquarrie, D.J. Supported metal nanoparticles on porous materials. Methods and applications. *Chem. Soc. Rev.* **2009**, *38*, 481–494. [CrossRef]
134. Nguyen, N.S.; Das, G.; Yoon, H.H. Nickel/cobalt oxide-decorated 3D graphene nanocomposite electrode for enhanced electrochemical detection of urea. *Biosens. Bioelectron.* **2016**, *77*, 372–377. [CrossRef]
135. Bai, J.; Zhou, B. Titanium dioxide nanomaterials for sensor applications. *Chem. Rev.* **2014**, *114*, 10131–10176. [CrossRef]
136. Malode, S.J.; Shetti, N.P.; Reddy, K.R. Highly sensitive electrochemical assay for selective detection of aminotriazole based on TiO_2/poly (CTAB) modified sensor. *Environ. Technol. Innov.* **2021**, *21*, 101222. [CrossRef]

137. Shetti, N.P.; Malode, S.J.; Nayak, D.S.; Reddy, K.R. Novel heterostructured Ru-doped TiO_2/CNTs hybrids with enhanced electrochemical sensing performance for cetirizine. *Mater. Res. Express* **2019**, *6*, 115085. [CrossRef]
138. Killedar, L.; Ilager, D.; Malode, S.J.; Shetti, N.P. Fast and facile electrochemical detection and determination of fungicide carbendazim at titanium dioxide designed carbon-based sensor. *Mater. Chem. Phys.* **2022**, *285*, 126131. [CrossRef]
139. Malode, S.J.; Shabhag, M.S.; Kumari, R.; Dkhar, D.S.; Chandra, P.; Shetti, N.P. Biomass-derived carbon nanomaterials for sensor applications. *J. Pharm. Biomed. Anal.* **2023**, *222*, 115102. [CrossRef] [PubMed]
140. Uzun, L.; Turner, A.P.F. Molecularly-imprinted polymer sensors: Realising their potential. *Biosens. Bioelectron.* **2016**, *76*, 131–144. [CrossRef] [PubMed]
141. Alqarni, S.A.; Hussein, M.A.; Ganash, A.A.; Khan, A. Composite Material–Based Conducting Polymers for Electrochemical Sensor Applications: A Mini Review. *BioNanoScience* **2020**, *10*, 351–364. [CrossRef]
142. Lapworth, D.J.; Baran, N.; Stuart, M.E.; Ward, R.S. Emerging organic contaminants in groundwater: A review of sources, fate and occurrence. *Environ. Pollut.* **2012**, *163*, 287–303. [CrossRef]
143. Vane, J.R.; Botting, R.M. Mechanism of action of nonsteroidal anti-inflammatory drugs. *Am. J. Med.* **1998**, *104*, 2S–8S, Discussion 21S. [CrossRef]
144. He, Y.; Wang, X.; Huang, W.; Chen, R.; Zhang, W.; Li, H.; Lin, H. Hydrophobic networked PbO2 electrode for electrochemical oxidation of paracetamol drug and degradation mechanism kinetics. *Chemosphere* **2018**, *193*, 89–99. [CrossRef]
145. Shokri, T.; Sadeghi, M.; Hadidi, S.; Mohammadi, S. Efficient fluorescence probe for detection of naproxen in pharmaceutical formulations and water samples using MPA-capped CdTe/ZnS core-shell nanocrystal-neutral red: Experimental and computational studies. *J. Photochem. Photobiol. A Chem.* **2024**, *452*, 115545. [CrossRef]
146. Tarahomi, S.; Rounaghi, G.H.; Daneshvar, L. A novel disposable sensor based on gold digital versatile disc chip modified with graphene oxide decorated with Ag nanoparticles/β-cyclodextrin for voltammetric measurement of naproxen. *Sens. Actuators B* **2019**, *286*, 445–450. [CrossRef]
147. Baj-Rossi, C.; Jost, T.R.; Cavallini, A.; Grassi, F.; De Micheli, G.; Carrara, S. Continuous monitoring of Naproxen by a cytochrome P450-based electrochemical sensor. *Biosens. Bioelectron.* **2014**, *53*, 283–287. [CrossRef] [PubMed]
148. Alagumalai, K.; Babulal, S.M.; Chen, S.; Shanmugam, R.; Yesuraj, J. Electrochemical evaluation of naproxen through Au@f-CNT/GO nanocomposite in environmental water and biological samples. *J. Ind. Eng. Chem.* **2021**, *104*, 32–42. [CrossRef]
149. Díaz, E.; Stożek, S.; Patiño, Y.; Ordóñez, S. Electrochemical degradation of naproxen from water by anodic oxidation with multiwall carbon nanotubes glassy carbon electrode. *Water Sci. Technol.* **2019**, *79*, 480–488. [CrossRef]
150. Kanagasabapathy, M.; Sekar, R. Chronopotentiometric/chronoamperometric transient analysis of naproxen via electrochemically synthesized nano spinel $ZnFe_2O_4$ films. *J. Electroanal. Chem.* **2019**, *832*, 59–68. [CrossRef]
151. Hung, C.M.; Huang, C.P.; Chen, S.K.; Chen, C.W.; Dong, C.D. Electrochemical analysis of naproxen in water using poly(l-serine)-modified glassy carbon electrode. *Chemosphere* **2020**, *254*, 126686. [CrossRef]
152. Afzali, M.; Jahromi, Z.; Nekooie, R. Sensitive voltammetric method for the determination of naproxen at the surface of carbon nanofiber/gold/polyaniline nanocomposite modified carbon ionic liquid electrode. *Microchem. J.* **2019**, *145*, 373–379. [CrossRef]
153. Roushani, M.; Shahdost-Fard, F. Fabrication of an ultrasensitive ibuprofen nanoaptasensor based on covalent attachment of aptamer to electrochemically deposited gold-nanoparticles on glassy carbon electrode. *Talanta* **2015**, *144*, 510–516. [CrossRef]
154. Nair, A.S.; Sooraj, M.P. Molecular imprinted polymer-wrapped AgNPs-decorated acid-functionalized graphene oxide as a potent electrochemical sensor for ibuprofen. *J. Mater. Sci.* **2020**, *55*, 3700–3711. [CrossRef]
155. Mutharani, B.; Rajakumaran, R.; Chen, S.; Ranganathan, P.; Chen, T.; Al Farraj, D.A.; Ali, M.A.; Al-Hemaid, F.M.A. Facile synthesis of 3D stone-like copper tellurate (Cu_3TeO_6) as a new platform for anti-inflammatory drug ibuprofen sensor in human blood serum and urine samples. *Microchem. J.* **2020**, *159*, 105378. [CrossRef]
156. Parlak, C.; Alver, Ö. Adsorption of ibuprofen on silicon decorated fullerenes and single walled carbon nanotubes: A comparative DFT study. *J. Mol. Struct.* **2019**, *1184*, 110–113. [CrossRef]
157. Kruanetr, S.; Pollard, P.; Fernandez, C.; Prabhu, R. Electrochemical oxidation of acetyl salicylic acid and its voltametric sensing in real samples at a sensitive edge plane pyrolytic graphite electrode modified with graphene. *Int. J. Electrochem. Sci.* **2014**, *9*, 5699–5711. [CrossRef]
158. Ghadimi, H.; Tehrani, M.A.; Basirun, W.J.; Aziz, N.J.A.; Mohamed, N.J.; Ghani, S.A. Electrochemical determination of aspirin and caffeine at MWCNTs-poly-4-vinylpyridine composite modified electrode, J. Taiwan Inst. *Chem. Eng.* **2016**, *65*, 101–109.
159. Diouf, A.; Aghoutane, Y.; Burhan, H.; Sen, F.; Bouchikhi, B.; El Bari, N. Tramadol sensing in non-invasive biological fluids using a voltammetric electronic tongue and an electrochemical sensor based on biomimetic recognition. *Int. J. Pharm.* **2021**, *593*, 120114. [CrossRef] [PubMed]
160. Xia, Y.; Bian, X.; Xia, Y.; Zhou, W.; Wang, L.; Fan, S.; Xiong, P.; Zhan, T.; Dai, Q.; Chen, J. Effect of indium doping on the PbO_2 electrode for the enhanced electrochemical oxidation of aspirin: An electrode comparative study. *Sep. Purif. Technol.* **2020**, *237*, 116321. [CrossRef]
161. Dandekar, A.A.; Kale, M.; Garimella, H.T.; Banga, A.K. Effect of compromised skin barrier on delivery of diclofenac sodium from brand and generic formulations via microneedles and iontophoresis. *Int. J. Pharm.* **2022**, *628*, 122271. [CrossRef]
162. Sataraddi, S.R.; Patil, S.M.; Bagoji, A.M.; Pattar, V.P.; Nandibewoor, S.T. Electrooxidation of Indomethacin at multiwalled carbon nanotubes-modified GCE and its determination in pharmaceutical dosage form and human biological fluids. *Anal. Chem.* **2014**, *2014*, 9. [CrossRef]

163. Arkan, E.; Karimi, Z.; Shamsipur, M.; Saber, R. Electrochemical determination of celecoxib on a graphene based carbon ionic liquid electrode modified with gold nanoparticles and its application to pharmaceutical analysis. *Anal. Sci.* **2013**, *29*, 855–860. [CrossRef]
164. Shalauddin, M.; Akhter, S.; Basirun, W.J.; Akhtaruzzaman, M.; Mohammed, M.A.; Rahman, N.M.M.A.; Salleh, N.M. Biosynthesized copper nanoparticle decorated multiwall carbon nanotube-nanocellulose nanocomposite: An electrochemical sensor for the simultaneous detection of acetaminophen and diclofenac sodium. *Surf. Interfaces* **2022**, *34*, 102385. [CrossRef]
165. Honakeri, N.C.; Malode, S.J.; Kulkarni, R.M.; Shetti, N.P. Electrochemical behavior of diclofenac sodium at coreshell nanostructure modified electrode and its analysis in human urine and pharmaceutical samples. *Sens. Int.* **2020**, *1*, 100002. [CrossRef]
166. Alizadeh, T.; Azizi, S. Graphene/graphite paste electrode incorporated with molecularly imprinted polymer nanoparticles as a novel sensor for differential pulse voltammetry determination of fluoxetine. *Biosens. Bioelectron.* **2016**, *81*, 198–206. [CrossRef]
167. Ardelean, M.; Pode, R.; Schoonman, J.; Pop, A.; Manea, F. Fast simultaneous electrochemical detection of tetracycline and fluoxetine in water, W.I.T. Trans. *Ecol. Environ.* **2017**, *216*, 213–220.
168. Ramos, D.L.O.; Freitas, J.M.; Munoz, R.A.A.; Richter, E.M. Simple and rapid voltammetric method for the detection of the synthetic adulterant fluoxetine in weight loss products. *J. Electroanal. Chem.* **2021**, *882*, 115028. [CrossRef]
169. Fasipe, O. Neuropharmacological classification of antidepressant agents based on their mechanisms of action. *Arch. Med. Health Sci. D* **2018**, *6*, 81–94. [CrossRef]
170. Oghli, A.H.; Soleymanpour, A. Polyoxometalate/reduced graphene oxide modified pencil graphite sensor for the electrochemical trace determination of paroxetine in biological and pharmaceutical media. *Mater. Sci. Eng. C Mater. Biol. Appl.* **2020**, *108*, 110407. [CrossRef] [PubMed]
171. Khosrokhavar, R.; Motaharian, A.; Hosseini, M.R.M.; Mohammadsadegh, S. Screen-printed carbon electrode (SPCE) modified by molecularly imprinted polymer (MIP) nanoparticles and graphene nanosheets for determination of sertraline antidepressant drug. *Microchem. J.* **2020**, *159*, 105348. [CrossRef]
172. Shoja, Y.; Rafati, A.A.; Ghodsi, J. Electropolymerization of Ni–LD metallopolymers on gold nanoparticles enriched multi-walled carbon nanotubes as nano-structure electrocatalyst for efficient voltammetric sertraline detection in human serum. *Electrochim. Acta* **2016**, *203*, 281–291. [CrossRef]
173. Craske, M.G.; Stein, M.B.; Eley, T.C.; Milad, M.R.; Holmes, A.; Rapee, R.M.; Wittchen, H.-U. Anxiety disorders. *Nat. Rev. Dis. Primers* **2017**, *3*, 17024. [CrossRef]
174. Sharafeldin, M.; Bishop, G.W.; Bhakta, S.; El-Sawy, A.; Suib, S.L.; Rusling, J.F. Fe_3O_4 nanoparticles on graphene oxide sheets for isolation and ultrasensitive amperometric detection of cancer biomarker proteins. *Biosens. Bioelectron.* **2017**, *91*, 359–366. [CrossRef]
175. Khalilzadeh, M.A.; Tajik, S.; Beitollahi, H.; Venditti, R.A. Green Synthesis of Magnetic Nanocomposite with Iron Oxide Deposited on Cellulose Nanocrystals with Copper (Fe_3O_4 @CNC/Cu): Investigation of Catalytic Activity for the Development of a Venlafaxine Electrochemical Sensor. *Ind. Eng. Chem. Res.* **2020**, *59*, 4219–4228. [CrossRef]
176. Kerr, G.W.; McGuffie, A.C.; Wilkie, S. Tricyclic antidepressant overdose: A review. *Emerg. Med. J.* **2001**, *18*, 236–241. [CrossRef]
177. Jankowska-Śliwińska, J.; Dawgul, M.; Pijanowska, D.G. DNA-based Electrochemical Biosensor for Imipramine Detection. *Procedia Eng.* **2015**, *120*, 574–577. [CrossRef]
178. Yamuna, A.; Sundaresan, P.; Chen, S.M. Sonochemical preparation of bismuth oxide nanotiles decorated exfoliated graphite for the electrochemical detection of imipramine. *Ultrason. Sonochem.* **2020**, *64*, 105014. [CrossRef]
179. Knihnicki, P.; Wieczorek, M.; Moos, A.; Kościelniak, P.; Wietecha-Posłuszny, R.; Woźniakiewicz, M. Electrochemical sensor for determination of desipramine in biological material. *Sens. Actuators B* **2013**, *189*, 37–42. [CrossRef]
180. Cincotto, F.H.; Golinelli, D.L.C.; Machado, S.A.S.; Moraes, F.C. Electrochemical sensor based on reduced graphene oxide modified with palladium nanoparticles for determination of desipramine in urine samples. *Sens. Actuators B* **2017**, *239*, 488–493. [CrossRef]
181. Sanghavi, B.J.; Srivastava, A.K. Adsorptive stripping voltammetric determination of imipramine, trimipramine and desipramine employing titanium dioxide nanoparticles and an Amberlite XAD-2 modified glassy carbon paste electrode. *Analyst* **2013**, *138*, 1395–1404. [CrossRef]
182. Li, Z.; Liu, C.; Sarpong, V.; Gu, Z. Multisegment nanowire/nanoparticle hybrid arrays as electrochemical biosensors for simultaneous detection of antibiotics. *Biosens. Bioelectron.* **2019**, *126*, 632–639. [CrossRef] [PubMed]
183. Li, Y.; Zhao, X.; Li, P.; Huang, Y.; Wang, J.; Zhang, J. Highly sensitive Fe_3O_4 nanobeads/graphene-based molecularly imprinted electrochemical sensor for 17β-estradiol in water. *Anal. Chim. Acta* **2015**, *884*, 106–113. [CrossRef]
184. Feier, B.; Ionel, I.; Cristea, C.; Săndulescu, R. Electrochemical behaviour of several penicillins at high potential. *New J. Chem.* **2017**, *41*, 12947–12955. [CrossRef]
185. Zhao, J.; Guo, W.; Pei, M.; Ding, F. GR-Fe_3O_4 NPs and PEDOT-AuNPs composite based electrochemical aptasensor for the sensitive detection of penicillin. *Anal. Methods* **2016**, *8*, 4391–4397. [CrossRef]
186. Wong, A.; Santos, A.M.; Cincotto, F.H.; Moraes, F.C.; Fatibello-Filho, O.; Sotomayor, M.D.P.T. A new electrochemical platform based on low cost nanomaterials for sensitive detection of the amoxicillin antibiotic in different matrices. *Talanta* **2020**, *206*, 120252. [CrossRef]
187. Kirchmann, E.; Earley, R.L.; Welch, L.E. The Electrochemical Detection of Penicillins in Milk. *J. Liq. Chromatogr.* **1994**, *17*, 1755–1772. [CrossRef]

188. Tang, Y.; Liu, P.; Xu, J.; Le Li, L.; Yang, L.; Liu, X.; Liu, S.; Zhou, Y. Electrochemical aptasensor based on a novel flower-like TiO_2 nanocomposite for the detection of tetracycline. *Sens. Actuators B* **2018**, *258*, 906–912. [CrossRef]
189. Liu, X.; Zheng, S.; Hu, Y.; Li, Z.; Luo, F.; He, Z. Electrochemical Immunosensor Based on the Chitosan-Magnetic Nanoparticles for Detection of Tetracycline. *Food Anal. Methods* **2016**, *9*, 2972–2978. [CrossRef]
190. Wang, H.; Zhao, H.; Quan, X.; Chen, S. Electrochemical Determination of Tetracycline Using Molecularly Imprinted Polymer Modified Carbon Nanotube-Gold Nanoparticles Electrode. *Electroanalysis* **2011**, *23*, 1863–1869. [CrossRef]
191. Qin, X.; Yin, Y.; Yu, H.; Guo, W.; Pei, M. A novel signal amplification strategy of an electrochemical aptasensor for kanamycin, based on thionine functionalized graphene and hierarchical nanoporous PtCu. *Biosens. Bioelectron.* **2016**, *77*, 752–758. [CrossRef]
192. Yao, Y.; Jiang, C.; Ping, J. Flexible freestanding graphene paper-based potentiometric enzymatic aptasensor for ultrasensitive wireless detection of kanamycin. *Biosens. Bioelectron.* **2019**, *123*, 178–184. [CrossRef]
193. Yi, W.; Li, Z.; Dong, C.; Li, H.W.; Li, J. Electrochemical detection of chloramphenicol using palladium nanoparticles decorated reduced graphene oxide. *Microchem. J.* **2019**, *148*, 774–783. [CrossRef]
194. Chen, H.Y.; Wang, J.; Meng, L.; Yang, T.; Jiao, K. Thin-layered MoS2/polyaniline nanocomposite for highly sensitive electrochemical detection of chloramphenicol. *Chin. Chem. Lett.* **2016**, *27*, 231–234. [CrossRef]
195. Rajaji, U.; Manavalan, S.; Chen, S.M.; Govindasamy, M.; Chen, T.W.; Maiyalagan, T. Microwave-assisted synthesis of europium(III) oxide decorated reduced graphene oxide nanocomposite for detection of chloramphenicol in food samples. *Compos. B Eng.* **2019**, *161*, 29–36. [CrossRef]
196. Aki, C.; Yilmaz, S.; Dilgin, Y.; Yagmur, S.; Suren, E. Electrochemical study of natamycin–analytical application to pharmaceutical dosage forms by differential pulse voltammetry. *Pharmazie* **2005**, *60*, 747–750.
197. Ye, Z.; Yang, L.; Wen, J.; Ye, B. Sensitive determination of natamycin based on a new voltammetric sensor: A single-walled carbon nanotube composite poly(l-serine) film modified electrode. *Anal. Methods* **2015**, *7*, 2855–2861. [CrossRef]
198. Yang, X.; Yu, X.; Heng, Y.; Wang, F. Facile fabrication of 3D graphene–multi walled carbon nanotubes network and its use as a platform for natamycin detection. *J. Electroanal. Chem.* **2018**, *816*, 54–61. [CrossRef]
199. Yousefi, A.; Babaei, A.; Delavar, M. Application of modified screen-printed carbon electrode with MWCNTs-Pt-doped CdS nanocomposite as a sensitive sensor for determination of natamycin in yoghurt drink and cheese. *J. Electroanal. Chem.* **2018**, *822*, 1–9. [CrossRef]
200. Zad, Z.R.; Davarani, S.S.H.; Taheri, A.; Bide, Y. A yolk shell Fe_3O_4 @PA-Ni@Pd/Chitosan nanocomposite -modified carbon ionic liquid electrode as a new sensor for the sensitive determination of fluconazole in pharmaceutical preparations and biological fluids. *J. Mol. Liq.* **2018**, *253*, 233–240. [CrossRef]
201. Nagatani, N.; Yamanaka, K.; Saito, M.; Koketsu, R.; Sasaki, T.; Ikuta, K.; Miyahara, T.; Tamiya, E. Semi-real time electrochemical monitoring for influenza virus RNA by reverse transcription loop-mediated isothermal amplification using a USB powered portable potentiostat. *Analyst* **2011**, *136*, 5143–5150. [CrossRef]
202. Mielech-Łukasiewicz, K.; Rogińska, K. Voltammetric determination of antifungal agents in pharmaceuticals and cosmetics using boron-doped diamond electrodes. *Anal. Methods* **2014**, *6*, 7912–7922. [CrossRef]
203. Khairy, M.; Khorshed, A.A. Inspection of electrochemical behavior of tolnaftate a topical antifungal agent and its active hydrolysis products by disposable screen-printed carbon electrode. *J. Electroanal. Chem.* **2020**, *871*, 114274. [CrossRef]
204. Kokulnathan, T.; Priya, T.S.; Wang, T.J. Surface Engineering Three-Dimensional Flowerlike Cerium Vanadate Nanostructures Used as Electrocatalysts: Real Time Monitoring of Clioquinol in Biological Samples. *ACS Sustain. Chem. Eng.* **2019**, *7*, 16121–16130. [CrossRef]
205. Kokulnathan, T.; Chen, S.M. Rational Design for the Synthesis of Europium Vanadate-Encapsulated Graphene Oxide Nanocomposite: An Excellent and Efficient Catalyst for the Electrochemical Detection of Clioquinol. *ACS Sustain. Chem. Eng.* **2019**, *7*, 4136–4146. [CrossRef]
206. Wang, P.; Gan, T.; Zhang, J.; Luo, J.; Zhang, S. Polyvinylpyrrolidone-enhanced electrochemical oxidation and detection of acyclovir. *J. Mol. Liq.* **2013**, *177*, 129–132. [CrossRef]
207. Dilgin, D.G.; Karakaya, S. Differential pulse voltametric determination of acyclovir in pharmaceutical preparations using a pencil graphite electrode. *Mater. Sci. Eng. C Mater. Biol. Appl.* **2016**, *63*, 570–576. [CrossRef] [PubMed]
208. Shetti, N.P.; Malode, S.J.; Nayak, D.S.; Naik, R.R.; Kuchinad, G.T.; Reddy, K.R.; Shukla, S.S.; Aminabhavi, T.M. Hetero-nanostructured iron oxide and bentonite clay composite assembly for the determination of an antiviral drug acyclovir. *Microchem. J.* **2020**, *155*, 104727. [CrossRef]
209. Uslu, B.; Doğan, B.; Özkan, S.A. Electrochemical studies of ganciclovir at glassy carbon electrodes and its direct determination in serum and pharmaceutics by square wave and differential pulse voltammetry. *Anal. Chim. Acta* **2005**, *537*, 307–313. [CrossRef]
210. Zhou, Y.; Zhi, J.; Zhang, X.; Xu, M. Electrochemical studies of ganciclovir at boron-doped nanocrystalline diamond electrodes. *Diam. Relat. Mater.* **2011**, *20*, 18–22. [CrossRef]
211. Gholivand, M.B.; Karimian, N. Fabrication of a highly selective and sensitive voltammetric ganciclovir sensor based on electropolymerized molecularly imprinted polymer and gold nanoparticles on multiwall carbon nanotubes/glassy carbon electrode. *Sens. Actuators B* **2015**, *215*, 471–479. [CrossRef]
212. Skrzypek, S. Electrochemical Studies of the Neuraminidase Inhibitor Zanamivir and its Voltammetric Determination in Spiked Urine. *Electroanalysis* **2010**, *22*, 2339–2346. [CrossRef]

213. Wahyuni, W.T.; Ivandini, T.A.; Jiwanti, P.K.; Saepudin, E.; Gunlazuardi, J.; Einaga, Y. Electrochemical Behavior of Zanamivir at Gold-Modified Boron-Doped Diamond Electrodes for an Application in Neuraminidase Sensing. *Electrochemistry* **2015**, *83*, 357–362. [CrossRef]
214. Adhikari, B.R.; Govindhan, M.; Schraft, H.; Chen, A. Simultaneous and sensitive detection of acetaminophen and valacyclovir based on two dimensional graphene nanosheets. *J. Electroanal. Chem.* **2016**, *780*, 241–248. [CrossRef]
215. Holgado, T.M.M.; Quintana, M.C.; Pinilla, J.M. Electrochemical study of taxol (paclitaxel) by cathodic stripping voltammetry: Determination in human urine. *Microchem. J.* **2003**, *74*, 99–104. [CrossRef]
216. Taei, M.; Hassanpour, F.; Salavati, H.; Sadeghi, Z.; Alvandi, H. Highly Selective Electrochemical Determination of Taxol Based on ds-DNA-Modified Pencil Electrode. *Appl. Biochem. Biotechnol.* **2015**, *176*, 344–358. [CrossRef]
217. Tajik, S.; Taher, M.A.; Beitollahi, H.; Torkzadeh-Mahani, M. Electrochemical determination of the anticancer drug taxol at a ds-DNA modified pencil-graphite electrode and its application as a label-free electrochemical biosensor. *Talanta* **2015**, *134*, 60–64. [CrossRef] [PubMed]
218. Hahn, Y.; Lee, H.Y. Electrochemical behavior and square wave voltammetric determination of doxorubicin hydrochloride. *Arch. Pharm. Res.* **2004**, *27*, 31–34. [CrossRef]
219. Bahner, N.; Reich, P.; Frense, D.; Menger, M.; Schieke, K.; Beckmann, D. An aptamer-based biosensor for detection of doxorubicin by electrochemical impedance spectroscopy. *Anal. Bioanal. Chem.* **2018**, *410*, 1453–1462. [CrossRef] [PubMed]
220. Guo, Y.; Chen, Y.; Zhao, Q.; Shuang, S.; Dong, C. Electrochemical Sensor for Ultrasensitive Determination of Doxorubicin and Methotrexate Based on Cyclodextrin-Graphene Hybrid Nanosheets. *Electroanalysis* **2011**, *23*, 2400–2407. [CrossRef]
221. Hatamluyi, B.; Es'haghi, Z. A layer-by-layer sensing architecture based on dendrimer and ionic liquid supported reduced graphene oxide for simultaneous hollow-fiber solid phase microextraction and electrochemical determination of anti-cancer drug imatinib in biological samples. *J. Electroanal. Chem.* **2017**, *801*, 439–449. [CrossRef]
222. Rodríguez, J.; Castañeda, G.; Lizcano, I. Electrochemical sensor for leukemia drug imatinib determination in urine by adsorptive striping square wave voltammetry using modified screen-printed electrodes. *Electrochim. Acta* **2018**, *269*, 668–675. [CrossRef]
223. Chen, H.; Luo, K.; Li, K. A facile electrochemical sensor based on NiO-ZnO/MWCNT-COOH modified GCE for simultaneous quantification of Imatinib and Itraconazole. *J. Electrochem. Soc.* **2019**, *166*, B697–B707. [CrossRef]
224. Tseng, T.W.; Rajaji, U.; Chen, T.W.; Chen, S.M.; Huang, Y.C.; Mani, V.; Jothi, A.I. Sonochemical synthesis and fabrication of perovskite type calcium titanate interfacial nanostructure supported on graphene oxide sheets as a highly efficient electrocatalyst for electrochemical detection of chemotherapeutic drug. *Ultrason. Sonochem.* **2020**, *69*, 105242. [CrossRef]
225. Diouf, A.; Moufid, M.; Bouyahya, D.; Osterlund, L.; Bari, N.E.; Bouchikhi, B. An electrochemical sensor based on chitosan capped with gold nanoparticles combined with a voltammetric electronic tongue for quantitative aspirin detection in human physiological fluids and tablets. *Mater. Sci. Eng. C* **2020**, *110*, 110665. [CrossRef]
226. Feyziazar, M.; Hasanzadeh, M.; Farshchi, F.; Saadati, A.; Hassanpour, S. An innovative method to electrochemical branching of chitosan in the presence of copper nanocubics on the surface of glassy carbon and its electrical behaviour study: A new platform for pharmaceutical analysis using elec trochemical sensors. *React. Funct. Polym.* **2020**, *146*, 104402. [CrossRef]
227. Afkhami, A.; Bahiraei, A.; Madrakian, T. Gold nanoparticle/multi-walled carbon nanotube modified glassy carbon electrode as a sensitive voltammetric sensor for the determination of diclofenac sodium. *Mater. Sci. Eng. C* **2016**, *59*, 168–176. [CrossRef] [PubMed]
228. Kimuam, K.; Rodthongkum, N.; Ngamrojanavanich, N.; Chailapakul, O.; Ruecha, N. Single step preparation of platinum nanoflowers/reduced gra phene oxide electrode as a novel platform for diclofenac sensor. *Microchem. J.* **2020**, *155*, 104744. [CrossRef]
229. Karuppiah, C.; Cheemalapati, S.; Chen, S.-M.; Palanisamy, S. Carboxyl-func tionalized graphene oxide-modified electrode for the electrochemical determination of nonsteroidal anti-inflammatory drug diclofenac. *Ionics* **2015**, *21*, 231–238. [CrossRef]
230. Qian, L.; Thiruppathi, A.R.; Elmahdy, R.; van der Zalm, J.; Chen, A. Graphene oxide based electrochemical sensors for the sensitive detection of pharmaceutical drug naproxen. *Sensors* **2020**, *20*, 1252. [CrossRef] [PubMed]
231. Shetti, N.P.; Nayak, D.S.; Malode, S.J.; Kulkarni, R.M.; Kulkarni, D.B.; Teggi, R.A.; Joshi, V.V. Electrooxidation and determination of flufenamic acid at graphene oxide modified carbon electrode. *Surf. Interfaces* **2017**, *9*, 107–113. [CrossRef]
232. Aguilar-Lira, G.Y.; Alvarez-Romero, G.A.; Zamora-Suarez, A.; Pardave, M.P.; Rojas-Hernandez, A.; Rodríguez-Avila, J.A.; Paez-Hernandez, M.E. New insights on diclofenac electrochemistry using graphite as working electrode. *J. Electroanal. Chem.* **2017**, *794*, 182–188. [CrossRef]
233. Okoth, O.K.; Yan, K.; Liu, L.; Zhang, J. Simultaneous electrochemical determi nation of paracetamol and diclofenac based on poly (diallyldimethylammonium chloride) functionalized graphene. *Electroanalysis* **2016**, *28*, 76–82. [CrossRef]
234. Bayraktepe, D.E.; Yazan, Z. Application of single-use electrode based on nano clay and MWCNT for simultaneous determination of acetaminophen, ascorbic acid and acetylsalicylic acid in pharmaceutical dosage. *Electro Anal.* **2020**, *32*, 1263–1272. [CrossRef]
235. Montes, R.H.O.; Lima, A.R.; Cunha, R.R.; Guedes, T.J.; Santos, W.T.P.D.; Nossol, E.; Richter, E.M.; Munoz, R.A.A. Size effects of multi-walled carbon nanotubes on the electrochemical oxidation of propionic acid derivative drugs: Ibuprofen and naproxen. *J. Electroanal. Chem.* **2016**, *775*, 342–349. [CrossRef]
236. Khaled, E.; Kamel, M.S.; Hassan, H.N.A.; Haroun, A.A.; Youssef, A.M.; Enein, H.Y.A. Novel multi walled carbon nanotubes/b-cyclodextrin based carbon paste electrode for flow injection potentiometric determination of piroxicam. *Talanta* **2012**, *97*, 96–102. [CrossRef]

237. Kong, F.-Y.; Li, R.-F.; Yao, L.; Wang, Z.-X.; Lv, W.-X.; Wang, W. Pt nanoparticles supported on nitrogen doped reduced graphene oxide-single wall carbon nanotubes as a novel platform for highly sensitive electrochemical sensing of piroxicam. *J. Electroanal. Chem.* **2019**, *832*, 385–391. [CrossRef]
238. Nigovic, B.; Juric, S.; Mornar, A. Electrochemical determination of nepafenac topically applied nonsteroidal anti-inflammatory drug using graphene nanoplatelets-carbon nanofibers modified glassy carbon electrode. *J. Electroanal. Chem.* **2018**, *817*, 30–35. [CrossRef]
239. Dondo, N.; Shumba, M.; Moyo, M.; Nyoni, S. Simultaneous non-steroidal anti inflammatory drug electrodetection on nitrogen doped carbon nanodots and nanosized cobalt phthallocyanine conjugate modified glassy carbon electrode. *Arab. J. Chem.* **2020**, *13*, 7809–7819. [CrossRef]
240. Sivakumar, M.; Sakthivel, M.; Chen, S.-M.; Cheng, Y.-H.; Pandi, K. One-step synthesis of porous copper oxide for electrochemical sensing of acetylsali cylic acid in the real sample. *J. Colloid Interface Sci.* **2017**, *501*, 350–356. [CrossRef] [PubMed]
241. Bukkitgar, S.D.; Shetti, N.P.; Kulkarni, R.M.; Halbhavi, S.B.; Wasim, M.; Mylar, M.; Durgi, P.S.; Chirmure, S.S. Electrochemical oxidation of nimesulide in aqueous acid solutions based on TiO2 nanostructure modified electrode as a sensor. *J. Electroanal. Chem.* **2016**, *778*, 103–109. [CrossRef]
242. Muthusankar, G.; Sasikumar, R.; Chen, S.-M.; Gopu, G.; Sengottuvelan, N.; Rwei, S.P. Electrochemical synthesis of nitrogen-doped carbon quantum dots decorated copper oxide for the sensitive and selective detection of non steroidal anti-inflammatory drug in berries. *J. Colloid Interface Sci.* **2018**, *523*, 191–200. [CrossRef]
243. Jain, R.; Shrivastava, S. A Graphene-polyaniline-Bi_2O_3 hybrid film sensor for voltammetric quantification of anti-inflammatory drug etodolac. *J. Electrochem. Soc.* **2014**, *161*, H189–H194. [CrossRef]
244. Sakthivel, M.; Ramaraj, S.; Chen, S.-M.; Dinesh, B. Synthesis of rose like struc tured $LaCoO_3$ assisted functionalized carbon nanofiber nanocomposite for efficient electrochemical detection of anti-inflammatory drug 4 aminoantipyrine. *Electrochim. Acta* **2018**, *260*, 571–581. [CrossRef]
245. Khoobi, A.; Soltani, N.; Aghaei, M. Computational design and multivariate statistical analysis for electrochemical sensing platform of iron oxide nano particles in sensitive detection of anti-inflammatory drug diclofenac in bio logical fluids. *J. Alloys Compd.* **2020**, *831*, 154715. [CrossRef]
246. Dehdashti, A.; Babaei, A. Highly sensitive electrochemical sensor based on Pt doped NiO Nanoparticles/MWCNTs nanocomposite modified electrode for simultaneous sensing of piroxicam and amlodipine. *Electroanalysis* **2020**, *32*, 1017–1024. [CrossRef]
247. Shetti, N.P.; Nayak, D.S.; Malode, S.J.; Reddy, K.R.; Shukla, S.S.; Aminabhavi, T.M. Electrochemical behavior of flufenamic acid at Amberlite XAD-4 resin and silver-doped titanium dioxide/Amberlite XAD-4resin modified carbon electrodes. *Colloids Surf. B* **2019**, *177*, 407–415. [CrossRef] [PubMed]
248. Shetti, N.P.; Nayak, D.S.; Malode, S.J.; Kakarla, R.R.; Shukla, S.S.; Aminabhavi, T.M. Sensors based on ruthenium-doped TiO_2 nanoparticles loaded into multi walled carbon nanotubes for the detection of flufenamic acid and mefenamic acid. *Anal. Chim. Acta* **2019**, *1051*, 58–72. [CrossRef] [PubMed]
249. Zhang, C.; Cao, Z.; Zhang, G.; Yan, Y.; Yang, X.; Chang, J.; Song, Y.; Jia, Y.; Pan, P.; Mi, W.; et al. An electrochemical sensor based on plasma treated zinc oxide nanoflowers for the simultaneous detection of dopa mine and diclofenac sodium. *Microchem. J.* **2020**, *158*, 105237. [CrossRef]
250. Monsef, R.; Salavati-Niasari, M. Hydrothermal architecture of $Cu_5V_2O_{10}$ nanostructures as new electro-sensing catalysts for voltammetric quantifi cation of mefenamic acid in pharmaceuticals and biological samples. *Biosens. Bioelectr.* **2021**, *178*, 113017. [CrossRef] [PubMed]
251. Parsaee, Z.; Karachi, N.; Abrishamifar, S.M.; Kahkha, M.R.R.; Razavi, R. Silver choline chloride modified graphene oxide: Novel nano-bioelectrochemical sensor for celecoxib detection and CCD-RSM model. *Ultrason. Sonochem.* **2018**, *45*, 106–115. [CrossRef]
252. Bahrani, S.; Razmi, Z.; Ghaedi, M.; Asfaram, A.; Javadian, H. Ultrasound-accel erated synthesis of gold nanoparticles modified choline chloride function alized graphene oxide as a novel sensitive bioelectrochemical sensor: Optimized meloxicam detection using CCD-RSM design and application for human plasma sample. *Ultrason. Sonochem.* **2018**, *42*, 776–786. [CrossRef]
253. Govindasamy, M.; Mani, V.; Chen, S.-M.; Maiyalagan, T.; Selvaraj, S.; Chen, T.-W.; Lee, S.-Y.; Chang, W.-H. Highly sensitive determination of non-steroidal anti inflammatory drug nimesulide using electrochemically reduced graphene oxide nanoribbons. *RSC Adv.* **2017**, *7*, 33043–33051. [CrossRef]
254. Mekassa, B.; Baker, P.G.L.; Chandravanshi, B.S.; Tessema, M. Synthesis, characterization, and preparation of nickel nanoparticles decorated electro chemically reduced graphene oxide modified electrode for electrochemical sensing of diclofenac. *J. Solid State Electrochem.* **2018**, *22*, 3607–3619. [CrossRef]
255. Shalauddin, M.; Akhter, S.; Basirun, W.J.; Bagheri, S.; Anuar, N.S.; Johan, M.R. Hybrid nanocellulose/f-MWCNTs nanocomposite for the electrochemical sensing of diclofenac sodium in pharmaceutical drugs and biological fluids. *Electrochim. Acta* **2019**, *304*, 323–333. [CrossRef]
256. Mohamed, M.A.; Hasan, M.M.; Abdullah, I.H.; Abdellah, A.M.; Yehia, A.M.; Ahmed, N.; Abbas, W.; Allam, N.K. Smart bi-metallic perovskite nanofibers as selective and reusable sensors of nano-level concentrations of non-steroidal anti-inflammatory drugs. *Talanta* **2018**, *185*, 344–351. [CrossRef]
257. Tarlekar, P.; Chatterjee, S. Enhancement in sensitivity of non-steroidal anti inflammatory drug mefenamic acid at carbon nanostructured sensor. *J. Electroanal. Chem.* **2017**, *803*, 51–57. [CrossRef]

258. Coldibeli, B.; Campos, N.S.M.; Salamanca-Neto, C.A.R.; Scremin, J.; Mattos, G.J.; Marcheafave, G.G.; Sartori, E.R. Feasibility of the use of boron-doped diamond electrode coupled to electroanalytical techniques for the individual deter mination of pravastatin and its association with acetylsalicylic acid. *J. Electroanal. Chem.* **2020**, *862*, 113987. [CrossRef]
259. Aguilar-Lira, G.Y.; Gutierrez-Salgado, J.M.; Rojas-Hernandez, A.; Avila, J.A.R.; Paez-Hernandez, M.E.; Alvarez-Romero, G.A. Artificial neural network for the voltamperometric quantification of diclofenac in presence of other nonsteroidal anti-inflammatory drugs and some commercial excipients. *J. Electroanal. Chem.* **2017**, *801*, 527–535. [CrossRef]
260. Bayraktepe, D.E.; Yazan, Z.; Onal, M. Sensitive and cost effective disposable composite electrode based on graphite, nanosmectite and multiwall carbon nanotubes for the simultaneous trace level detection of ascorbic acid and acetylsalicylic acid in pharmaceuticals. *Talanta* **2019**, *203*, 131–139. [CrossRef] [PubMed]
261. Atta, N.F.; Galal, A.; El-Ads, E.H.; Galal, A.E. New insight in fabrication of a sensitive nano-magnetite/glutamine/carbon based electrochemical sensor for determination of aspirin and omeprazole. *J. Electrochem. Soc.* **2019**, *166*, B161–B172. [CrossRef]
262. Zhang, J.-W.; Li, R.-F.; Yao, L.; Wang, Z.-X.; Lv, W.-X.; Kong, F.-Y.; Wang, W. Highly sensitive determination of piroxicam using a glassy carbon electrode modified with silver nanoparticles dotted single walled carbon nanotubes-reduced graphene oxide nanocomposite. *J. Electroanal. Chem.* **2018**, *823*, 1–8. [CrossRef]
263. Lima, A.P.; Nunes, G.L.; Franco, R.G.; Mariano-Neto, R.; Oliveira, G.S.; Richter, E.M.; Nossol, E.; Munoz, R.A.A. Al2O3 microparticles immobilized on glassy-carbon electrode as catalytic sites for the electrochemical oxidation and high detectability of naproxen: Experimental and simulation insights. *J. Electroanal. Chem.* **2021**, *882*, 114988. [CrossRef]
264. Prado, T.M.D.; Badaro, C.C.; Machado, R.G.; Fadini, P.S.; Fatibello-Filho, O.; Moraes, F.C. Using bismuth vanadate/copper oxide nanocomposite as pho toelectrochemical sensor for naproxen determination in sewage. *Electro Anal.* **2020**, *32*, 1930–1937. [CrossRef]
265. Sarhangzadeh, K.; Khatami, A.A.; Jabbari, M.; Bahari, S. Simultaneous deter mination of diclofenac and indomethacin using a sensitive electrochemical sensor based on multiwalled carbon nanotube and ionic liquid nano composite. *J. Appl. Electrochem.* **2013**, *43*, 1217–1224. [CrossRef]
266. Farshchi, F.; Hasanzadeh, M.; Feyziazar, M.; Saadati, A.; Hassanpour, S. Elec tropolymerization of chitosan in the presence of CuNPs on the surface of a copper electrode: An advanced nanocomposite for the determination of mefenamic acid and indomethacin in human plasmasamples and prevention of drug poisoning. *Anal. Methods* **2020**, *12*, 1212–1217. [CrossRef]
267. Torrinha, A.; Martins, M.; Tavares, M.; Delerue-Matos, C.; Morais, S. Carbon paper as a promising sensing material: Characterization and electroanalysis of ketoprofen in wastewater and fish. *Talanta* **2021**, *226*, 122111. [CrossRef] [PubMed]
268. Mostafavi, M.; Yaftian, M.R.; Piri, F.; Shayani-Jam, H. A new diclofenac molec ularly imprinted electrochemical sensor based upon a polyaniline/reduced graphene oxide nano-composite. *Biosens. Bioelectr.* **2018**, *122*, 160–167. [CrossRef] [PubMed]
269. Puangjan, A.; Chaiyasith, S.; Wichitpanya, S.; Daengduang, S.; Puttota, S. Elec trochemical sensor based on PANI/MnO_2-Sb_2O_3 nanocomposite for selective simultaneous voltammetric determination of ascorbic acid and acetylsali cylic acid. *J. Electroanal. Chem.* **2016**, *782*, 192–201. [CrossRef]
270. Jaramillo-Aguirre, A.; Espitia-H, J.; Castro-Narvaez, S.; Rojas, G. Voltammetric determination of diclofenac at a PEDOT modified glassy carbon electrode. *J. Phys. Conf. Ser* **2020**, *1541*, 12002. [CrossRef]
271. Wong, A.; Santos, A.M.; Fatibello-Filho, O. Determination of piroxicam and nimesulide using an electrochemical sensor based on reduced graphene oxide and PEDOT: PSS. *J. Electroanal. Chem.* **2017**, *799*, 547–555. [CrossRef]
272. Thiagarajan, S.; Rajkumar, M.; Chen, S.-M. Nano TiO_2-PEDOT film for the simultaneous detection of ascorbic acid and diclofena. *Int. J. Electrochem. Sci.* **2012**, *7*, 2109–2122. [CrossRef]
273. Farghali, R.A.; Ahmed, R.A.; Alharthi, A.A. Synthesis and characterization of electrochemical sensor based on polymeric/TiO_2 nanocomposite modified with imidizolium ionic liquid for determination of diclofenac. *Int. J. Elec Trochem. Sci.* **2018**, *13*, 10390–10414. [CrossRef]
274. Vernekar, P.R.; Purohit, B.; Shetti, N.P.; Chandra, P. Glucose modified carbon paste sensor in the presence of cationic surfactant for mefenamic acid detection in urine and pharmaceutical samples. *Microchem. J.* **2021**, *160*, 105599. [CrossRef]
275. Bukkitgar, S.D.; Shetti, N.P.; Kulkarni, R.M.; Churmure, S. Nano-silica modified electrode as a sensor for the determination of mefenamic acid-A voltam metric sensor. *Mater. Today* **2018**, *5*, 21466–21473.
276. Hasanzadeh, M.; Shadjou, N.; Saghatforoush, L.; Dolatabadi, J.E.N. Preparation of a new electrochemical sensor based on iron (III) complexes modified carbon paste electrode for simultaneous determination of mefenamic acid and indomethacin. *Colloids Surf. B* **2012**, *92*, 91–97. [CrossRef]
277. Ghobadpour, G.; Farjami, F.; Fasihi, F. Sensitive Electrochemical monitoring of piroxicam in pharmaceuticals using carbon ionic liquid electrode. *Curr. Pharm. Anal* **2019**, *15*, 45–50. [CrossRef]
278. Shetti, N.P.; Malode, S.J.; Nayak, D.S.; Bukkitgar, S.D.; Bagihalli, G.B.; Kulkarni, R.M.; Reddy, K.R. Novel nanoclay-based electrochemical sensor for highly efficient electrochemical sensing nimesulide. *J. Phys. Chem. Solids* **2020**, *137*, 109210. [CrossRef]
279. Oliveira, T.M.B.; Pessoa, G.D.P.; dos Santos, A.B.; de Lima-Neto, P.; Correia, A.N. Simultaneous electrochemical sensing of emerging organic contaminants in full-scale sewage treatment plants. *Chem. Eng. J.* **2015**, *267*, 347–354. [CrossRef]
280. Zhang, R.; Liu, J.; Li, Y. MXene with great adsorption ability toward organic dye: An excellent material for constructing a ratiometric electrochemical sensing platform. *ACS Sens.* **2019**, *4*, 2058–2064. [CrossRef]

281. Roushani, M.; Shahdost-fard, F. Covalent attachment of aptamer onto nano composite as a high performance electrochemical sensing platform: Fabri cation of an ultra-sensitive ibuprofen electrochemical aptasensor. *Mater. Sci. Eng. C* **2016**, *68*, 128–135. [CrossRef]
282. Roushani, M.; Shahdost-fard, F. Ultra-sensitive detection of ibuprofen (IBP) by electrochemical aptasensor using the dendrimer-quantum dot (Den-QD) bioconjugate as an immobilization platform with special features. *Mater. Sci. Eng. C* **2017**, *75*, 1091–1096. [CrossRef]
283. Azadbakht, A.; Derikvandi, Z. Aptamer-based sensor for diclofenac quantifi cation using carbon nanotubes and graphene oxide decorated with magnetic nanomaterials. *J. Iran. Chem. Soc.* **2018**, *15*, 595–606. [CrossRef]
284. Nguyen, T.T.K.; Vu, T.T.; Anquetin, G.; Tran, H.V.; Reisberg, S.; Noel, V.; Mattana, G.; Nguyen, Q.V.; Lam, T.D.; Pham, M.C.; et al. Enzyme-less electrochemical displacement heterogeneous immunosensor for diclofenac detection. *Biosens. Bioelectron.* **2017**, *97*, 246–252. [CrossRef]
285. Derikvand, H.; Roushani, M.; Abbasi, A.R.; Derikvand, Z.; Azadbakht, A. Design of folding-based impedimetric aptasensor for determination of the nonste roidal anti-inflammatory drug. *Anal. Biochem.* **2016**, *513*, 77–86. [CrossRef]
286. Kashefi-Kheyrabadi, L.; Mehrgardi, M.A. Design and construction of a label free aptasensor for electrochemical detection of sodium diclofenac. *Biosens. Bioelectron.* **2012**, *33*, 184–189. [CrossRef]
287. Shahdost-fard, F.; Roushani, M. An impedimetric aptasensor based on water soluble cadmium telluride (CdTe) quantum dots (QDs) for detection of ibuprofen. *J. Electroanal. Chem.* **2016**, *763*, 18–24. [CrossRef]
288. Kassahun, G.S.; Griveau, S.; Juillard, S.; Champavert, J.; Ringuede, A.; Bresson, B.; Tran, Y.; Bedioui, F.; Slim, C. Hydrogel matrix-grafted impedimetric apta sensors for the detection of diclofenac. *Langmuir* **2020**, *36*, 827–836. [CrossRef] [PubMed]
289. Roushani, M.; Shahdost-Fard, F. Applicability of AuNPs@N-GQDs nano composite in the modeling of the amplified electrochemical ibuprofen aptasensing assay by monitoring of riboflavin. *Bioelectrochemistry* **2019**, *126*, 38–47. [CrossRef] [PubMed]

chemosensors

Review

Investigating Sepsis-Associated Delirium Through Optical Neuroimaging: A New Frontier in Critical Care Research

Shixie Jiang [1,*], Matthew Gunther [2], Jose R. Maldonado [2], Philip A. Efron [3], Steven T. DeKosky [4] and Huabei Jiang [5]

1 Department of Psychiatry, University of Florida College of Medicine, Gainesville, FL 32610, USA
2 Department of Psychiatry and Behavioral Sciences, School of Medicine, Stanford University, Stanford, CA 94305, USA; guntherm@stanford.edu (M.G.); jrm@stanford.edu (J.R.M.)
3 Department of Surgery, University of Florida College of Medicine, Gainesville, FL 32610, USA; philip.efron@surgery.ufl.edu
4 Department of Neurology, University of Florida College of Medicine, Gainesville, FL 32610, USA; steven.dekosky@neurology.ufl.edu
5 Department of Medical Engineering, University of South Florida, Tampa, FL 33620, USA; hjiang1@usf.edu
* Correspondence: mjiang1@ufl.edu

Abstract: Sepsis is a life-threatening syndrome consisting of physiological, pathological, and biochemical abnormalities induced by infection which continues to be a major public health burden. It remains one of the most common reasons for intensive care unit (ICU) admission. Delirium precipitated by sepsis in the intensive care setting is one of its most common neuropsychiatric complications that leads to prolonged hospitalization, increased mortality, and an increased risk of incident dementia. Understanding the pathophysiology and neurobiological mechanisms of sepsis-associated delirium is difficult; neuroimaging biomarkers are lacking due to difficulties with imaging critically ill patients. Optical imaging techniques, including near-infrared spectroscopy and diffuse optical tomography are potentially promising approaches for investigating this pathophysiology due to their portability and high spatiotemporal resolution. In this review, we examine the emergence of optical neuroimaging techniques for the study of sepsis-associated delirium in the ICU and how they can further advance our knowledge and lead to the development of improved preventative, predictive, and therapeutic strategies.

Keywords: optical imaging; functional neuroimaging; near-infrared spectroscopy; diffuse optical tomography; sepsis; delirium; encephalopathy

1. Introduction

Sepsis is a life-threatening syndrome consisting of physiological, pathologic, and biochemical abnormalities induced by infection which remains a major public health burden [1]. In the United States, sepsis is responsible for 6.2% of the aggregate costs for all hospitalizations, approximately USD 23.7 billion annually [2]. It is the leading cause of mortality and critical illness worldwide in the intensive care unit (ICU) setting, with an estimated worldwide prevalence of 29.5% and a mortality level of 25.8% [3–5]. Survivors of sepsis commonly suffer from various long-term physical, psychological, and cognitive disabilities with significant health care and psychosocial implications [6]. The main mechanism causing such disability and complications from sepsis is the presence of delirium. Delirium is a neuropsychiatric syndrome that typically manifests acutely or subacutely, with a fluctuating course. It involves disturbances in attention, alertness, various cognitive functions, psychomotor activity, emotional regulation, and the sleep–wake cycle. The three major subtypes of delirium are hyperactive (agitation), hypoactive (psychomotor slowing), and mixed [7]. It is always caused by a medical insult, with sepsis being one of its most common precipitants, particularly in the ICU [8]. Delirium is exceedingly common in the critically ill, with rates as high as 83% in mechanically ventilated patients [9]. Irrespective even of sepsis, delirium is independently associated with a higher risk of mortality, institutionalization after hospital discharge, and cognitive impairment [10–12]. At present, there is no definitive treatment for any type of delirium, and managing the underlying medical condition causing the delirium remains the priority. To make real progress in preventing and treating sepsis-associated delirium, it is essential to enhance our ability to investigate its underlying neural mechanisms and identify reliable biomarkers.

1.1. Sepsis-Associated Delirium Pathophysiology

Sepsis is defined as a life-threatening organ dysfunction caused by a dysregulated host response to infection [1]. The immune response to a pathogen starts with the activation of innate immune cells, such as macrophages, monocytes, neutrophils, and natural killer cells. This activation occurs when pathogen-associated molecular patterns (PAMPs), like bacterial endotoxins and fungal β-glucans, interact with pattern recognition receptors [13]. Additionally, damage-associated molecular patterns (DAMPs), which consist of intracellular substances or molecules released by damaged or dying cells (like ATP and mitochondrial DNA), can also engage specific receptors on monocytes, macrophages, and myeloid-derived suppressor cells (MDSCs) [14], including toll-like receptors (TLRs), C-type lectin receptors, nucleotide-binding oligomerization domain-like (NOD-like) receptors, and retinoic acid-inducible gene I (RIG-I-like) receptors. This interaction activates intracellular signaling pathways that lead to the transcription and release of proinflammatory cytokines, such as TNFα, IL-1, and IL-6 [15,16]. Some pattern recognition receptors, like the NOD-like receptor family, can form larger protein complexes called inflammasomes, which contribute to the production of cytokines like IL-1β and IL-18, as well as caspases involved in programmed cell death [17]. The resulting proinflammatory cytokines trigger leukocyte activation and proliferation and complement system activation, endothelial adhesion molecule expression, and chemokine production [18]. In sepsis, this immune response becomes dysregulated and exaggerated, leading to significant inflammatory damage to host cells and tissues.

In addition to proinflammatory pathway dysregulation, there is also the simultaneous dysregulation of hemostatic and coagulation cascades. The disruption of coagulation in sepsis arises from multiple contributing factors. One key driver of the hypercoagulable state in sepsis is the release of tissue factor, primarily from damaged endothelial cells, but also from monocytes and polymorphonuclear cells [19]. This tissue factor triggers widespread activation of the coagulation cascade, leading to thrombin production, platelet activation, and the formation of platelet–fibrin clots. These clots can cause microthrombosis, which impairs local blood flow, resulting in tissue hypoxia and organ dysfunction [20]. Additionally, sepsis is associated with a decrease in fibrinolysis. Elevated levels of TNFα and IL-1β prompt the release of tissue plasminogen activators from endothelial cells, increasing plasmin activation. However, this process is counteracted by a sustained rise in plasminogen activator inhibitor type 1 (PAI-1), leading to reduced fibrinolysis and the impaired removal of fibrin. This combination of hypercoagulability and reduced fibrinolysis contributes to ongoing microvascular thrombosis [21].

The blood–brain barrier (BBB) is composed of endothelial cells and is responsible for the regulation of nutrients and the prevention of neurotoxins from entering the central nervous system (CNS) [22]. Sepsis induces profound alterations in the BBB endothelium through the mechanisms described above, thus causing improper leukocyte adhesion, coagulation, vasodilation, and a loss of barrier function [23]. Macroscopically, this leads to hypoperfusion, impaired cerebral autoregulation of blood flow, and most critically, oxygenation deficits throughout various brain networks. Reduced cerebral oxygen levels have been closely linked to the disruption of ionic gradients, impaired cellular depolarization, and the accumulation of neurotoxic free radicals [24]. Furthermore, inadequate oxygenation disrupts normal neurotransmitter metabolism, leading to a significant increase in glutamate and dopamine levels, along with decreased acetylcholine production—all of which are strongly associated with the development of delirium, even in non-septic cases [25–27]. Additionally, poor oxygenation contributes to decreased cerebral perfusion and heightened brain inflammation, perpetuating a cycle of dysfunction [28]. In combination, immune, inflammatory, and coagulation dysregulation leads to hypoperfusion and oxygenation deficits in the brain which can ultimately cause delirium (Figure 1).

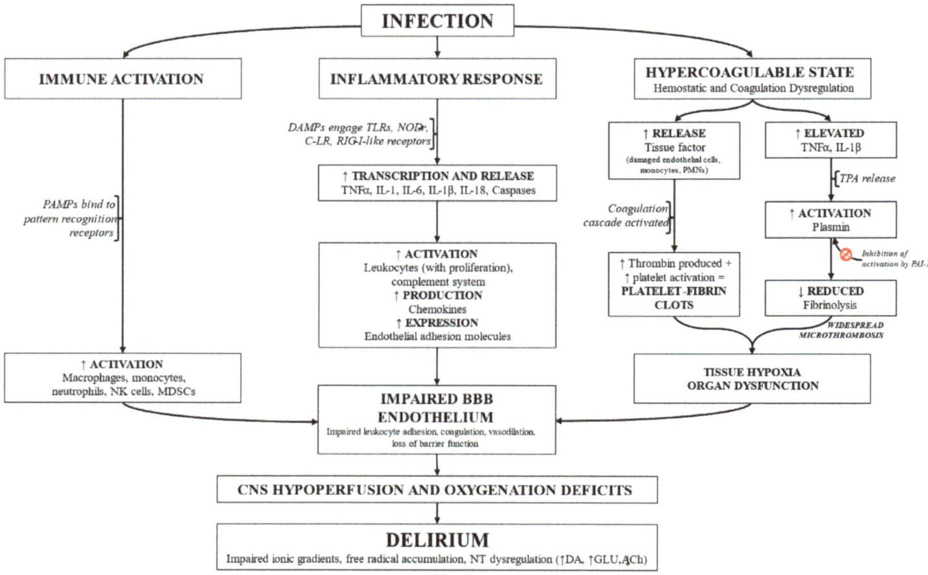

Figure 1. Sepsis-associated delirium pathophysiology. Abbreviations: PAMP = pathogen-associated molecular patterns; TLR = toll-like receptor; NODR = nod-like receptors; C-LR = c-type lectin receptors; TNF-α = tumor necrosis factor alpha; PMN = polymorphonuclear cells; TPA = tissue plasminogen activator; PAI-1 = plasminogen activator inhibitor-1; MDSC = myeloid-derived suppressor cells; NK = natural killer cells; BBB = blood–brain barrier; CNS = central nervous system.

1.2. Delirium Neuroimaging Studies

To fully appreciate and investigate the underlying neural mechanisms of delirium, validating neuroimaging biomarkers is critically important. Previous structural neuroimaging studies using magnetic resonance imaging (MRI) and computer tomography (CT) have shown that delirium is linked to grey matter volume reduction and white matter hyperintensities, along with tract disruptions in various brain regions [29–31]. However, these results are not exclusive to delirium, and are largely due to non-specific findings, diverse patient populations, and small sample sizes. More recent functional imaging studies have identified significant hypoactivity in several cortical regions and disruptions in connectivity within the default mode and central executive networks [32,33]. The frontal and cingulate cortices are frequently implicated in delirium, along with subcortical structures like the thalamus and caudate, which are crucial for arousal regulation via the ascending reticular activating system [34,35]. Functional MRI (fMRI) and positron emission tomography (PET) have been used in these studies, though they often involve even smaller sample sizes than structural imaging research, given the operational difficulties in doing such scans. Moreover, PET imaging requires fasting and a long uptake period (approximately 45 min depending on the radioligand), making it impractical for many delirious patients. A common limitation across MRI, CT, and PET techniques is the lack of portability and low patient tolerance due to the patient's acute illness and cognitive impairments. This is particularly cumbersome and non-feasible in the ICU population where patients are even more seriously ill and unable even to be transported readily. Moreover, in cases of hyperactive or mixed delirium, the severity of agitation often prevents the patient from being able to safely undergo imaging with standard techniques, as they are required to remain still in an enclosed space. While electroencephalography (EEG) is more portable and widely used, its low spatial resolution limits its ability to conduct anatomical localization of brain activity and advanced regional and network analyses (Table 1) [36]. The emergence of optical imaging techniques offers a potential solution to the challenges of neuroimaging in delirium.

Table 1. Characteristics of functional imaging techniques. Abbreviations: DOT = diffuse optical tomography; fNIRS = functional near-infrared spectroscopy; fMRI = functional magnetic resonance imaging; EEG = electroencephalography; PET = positron emission tomography; SPECT = single-photon emission computed tomography.

Techniques	Spatial Resolution	Temporal Resolution	Bedside Capabilities	Patient and Safety Considerations
DOT	mm	ms	Yes	None
fNIRS	cm	ms	Yes	None
fMRI	mm	s	No	Ferromagnetic material
EEG	cm	ms	Yes	None
PET	mm	min	No	Fasting requirement
SPECT	cm	min	No	Ionizing radiation

1.3. Optical Neuroimaging

In 1977, Jöbsis demonstrated the potential to measure blood and tissue oxygenation levels in the brain of a cat with near-infrared (NIR) light [37]. In the decades since, optical neuroimaging has expanded into a diverse research area, with many scientific and clinical studies utilizing the distinctive properties of light for brain imaging [38]. NIR light can provide valuable functional imaging information by capturing intrinsic changes in absorption, fluorescence, or the scattering of light within soft tissues. Additionally, various exogenous contrast agents can be used to obtain further insights [39–41]. Commonly measured chromophores include oxyhemoglobin, deoxyhemoglobin, cytochromes, and metabolites, which serve as indicators of brain activation, similar to traditional functional imaging techniques. A typical setup focused on portability will often include a cart that holds the light source (laser-emitting diodes or pulsed lasers), data acquisition system, computer, and timing electronics that connect to a flexible head interface via optical fibers. The interface itself contains the source–detector pairs and optodes that physically contact the hair and scalp, similar to how an EEG cap is designed.

Optical imaging offers several advantages over conventional functional imaging, including real-time data acquisition, greater portability, fewer movement restrictions, no exposure to ionizing radiation, a wider range of contrast agents, and lower costs [42]. These benefits are notable, particularly for use in ICU patients given their many restrictions due to their critically ill status. For applications in delirium, two key optical imaging techniques of interest are functional near-infrared spectroscopy (fNIRS) and diffuse optical tomography (DOT).

Functional near-infrared spectroscopy (fNIRS) is based on the core principles of NIR spectroscopy, with the term "functional" added after its initial use in human studies [43]. fNIRS allows for the simultaneous measurement of changes in the optical properties of the human cortex across multiple sites, presenting results as a topographical map or image of the region of interest [44]. The technique leverages the fact that human tissues are transparent to NIR light in the 650–1000 nm spectral range, where chromophores like hemoglobin in small blood vessels absorb or scatter the light [45]. By measuring increases in oxyhemoglobin and decreases in deoxyhemoglobin, fNIRS detects real-time markers of local arteriolar vasodilation, which corresponds to increased oxygenation, cerebral blood flow, and volume in specific brain areas. This hemodynamic response is linked to neurovascular coupling, serving as an indirect indicator of neuronal activity [46]. Many companies now offer multi-channel fNIRS devices at a much lower cost than fMRI machines. These devices are compact, easy to set up, and can be quickly transferred between patients, making them highly practical for clinical use [47].

Diffuse optical tomography (DOT) is a modern noninvasive imaging technique based on near-infrared (NIR) light, similar to how magnetic resonance spectroscopy relates to magnetic resonance imaging (MRI) [48]. In contrast to the two-dimensional capabilities of fNIRS, DOT utilizes multiple wavelengths and dense, overlapping channels with different source–detector distances to gather data at various depths. This allows for the measurement of hemodynamic responses at different brain depths and the generation of high-resolution three-dimensional images (Figure 2) [49]. As a result, DOT provides a strong alternative for 3D functional neuroimaging, even compared to fMRI. While both DOT and fMRI detect blood-oxygen-level dependent (BOLD) signals, fMRI primarily measures deoxyhemoglobin [50]. In contrast, DOT can simultaneously capture all hemoglobin signals, enabling better differentiation of the timing, location, and magnitude of neurovascular coupling, which provides a more detailed view of dynamic brain activity [51–53]. Like fNIRS, DOT is affordable, portable, and mobile, and the development of wearable DOT systems with flexible interfaces is progressing rapidly [54–58].

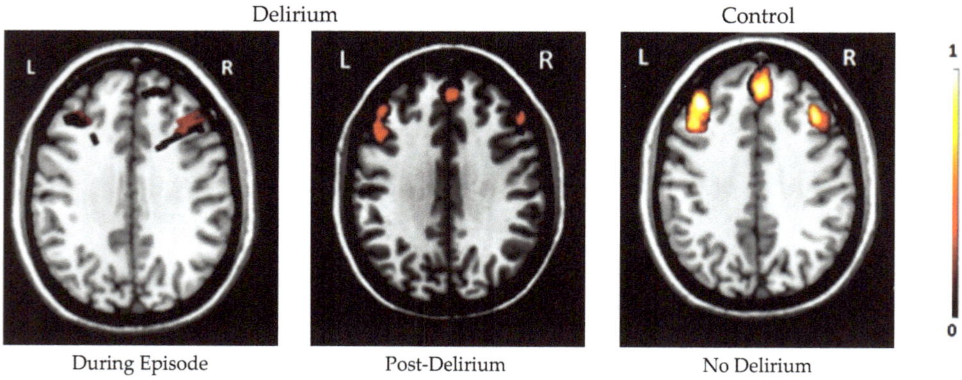

Figure 2. An example of a DOT image reconstruction comparing a delirious subject to a non-delirious subject. The darker (more red) colors represent lower areas of cerebral oxygenation.

In addition to the technical parameters that highlight the potential strengths of optical imaging for sepsis-associated delirium, another critical advantage is the focus on measuring oxygenation changes through the evaluation of hemoglobin signals. This concurrently measures cerebral hemodynamic and perfusion states, thus providing a high-resolution map of various regions involving dysconnectivity. Based on sepsis pathophysiology, as described above, cerebral oxygenation changes are hypothesized to be the penultimate pathway in the development of delirium. Thus, the capability to measure this directly and dynamically at the bedside is highly important for advancing our understanding of delirium pathophysiology and how it aligns with sepsis pathophysiology.

2. Optical Neuroimaging in Sepsis-Associated Delirium

In 2008, Pfister and colleagues were the first to explore the potential of optical neuroimaging in studying the pathophysiology of sepsis-associated delirium (Table 2) [59]. They enrolled 23 septic patients, with 16 included in the final analysis, of whom 12 were diagnosed with delirium using the Confusion Assessment Method for the Intensive Care Unit (CAM-ICU) [9]. To assess cerebral oxygenation, the researchers used a tissue oxygenation index (TOI) as a proxy, measured via bilateral NIRS over the frontal to frontoparietal regions for one hour within 48 h of ICU admission. No significant differences in the TOI were observed between delirious and non-delirious patients. However, separate transcranial Doppler measurements revealed significant differences in blood flow velocity and regulation between the two groups. The authors suggested several factors that may have contributed to the inconclusive TOI results, such as a small sample size, a lack of simultaneous Doppler and NIRS recordings, and limited optode placement (two channels; an optode is similar to an EEG electrode).

Table 2. Summary of published sepsis-associated delirium optical imaging studies.

Reference	Number of Patients	Optical Imaging Technique	Imaging Site(s)	Results
Pfister et al., 2008 [59].	23	NIRS	Frontal lobe and frontoparietal	No difference in oxygenation levels during delirium; however, Doppler-based blood flow velocity was diminished in delirious patients.
Funk et al., 2016 [60].	15	NIRS	Frontal lobe	No difference in cerebral oxygenation in delirious patients.
Wood et al., 2016 [61].	10	NIRS	Single forehead optode	Higher saturated oxygenation levels were observed in delirium.
Vasko et al., 2014 [62].	25	NIRS	Frontal lobe	Lower cerebral oxygenation was reported in delirious patients consistently.
Wood et al., 2017 [63].	88	NIRS	Single forehead optode	Longer duration of delirium was correlated with worse cerebral oxygenation values.
Lee et al., 2019 [64].	40	NIRS	Single forehead optode	Duration of delirium and worse COx values associated with the development of delirium.
Rosenblatt et al., 2020 [65].	6	NIRS	Frontal lobe	Severity of delirium was associated with COx values.
Jiang et al., 2024 [66].	12	DOT	Dorsolateral and dorsomedial prefrontal cortex	During delirium and post-delirium exhibited lower oxygenation levels compared to controls. Higher severity of delirium correlated with lower oxygenation levels.

Subsequent studies from other research groups helped shed more light on the potential mechanisms linking sepsis to delirium. Funk et al. conducted a similar study, enrolling 15 patients, 7 of whom were CAM-ICU positive for delirium [60]. By employing bilateral frontal NIRS, the researchers assessed tissue oxygen saturation for 24 to 48 h within 12 h of ICU admission. Their results indicated no definitive link between tissue oxygen saturation and the onset of delirium. However, the authors expressed concerns about the sensitivity of their chosen saturation threshold (65%) in detecting delirium and proposed that cerebral edema in their critically ill patients could have obfuscated the findings as well. In contrast, Wood et al. performed a smaller study using single-forehead NIRS on 10 septic patients, 5 of whom were delirious [61]. They found that the non-delirious patients had higher brain tissue oxygenation (BtO2) levels compared to those with delirium. Unlike previous studies, Wood et al. extended the monitoring period, using continuous NIRS over the first 72 h of sepsis onset. They proposed that the timing of the NIRS measurements—particularly during the early treatment phase—could be important due to fluctuations in oxygenation levels linked to delirium. These findings were later corroborated by Vasko et al., who compared cerebral oxygenation between 15 septic patients and 10 age- and sex-matched controls [62]. Their results showed significantly lower oxygen saturation levels in patients with sepsis-associated delirium, as measured by bilateral frontal NIRS.

The first major prospective cohort study using NIRS to track the development of delirium was carried out by Wood et al. as part of their subsequent trial, the Cerebral Oxygenation and Neurological Outcomes Following Critical Illness (CONFOCAL) study [63]. This trial included 88 adult ICU patients, who were monitored with a single forehead NIRS sensor during the first 24 h of their admission. Delirium screenings were performed daily, with a maximum enrollment period of 30 days. The study confirmed and expanded upon their earlier pilot findings, showing a significant inverse relationship between brain tissue oxygenation (BtO2) and the proportion of time patients spent in delirium while in the ICU. BtO2 was also identified as an independent predictor of delirium, regardless of other variables. A significant additional finding showed that BtO2 levels were not correlated with peripheral hemodynamic measures, suggesting that cerebral autoregulation operates through an independent mechanism. In a subsequent study using data from the CONFOCAL trial, researchers examined cerebral autoregulation by computing the cerebral oximetry index (COx). COx was defined as the time-varying correlation between the mean arterial pressure (MAP) and NIRS-derived BtO2, with positive values indicating impaired autoregulation. NIRS measurements were taken from 40 patients using a single forehead sensor, and COx values were calculated during the first 72 h of ICU admission. The findings showed that prolonged dysfunction of cerebral autoregulation during the early treatment phase was an independent risk factor for developing delirium. The authors suggested that future research should explore optimizing MAP to maintain healthy COx levels.

Building on the findings from the CONFOCAL study, Rosenblatt et al. published results examining the link between optimizing MAP based on cerebral oximetry index (COx) values and the severity of delirium [65]. In this study, six patients with sepsis-associated delirium underwent 12 h of bilateral frontal NIRS monitoring within the first 48 h of ICU admission. The severity of delirium was assessed using Glasgow Coma Scale (GCS) scores. The results showed that patients with lower GCS scores had consistently higher COx measurements, indicating greater impairment in cerebral autoregulation. Furthermore, there was significant variability in MAP values among patients, highlighting the need for personalized, continuous monitoring. The authors suggested that the standard MAP target of $\geq$65 mm Hg in sepsis may not be suitable for every patient and should be tailored based on individual COx data.

The first study to investigate the use of diffuse optical tomography (DOT) in delirium and sepsis-associated delirium was published in 2024 by Jiang et al. [66]. This was the largest functional neuroimaging study on delirium to date, involving 50 participants (12 with sepsis), with matched controls based on age, gender, handedness, and admission setting. A custom-designed 48-channel DOT system was developed, featuring a lighter mesh and lower-density optical fibers to enable bedside use in delirious patients, both in the

ICU and in medical inpatient services. The DOT interface focused on the prefrontal cortex, particularly the bilateral dorsolateral and dorsomedial regions. To assess brain activation, the Months Backwards Test [67], validated for measuring attention, working memory, executive function, and processing speed in delirium and dementia, was administered during imaging. Patients were scanned both during their initial delirium episode and after delirium resolution, with Delirium Rating Scale-Revised-98 (DRS-R-98) [68] scores recorded at both timepoints to evaluate clinical severity. The study found significantly lower total and oxygenated hemoglobin levels during delirium, which remained low even after resolution when compared to matched controls. Additionally, lower hemoglobin levels were associated with higher, more severe DRS-R-98 scores. These findings suggest that DOT's three-dimensional, bedside capabilities could play a key role in validating optical neuroimaging biomarkers for sepsis-associated delirium and potentially studying the long-term cognitive decline that can follow delirium.

3. Challenges and Limitations

The complexity of depth sensitivity and the penetration limits of near-infrared (NIR) light are challenging issues influenced by various factors in NIRS applications, including the technology, parameters, and neuroanatomical characteristics of the tissue being examined. These factors significantly affect how light is absorbed and scattered within the brain, with different depths exhibiting variable absorption and scattering coefficients that require specific calculations [45,46]. In commercial NIRS devices, the typical imaging depth is estimated to be around 2–3 cm beneath the scalp [69–71]. However, it has been reported that employing wavelengths of 808 nm or greater allows for imaging depths of 4 to 5 cm reliably [72–74]. Unlike standard fNIRS, DOT, with its advanced signal processing and sophisticated software, consistently shows the capability to image at these deeper depths [75,76]. Additionally, recent advancements in time- or frequency-domain detection modes offer potential improvements to the depth limitations of the conventional continuous-wave approach [77]. Despite these advances, the challenge of limited depth penetration remains a constraint for using NIR light to image deeper brain structures, which we postulate is important for fully understanding the pathophysiology of delirium. For example, subcortical regions like the thalamus and caudate are believed to play a role in disturbances of arousal in delirium, particularly the hypoactive subtype, due to their connection to the ascending reticular activating system [35].

A common challenge across all functional neuroimaging techniques is their vulnerability to motion artifacts. The subtle variations in blood oxygenation and flow associated with neural activity can be difficult to distinguish from motion-induced signal fluctuations, complicating the interpretation of hemodynamic responses in specific brain regions [78]. These artifacts can degrade image quality, skew statistical analyses, and lead to inaccurate conclusions [79]. In optical neuroimaging, movement between the optical fibers and the scalp can interfere with data collection, causing signal disruptions and fluctuations [80]. The most frequent motion artifact appears as a brief, high-amplitude intensity spike that quickly diminishes once the motion stops. In fMRI, such artifacts can render entire datasets unusable if the motion is significant during data acquisition. However, NIRS and DOT are generally more tolerant of head and scalp movement due to their flexible interface design, allowing for the capture of unaffected data segments despite brief motion [81]. This greater tolerance is likely due to differences in algorithms and the use of mesh-based headgear that adjusts to the scalp, as opposed to fMRI's fixed setup. Traditional methods used to minimize motion artifacts include the careful design of the optode array, reducing subject movement through visual fixation, limiting stimuli, ensuring patient comfort, and applying advanced post-processing techniques [46,48]. New computational methods, extending beyond traditional filters and channel regression, include techniques such as temporal derivative distribution repair, transient artifact reduction algorithms, and dual-stage median filters. In the context of delirium research, optical imaging holds promise for examining hyperactive delirium or delirious agitation, owing to its lower sensitivity to motion artifacts. This would additionally allow for imaging such patients in a naturalistic manner (at the bedside), which would lead to a more realistic assessment of brain activity [82]. Previous research has primarily focused on hypoactive delirium, as patients with behavioral agitation often cannot endure prolonged neuroimaging sessions without inciting further agitation. The pathophysiology and neural mechanisms of different delirium subtypes likely differ considerably as they exhibit entirely different symptoms, making this a promising area for further investigation using techniques like NIRS and DOT.

Given the prominent hypoperfusion, coagulation cascade dysregulation, and oxygenation deficits in sepsis, the occurrence of brain lesions is not uncommon. Longer durations and higher severity of sepsis have been correlated with the development of white matter, ischemic, and hemorrhagic lesions [83–85]. These tend to occur in areas of the brain sensitive to ischemia and hypoperfusion, such as the hippocampus, basal ganglia, cerebellum, and amygdala [86]. Large enough lesions (>5 cm) may obfuscate optical imaging results given serious structural changes that could occur during sepsis. There has been some success in using fNIRS and DOT for stroke detection [87–90]; however, these data remain preliminary and have not been validated well in large-scale trials yet, especially in comparison to CT or MRI. Pairing optical neuroimaging with CT or MRI may be a strategy to overcome this specific obstacle. Otherwise, smaller lesions caused as a complication of sepsis should not be a contraindication for optical neuroimaging. Furthermore, since the cortex is the predominant region of interest captured by fNIRS and DOT currently, the presence of lesions is likely not a hindrance as they likely occur in more subcortical locations susceptible to ischemia.

4. Future Directions

Most studies to date have concentrated on NIRS, rather than on fNIRS or DOT, and this distinction is significant. NIRS typically uses a limited number of channels, which restricts data collection to a small portion of the target region. In all published studies on sepsis-associated delirium, one or two-channel NIRS was applied to the forehead, meaning the data on cerebral oxygenation and functional activity were limited to a small section of the frontal cortex. In contrast, the denser optode arrays used in fNIRS and DOT allow for the simultaneous assessment of larger brain areas and facilitate connectivity analyses, similar to fMRI [91,92]. Network analyses are essential for progressing delirium research, as it is improbable that only the frontal lobe is impacted. Previous studies using EEG, fMRI, and PET have indicated that the parietal and temporal lobes may also contribute significantly given their roles in regulating attention, sensations, memory, and language [32,34,35]. For instance, in order to map attention as a cognitive domain, multiple areas of the brain would have to be analyzed, including the medial and lateral prefrontal cortices, precuneus, and inferior parietal lobule [93]. Such a network connectivity-based approach would allow for further studies characterizing different networks involved in various subtypes of delirium and would also lead to personalized interventions targeting abnormal neurocircuitry, depending on the type of delirium and individual patient. Recently developed whole cortex fNIRS and DOT devices, featuring over 100 channels, offer an ideal solution for studying these brain regions and their network connectivity in delirium. Despite their advanced capabilities, these devices remain lightweight and portable for use in human research [54,94,95].

In clinical research, neuroimaging studies on sepsis-associated delirium and other forms of delirium have been largely constrained by their focus on hypoactive delirium. This is likely because patients with hypoactive delirium experience marked psychomotor slowing, making them easier to image. In contrast, hyperactive delirium, characterized by severe agitation and an inability to tolerate routine medical care, creates significant challenges for imaging procedures like MRI or CT scans [7]. The mixed subtype of delirium poses additional questions regarding the underlying pathophysiology and neural circuits affected, as these patients exhibit periods of psychomotor slowing intermixed with episodes of agitation as well. The brain regions and underlying mechanisms of these different delirium subtypes are likely to vary significantly, and improving our understanding of the neurocircuitry may lead to improvements in the prevention and management of delirium.

Optical imaging offers significant advantages for studying all delirium subtypes, especially hyperactive and mixed delirium, for several reasons. The ability to conduct bedside imaging allows for more naturalistic observations, avoiding the logistical challenges and tolerability issues associated with transporting critically ill patients to a designated scanner room or requiring the administration of extra sedation to facilitate imaging. This is especially important in ICU settings, where patients often have even stricter medical limitations and further administration of sedatives may prolong or worsen delirium [96]. However, it is important to acknowledge that in severe cases, standard optical imaging systems using fiber optics may still encounter significant motion artifacts. Advances in technology have introduced fiberless systems, incorporating cabled designs, flex-rigid printed circuit boards, and modular setups [94]. Although these systems may have fewer channels compared to fiber-based arrays, several wireless devices have been developed and validated for advanced functional data collection. These truly wireless systems are ideal for investigating delirium with agitation and can be used to assess the impact of interventions such as physical and occupational therapy on delirium outcomes, enabling functional analyses during activity. This could lead to more personalized and refined delirium treatment approaches.

The development of alternative optical imaging biomarkers could significantly contribute to understanding sepsis-associated delirium pathophysiology. Most optical neuroimaging studies on delirium have focused on absorption-based techniques to measure hemoglobin as the primary chromophore. However, other chromophores may also be useful in evaluating brain function. One such example is cytochrome c oxidase (COX), the final enzyme in the mitochondrial electron transport chain, which maintains the proton gradient essential for adenosine triphosphate (ATP) production, the cell's main energy source [97]. Notably, mitochondrial dysfunction has been highly linked to sepsis-associated organ failure and has also been implicated in Alzheimer's disease and other neurodegenerative conditions [98–100]. A 2019 study by Samuels et al. found that mitochondrial DNA variations were connected to both the risk of and protection from delirium in specific ethnic groups [101]. These findings suggest a new direction for using fNIRS and DOT to examine COX activity in relation to sepsis-associated delirium progression, especially considering the role of mitochondria in oxygen regulation.

Finally, resting-state and task-based approaches in optical neuroimaging require further exploration in sepsis-associated delirium. All previous NIRS studies essentially relied on a resting-state measurement, which offers the benefits of simplicity, easier baseline measurements for generalization, and the opportunity to study the default-mode network [102] (which is most active at rest and highly implicated in self-reference, social cognition, memory, and language). However, resting-state approaches involve less control over activated brain regions, a lack of behavioral correlations to specific cognitive processes, and interpretation difficulties given the presence of spontaneous physiological activity or background neural noise [103]. These weaknesses may be particularly problematic in the assessment of delirium, as patients are already unable to participate as readily in bedside neurocognitive evaluations (e.g., structured interviews and questionnaires). In the Jiang et al. DOT delirium study, a task-based approach using the Months Backwards Test was employed for brain activation. With this type of approach, brain activity can be more directly and confidently correlated to behaviors, further localized, and linked to specific deficits. Disadvantages include the requirement of patient cooperation, specific task-dependent results, a lack of generalizability, and the complexity of the design choice [104]. Both approaches have their merits, and utilizing them further in future studies would lead to the most consummate and expeditious improvements in our understanding of sepsis-associated delirium pathophysiology and neural mechanisms.

5. Conclusions

Sepsis-associated delirium remains exceedingly common yet poorly understood. Optical neuroimaging technologies hold significant promise for advancing the study of sepsis and delirium and enhancing our understanding of underlying mechanisms. Their key advantage lies in the distinctive combination of high-resolution imaging, portability, real-time data acquisition, and affordability. At present, no other imaging techniques provide all these benefits simultaneously, especially when applied in the ICU environment with patients experiencing delirium. Early research has demonstrated the effective use of NIRS and DOT in sepsis-associated delirium studies. With further investments, these methods are poised to play a crucial role in deepening our knowledge of sepsis and delirium pathophysiology and fostering the development of preventive, diagnostic, and therapeutic approaches.

Author Contributions: S.J. conceived and drafted the manuscript in its entirety. M.G. assisted with editing, writing, and creating figures. J.R.M., P.A.E., S.T.D. and H.J. provided supervision and contributed revisions to the manuscript. All authors have read and agreed to the published version of the manuscript.

Funding: This research received no external funding.

Conflicts of Interest: The authors declare no conflicts of interest.

References

1. Singer, M.; Deutschman, C.S.; Seymour, C.W.; Shankar-Hari, M.; Annane, D.; Bauer, M.; Bellomo, R.; Bernard, G.R.; Chiche, J.-D.; Coopersmith, C.M.; et al. The Third International Consensus Definitions for Sepsis and Septic Shock (Sepsis-3). *JAMA* **2016**, *315*, 801–810. [CrossRef]
2. Torio, C.M.; Andrews, R.M. National Inpatient Hospital Costs: The Most Expensive Conditions by Payer, 2011. In *Healthcare Cost and Utilization Project (HCUP) Statistical Briefs*; Agency for Healthcare Research and Quality (US): Rockville, MD, USA, 2006. Available online: http://www.ncbi.nlm.nih.gov/books/NBK169005/ (accessed on 7 September 2024).
3. Vincent, J.-L.; Marshall, J.C.; Namendys-Silva, S.A.; François, B.; Martin-Loeches, I.; Lipman, J.; Reinhart, K.; Antonelli, M.; Pickkers, P.; Njimi, H.; et al. Assessment of the worldwide burden of critical illness: The intensive care over nations (ICON) audit. *Lancet Respir. Med.* **2014**, *2*, 380–386. [CrossRef] [PubMed]
4. Fleischmann, C.; Scherag, A.; Adhikari, N.K.J.; Hartog, C.S.; Tsaganos, T.; Schlattmann, P.; Angus, D.C.; Reinhart, K. Current Estimates and Limitations. *Am. J. Respir. Crit. Care Med.* **2016**, *193*, 259–272. [CrossRef] [PubMed]
5. Sakr, Y.; Jaschinski, U.; Wittebole, X.; Szakmany, T.; Lipman, J.; Ñamendys-Silva, S.A.; Martin-Loeches, I.; Leone, M.; Lupu, M.-N.; Vincent, J.-L.; et al. Sepsis in Intensive Care Unit Patients: Worldwide Data From the Intensive Care over Nations Audit. *Open Forum Infect. Dis.* **2018**, *5*, ofy313. [CrossRef]
6. Iwashyna, T.J.; Ely, E.W.; Smith, D.M.; Langa, K.M. Long-term cognitive impairment and functional disability among survivors of severe sepsis. *JAMA* **2010**, *304*, 1787–1794. [CrossRef] [PubMed]
7. Maldonado, J.R. Acute Brain Failure: Pathophysiology, Diagnosis, Management, and Sequelae of Delirium. *Crit. Care Clin.* **2017**, *33*, 461–519. [CrossRef] [PubMed]
8. Stollings, J.L.; Kotfis, K.; Chanques, G.; Pun, B.T.; Pandharipande, P.P.; Ely, E.W. Delirium in critical illness: Clinical manifestations, outcomes, and management. *Intensive Care Med.* **2021**, *47*, 1089–1103. [CrossRef]

9. Ely, E.W.; Inouye, S.K.; Bernard, G.R.; Gordon, S.; Francis, J.; May, L.; Truman, B.; Speroff, T.; Gautam, S.; Margolin, R.; et al. Delirium in mechanically ventilated patients: Validity and reliability of the confusion assessment method for the intensive care unit (CAM-ICU). *JAMA* **2001**, *286*, 2703–2710. [CrossRef] [PubMed]
10. Goldberg, T.E.; Chen, C.; Wang, Y.; Jung, E.; Swanson, A.; Ing, C.; Garcia, P.S.; Whittington, R.A.; Moitra, V. Association of Delirium With Long-term Cognitive Decline: A Meta-analysis. *JAMA Neurol.* **2020**, *77*, 1373–1381. [CrossRef] [PubMed]
11. Leighton, S.P.; Herron, J.W.; Jackson, E.; Sheridan, M.; Deligianni, F.; Cavanagh, J. Delirium and the risk of developing dementia: A cohort study of 12 949 patients. *J. Neurol. Neurosurg. Psychiatry* **2022**, *93*, 822–827. [CrossRef]
12. Inouye, S.K.; Westendorp, R.G.J.; Saczynski, J.S. Delirium in elderly people. *Lancet* **2014**, *383*, 911–922. [CrossRef] [PubMed]
13. Moine, P.; Abraham, E. Immunomodulation and sepsis: Impact of the pathogen. *Shock* **2004**, *22*, 297–308. [CrossRef]
14. Mathias, B.; Delmas, A.L.; Ozrazgat-Baslanti, T.; Vanzant, E.L.; Szpila, B.E.; Mohr, A.M.; Moore, F.A.; Brakenridge, S.C.; Brumback, B.A.; Moldawer, L.L.; et al. Human Myeloid-derived Suppressor Cells are Associated With Chronic Immune Suppression After Severe Sepsis/Septic Shock. *Ann. Surg.* **2017**, *265*, 827–834. [CrossRef]
15. Takeuchi, O.; Akira, S. Pattern recognition receptors and inflammation. *Cell* **2010**, *140*, 805–820. [CrossRef]
16. Schulte, W.; Bernhagen, J.; Bucala, R. Cytokines in sepsis: Potent immunoregulators and potential therapeutic targets--an updated view. *Mediators Inflamm.* **2013**, *2013*, 165974. [CrossRef] [PubMed]
17. Schroder, K.; Tschopp, J. The inflammasomes. *Cell* **2010**, *140*, 821–832. [CrossRef]
18. Ward, P.A.; Gao, H. Sepsis, complement and the dysregulated inflammatory response. *J. Cell Mol. Med.* **2009**, *13*, 4154–4160. [CrossRef]
19. Remick, D.G. Pathophysiology of sepsis. *Am. J. Pathol.* **2007**, *170*, 1435–1444. [CrossRef]
20. van der Poll, T.; Opal, S.M. Host-pathogen interactions in sepsis. *Lancet Infect. Dis.* **2008**, *8*, 32–43. [CrossRef] [PubMed]
21. Taylor, F.B.; Chang, A.; Ruf, W.; Morrissey, J.H.; Hinshaw, L.; Catlett, R.; Blick, K.; Edgington, T.S. Lethal *E. coli* septic shock is prevented by blocking tissue factor with monoclonal antibody. *Circ. Shock* **1991**, *33*, 127–134.
22. Sweeney, M.D.; Zhao, Z.; Montagne, A.; Nelson, A.R.; Zlokovic, B.V. Blood-Brain Barrier: From Physiology to Disease and Back. *Physiol. Rev.* **2019**, *99*, 21–78. [CrossRef]
23. Aird, W.C. The role of the endothelium in severe sepsis and multiple organ dysfunction syndrome. *Blood* **2003**, *101*, 3765–3777. [CrossRef] [PubMed]
24. Maldonado, J.R. Delirium pathophysiology: An updated hypothesis of the etiology of acute brain failure. *Int. J. Geriatr. Psychiatry* **2018**, *33*, 1428–1457. [CrossRef] [PubMed]
25. Katayama, Y.; Kawamata, T.; Tamura, T.; Hovda, D.A.; Becker, D.P.; Tsubokawa, T. Calcium-dependent glutamate release concomitant with massive potassium flux during cerebral ischemia in vivo. *Brain Res.* **1991**, *558*, 136–140. [CrossRef] [PubMed]
26. Broderick, P.A.; Gibson, G.E. Dopamine and serotonin in rat striatum during in vivo hypoxic-hypoxia. *Metab. Brain Dis.* **1989**, *4*, 143–153. [CrossRef] [PubMed]
27. Gibson, G.E.; Blass, J.P. Impaired synthesis of acetylcholine in brain accompanying mild hypoxia and hypoglycemia. *J. Neurochem.* **1976**, *27*, 37–42. [CrossRef] [PubMed]
28. Xu, F.; Liu, P.; Pascual, J.M.; Xiao, G.; Lu, H. Effect of hypoxia and hyperoxia on cerebral blood flow, blood oxygenation, and oxidative metabolism. *J. Cereb. Blood Flow. Metab.* **2012**, *32*, 1909–1918. [CrossRef] [PubMed]
29. Morandi, A.; Rogers, B.P.; Gunther, M.L.; Merkle, K.; Pandharipande, P.; Girard, T.D.; Jackson, J.C.; Thompson, J.; Shintani, A.K.; Geevarghese, S.; et al. The relationship between delirium duration, white matter integrity, and cognitive impairment in intensive care unit survivors as determined by diffusion tensor imaging: The VISIONS prospective cohort magnetic resonance imaging study. *Crit. Care Med.* **2012**, *40*, 2182–2189. [CrossRef]
30. Kant, I.M.J.; de Bresser, J.; van Montfort, S.J.T.; Witkamp, T.D.; Walraad, B.; Spies, C.D.; Hendrikse, J.; van Dellen, E.; Slooter, A.J.C. BioCog consortium Postoperative delirium is associated with grey matter brain volume loss. *Brain Commun.* **2023**, *5*, fcad013. [CrossRef] [PubMed]
31. Hatano, Y.; Narumoto, J.; Shibata, K.; Matsuoka, T.; Taniguchi, S.; Hata, Y.; Yamada, K.; Yaku, H.; Fukui, K. White-matter hyperintensities predict delirium after cardiac surgery. *Am. J. Geriatr. Psychiatry* **2013**, *21*, 938–945. [CrossRef] [PubMed]
32. Nitchingham, A.; Pereira, J.V.-B.; Wegner, E.A.; Oxenham, V.; Close, J.; Caplan, G.A. Regional cerebral hypometabolism on 18F-FDG PET/CT scan in delirium is independent of acute illness and dementia. *Alzheimer's Dement.* **2023**, *19*, 97–106. [CrossRef] [PubMed]
33. van Montfort, S.J.T.; van Dellen, E.; Stam, C.J.; Ahmad, A.H.; Mentink, L.J.; Kraan, C.W.; Zalesky, A.; Slooter, A.J.C. Brain network disintegration as a final common pathway for delirium: A systematic review and qualitative meta-analysis. *Neuroimage Clin.* **2019**, *23*, 101809. [CrossRef]
34. Oh, J.; Shin, J.E.; Yang, K.H.; Kyeong, S.; Lee, W.S.; Chung, T.-S.; Kim, J.-J. Cortical and subcortical changes in resting-state functional connectivity before and during an episode of postoperative delirium. *Aust. N. Z. J. Psychiatry* **2019**, *53*, 794–806. [CrossRef]

35. Choi, S.-H.; Lee, H.; Chung, T.-S.; Park, K.-M.; Jung, Y.-C.; Kim, S.I.; Kim, J.-J. Neural network functional connectivity during and after an episode of delirium. *Am. J. Psychiatry* **2012**, *169*, 498–507. [CrossRef] [PubMed]
36. Wiegand, T.L.T.; Rémi, J.; Dimitriadis, K. Electroencephalography in delirium assessment: A scoping review. *BMC Neurol.* **2022**, *22*, 86. [CrossRef] [PubMed]
37. Jöbsis, F.F. Noninvasive, infrared monitoring of cerebral and myocardial oxygen sufficiency and circulatory parameters. *Science* **1977**, *198*, 1264–1267. [CrossRef] [PubMed]
38. Luker, G.D.; Luker, K.E. Optical imaging: Current applications and future directions. *J. Nucl. Med.* **2008**, *49*, 1–4. [CrossRef]
39. Hillman, E.M.C. Optical brain imaging in vivo: Techniques and applications from animal to man. *J. Biomed. Opt.* **2007**, *12*, 051402. [CrossRef] [PubMed]
40. Wen, Y.; Guo, D.; Zhang, J.; Liu, X.; Liu, T.; Li, L.; Jiang, S.; Wu, D.; Jiang, H. Clinical photoacoustic/ultrasound dual-modal imaging: Current status and future trends. *Front. Physiol.* **2022**, *13*, 1036621. [CrossRef]
41. Wu, D.; Huang, L.; Jiang, M.S.; Jiang, H. Contrast agents for photoacoustic and thermoacoustic imaging: A review. *Int. J. Mol. Sci.* **2014**, *15*, 23616–23639. [CrossRef]
42. Morone, K.A.; Neimat, J.S.; Roe, A.W.; Friedman, R.M. Review of functional and clinical relevance of intrinsic signal optical imaging in human brain mapping. *Neurophotonics* **2017**, *4*, 031220. [CrossRef]
43. Hoshi, Y.; Tamura, M. Detection of dynamic changes in cerebral oxygenation coupled to neuronal function during mental work in man. *Neurosci. Lett.* **1993**, *150*, 5–8. [CrossRef]
44. Okada, E.; Delpy, D.T. Near-infrared light propagation in an adult head model. II. Effect of superficial tissue thickness on the sensitivity of the near-infrared spectroscopy signal. *Appl. Opt.* **2003**, *42*, 2915–2922. [CrossRef]
45. Delpy, D.T.; Cope, M. Quantification in tissue near-infrared spectroscopy. *Philos. Trans. R. Soc. Lond. B Biol. Sci.* **1997**, *352*, 649–659. [CrossRef]
46. Elwell, C.E.; Cooper, C.E. Making light work: Illuminating the future of biomedical optics. *Philos. Trans. A Math. Phys. Eng. Sci.* **2011**, *369*, 4358–4379. [CrossRef] [PubMed]
47. Ferrari, M.; Quaresima, V. A brief review on the history of human functional near-infrared spectroscopy (fNIRS) development and fields of application. *NeuroImage* **2012**, *63*, 921–935. [CrossRef] [PubMed]
48. Jiang, H. *Diffuse Optical Tomography*; CRC Press: Boca Raton, FL, USA, 2018. [CrossRef]
49. Hoshi, Y.; Yamada, Y. Overview of diffuse optical tomography and its clinical applications. *J. Biomed. Opt.* **2016**, *21*, 091312. [CrossRef] [PubMed]
50. Obata, T.; Liu, T.T.; Miller, K.L.; Luh, W.M.; Wong, E.C.; Frank, L.R.; Buxton, R.B. Discrepancies between BOLD and flow dynamics in primary and supplementary motor areas: Application of the balloon model to the interpretation of BOLD transients. *NeuroImage* **2004**, *21*, 144–153. [CrossRef] [PubMed]
51. Culver, J.P.; Durduran, T.; Furuya, D.; Cheung, C.; Greenberg, J.H.; Yodh, A.G. Diffuse optical tomography of cerebral blood flow, oxygenation, and metabolism in rat during focal ischemia. *J. Cereb. Blood Flow. Metab.* **2003**, *23*, 911–924. [CrossRef]
52. Culver, J.P.; Siegel, A.M.; Franceschini, M.A.; Mandeville, J.B.; Boas, D.A. Evidence that cerebral blood volume can provide brain activation maps with better spatial resolution than deoxygenated hemoglobin. *NeuroImage* **2005**, *27*, 947–959. [CrossRef]
53. Wolf, M.; Wolf, U.; Toronov, V.; Michalos, A.; Paunescu, L.A.; Choi, J.H.; Gratton, E. Different time evolution of oxyhemoglobin and deoxyhemoglobin concentration changes in the visual and motor cortices during functional stimulation: A near-infrared spectroscopy study. *NeuroImage* **2002**, *16*, 704–712. [CrossRef] [PubMed]
54. Vidal-Rosas, E.E.; Zhao, H.; Nixon-Hill, R.W.; Smith, G.; Dunne, L.; Powell, S.; Cooper, R.J.; Everdell, N.L. Evaluating a new generation of wearable high-density diffuse optical tomography technology via retinotopic mapping of the adult visual cortex. *Neurophotonics* **2021**, *8*, 025002. [CrossRef]
55. Jiang, S.; Huang, J.; Yang, H.; Wagoner, R.; Kozel, F.A.; Currier, G.; Jiang, H. Neuroimaging of depression with diffuse optical tomography during repetitive transcranial magnetic stimulation. *Sci. Rep.* **2021**, *11*, 7328. [CrossRef] [PubMed]
56. Jiang, S.; Carpenter, L.L.; Jiang, H. Optical neuroimaging: Advancing transcranial magnetic stimulation treatments of psychiatric disorders. *Vis. Comput. Ind. Biomed. Art.* **2022**, *5*, 22. [CrossRef] [PubMed]
57. Huang, J.; Jiang, S.; Wagoner, R.; Yang, H.; Currier, G.; Jiang, H. Three-dimensional optical imaging of brain activation during transcranial magnetic stimulation. *J. Xray Sci. Technol.* **2021**, *29*, 891–902. [CrossRef] [PubMed]
58. Huang, J.; Jiang, S.; Yang, H.; Czuma, R.; Yang, Y.; Kozel, F.A.; Jiang, H. Portable Diffuse Optical Tomography for Three-Dimensional Functional Neuroimaging in the Hospital. *Photonics* **2024**, *11*, 238. [CrossRef]
59. Pfister, D.; Siegemund, M.; Dell-Kuster, S.; Smielewski, P.; Rüegg, S.; Strebel, S.P.; Marsch, S.C.U.; Pargger, H.; Steiner, L.A. Cerebral perfusion in sepsis-associated delirium. *Crit. Care* **2008**, *12*, R63. [CrossRef]
60. Funk, D.J.; Kumar, A.; Klar, G. Decreases in cerebral saturation in patients with septic shock are associated with increased risk of death: A prospective observational single center study. *J. Intensive Care* **2016**, *4*, 42. [CrossRef] [PubMed]
61. Wood, M.; Song, A.; Maslove, D.; Ferri, C.; Howes, D.; Muscedere, J.; Boyd, J.G. Brain Tissue Oxygenation in Patients with Septic Shock: A Feasibility Study. *Can. J. Neurol. Sci.* **2016**, *43*, 65–73. [CrossRef]

62. Vaskó, A.; Siró, P.; László, I.; Szatmári, S.; Molnár, L.; Fülesdi, B.; Molnár, C. Assessment of cerebral tissue oxygen saturation in septic patients during acetazolamide provocation—A near infrared spectroscopy study. *Acta Physiol. Hung.* **2014**, *101*, 32–39. [CrossRef] [PubMed]
63. Cerebral Oxygenation and Neurological Outcomes Following Critical Illness (CONFOCAL) Research Group; Canadian Critical Care Trials Group; Wood, M.; Maslove, D.M.; Muscedere, J.G.; Day, A.G.; Gordon Boyd, J. Low brain tissue oxygenation contributes to the development of delirium in critically ill patients: A prospective observational study. *J. Crit. Care* **2017**, *41*, 289–295. [CrossRef] [PubMed]
64. Lee, K.F.; Wood, M.D.; Maslove, D.M.; Muscedere, J.G.; Boyd, J.G. Dysfunctional cerebral autoregulation is associated with delirium in critically ill adults. *J. Cereb. Blood Flow. Metab.* **2019**, *39*, 2512–2520. [CrossRef]
65. Rosenblatt, K.; Walker, K.A.; Goodson, C.; Olson, E.; Maher, D.; Brown, C.H.; Nyquist, P. Cerebral Autoregulation-Guided Optimal Blood Pressure in Sepsis-Associated Encephalopathy: A Case Series. *J. Intensive Care Med.* **2020**, *35*, 1453–1464. [CrossRef] [PubMed]
66. Jiang, S.; Huang, J.; Yang, H.; Czuma, R.; Farley, L.; Cohen-Oram, A.; Hartney, K.; Chechotka, K.; Kozel, F.A.; Jiang, H. Diffuse optical tomography for mapping cerebral hemodynamics and functional connectivity in delirium. *Alzheimer's Dement.* **2024**, *20*, 4032–4042. [CrossRef] [PubMed]
67. Meagher, J.; Leonard, M.; Donoghue, L.; O'Regan, N.; Timmons, S.; Exton, C.; Cullen, W.; Dunne, C.; Adamis, D.; Maclullich, A.J.; et al. Months backward test: A review of its use in clinical studies. *World J. Psychiatry* **2015**, *5*, 305–314. [CrossRef] [PubMed]
68. Trzepacz, P.T.; Mittal, D.; Torres, R.; Kanary, K.; Norton, J.; Jimerson, N. Validation of the Delirium Rating Scale-revised-98: Comparison with the delirium rating scale and the cognitive test for delirium. *J. Neuropsychiatry Clin. Neurosci.* **2001**, *13*, 229–242. [CrossRef] [PubMed]
69. Okada, F.; Tokumitsu, Y.; Hoshi, Y.; Tamura, M. Gender- and handedness-related differences of forebrain oxygenation and hemodynamics. *Brain Res.* **1993**, *601*, 337–342. [CrossRef] [PubMed]
70. Strangman, G.E.; Zhang, Q.; Li, Z. Scalp and skull influence on near infrared photon propagation in the Colin27 brain template. *NeuroImage* **2014**, *85 Pt 1*, 136–149. [CrossRef] [PubMed]
71. Hamblin, M.R. Shining light on the head: Photobiomodulation for brain disorders. *BBA Clin.* **2016**, *6*, 113–124. [CrossRef] [PubMed]
72. Tedford, C.E.; DeLapp, S.; Jacques, S.; Anders, J. Quantitative analysis of transcranial and intraparenchymal light penetration in human cadaver brain tissue. *Lasers Surg. Med.* **2015**, *47*, 312–322. [CrossRef]
73. Yaroslavsky, A.N.; Schulze, P.C.; Yaroslavsky, I.V.; Schober, R.; Ulrich, F.; Schwarzmaier, H.J. Optical properties of selected native and coagulated human brain tissues in vitro in the visible and near infrared spectral range. *Phys. Med. Biol.* **2002**, *47*, 2059–2073. [CrossRef]
74. Pitzschke, A.; Lovisa, B.; Seydoux, O.; Zellweger, M.; Pfleiderer, M.; Tardy, Y.; Wagnières, G. Red and NIR light dosimetry in the human deep brain. *Phys. Med. Biol.* **2015**, *60*, 2921–2937. [CrossRef] [PubMed]
75. Eggebrecht, A.T.; Ferradal, S.L.; Robichaux-Viehoever, A.; Hassanpour, M.S.; Dehghani, H.; Snyder, A.Z.; Hershey, T.; Culver, J.P. Mapping distributed brain function and networks with diffuse optical tomography. *Nat. Photonics* **2014**, *8*, 448–454. [CrossRef] [PubMed]
76. Habermehl, C.; Holtze, S.; Steinbrink, J.; Koch, S.P.; Obrig, H.; Mehnert, J.; Schmitz, C.H. Somatosensory activation of two fingers can be discriminated with ultrahigh-density diffuse optical tomography. *NeuroImage* **2012**, *59*, 3201–3211. [CrossRef]
77. Lange, F.; Tachtsidis, I. Clinical Brain Monitoring with Time Domain NIRS: A Review and Future Perspectives. *Appl. Sci.* **2019**, *9*, 1612. [CrossRef]
78. Havsteen, I.; Ohlhues, A.; Madsen, K.H.; Nybing, J.D.; Christensen, H.; Christensen, A. Are Movement Artifacts in Magnetic Resonance Imaging a Real Problem?—A Narrative Review. *Front. Neurol.* **2017**, *8*, 232. [CrossRef] [PubMed]
79. Van Dijk, K.R.A.; Sabuncu, M.R.; Buckner, R.L. The influence of head motion on intrinsic functional connectivity MRI. *NeuroImage* **2012**, *59*, 431–438. [CrossRef] [PubMed]
80. Brigadoi, S.; Ceccherini, L.; Cutini, S.; Scarpa, F.; Scatturin, P.; Selb, J.; Gagnon, L.; Boas, D.A.; Cooper, R.J. Motion artifacts in functional near-infrared spectroscopy: A comparison of motion correction techniques applied to real cognitive data. *NeuroImage* **2014**, *85*, 10.1016. [CrossRef] [PubMed]
81. Scarapicchia, V.; Brown, C.; Mayo, C.; Gawryluk, J.R. Functional Magnetic Resonance Imaging and Functional Near-Infrared Spectroscopy: Insights from Combined Recording Studies. *Front. Hum. Neurosci.* **2017**, *11*, 419. [CrossRef]
82. Huang, R.; Hong, K.-S.; Yang, D.; Huang, G. Motion artifacts removal and evaluation techniques for functional near-infrared spectroscopy signals: A review. *Front. Neurosci.* **2022**, *16*, 878750. [CrossRef]
83. Sharshar, T.; Carlier, R.; Bernard, F.; Guidoux, C.; Brouland, J.-P.; Nardi, O.; de la Grandmaison, G.L.; Aboab, J.; Gray, F.; Menon, D.; et al. Brain lesions in septic shock: A magnetic resonance imaging study. *Intensive Care Med.* **2007**, *33*, 798–806. [CrossRef] [PubMed]

84. Heming, N.; Mazeraud, A.; Verdonk, F.; Bozza, F.A.; Chrétien, F.; Sharshar, T. Neuroanatomy of sepsis-associated encephalopathy. *Crit. Care* **2017**, *21*, 65. [CrossRef]
85. Orhun, G.; Esen, F.; Özcan, P.E.; Sencer, S.; Bilgiç, B.; Ulusoy, C.; Noyan, H.; Küçükerden, M.; Ali, A.; Barburoğlu, M.; et al. Neuroimaging Findings in Sepsis-Induced Brain Dysfunction: Association with Clinical and Laboratory Findings. *Neurocrit Care* **2019**, *30*, 106–117. [CrossRef]
86. Ahad, M.A.; Kumaran, K.R.; Ning, T.; Mansor, N.I.; Effendy, M.A.; Damodaran, T.; Lingam, K.; Wahab, H.A.; Nordin, N.; Liao, P.; et al. Insights into the neuropathology of cerebral ischemia and its mechanisms. *Rev. Neurosci.* **2020**, *31*, 521–538. [CrossRef] [PubMed]
87. Giacalone, G.; Zanoletti, M.; Re, R.; Germinario, B.; Contini, D.; Spinelli, L.; Torricelli, A.; Roveri, L. Time-domain near-infrared spectroscopy in acute ischemic stroke patients. *Neurophotonics* **2019**, *6*, 015003. [CrossRef]
88. Park, J.J.; Kim, Y.; Chai, C.L.; Jeon, J.P. Application of Near-Infrared Spectroscopy for the Detection of Delayed Cerebral Ischemia in Poor-Grade Subarachnoid Hemorrhage. *Neurocrit Care* **2021**, *35*, 767–774. [CrossRef]
89. Liu, Y.-C.; Yang, Y.-R.; Tsai, Y.-A.; Wang, R.-Y.; Lu, C.-F. Brain Activation and Gait Alteration During Cognitive and Motor Dual Task Walking in Stroke-A Functional Near-Infrared Spectroscopy Study. *IEEE Trans. Neural Syst. Rehabil. Eng.* **2018**, *26*, 2416–2423. [CrossRef]
90. Yang, J.; Wu, D.; Zhang, G.; Zhao, Y.; Jiang, M.; Yang, X.; Xu, Q.; Jiang, H. Intracerebral haemorrhage-induced injury progression assessed by cross-sectional photoacoustic tomography. *Biomed. Opt. Express* **2017**, *8*, 5814–5824. [CrossRef] [PubMed]
91. White, B.R.; Snyder, A.Z.; Cohen, A.L.; Petersen, S.E.; Raichle, M.E.; Schlaggar, B.L.; Culver, J.P. Resting-state functional connectivity in the human brain revealed with diffuse optical tomography. *NeuroImage* **2009**, *47*, 148–156. [CrossRef]
92. Eggebrecht, A.T.; White, B.R.; Ferradal, S.L.; Chen, C.; Zhan, Y.; Snyder, A.Z.; Dehghani, H.; Culver, J.P. A quantitative spatial comparison of high-density diffuse optical tomography and fMRI cortical mapping. *NeuroImage* **2012**, *61*, 1120–1128. [CrossRef] [PubMed]
93. Williams, L.M. Precision psychiatry: A neural circuit taxonomy for depression and anxiety. *Lancet Psychiatry* **2016**, *3*, 472–480. [CrossRef] [PubMed]
94. Zhao, H.; Cooper, R.J. Review of recent progress toward a fiberless, whole-scalp diffuse optical tomography system. *Neurophotonics* **2018**, *5*, 011012. [CrossRef]
95. Khan, A.F.; Zhang, F.; Yuan, H.; Ding, L. Brain-wide functional diffuse optical tomography of resting state networks. *J. Neural Eng.* **2021**, *18*, 046069. [CrossRef] [PubMed]
96. Pandharipande, P.; Shintani, A.; Peterson, J.; Pun, B.T.; Wilkinson, G.R.; Dittus, R.S.; Bernard, G.R.; Ely, E.W. Lorazepam is an independent risk factor for transitioning to delirium in intensive care unit patients. *Anesthesiology* **2006**, *104*, 21–26. [CrossRef] [PubMed]
97. Wikström, M.; Krab, K.; Sharma, V. Oxygen Activation and Energy Conservation by Cytochrome c Oxidase. *Chem. Rev.* **2018**, *118*, 2469–2490. [CrossRef] [PubMed]
98. Wang, W.; Zhao, F.; Ma, X.; Perry, G.; Zhu, X. Mitochondria dysfunction in the pathogenesis of Alzheimer's disease: Recent advances. *Mol. Neurodegener.* **2020**, *15*, 30. [CrossRef]
99. Wang, Y.; Xu, E.; Musich, P.R.; Lin, F. Mitochondrial dysfunction in neurodegenerative diseases and the potential countermeasure. *CNS Neurosci. Ther.* **2019**, *25*, 816–824. [CrossRef]
100. Singer, M. The role of mitochondrial dysfunction in sepsis-induced multi-organ failure. *Virulence* **2014**, *5*, 66–72. [CrossRef] [PubMed]
101. Samuels, D.C.; Hulgan, T.; Fessel, J.P.; Billings, F.T.; Thompson, J.L.; Chandrasekhar, R.; Girard, T.D. Mitochondrial DNA Haplogroups and Delirium During Sepsis. *Crit. Care Med.* **2019**, *47*, 1065–1071. [CrossRef]
102. Menon, V. 20 years of the default mode network: A review and synthesis. *Neuron* **2023**, *111*, 2469–2487. [CrossRef]
103. Lemée, J.-M.; Berro, D.H.; Bernard, F.; Chinier, E.; Leiber, L.-M.; Menei, P.; Ter Minassian, A. Resting-state functional magnetic resonance imaging versus task-based activity for language mapping and correlation with perioperative cortical mapping. *Brain Behav.* **2019**, *9*, e01362. [CrossRef] [PubMed]
104. Zhao, W.; Makowski, C.; Hagler, D.J.; Garavan, H.P.; Thompson, W.K.; Greene, D.J.; Jernigan, T.L.; Dale, A.M. Task fMRI paradigms may capture more behaviorally relevant information than resting-state functional connectivity. *NeuroImage* **2023**, *270*, 119946. [CrossRef]

chemosensors

MDPI

Review

Sustainable Biopolymer-Based Electrochemical Sensors for Trace Heavy Metal Determination in Water: A Comprehensive Review

Rabiaa Helim [1,2], Ali Zazoua [2,3] and Hafsa Korri-Youssoufi [1,*]

[1] Université Paris-Saclay, CNRS, Institut de Chimie Moléculaire et des Matériaux d'Orsay (ICMMO), ECBB, Site Henri Moisson, 17 Avenue des Sciences, 91400 Orsay, France; rabiaa.helim@univ-jijel.dz
[2] Laboratory of Applied Energetics and Materials, Faculty of Science and Technology, University of Jijel, Ouled Aissa, P.O. Box 98, Jijel 18000, Algeria; a_zazoua@univ-jijel.dz
[3] Laboratory of Process Engineering for Sustainable Development and Health Products, Ecole Nationale Polytechnique of Constantine, Constantine 25000, Algeria
* Correspondence: hafsa.korri-youssoufi@universite-paris-saclay.fr

Abstract: The growing concern over heavy metal contamination in environmental and industrial settings has intensified the need for sensitive, selective, and cost-effective detection technologies. Electrochemical sensors, due to their high sensitivity, rapid response, and portability, have emerged as promising tools for detecting heavy metals. Recent years have seen significant progress in utilizing biopolymer-based materials to enhance the performance of these sensors. Biopolymers, derived from renewable raw materials, have garnered considerable interest in both science and industry. These biopolymer-based composites are increasingly recognized as superior alternatives to conventional non-biodegradable materials because of their ability to degrade through environmental exposure. This review provides a comprehensive overview of recent advancements in biopolymer-based electrochemical sensors for heavy metal detection. It discusses various types of biopolymers and bio-sourced polymers, their extraction methods, and chemical properties. Additionally, it highlights the state of the art in applying biopolymers to electrochemical sensor development for heavy metal detection, synthesizing recent advances and offering insights into design principles, fabrication strategies, and analytical performance. This review underscores the potential of biopolymer-based sensors as cost-effective, eco-friendly, and efficient tools for addressing the pressing issue of heavy metal contamination in water and discusses their advantages and limitations. It also outlines future research directions to further enhance the performance and applicability of these sensors.

Keywords: biopolymers; electrochemical sensors; heavy metals; detection; water pollution; sustainability; environmental; green technology; polysaccharides

1. Introduction

Heavy metal contamination in water has become a growing concern, with pollution levels rising dramatically over recent decades [1]. To mitigate the harmful effects on human health and the environment, it is essential to develop strategies, policies, technologies, and materials to control this problem [2]. Developing cost-effective, sustainable, and environmentally friendly materials is crucial to addressing these challenges [3]. Although nanomaterials have been extensively studied for sensor applications due to their unique physicochemical properties, concerns about their potential toxicological effects have shifted attention toward biopolymers [4].

Biopolymers, or bio-sourced polymers derived from renewable resources, have gained increasing importance in sensing applications. These materials, produced from plants, animals, and algae, are seeing a steady rise in production and use. Biopolymers from renewable raw materials can be categorized into four main groups based on their chemical structure and properties:

- Proteins (e.g., gelatin and collagen), known for their high mechanical strength;
- Poly(lactic acid) and poly(hydroxyalkanoates);
- Natural rubber latex, offering flexibility and conductivity;
- Polysaccharides (e.g., cellulose, chitosan, lignin), valued for their biocompatibility, biodegradability, and versatile functional groups [5].

Biopolymers are increasingly being applied in environmental remediation, particularly in the removal of metal ions. Recent research has focused on their potential to replace synthetic materials in electrochemical sensors for detecting heavy metals, aligning with sustainability goals. These biopolymers can be included into the content of the electrode, modifying layers, films, or composites to form functionalized detection surfaces with enhanced electrochemical properties. Their chemical structures also offer opportunities for modification, such as grafting functional groups to improve performance [5].

This review summarizes recent advances in the use of low-cost biopolymers and their chemical and physical modifications to enhance metal removal and electrochemical sensing capabilities. It begins by emphasizing the importance of heavy metal detection and the limitations of traditional methods. Next, this review explores the characteristics of biopolymers, highlighting their renewability, biocompatibility, and multifunctionality, which make them ideal for sensor development. Biopolymers are categorized by their source, structure, and properties, and their roles as sensing elements in electrochemical sensors for heavy metal detection are discussed.

This review further analyzes the integration of biopolymers into various electrochemical sensor platforms, such as amperometric, potentiometric, and impedimetric systems, focusing on strategies like nanocomposite fabrication and surface modification to improve the sensor selectivity, sensitivity, and stability. It also evaluates the performance of biopolymer-based electrochemical sensors in detecting heavy metals, including lead, mercury, cadmium, arsenic, and chromium, addressing key factors such as detection limits, response times, and interference effects. Finally, this review assesses the real-world applicability of these sensors in environmental monitoring, industrial processes, and point-of-care diagnostics and discusses the research directions that should be realized in the future to improve their performance and applicability.

2. Heavy Metals

2.1. Heavy Metals Definition and Sources

Although the definition of heavy metals is controversial and not entirely clear, an element can be classified as a heavy metal if it has a much higher density than water, occurs naturally, and is present primarily in the earth's crust. Approximately 40% of the lakes and rivers of the planet have been polluted by heavy metals [6]. The main heavy metal pollutants in surface waters are Lead Pb(II), Zinc Zn(II), Cadmium Cd(II), Copper Cu(II), Nickel Ni(II), Arsenic As(II), Cobalt Co(II), Iron Fe(II), Manganese Mn(II), Mercury Hg(II), Chromium Cr(IV), Silver Ag(I), Gold Au(III), Palladium Pd(II), Platinum Pt(III), Uranium U(VI), and Cesium Cs(I). Cr(VI), Ni(II), Cd(II), Pb(II), and Hg(II) are among the most toxic ions to be found in nature, particularly in wastewater [7].

The sources of heavy metals can be natural or anthropogenic. Natural sources include interactions with meta-bearing rocks normally present in the environment and volcanic eruptions [8]. Anthropogenic sources include those associated with industrial (e.g., fossil fuel combustion, metal processing), agricultural (pesticides), and domestic activities (e.g., garbage, cleaning products) [9]. Mining is one of the most important sectors to consider, particularly because it plays a central role in the economies of both developed and developing countries. This activity releases large quantities of heavy metals, which are released through mineral extraction and transported through rivers and streams, where they may be dissolved in the water or as part of the sediments [10]. These metals typically seep into groundwater and can also cause water shortages, prevent crop growth through soil erosion, and cause serious health problems for local animals and people [11]. The other main sources of heavy metals are also industries such as tanneries, pharmaceutical and chemical industries, electroplating, alloy production, fertilizers, etc. (see Table 1).

2.2. Toxicological Effects

Heavy metals are among the most dangerous pollutants because they are toxic, non-biodegradable, and accumulate in ecological systems. Determining heavy metals is therefore crucial for monitoring environmental quality, which is currently under pressure due to increasing pollution from industrial, agricultural, and domestic activities. When heavy metals enter and accumulate in the environment, plants and animals living in contaminated areas can take them up. Through the food chain, they eventually become biomagnified in the human body through consumption of contaminated plants, animals, and water [12]. A natural mechanism for controlling heavy metals' removal from the human body is not yet known. Therefore, traces of toxic heavy metals can have harmful effects on human health, including damage to multiple organs and the nervous system [13].

Heavy metal ions in water are involved in the environment and ecological cycles in a variety of forms, along with other inorganic metal ions, hydrated metal ions, hydroxyl complexes, carbonate complexes, and complexes mixed with natural substances. Also, they are taken up and enriched by aquatic plants, animals, and microorganisms. They can also interact with several inorganic or organic colloids and organic–inorganic complexes in the water or sediment and then settle to the bottom of the water body [1].

The World Health Organization (WHO) sets a guideline and recommendation regarding the maximum allowed level of various heavy metal in drinking water. Table 1 summarizes the main sources of heavy metals, their toxicological effects, and the permissible limits in drinking water recommended by WHO.

Table 1. Limits, sources, and effects of various heavy metal ion contaminations in human health.

Metal	WHO (mg L^{-1})	Toxicity		Anthropogenic Sources	Effects	Refs.
		Tolerable Daily Intake (mg/per day)	Lethal Dose mg kg^{-1} Body Weight			
Lead (Pb)	0.05	0.025–0.052	94–158	PVC pipes in sanitation, agriculture, recycled PVC, lead paint, jewelry, lead batteries, lunch boxes.	Alzheimer's disease and senile dementia, damage to the nervous system, also leads to neurodegenerative diseases, lower IQ, kidney damage, reduced bone growth, behavioral problems, digestive problems, urinary insufficiency.	[11,14–16]
Cadmium (Cd)	0.005	0.018–0.052	4.4–6.2	Paints, pigments, batteries, plastics rubbers, engraving process, photoconductors, and photovoltaic cells.	Renal toxicity, hypertension, weight loss, fatigue, microcytic hypochromic anemia, lymphocytosis, pulmonary fibrosis, lung cancer.	[15,17]
Mercury (Hg)	0.001	0.03	5.1–10.0	Combustion of coal, municipal solid waste incineration, and volcanic emissions.	Impaired neurologic development, effects on digestive system, immune system, lungs, kidneys, skin and eyes, hypertension.	[18,19]

Table 1. *Cont.*

Metal	WHO (mg L^{-1})	Toxicity: Tolerable Daily Intake (mg/per day)	Toxicity: Lethal Dose mg kg^{-1} Body Weight	Anthropogenic Sources	Effects	Refs.
Arsenic (Ar)	0.05	0.03	41	Wooden electricity poles that are treated with arsenic-based preservatives, pesticides, fertilizers.	Affects the cardiovascular system, pulmonary diseases, gastrointestinal tract, genitourinary system, hematopoietic system, dermatology, fetal and teratogenic diseases, anorexia, brown pigmentation, hyperpigmentation, local edema, and skin cancer.	
Chromium (Cr)	0.05	0.013–0.099	-	Leather industry, tanning, and chrome plating industries.	Gastrointestinal diseases, hepatic encephalopathy, respiratory and cardiovascular problems, renal and endocrine systems defects, hematological, ocular problems.	[15,20]
Silver (Ag)	0.1	-	-	Refining of copper, gold, nickel, zinc, jewelry, and electroplating industries.	Argyria, gastroenteritis, neuronal disorders, mental fatigue, rheumatism, knotting of cartilage, cytopathological effects in fibroblast, keratinocytes, and mast cells.	[4,17]
Zinc (Zn)	5	15–16.2	1–25.3	Soldering, cosmetics and pigments, respiratory disorders, metal fume fever, bronchiolar.	leucocytes, neuronal disorder, prostate cancer risks, macular degeneration, and impotence.	[9,15]
Copper (Cu)	1.3	10	4.0–7.2	Fertilizers, tanning, and photovoltaic cells.	Adrenocortical hyperactivity, allergies, anemia, alopecia, arthritis, autism, cystic fibrosis, diabetes, hemorrhaging, and kidney disorders.	[20,21]
Nickel (Ni)	0.07	0.089–0.231	-	Coal burning, diesel and fuel oil burning, tobacco smoking, wind dust, volcanic activity, garbage burning, cheap jewelry, stainless steel appliances.	Dermatitis, pulmonary fibrosis, asthma, respiratory and cardiovascular diseases, immune system failure, carcinogenic, DNA damage.	[22,23]

2.3. Conventional Methods for Heavy Metal Detection

It is essential to frequently determine and measure the concentration of heavy metals in tap water to ensure human safety. The selected technique must be sensitive enough to detect low concentrations of these metals accurately [17]. Although meeting all these criteria is challenging, the development and combination of various techniques have enabled accurate detection of heavy metals [3].

Conventional methods for determining heavy metals involve sample treatment, analytical techniques, and heavy instrumentation. The most commonly used methods are as follows:

Atomic Absorption Spectroscopy (AAS);

Inductively Coupled Plasma Mass Spectrometry (ICP-MS);

Inductively Coupled Plasma Atomic Emission Spectroscopy (ICP-AES);

Flame Atomic Emission Spectroscopy (FAES);

X-Ray Fluorescence (XRF), primarily used for solid sample analysis such as soil and sediments.

Colorimetric methods are less common but are still used for detecting specific heavy metals.

ICP-MS and ICP-AES are the most widely used methods because of their high sensitivity and the ability of simultaneous determination of multiple heavy metals and isotopes. Table 2 summarizes a comparison of traditional heavy metal detection methods with their advantages and disadvantages [24,25].

Table 2. Advantages and disadvantages of traditional heavy metal detection methods.

Method	Advantages	Disadvantages
Atomic Absorption Spectroscopy (AAS)	High sensitivity and specificity, simple sample preparation, wide range of applications.	Requires individual measurements for each element, susceptible to interference from other elements.
Inductively Coupled Plasma Optical Emission	Simultaneous multi-element analysis, high sensitivity and precision, wide linear dynamic range.	Complex instrumentation, expensive, requires skilled operators.
Spectroscopy (ICP-OES) Inductively Coupled Plasma Mass Spectrometry (ICP-MS)	Extremely high sensitivity, excellent detection limits, isotopic analysis capability.	
Colorimetric Methods	Simple, inexpensive, and rapid.	Low sensitivity, susceptible to interference, limited dynamic range.

Electrochemical techniques are also used to measure heavy metals in solution by monitoring the change in electrochemical properties of redox reactions of metal ions. Electrochemical methods also offer the advantages of simultaneous determination, high sensitivity, and cost-effectiveness, while also being environmentally friendly.

2.4. Electrochemical Sensors

Electrochemical sensors have emerged as powerful tools for environmental analysis control. They offer several advantages over traditional methods, including on-site detection, rapid response, and low cost. Electrochemical sensors can detect various pollutants, including metals, pharmaceuticals, agrochemicals, and illicit drugs [26].

The development of electrochemical sensors for the detection of metal pollution in the environment has received considerable attention in recent years. Such sensors can be used to detect low levels of metal pollutants in complex environments. Electrochemical sensors are also miniaturized systems that allow the development of portable instruments capable of monitoring the contamination on site. Sensors for metal ions detection can use a wide range of recognition elements, including biomolecules and macromolecules such as antibodies, enzymes, DNA aptamers, DNAzymes, and whole cells, as well as molecularly imprinted polymers (MIPs), macrocycles, and biopolymers. The use of recognition elements for capturing heavy metals have been considered as innovative tools in metal monitoring because of their stable interaction, low detection limit, and high selectivity [27,28]. The use of bio-sourced polymers in electrochemical sensors for metal detection is rapidly gaining traction in this field of research due to their potential properties. Biopolymers also offer the dual advantages of reliable detection and the potential for removal of metal pollutants.

2.5. Electrochemical Methods of Detection

Electrochemical techniques are cost effective, user friendly, and dependable. They can provide analytical results with lower detection limits compared to spectroscopic and optical methods. Electrochemical techniques, which are widely used in heavy metal detection, include potentiometry, amperometry, voltammetry, coulometry, impedance, and electrochemiluminescence. Voltammetry and potentiometry techniques are preferred due to their simplicity and capacity to track the redox signals of metal ions. Various techniques in voltammetry are employed to improve the sensitivity of detection and are widely used, such as linear sweep anodic stripping voltammetry (LSASV), square wave anodic stripping voltammetry (SWASV), and differential pulse anodic stripping voltammetry (DPASV). Chronoamperometry (CA) can be applied for real-time monitoring of the metal ions in real samples (Figure 1). However, detection with cyclic voltammetry (CV) and potentiometric electrochemical analysis methods suffer from low selectivity [29].

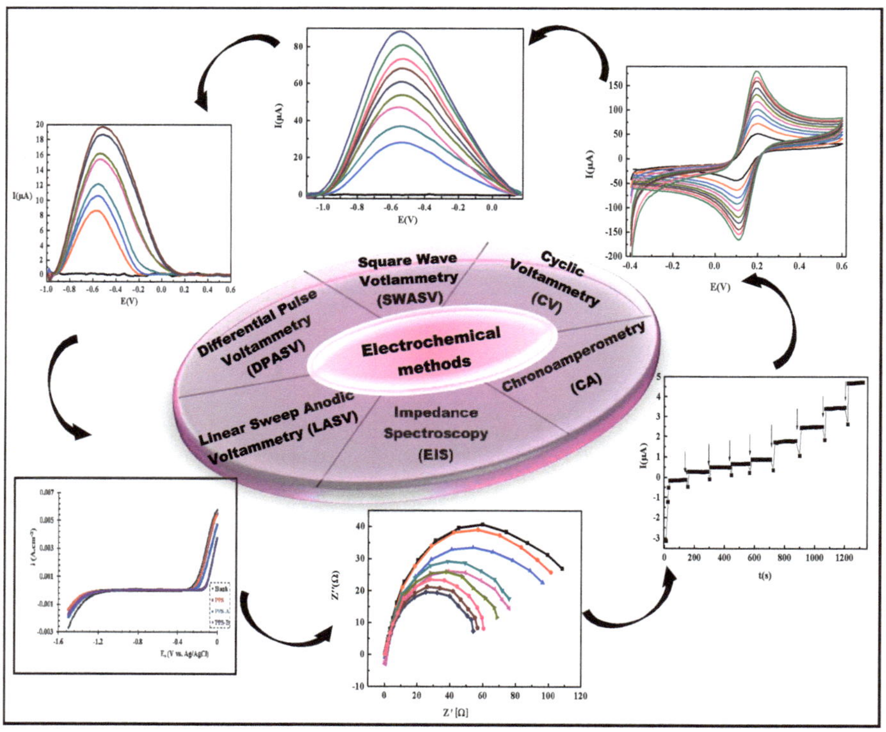

Figure 1. Presentation of the different electrochemical methods for heavy metal detection.

Electrochemical detection could be improved by modified electrodes where a selection of scaffold of metal ions improves their stability on the surface and then their sensitivity and selectivity of electrochemical signal detection.

Biopolymers and bio-sourced polymers modified electrodes present an interesting way to improve the attachment and stability of metal ions on the surface of the electrode, leading to an increased sensitivity and selectivity of detection. Another parameter in the development of sensor technology that has recently been considered is the use of renewable-source materials.

3. Polymers and Biopolymers as Sensing Layers

3.1. Definition and Characteristics

Polymers play a crucial role in the biological world as well as in today's industry. Some natural polymers, such as proteins and nucleic acids, possess and utilize their essential biological properties, while other polymers, such as polysaccharides, contribute to cellular functions and serve as structural components in living systems.

Biopolymers are a versatile category in their own right. The terms biodegradable polymers and biopolymers (or biologically based polymers) are sometimes used interchangeably in the literature, but there is a significant difference between the two types of polymers. Biodegradable polymers are materials whose chemical and physical properties deteriorate and completely degrade when exposed to microorganisms and aerobic and anaerobic processes. Bio-based polymers are a raw material-related term applied to polymers from renewable sources. Raw materials are defined as renewable if they are renewed by natural processes at a comparable rate or faster than they are consumed [30].

The definition of biopolymers is based on two different criteria: the source of the raw materials and the biodegradability of the polymer. They can be the following:

- Biopolymers produced from renewable (biological) and biodegradable raw materials.
- Biopolymers produced from sustainable (biological), non-biodegradable raw materials.
- Biodegradable biopolymers based on fossil fuels [30].

3.2. Synthetic Biopolymers

Synthetic biopolymers are polymers that have either been chemically synthesized from synthetic monomers or modified from natural polymers, enabling them to degrade naturally without leaving harmful residues in ecosystems. Due to their advantages over natural polymers in terms of stability and flexibility for a wide range of applications, synthetic biopolymers have garnered significant attention in recent years. These biopolymers are favored over conventional synthetic polymers due to their environmental safety and biodegradability. Figure 2 shows the structure of some synthetic biopolymers.

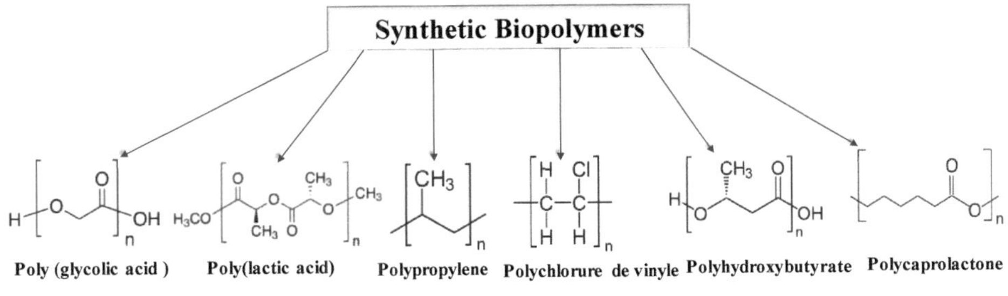

Figure 2. Examples of some structural units of synthetic biopolymers.

Advances in molecular design and polymer chemistry now allow the synthesis of synthetic biopolymers tailored to meet specific needs. Synthetic biopolymers are generally divided into two categories:

- Non-biodegradable synthetic biopolymers, which resist environmental degradation and contribute to waste (e.g., polyamide, polyvinylchloride, polypropylene)
- Biodegradable synthetic biopolymers, which break down when exposed to environmental factors, such as poly(glycolic acid), poly(lactic acid), polycaprolactone, and polyhydroxy butyrate [2].

These synthetic biopolymers can be synthesized using various techniques, including esterification, dehydration, polycondensation, hydrolysis, and granulation, to achieve specific structural and mechanical properties [31].

3.3. Natural Biopolymers (Bio-Sourced Polymers)

Natural polymers are macromolecules produced or occurring naturally in living organisms. "Biopolymers" is a broad term that includes both biodegradable and bio-based polymers, regardless of whether they are natural or manufactured. Natural polymers are derived from bacteria, plants, or animals.

Natural polymers are formed by covalently bonding monomer units. The specific monomers and their arrangement determine the properties of the polymer. Biopolymers, unlike synthetic polymers with simpler, random structures, have well-defined three-dimensional structures, which is essential for their function [32].

Natural polymers are classified into three main categories based on their monomer units:

- Polynucleotides: polymers composed of nucleotide monomers (e.g., RNA, DNA);
- Polypeptides: polymers made of amino acids (e.g., proteins);
- Polysaccharides: polymers made of carbohydrates (e.g., cellulose, hemicellulose, pectin) [33].

Polysaccharides consist of monosaccharide units linked by glycosidic bonds, which can be either linear or branched. Similarly, polynucleotides are made of nucleotide units linked by phosphodiester bonds, and polypeptides are chains of amino acids linked by peptide bonds (see Figure 3) [33].

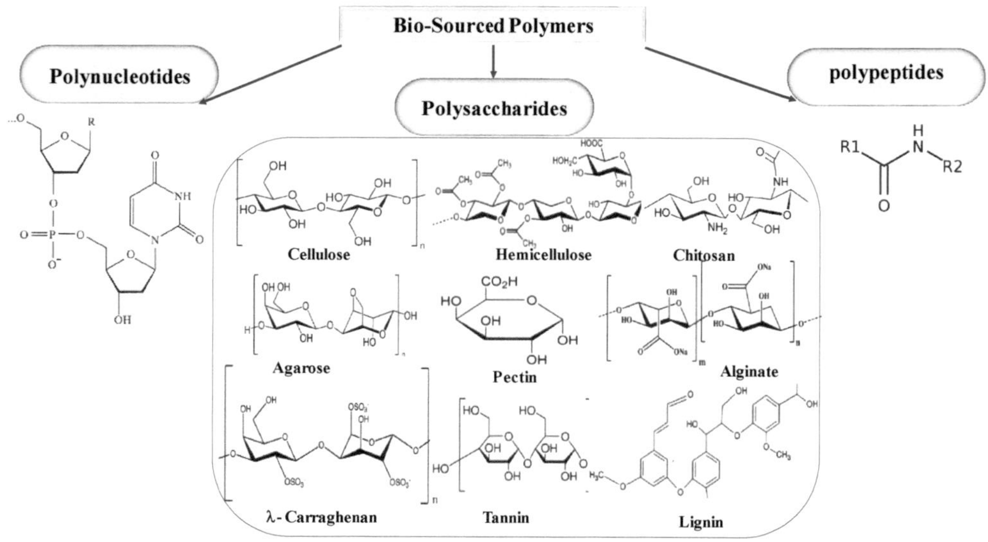

Figure 3. Structure of bio-sourced polymers formed with three family polynucleotides, polysaccharides and polypeptides.

3.4. Properties of Bio−Sourced Polymers

Bio-sourced polymers are environmentally friendly because they can be broken down into elemental units through natural processes using enzymes or microorganisms. The final products of this decomposition can re-enter the environment, leaving a minimal carbon footprint. Another advantage of bio-sourced polymers is their chemical and structural diversity, as they are sourced from various plants and living organisms.

Bio-sourced polymers such as chitosan, alginate, cellulose, pectin, gelatin, and acacia gum are widely used in the development of biosensors due to their inherent properties [34]. They are especially valued for these properties, such as the following:

- Biocompatibility: ability to interact harmoniously with biological systems.
- High adsorption capacity: enhanced ability to absorb or adsorb molecules.
- Hydrophilicity: affinity for water, which can improve performance in sensing applications.
- Relative thermostability: ability to withstand moderate thermal variations [35].

These properties make the biopolymers an ideal matrix for sensor applications, particularly in the development of selective and sensitive detection of heavy metals. Additionally, biopolymers possess functional groups such as hydroxyl, amine, and carboxyl groups that allow them to bind chemically and physically to various molecules [36,37].

4. Application of Biopolymers for the Removal of Heavy Metals from Water

Several technologies have been explored for the removal of heavy metals from water, for instance, ion exchange [38], coagulation–flocculation [39], precipitation, and membrane filtration [40], using biomaterials. Although these techniques reduce the concentration of residual metal ions in treated wastewater, their high operating costs, material costs, and limited absorption efficiency have restricted their large-scale application. Research shows that using low-cost adsorbents for heavy metal removal is both effective and economically viable. Various carbohydrate-based biopolymers have been extensively used for the removal of heavy metals from water [7]. Over the years, various natural polysaccharides, such as cellulose, hemicellulose, and chitosan [41–43], along with phenolic compounds (lignin) [44,45], chelators, activated carbon, and clay, have been used as adsorbents for removing heavy metals [46]. These biopolymers contain numerous functional groups that interact with metal ions by chelating metal ions and forming complexes improving the removal of heavy metals from water. To achieve high removal efficiency, adsorption relies on the attraction of the heavy metal ions present in wastewater by an adsorbent with a porous structure and a large surface area. The active functional groups found in natural biopolymers (such as aromatic, phenolic, alcoholic, carbonyl, methoxy, carboxyl, and amino groups) serve as adsorption sites for heavy metal ions [47,48]. Due to their abundance and accessibility, bio-sourced polymers are also cost-effective, making them a practical choice for long-term adsorption system design and maintenance, and can now be applied in some processes of decontamination.

Table 3 summarizes the most recent studies on adsorption efficiency, highlighting the use of natural and synthetic biopolymers and their composites with organic and inorganic materials for metal removal. Special attention is given to polysaccharide-based biopolymers, such as lignocellulose, cellulose, hemicellulose, chitosan, and alginate.

Table 3. Summary of the polymers and biopolymers developed for metal ion removal with the value of the maximum adsorption capacity.

Biopolymers Used for Removal	Metal Ions	Adsorption Capacity (mg g^{-1})	Ref.
Nano-sized TiO_2/carboxymethyl chitosan hemicellulose composites	Ni(II)	370.4	[49]
	Cd(II)	555.6	
	Cu(II)	526.3	
	Hg(II)	18.6	
	Mn(VII)	29.9	
	Cr(VI)	32.1	

Table 3. *Cont.*

Biopolymers Used for Removal	Metal Ions	Adsorption Capacity (mg g^{-1})	Ref.
Phosphorylated cellulose microsphere	Pb(II)	139.38	[50]
Porous carboxymethyl chitosan (PCMC)	Co(II)	46.25	[51]
Cellulose/N-isopropylacrylamide-glycidyl methacrylate Cell-*g*-NIPAM-*co*-GMA	Ni(II) Cu(II) Pd(II)	74.68 82.92 119.76	[52]
Carboxymethylated cellulose fiber (CMF)	Cu(II)	23.48	[53]
Glucan/chitosan (GL/CS) hydrogels	Cu(II) Co(II) Ni(II) Pb(II) Cd(II)	342 232 184 395 269	[54]
Chitosan/calcium alginate/bentonite composite hydrogel	Pb(II) Cu(II) Cd(II)	434.89 115.30 102.38	[55]
Carboxylated chitosan/carboxylated nanocellulose hydrogel beads	Pb(II)	334.9	[56]
Cellulose nanofiber and sodium alginate	Pb(II)	318.47	[57]
Picea smithiana sawdust	Pb(II) Cr(VI) Cd(II)	6.35 3.37 2.87	[58]
Sodium alginate@ polyethyleneimine-carbon dots	Pb(II)	380.39	[59]
Hemicellulose-based hydrogel	Pb(II)	5.88	[60]
Microwave-functionalized cellulose	Pb(II) Cd(II) Ni(II)	5.43 3.14 2.77	[61]
Thiol-functionalized cellulose nanofiber	Cu(II) Cd(II) Pb(II)	49.0 45.9 22.0	[62]
Lignin-based hybrid magnetic nanoparticles	Pb(II) Cu(II)	150.33 70.69	[63]
Three-dimensional porous graphene/lignin/sodium alginate nanocomposite (denoted as 3D PG/L/SA)	Cd(II) Pb(II)	79.88 226.24	[64]
Chitosan/nanoclay composite	Cu(II) Ni(II)	176 144	[65]
Chitosan/Two-Dimensional Metal-Organic Frameworks ($Ni_3(HITP)_2$) and MXene ($Ni_3(HITP)_2$/MXene/CS)	Pb(II)	448.93	[66]
Chitosan/4-hydroxy-3-methoxybenzaldehyde (VAN)-Epichlorohydrin (Fe_3O_4@CTS-VAN)	Cr(VI)	188.68	[67]
Xylan hemicellulose modified with sulfonic acid 30% content HA3	Pb(II) Cd(II) Cu(II)	193 182 66	[68]
Xylan hemicellulosemodified with sulfonate 50% content of Xylan	Pb(II) Cd(II) Cu(II)	273 143 45	

5. Applications of Bio-Sourced Polymers in Electrochemical Sensing of Heavy Metals

Lignocellulosic biomass has emerged as a promising tool for heavy metal detection. This efficiency can be partly attributed to the composition of the biomass, particularly the ratio of its key components: cellulose, hemicellulose, and lignin. Each component plays a critical role in the adsorption process, with functional groups providing binding sites for metal ions. Considerable research has explored the potential of lignocellulosic biomass in developing electrochemical sensors based on modified electrodes incorporating biopolymers and bio-sourced polymers derived from this biomass [69].

This section discusses several relevant electrochemical sensors for heavy metal detection based on polysaccharide derivatives (e.g., cellulose, sodium alginate, chitosan, chitin, and pectin) and polyphenols. We also explore their association with other organic and inorganic nanomaterials.

Polysaccharides are long chains of monosaccharides linked by glycosidic bonds, and their specific sugar types and linkages define their properties, such as solubility and rigidity. Additionally, the linear or branched structure of a polysaccharide influences these characteristics. Among these polymers, cellulose and its composites stand out due to their stability, conductivity, and affinity for heavy metals, making them particularly valuable for designing electrochemical sensors for heavy metal detection [70].

5.1. Cellulose and Cellulose Composite-Based Sensors

Cellulose, one of the most common polysaccharides in plants, is widely used in biosensors. It is an oxygen-rich polysaccharide with glucose units linked by oxygen bonds [71]. Plants produce cellulose in a fibrous form, which strengthens cell walls. Cellulose has a fibril structure with high resistance, allowing it to form durable polysaccharide-based walls. Its carbon structure enables cellulose to be both crystalline and amorphous.

Cellulose can be modified to produce conductive forms, such as carboxymethylcellulose (CMC), cellulose nanocrystals (CNC), and cellulose nanofibers (CNF); all possess high adsorption capacities and porous surfaces [72]. Hydroxyethyl cellulose, while not directly used for heavy metal uptake, is employed as a supporting matrix or immobilization platform in sensor systems.

Several studies have reported using cellulose and its derivatives to construct heavy metal electrochemical sensors. For example, sodium carboxymethylcellulose has been used to modify GCE to detect cadmium ions using DPASV. Under optimal conditions, the proposed CMC/GCE sensor showed a strong linear response to cadmium ions and achieved a detection limit of 0.75 nM [73].

Bacterial cellulose has also been employed in heavy metal sensing due to its highly porous network and large surface. A notable example is an electrochemical sensor developed by Qin et al. to detect cadmium Cd(II) and lead Pb(II) in drinking water. This sensor used a GCE modified by a composite combining carbonated bacterial cellulose (CBC) with gamma-alumina (γ-AlOOH) and used DPASV for detection. The unique structure of this composite provided a highly porous network and strong affinity for heavy metals, resulting in detection limits of 0.17 μg/L (1.5 nM) for Cd(II) and 0.1 μg/L for Pb(II)(0.48 nM). The authors compared these results to those obtained through the more established method of ICP-MS, demonstrating the sensor's reliability and accuracy [74].

Cellulose nanofibers have also emerged as a highly sensitive material for detecting heavy metals due to their ability to adsorb large amounts of metal ions. Zinoubi et al. reported the development of a GCE modified with nanocellulose fibers derived from eucalyptus for detecting traces of Cd(II), Cu(II), Pb(II), and Hg(II) using DPASV. This modified electrode CNF/GCE demonstrated high sensitivity, stability, and low detection limits of 5 nM for Cd(II) and Hg(II) and 0.5 nM for Cu(II) and Pb(II) [75].

Combining cellulose derivatives as scaffolds with other components, such as biomolecules or nanomaterials, leads to improved heavy metal sensing properties. Many developed sensors include various cellulose derivatives with carbon nanomaterials or metal oxide. For example, nanocellulose has been combined with biomolecules to enhance sensors sensitivity. Taheri et al. demonstrated that a nanocellulose composite modified with d-penicillamine (DPA-NC) significantly improves the detection of Cu(II) in tap and river water (Figure 4). A pencil-shaped graphite electrode modified with DPA-NC exhibited amperometric detection of Cu(II) measured by SWASV, with a sensitivity of 0.2 μA/μmol and a detection limit of 0.048 pM [76]. This result demonstrated the ability of sensors based on biopolymers to detect the presence of metal ions in real samples.

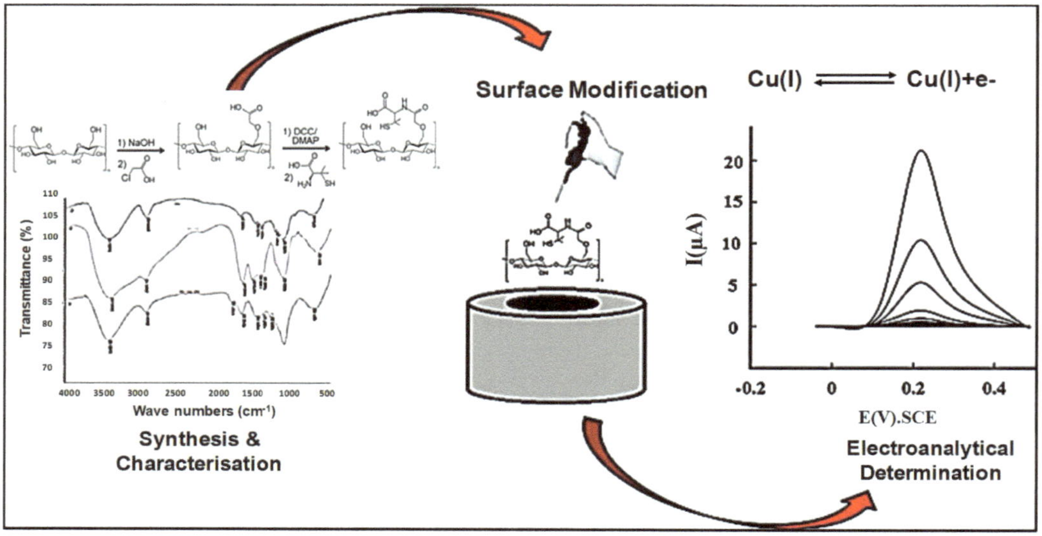

Figure 4. Nanocellulose functionalized with d-penicillamine used as electrochemical transducers for copper detection, the scheme shows the composition of the nanocomposite and them the deposition on surface electrode by drop casting followed by detection of copper using SWASV for electroanalytical determination (reproduced with permission from Taheri et al., *J. Phys. Chem. Solids*, publisher Elsevier2018, ref. [76].

In the same way, the association of carboxymethylcellulose (CMC) with carbon nanomaterials has been explored for the detection of cadmium and lead. A study by Prya et al. has demonstrated the simultaneous detection of trace levels of Cd(II) and Pb(II) using a nanocomposite made with porous graphene, CMC, and fondaparinux, a penta-saccharide, to form a composite (PrGO/CMC/Fonda). After deposition on GCE, this nanocomposite allows the detection of various heavy metals using SWASV with a high sensitivity and detection limits of 0.28 nM for Cd(II) and 0.17 nM for Pb(II). The composite's components worked synergistically to improve electron transfer and immobilization of metal ions [77].

Cellulose nanocrystals, known as nano-whiskers (CNWs), are rod-like nanoparticles derived from cellulose fibers through various mechanical and chemical treatments. CNWs are often used in combination with other nanomaterials for enhanced functionality. They can be obtained from cellulose via conventional acid hydrolysis of white cotton fibers. Teodoro et al. combined cellulose nanocrystals with reduced graphene oxide (rGO) and polyamide 6 through an electrospinning synthesis approach, creating a hybrid composite designed for electrochemical mercury detection. This composite exhibited improved charge transfer properties, as evaluated by cyclic voltammetry, due to the excellent electrical properties of graphene. The nanocomposite allows the electrochemical detection of mercury in water samples, achieving a limit of detection of 0.52 μM and a wide dynamic linear range of 2.5–200 μM [78].

Additionally, metal oxide nanomaterials are also associated with cellulose to improve the conductivity of the nanocomposite. Padmalaya et al. developed a cellulose-based composite using cellulose acetate, in combination with zinc oxide. This nanocomposite served as an electrochemical sensor for cadmium quantification. Square wave voltammetry was employed to assess cadmium presence, with a LOD of 0.41 μM within a linear concentration range of 0.1–0.5 mM. The conductive nature of zinc oxide, its stability, and the hydroxyl groups in the cellulose acetate's structure endowed the nanocomposite with electrical and chemical properties well-suited for lead detection [79].

Cellulose can also serve as an electrode and supporting matrix for the immobilization of chelating agents of metal ions. For example, hierarchical porous metal organic framework zeolitic imidazolate framework (ZIF-8s) was integrated into cellulose paper for removal and detection of metal ions (Figure 5). The modified cellulose was used in working electrodes for the selective electrochemical detection of lead ions (Pb(II)) with an LOD of 8 μM [80].

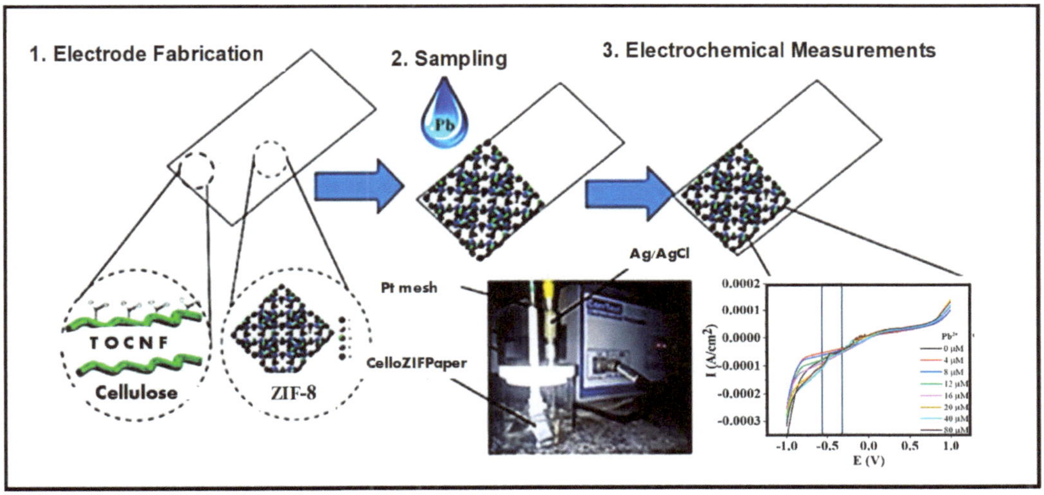

Figure 5. Schematic representation of electrode fabrication, sampling from cellulose, and electrochemical measurements of CelloZIFPaper for detection of lead ions. The inset camera image shows the setup of the cell electrodes and potentiostat. Reproduced with permission from Abdelhamid et al., *Chem. Eng. J.*; publisher by Elsevier 2022 ref. [80].

Table 4 summarizes the sensors developed based on other cellulose derivatives and composites with other materials and highlights the methods of detection used as well as the limit of detection and linear range.

Table 4. Different polymeric materials as the modifying layers of the sensors for heavy metals determination.

Electrode	Method	Analyte	LOD	Linear Range	Applications	Ref
Au/Agarose-Hemicellulose	SWASV	Pb(II)	1.3 fM	1 μM–1 fM	Tap, spring, and sea water	[27]
GCE/Cellulose nanofiber	DPASV	Cd(II) Cu(II) Pb(II) Hg(II)	5 nM 0.5 nM 0.5 nM 5 nM	0.1 nM–10 μM	Sea water	[75]
Penicillamine functionalized nano-cellulose modified pencil graphite electrode	SWASV	Cu(II)	0.048 pM	0.2–50 pM	Tap and river water	[76]
PA_6/Cellulose nanowhiskers /rGO	DPASV	Hg(II)	0.52 μM	2.5–75 μM	River and tap water	[78]
AuNPs/Cellulose nanofiber/GCE	SWASV	Cd(II) Pb(II) Cu(II)	0.1 μM	0.1–1.0 μM	-	[81]
γ-AlOOH-carbonated bacterial cellulose	DPASV	Cd(II) Pb(II)	1.5 nM 0.5 nM	4.4–2200 nM 2–1200 nM	Drinking water	[74]

Table 4. *Cont.*

Electrode	Method	Analyte	LOD	Linear Range	Applications	Ref
Carbon nanodots Dot (CNDS)	DPASV	Hg(II) Pb(II)	124 nM 551 nM	-	Drinking water	[82]
Hydroxyethylcellulose-CA	EIS	Pb(II)	1.8 nM	-	Leachates from detonation chamber dust (DCD) and galvanic sludge from the plating industry (GS)	[83]

Au: gold; PA6: Polyamide 6; rGO: reduced graphene oxide; AuNPs: gold nanoparticles; CPE: screen-printed electrode; CA: citric acid.

5.2. Alginate-Based Sensors

Sodium alginate (SA) is a linear polyanionic polysaccharide derived from brown algae, consisting of α-L-guluronic acid (G) and β-D-mannuronic acid (M) residues linked by glycosidic bonds [7,8]. Due to its abundance, antibacterial properties, and high ionic absorption capacity, sodium alginate has wide applications in environmental remediation, particularly in water treatment [84]. Its biocompatibility and ability to bind metal ions make it suitable for electrochemical sensors for heavy metal detection.

Sodium alginate's mechanical properties can be improved by forming composites with other materials. For example, combining alginate with chitosan, another biopolymer, can result in stable hydrogels easily deposited on sensor surfaces. The richness of these biopolymers' functional groups such as carboxyl (-COOH) and nitrogen-containing groups allows selective heavy metal detection. This is demonstrated in the work of Chen et al. where a nanocomposite of sodium alginate and chitosan was applied to a glassy carbon electrode (GCE) for the detection of copper ions (Cu(II)) using DPASV. The sensor achieved a linear detection range between 1 and 100 μM, with a detection limit of 0.9545 μM [85].

To further enhance performance and electron transfer ability, sodium alginate can be combined with carbon-based materials such as single-walled carbon nanotubes (SWCNTs). This approach leverages SWCNTs' large surface area and high conductivity, leading to improved adsorption and faster sensor response times. Thus, Chrouda et al. demonstrated a biopolymer sensor based on sodium alginate decorated with SWCNTs for the detection of Pb(II), Cd(II), and Cu(II) using DPASV. The sensor achieved detection limits of 0.1 nM for Pb(II), 31 nM for Cd(II), and 1 nM for Cu(II) [86].

5.3. Chitosan-Based Sensors

Chitosan is a linear biopolymer composed of randomly arranged D-glucosamine and N-acetyl-D-glucosamine units linked by β(1–4) glycosidic bonds. Its structure contains amine (-NH_2) groups at the C2 carbon, and numerous hydroxyl (-OH) groups, which impart strong hydrophilic properties to the molecule. Chitosan is derived by deacetylating chitin in an alkaline medium [87], leading to amino groups. The chitosan is particularly valuable due to the free amine groups that are active sites for chemical reactions as well as metal chelation. Primary amino groups (-NH_2) have been extensively exploited for heavy metal ion detection due to the favorable acid–base interaction between these electron-rich amino ligands and electron-deficient heavy metal ions. Thus, chitosan is widely used across various industries, including wastewater treatment and environmental monitoring [88].

Chitosan membranes or films form effective matrices for sensing heavy metals due to their strong mechanical strength, hydrophilic properties, and ability to bind metals through chelation. Various studies have demonstrated the effectiveness of chitosan as a sensing material for detecting heavy metals.

For example, a flat carbon electrode coated with chitosan has been used to detect zinc (Zn(II)) and lead (Pb(II)) without any prior extraction or treatment. Using SWASV, two distinct peaks were obtained at various potentials corresponding to Zn(II) and Pb(II), with detection limits of 0.6 and 1 ppb, respectively [89].

Another study by Hadnine et al. developed an electrochemical sensor based on a carbon paste electrode modified with chitosan-based chelating thiourea and glutaraldehyde. This composite is used to detect mercury ions and showed sensitivity to Hg(II) ions in the range of 5 nM to 1 μM, with a detection limit of 1.61 nM [90]. The synergistic effect of thiourea's sulfur atoms and chitosan's nitrogen and hydroxyl groups contributed to the sensor's sensitivity.

Chitosan has also been employed as a matrix for immobilizing other molecules. Fort et al. developed a modified electrode using doubly doped mesoporous carbon xerogel confined within a chitosan hydrogel, deposited on a GCE. This electrode was investigated to detect trace amounts of Pb(II) and Cd(II) using SWASV. The sensor exhibited a detection limit of 0.07 ppb (0.07 nM) for Pb(II) and 5.06 ppm (5 μM) for Cd(II) [91].

Chitosan's ability to form composites with metal nanomaterials has enhanced the sensitivity of heavy metal sensors. For instance, Pathak et al. developed a flexible electrochemical sensor based on a copper–chitosan nanocomposite. The sensor, fabricated through a low-cost screen-printing technique, was used to detect Pb(II) ions in water samples. The sensor exhibited a detection limit of 0.72 ppb (0.72 nM) in tap water [92]. This work demonstrates the potential of the chitosan to be printed and gives electrodes with high detection efficiency. However, the stability of these devices over time and in challenging conditions still needs further development.

Chitosan can also be combined with magnetic materials, such as Fe_3O_4 nanoparticles, to improve detection performance. Zhou et al. synthesized Fe_3O_4-chitosan nanoparticles through a one-step in situ co-precipitation method. These nanoparticles were used as a sensor for Pb(II) ions using SWASV, achieving a detection limit of 0.04 μM [93].

Chitosan and metal oxides are widely employed in fabricating electrochemical sensors for heavy metal detection. The oxygen atoms in metal oxides can donate electron pairs, forming covalent bonds with transition metals, and their porous structure further increases the available surface area, enhancing metal ion interaction. For example, Shang et al. presented a novel strategy that utilizes nickel oxide, molybdenum oxide, and chitosan to construct a 3D Ni/NiO/MoO_3/chitosan interface, acting as a sensing element for Cu(II). The electrochemical response arises from a reduction in barrier height at the interface due to Cu(II) uptake, with a linear detection range of 0–25 μM and a low detection limit of 5.69 nM. Chitosan (CS) demonstrates excellent Cu(II) adsorption capacity due to its abundance of reactive hydroxyl and carboxyl groups. Additionally, the wide band gaps of NiO and MoO_3 allow for a tunable electronic range, while the nanostructured oxides provide active surface sites for metal ion binding [94].

Chitosan can also be combined with carbon nanomaterials, such as carbon nanotubes or graphene, as a sensing layer for heavy metal detection. These carbon nanomaterials offer several advantages: increased surface area, enhanced electrical conductivity, and the ability to be functionalized with chemical groups that selectively attract certain heavy metals. For instance, a composite of chitosan, reduced graphene oxide (rGO), and poly-L-lysine (PLL) was developed through electropolymerization, achieving detection limits for Cd(II), Pb(II), and Cu(II) at 0.01, 0.02, and 0.02 μg/L (0.09, 0.1, 0.3 nM), respectively [95].

Ion-imprinting techniques have gained attention in the selective detection of metal ions. Wei et al. developed an electrochemical sensor based on a chitosan–graphene oxide composite with a polymer-modified GCE (CS/GO-IIP) for Cu(II) detection via an immersion coating method. Cu(II) ions were imprinted by chemical crosslinking with epichlorohydrin after the CS/GO/Cu(II) composite was applied to the glassy carbon electrode. A linear response was observed from 0.5 to 100 μM, with a detection limit of 0.15 μM [96].

In similar work, Yin et al. developed an electrochemical sensor composed from a covalent organic framework (COF), calcium lignosulfonate (CLS)-multiwalled carbon nanotubes (MWCNTs), and nafion for the simultaneous analysis of Cu(II), Pb(II), and Cd(II). The nanocomposite porous and 3D structure with the abundance of amino groups allows the efficient accumulation of heavy metal ions. The MWCNTs enhanced the sensor's conductivity, while the CLS's hydrophilic groups prevented MWCNT aggregation. Under optimal conditions, this sensor demonstrated broad linear responses for Cu(II), Pb(II), and Cd(II) within the ranges of 0.6–63.5, 2.1–207.2, and 1.1–112.4 μg/L, respectively, and low detection limits of 0.2, 0.7, and 0.4 μg/L (3 nM, 3.3 nM, 3.5 nM) [97].

Researchers also combine chitosan with conductive polymers to form composite materials with enhanced sensitivity, selectivity, and charge transfer capabilities, improving sensor performance and design robustness. Since chitosan is a non-conductive material, it has been paired with various conductive polymers to improve its electron transfer ability. Xu et al. reported a chitosan–polypyrrole hybrid polymer used in constructing sensors for Pb(II) detection in wastewater, effectively measuring Pb(II) concentrations via electrochemical methods [98].

Chitin, like chitosan, is a long-chain, biodegradable biopolymer that can be sourced from crustaceans. The NHCO group in each glucose ring of chitin facilitates metal ion trapping via complexation. Singh et al. demonstrated a chitin-based sensor with a chemically interactive polyaniline electrode grafted with chitin (Cs-g-PANI) for copper ion detection. The electrode's potentiometric response to Cu(II) ions followed the Nernst relationship within a range of 1 to 103 ppm (103 μM), with a detection limit of 13.7 ppm (13.7 μM) and minimal interference from other cations and anions [99].

The literature data regarding chitosan-based sensors for heavy metals detection are extensive. Table 5 summarizes some relevant papers regarding the detection of heavy metals where detection is performed in real samples for water environment control.

Table 5. The summary of the relevant sensors based on chitosan for heavy metal determination.

Electrode	Method	Metal	LOD	Linear Range	Application	Ref.
Thymine-Hg^{2+}-Thymine/AuNPs/Chitosane (Aptamer/$(AuNPs/CS)_2$/GCE)	DPASV	Hg(II)	0.005 nM	0.01–500 nM	Tap water	[100]
GC/Chitisane–(Bi–CX)	SWASV	Pb(II) Cd(II)	0.07 nM 5.06 μM	0.2–2 nM 11.2–124 μM	Drilled well water	[91]
AuNPs/CS-Aptamer/GCE	DPASV	Cd(II)	0.05 pM	0.001–100 nM	Tap water	[101]
Amino-functionalized graphene/chitosan (NH_2–G/CS)	DPASV	Cu(II)	0.064 μM^{-1}	0.4–40 μM	Tap water	[102]
CS/AuNPs/GR/GCE	DPASV	Cd(II)	16.2 nM	0.1–0.9 μM	River water, tap water, and pure milk	[103]
Biochar-nanodiamond-chitosan electrode ND-BC-CS	SWASV	Cd(II) Pb(II)	0.11 μM 0.056 μM	1.0–75 μM 0.25–6 μM	-	[104]
Chitosan–graphene oxide composites (CS/GO-IIP)	DPASV	Cu(II)	0.15 μM	0.5–100 μM	Tap and river water	[96]
rGO/MoS_2/CS (GCE)	SWASV	Pb(II)	1.6 nM	0.005–2.0 μM	Tobacco leaves	[105]
NiO-CS/CPE	EIS	Pb(II)	0.3 μM	1 μM–0.1 mM	Waste water	[106]

5.4. Polyphenols as Sensing Platforms

Polyphenols, also known as phenolic compounds, are characterized by at least one aromatic ring in their structure, which bears a variable number of hydroxyl (OH) groups with high affinity for metal ions. Polyphenols can be monomers, polymers, or complexes, with molecular weight up to 9000 Daltons. Due to their unique properties, polyphenols hold promise for heavy metal detection applications.

One example is the use of tannins, a type of polyphenol, for developing composite materials. Bouraoui et al. modified a gold electrode with tannin extracted from pomegranate peel (*Punica granatum* L.) to detect heavy metals in water. The adjacent hydroxyl groups in the tannin's aromatic ring allowed for chelation of metal ions. Using square wave voltammetry (SWV) and electrochemical impedance spectroscopy (EIS), the modified electrode demonstrated detection limits of 6 ng/L (0.094 nM) for Cu(II), 35 ng/L (0.31 nM) for Cd(II), and 11 ng/L (0.05 nM) for Pb(II) [107].

Polyphenols from various plants have been explored for metal ion detection. Zazoua et al. studied sensors based on a boron-doped diamond electrode modified with a polyphenol-polyvinyl chloride membrane using polyphenols extracted from acorn shells. The modified electrode demonstrated sensitivity to Cd(II), Pb(II), and Ni(II), with detection limits of 0.0221 nM, 0.25 nM, and 0.00424 nM, respectively [108].

The combination of polyphenols with nanomaterials can further improve sensing performance. Suherman et al. reported an electrochemical sensor based on a screen-printed electrode modified with gold nanoparticles capped with tannic acid (AuNP@TA). This sensor demonstrated an exceptionally low detection limit of 100.0 fM for Hg(II), far below the World Health Organization (WHO) allowable limit for mercury in drinking water [109]. Integrating phenolic compounds with carbon-based materials exemplifies an innovative approach to enhancing the performance of electrochemical sensors, especially for applications in heavy metal detection. The unique properties imparted by these composites—such as increased conductivity, stability, sensitivity, and specific ion detection sites—make them particularly valuable for environmental monitoring, where rapid and accurate heavy metal detection is critical.

For example, the work by Gonçalves et al. underscores the effectiveness of lignin–polyurethane copolymer composites in achieving high selectivity and stability in Cu(II) ion detection. The MWCNTs enhance conductivity and introduce a robust framework that retains essential mechanical and viscoelastic properties, demonstrating the feasibility of creating durable sensors for field applications. The presence of polyphenolic groups in lignin, attributed to tannins, adds another layer of functionality by improving specificity towards target metal ions. This multi-functional approach could pave the way for designing materials that respond selectively to specific pollutants while maintaining structural integrity over extended periods, an essential factor for practical use in real-world environmental monitoring [110].

Similarly, Mahfoud et al. demonstrated the role of lignin derived from olive pits combined with polyvinyl chloride for Pb(II) detection. The low detection limit achieved (5 nM) through electrochemical impedance spectroscopy (EIS) highlights the potential of lignin as a sustainable and efficient material for heavy metal ion sensing. The underlying mechanism of lignin interaction with heavy metals chelation, ion exchange, adsorption, and surface modification suggest that lignin and similar biopolymers could serve as versatile agents in various environmental sensing applications. This versatility is crucial for developing cost-effective, biodegradable materials for heavy metal removal and sensing, aligning with the growing demand for sustainable environmental technologies [111].

Moreover, the research by Xin Bao et al. emphasizes the use of naturally occurring polyphenols from tea in fabricating composites with zero-valent iron (ZVI) and reduced graphene oxide (rGO) (rGO–ZVI), which showed remarkable sensitivity toward Hg(II) detection. Applying green chemistry methods, for synthesis by using tea polyphenols as reducing agents, aligns with a sustainable approach for sensor development by reducing the environmentally damaging chemicals while enhancing material performance. The synergy between zero-valent iron (ZVI) and reduced graphene oxide (rGO) offers an efficient ion accumulation and electron transfer platform, with a detection limit of 1.2 nM, making it highly effective for mercury detection in aqueous environments. This approach suggests a pathway for developing sensors with rapid response times and high accuracy for a range of heavy metals, leveraging natural compounds as mediating agent to improve detection performance [112].

5.5. Other Biopolymers in Heavy Metal Detection

Starch, a widely consumed carbohydrate and a staple of the human diet consists of two distinct polysaccharides: amylose and amylopectin. Amylose is a linear polysaccharide with D-glucose units linked by (1–4) glycosidic bonds, while amylopectin is highly branched with similar D-glucose backbones but features about 5% (1–6) linkages. These structural features of starch have significant implications for various properties, including its potential in sensor applications [113].

Pectin, a polysaccharide rich in carboxyl groups, can be associated with other nanomaterials for sensing heavy metals. In a study by Murilo Alves et al. (2021), a citrus pectin-modified carbon paste electrode (PEC/CPE) was used for the sensitive electrochemical detection of copper in biofuels. The carboxylic acid groups in the pectin increased the current response by 32% compared to the unmodified electrode. Using differential pulse anodic stripping voltammetry, the analytical curve for copper detection showed a linear range from 50 nM to 0.01 M, with a detection limit of 25 nM and a quantification limit of 83 nM [114].

To address the low conductivity of biopolymers, they can be copolymerized with conductive polymers to create composites with novel and beneficial properties. Polypyrrole, a conducting polymer, is particularly suitable for such applications because of its stability, conductivity, and amine functionalities. Combining polypyrrole with pectin has been shown to enhance detection performance significantly. For example, Arulraj et al. fabricated an electrochemical sensor using a composite of pectin, polypyrrole, and graphene (PPy/Pct/GR) for the detection of mercury (Hg(II)). The sensor demonstrated excellent performance, with a detection limit as low as 4 (fM) [115].

Another promising biopolymer for metal sensing applications is walnut shell biochar (WS-BC), which is both environmentally friendly and readily available. El Hamdouni et al. incorporated biochar derived from walnut shells into a carbon paste electrode (CPE) and electrochemically deposited polytyrosine on the surface of the biochar-doped electrode. This modified platform was tested for the detection of Cd(II), Pb(II), Cu(II), and Hg(II) ions in water and soil samples using square wave voltammetry (SWASV), achieving excellent sensitivity with detection limits of 0.086 nM, 0.175 nM, 0.246 nM, and 0.383 nM for Cd(II), Pb(II), Cu(II), and Hg(II), respectively [116].

Biopolymers extracted from red algae, such as agar and carrageenan, have also shown potential in heavy metal detection. De Oliveira Farias et al. applied a novel method to create thin films of these polysaccharides using layer-by-layer self-assembly. Alternating agar, carrageenan, and polyaniline (PANI) layers were coated onto tin-doped indium oxide (ITO) electrodes. Cyclic voltammetry revealed that these films enhanced electrochemical resistance in acidic media, allowing for the electrochemical detection of chromium (Cr(VI)) [117].

Table 6 summarizes various biopolymers derived from natural sources, combined with different polymeric materials, and their applications in heavy metal sensing. This table highlights the versatility of these biopolymers and their composites, demonstrating their wide-ranging potential for improving the sensitivity, selectivity, and efficiency of electrochemical sensors for heavy metal detection.

Table 6. The summary of the sensors based on polyphenols derivatives for heavy metal determination.

Electrode	Method	Analyte	LOD	Linear Range	Application	Ref.
Tea polyphenols mediated zero-valent iron/reduced graphene oxide nanocomposites (rGO-ZVI-P)	SWASV	Hg(II)	1.2 nM	-	River	[112]
Tannic acid capped gold nanoparticle (AuNPs@TA) complexes	SWASV	Hg(II)	100.0 fM	100 fM–100 nM	Tap	[109]
Crosslinked Sodium alginate (SA) and chitosan (CS)SA-CS/GCE	DPASV	Cu(II)	0.95 μM	1–100 μM	Tap/river	[85]
Sodium alginate-decorated single-walled carbon nanotube	DPASV	Pb(II) Cd(II) Cu(II)	0.1 nM 31 nM 1 nM	-	Tap	[86]
AuNPs-biopolymer-coated carbon SPE sensor	SWASV	Hg(II)	1.7 nM	10–100 nM	Landfill leachate.	[118]
Grafted *Tricholoma* mushroom polysaccharide–silver composite nanoparticles (TMPSGP-Ag NPs)	CA	Zn(II)	0.5 nM	1 nM	River	[119]
Cork–graphite electrodes	DPASV	Pb(II)	0.3 μM	1–25 μM	Tap Ground "produced water" (a brackish water)	[120]
Bi/AgNPs/Nafion-SPGE with Pectin of Citrofortunella Microcarpa	ASV	Pb(II)	267 nM	-	River	[121]
β-cyclodextrin (β-CD)-graphene hybrids (AuNPs-CD-GS)	DPASV	Cd(II) Pb(II)	0.21 μM 0.05 μM	0.035–10 μM 0.2–6 μM	River	[122]
Green nanoparticles based on gum Arabic	DPASV	Zn(II) Hg(II) Pb(II) Cu(II)	1.9 nM 0.9 nM 4.2 nM 9.6 nM	2–150 nM 1–100 nM 5–300 nM 10–300 nM	Lake	[123]

5.6. Discussion: Pros and Cons of Using Biopolymers in Heavy Metal Detection

These studies underscore sustainable, biopolymer-based materials' role in environmental heavy metal detection. The ability of these composites to detect trace levels of heavy metals in complex matrices, such as soil and water, is crucial for environmental health, as even low concentrations of heavy metals can accumulate and pose severe risks to ecosystems and human health. Using abundant natural resources, such as lignin from agricultural by-products or tea polyphenols, also addresses sustainability concerns, as these materials can be sourced without adverse environmental impact.

The advantages of biopolymers are related to their biodegradability and sustainability.

Biopolymers are typically derived from renewable resources; they are biodegradable and environmentally friendly, reducing the ecological footprint associated with sensor production and disposal. This is especially important for environmental applications, where sustainable monitoring solutions are preferable. In addition, the high metal binding affinity of biopolymers is an advantage compared to synthetic macrocycles, as they offer various functional groups (hydroxyl, amine, carboxyl groups) that can readily bind to metal ions through chelation or adsorption. This natural affinity for metal ions enhances their ability to detect heavy metals, even at trace levels, making them highly sensitive in low-concentration environmental settings.

One advantage of biopolymers is their low toxicity and green synthesis ability regarding conventional-based sensors, which can involve harmful synthetic chemicals. The cost-effectiveness is also an advantage of biopolymers, as many biopolymers are by-products of agricultural or industrial processes (e.g., lignin from paper production, chitosan from seafood waste, or pectin from agricultural waste), making them relatively low-cost materials. This cost-effectiveness is advantageous when producing large-scale sensors for widespread environmental monitoring. The surface functionalization flexibility and their easy modification or combination with other materials are also advantages of these biopolymers. Biopolymers can be combined with carbon nanomaterials or metal oxides to enhance conductivity, selectivity, and sensitivity. This versatility allows for the development of custom sensors that are tailored to detect specific heavy metals in complex environmental samples.

Printing compatibility is an advantage for their application as devices, as many biopolymers, such as lignin, chitosan, and cellulose, can be processed into printable inks, enabling sensor fabrication via low-cost techniques like screen printing, inkjet printing, or roll-to-roll printing. This printing compatibility leads to significant cost savings by enabling large-scale, efficient production processes. Furthermore, the flexibility of printed biopolymer-based sensors makes them ideal for developing lightweight, portable devices suitable for environmental applications.

However, while the biopolymers present numerous advantages, some limitations need to be addressed for broader applications and commercialization. The low electrical conductivity is a limitation, as many biopolymers, such as polysaccharides, are non-conductive or have limited conductivity, which can impede electron transfer and reduce sensor efficiency. Biopolymers often require integration with conductive materials such carbon nanotubes or graphene, which can complicate the fabrication process and increase costs. In addition, the potential for degradation in complex conditions could be a limitation in their applications. While biopolymers are biodegradable, this can also be a limitation. In challenging environmental conditions (high temperatures, extreme pH, or prolonged exposure to water), biopolymers may degrade, which could limit their durability and lifespan as sensors. In addition, biopolymers can have a shorter shelf life than synthetic polymers, especially in environments prone to microbial growth or moisture. This short shelf life can lead to decreased long-term sensor stability, making it necessary to store or use biopolymer-based sensors under controlled conditions. The variable quality and consistency of bio-sourced biopolymers can be a limitation, as the properties of biopolymers can vary depending on their source and extraction methods, leading to inconsistent sensor performance. Standardizing biopolymer quality can be challenging, as natural variations might affect metal binding affinity, mechanical strength, and stability. In addition, the fabrication and functionalization processes to modify biopolymers or to improve their conductivity and selectivity require multiple fabrication processes, such as functionalization or integration with nanomaterials. These additional steps can increase the time, expertise, and resources needed to produce biopolymer-based sensors, which may limit scalability for widespread environmental deployment.

While biopolymers present a promising, eco-friendly alternative for electrochemical heavy metal detection in environmental applications, conductivity, durability, and production consistency must be addressed to leverage their benefits fully. The development of hybrid materials and improvements in biopolymer processing can help mitigate these limitations, making biopolymer-based sensors a viable option for sustainable and effective environmental monitoring.

6. Future Research Directions

While current developments in biopolymer-based electrochemical sensors are promising, there are several key areas where future research should focus to improve their performance and applicability further:

1. Exploring new methods for biopolymer production using biological methods such as enzymatic or bacterial production that can give reproducible biopolymers.
2. Enhancing biopolymer functionalization by exploring more efficient methods of functionalizing biopolymers to improve their metal ion binding capacities. This could include advanced chemical modification techniques and the development of new biopolymer–nanomaterial composites.
3. Sensor stability and durability: Long-term sensor stability remains a challenge, and future research should aim to enhance the durability of biopolymer-based sensors under different environmental conditions, ensuring consistent performance in real-world applications by developing cross-linking techniques or nanocomposite formulations. These modifications should enhance the mechanical and chemical stability of biopolymer sensors under prolonged exposure to challenging environments (pH fluctuations, temperature variations, salinity) and evaluate the degradation rates of biopolymer-based sensors, optimizing their durability while maintaining biodegradability.
4. Real-time sensing and multi-metal detection: Current sensors often target specific metals, but future research should aim to develop sensors capable of simultaneously detecting multiple heavy metals in real-time.
5. Exploring wireless sensor networks and portable detection systems can provide real-time data transmission for the remote monitoring of aquatic environments. This would provide a more comprehensive solution for environmental monitoring.
6. Developing new biopolymer sources: Exploring less common biopolymer sources could lead to materials with novel properties that enhance sensor performance, and future research could explore the following:
    - Investigating biopolymers from algae, fungi, or microorganisms may offer unique structural advantages or metal-binding capacities.
    - Using genetic engineering or synthetic biology to design biopolymers with optimized electrochemical properties and metal ion selectivity.
    - Assessing the environmental impact of harvesting new biopolymer sources to ensure they align with sustainability goals.
7. Scalability and commercialization: Although biopolymer-based sensors show great potential in laboratory settings, their scalability for mass production and commercialization remains challenging. Further research should focus on cost-effective manufacturing processes and material sourcing to facilitate the widespread adoption of these sensors.
8. Integrating biopolymer-based sensors with internet of things (IoT) and wireless technologies significantly enhances their capabilities for environmental monitoring. Connecting these sensors to IoT systems makes continuous, real-time monitoring of heavy metal concentrations in water and soil possible. Wireless modules enable remote data transmission to cloud platforms, facilitating a faster response to pollution events and

informed decision-making. These sensors' lightweight and flexible nature allows their deployment in remote and inaccessible areas, while wireless connectivity ensures data transmission without direct physical access. This enables the creation of comprehensive contamination maps, supporting large-scale environmental assessment and remediation efforts. Additionally, integrating low-cost, printed biopolymer sensors with IoT systems reduces infrastructure costs and enables large-scale, dense sensor networks for improved spatial resolution in environmental data.

9. Biopolymer-based sensors are generally low-power, making them compatible with energy-efficient wireless protocols like LoRaWAN and NB-IoT. When combined with solar-powered or other renewable energy sources, these sensors form sustainable, self-sufficient monitoring systems that can be well-suited for long-term environmental monitoring. This also helps reduce the ecological impact of continuous heavy metal monitoring operations.

7. Conclusions

In recent years, significant advances have been made in the development of biopolymer-based electrochemical sensors for detecting heavy metals in aquatic environments. These sensors offer numerous advantages over conventional methods, including cost-effectiveness, eco-friendliness, and high sensitivity. By utilizing natural, renewable resources, biopolymers provide an excellent alternative to synthetic materials, aligning with the global push toward sustainability and environmental protection.

Biopolymers, such as cellulose, chitosan, alginate, and other polysaccharides, have shown considerable potential in enhancing the performance of electrochemical sensors. These materials exhibit high adsorption capacities and can be functionalized with nanomaterials, further improving their ability to detect trace amounts of heavy metals. Additionally, their chemical versatility allows for modifications that enhance sensor stability, sensitivity, and selectivity.

The integration of biopolymers with nanomaterials, such as carbon nanotubes, graphene, and metallic nanoparticles, has opened new pathways for improving sensor performance. These hybrid materials combine the high surface area, conductivity, and mechanical strength of nanomaterials with the biocompatibility and biodegradability of biopolymers. As a result, sensors based on biopolymer–nanomaterial composites are becoming increasingly effective for detecting metal ions such as lead (Pb), cadmium (Cd), mercury (Hg), and copper (Cu), with low detection limits and high selectivity.

Despite these advances, there are still challenges that need to be addressed. The scalability of biopolymer-based sensors for large-scale industrial applications remains a key area of focus. Additionally, the long-term stability and reproducibility of the sensors under various environmental conditions must be further investigated. Future research should focus on optimizing biopolymer synthesis, improving electrode modification techniques, and exploring new biopolymer sources for sensor development.

In conclusion, biopolymer-based electrochemical sensors represent a promising solution for the detection of heavy metal contamination in aquatic environments. As the research continues to evolve, these sensors are expected to play a crucial role in environmental monitoring, industrial applications, and public health protection.

Author Contributions: Conceptualization, R.H., A.Z. and H.K.-Y.; methodology, R.H., A.Z. and H.K.-Y.; software, R.H.; validation, A.Z. and H.K.-Y.; formal analysis, R.H.; investigation, R.H.; writing—original draft preparation, R.H.; writing—review and editing, R.H., A.Z. and H.K.-Y.; visualization, R.H.; supervision, H.K.-Y. and A.Z.; project administration, H.K.-Y.; funding acquisition, H.K.-Y. All authors have read and agreed to the published version of the manuscript.

Funding: This research was funded by Ministries of Europe and Foreign affairs and of the superior teaching and the scientific research in France and ministry of the superior teaching and the scientific research in Algeria within PHC program, grant number 22MAG20.

Informed Consent Statement: Not applicable.

Data Availability Statement: Not applicable.

Conflicts of Interest: The authors declare no conflicts of interest.

References

1. Zhao, C.; Liu, G.; Tan, Q.; Gao, M.; Chen, G.; Huang, X.; Xu, X.; Li, L.; Wang, J.; Zhang, Y. Polysaccharide-Based Biopolymer Hydrogels for Heavy Metal Detection and Adsorption. *J. Adv. Res.* **2023**, *44*, 53–70. [CrossRef]
2. Bilge, S.; Karadurmus, L.; Sınağ, A.; Ozkan, S.A. Green Synthesis and Characterization of Carbon-Based Materials for Sensitive Detection of Heavy Metal Ions. *TrAC Trends Anal. Chem.* **2021**, *145*, 116473. [CrossRef]
3. Zamora-Ledezma, C.; Negrete-Bolagay, D.; Figueroa, F.; Zamora-Ledezma, E.; Ni, M.; Alexis, F.; Guerrero, V.H. Heavy Metal Water Pollution: A Fresh Look about Hazards, Novel and Conventional Remediation Methods. *Environ. Technol. Innov.* **2021**, *22*, 101504. [CrossRef]
4. Langari, M.M.; Antxustegi, M.M.; Labidi, J. Nanocellulose-Based Sensing Platforms for Heavy Metal Ions Detection: A Comprehensive Review. *Chemosphere* **2022**, *302*, 134823. [CrossRef]
5. Imre, B.; Pukánszky, B. Compatibilization in Bio-Based and Biodegradable Polymer Blends. *Eur. Polym. J.* **2013**, *49*, 1215–1233. [CrossRef]
6. Zhou, Q.; Yang, N.; Li, Y.; Ren, B.; Ding, X.; Bian, H.; Yao, X. Total Concentrations and Sources of Heavy Metal Pollution in Global River and Lake Water Bodies from 1972 to 2017. *Glob. Ecol. Conserv.* **2020**, *22*, e00925. [CrossRef]
7. Fouda-Mbanga, B.; Prabakaran, E.; Pillay, K. Carbohydrate Biopolymers, Lignin Based Adsorbents for Removal of Heavy Metals (Cd^{2+}, Pb^{2+}, Zn^{2+}) from Wastewater, Regeneration and Reuse for Spent Adsorbents Including Latent Fingerprint Detection: A Review. *Biotechnol. Rep.* **2021**, *30*, e00609. [CrossRef]
8. Ali, H.; Khan, E.; Ilahi, I. Environmental Chemistry and Ecotoxicology of Hazardous Heavy Metals: Environmental Persistence, Toxicity, and Bioaccumulation. *J. Chemother.* **2019**, *2019*, 1–14. [CrossRef]
9. Vareda, J.P.; Valente, A.J.; Durães, L. Assessment of Heavy Metal Pollution from Anthropogenic Activities and Remediation Strategies: A Review. *J. Environ. Manag.* **2019**, *246*, 101–118. [CrossRef]
10. Vélez-Pérez, L.; Ramirez-Nava, J.; Hernández-Flores, G.; Talavera-Mendoza, O.; Escamilla-Alvarado, C.; Poggi-Varaldo, H.; Solorza-Feria, O.; López-Díaz, J. Industrial Acid Mine Drainage and Municipal Wastewater Co-Treatment by Dual-Chamber Microbial Fuel Cells. *Int. J. Hydrogen Energy* **2020**, *45*, 13757–13766. [CrossRef]
11. Birn, A.-E.; Shipton, L.; Schrecker, T. Canadian Mining and Ill Health in Latin America: A Call to Action. *Can. J. Public Health* **2018**, *109*, 786–790. [CrossRef] [PubMed]
12. Malik, L.A.; Bashir, A.; Qureashi, A.; Pandith, A.H. Detection and Removal of Heavy Metal Ions: A Review. *Environ. Chem. Lett.* **2019**, *17*, 1495–1521. [CrossRef]
13. Ding, R.; Cheong, Y.H.; Ahamed, A.; Lisak, G. Heavy Metals Detection with Paper-Based Electrochemical Sensors. *Anal. Chem.* **2021**, *93*, 1880–1888. [CrossRef]
14. Fu, Z.; Xi, S. The Effects of Heavy Metals on Human Metabolism. *Toxicol. Mech. Methods* **2020**, *30*, 167–176. [CrossRef]
15. Hasanpour, M.; Hatami, M. Application of Three Dimensional Porous Aerogels as Adsorbent for Removal of Heavy Metal Ions from Water/Wastewater: A Review Study. *Adv. Colloid Interface Sci.* **2020**, *284*, 102247. [CrossRef]
16. Qadri, H.; Bhat, R.A.; Mehmood, M.A.; Dar, G.H. *Fresh Water Pollution Dynamics and Remediation*; Springer: Berlin/Heidelberg, Germany, 2020; ISBN 9811382778.
17. Gumpu, M.B.; Sethuraman, S.; Krishnan, U.M.; Rayappan, J.B.B. A Review on Detection of Heavy Metal Ions in Water–an Electrochemical Approach. *Sens. Actuators B Chem* **2015**, *213*, 515–533. [CrossRef]
18. Kinuthia, G.K.; Ngure, V.; Beti, D.; Lugalia, R.; Wangila, A.; Kamau, L. Levels of Heavy Metals in Wastewater and Soil Samples from Open Drainage Channels in Nairobi, Kenya: Community Health Implication. *Sci. Rep.* **2020**, *10*, 8434. [CrossRef]
19. Zhang, M.; Zhang, L.; Tian, H.; Lu, A. Universal Preparation of Cellulose-Based Colorimetric Sensor for Heavy Metal Ion Detection. *Carbohydr. Polym.* **2020**, *236*, 116037. [CrossRef]
20. Balusamy, B.; Senthamizhan, A.; Uyar, T. Functionalized Electrospun Nanofibers as a Versatile Platform for Colorimetric Detection of Heavy Metal Ions in Water: A Review. *Materials* **2020**, *13*, 2421. [CrossRef]
21. Vardhan, K.H.; Kumar, P.S.; Panda, R.C. A Review on Heavy Metal Pollution, Toxicity and Remedial Measures: Current Trends and Future Perspectives. *J. Mol. Liq.* **2019**, *290*, 111197. [CrossRef]
22. Cempel, M.; Nikel, G. Nickel: A Review of Its Sources and Environmental Toxicology. *Pol. J. Environ. Stud.* **2006**, *15*, 375–382.

23. Genchi, G.; Carocci, A.; Lauria, G.; Sinicropi, M.S.; Catalano, A. Nickel: Human Health and Environmental Toxicology. *Int. J. Environ. Res. Public Health* **2020**, *17*, 679. [CrossRef] [PubMed]
24. He, S.; Niu, Y.; Xing, L.; Liang, Z.; Song, X.; Ding, M.; Huang, W. Research Progress of the Detection and Analysis Methods of Heavy Metals in Plants. *Front. Plant Sci.* **2024**, *15*, 1310328. [CrossRef] [PubMed]
25. Nadakuditi, A.; Reddy-Vangala, V. An Overview of Analytical Techniques for Heavy Metal Ion Detection and Removal from Industrial Sewage. *AiBi Rev. Investig. Adm. E Ing.* **2024**, *12*, 29–37. [CrossRef]
26. Maciel, J.V.; Durigon, A.M.M.; Souza, M.M.; Quadrado, R.F.; Fajardo, A.R.; Dias, D. Polysaccharides Derived from Natural Sources Applied to the Development of Chemically Modified Electrodes for Environmental Applications: A Review. *Trends Environ. Anal. Chem.* **2019**, *22*, e00062. [CrossRef]
27. Helim, R.; Zazoua, A.; Jaffrezic-Renault, N.; Korri-Youssoufi, H. Label Free Electrochemical Sensors for Pb(II) Detection Based on Hemicellulose Extracted from Opuntia *Ficus indica* Cactus. *Talanta* **2023**, *265*, 124784. [CrossRef] [PubMed]
28. Ejeian, F.; Etedali, P.; Mansouri-Tehrani, H.-A.; Soozanipour, A.; Low, Z.-X.; Asadnia, M.; Taheri-Kafrani, A.; Razmjou, A. Biosensors for Wastewater Monitoring: A Review. *Biosens. Bioelectron.* **2018**, *118*, 66–79. [CrossRef] [PubMed]
29. Chen, Q.; Yao, Y.; Li, X.; Lu, J.; Zhou, J.; Huang, Z. Comparison of Heavy Metal Removals from Aqueous Solutions by Chemical Precipitation and Characteristics of Precipitates. *J. Water Process Eng.* **2018**, *26*, 289–300. [CrossRef]
30. Abhilash, M.; Thomas, D. Biopolymers for Biocomposites and Chemical Sensor Applications. In *Biopolymer Composites in Electronics*; Elsevier: Amsterdam, The Netherlands, 2017; pp. 405–435.
31. Francis, R.; Sasikumar, S.; Gopalan, G.P. Synthesis, Structure, and Properties of Biopolymers (Natural and Synthetic). In *Polymer Composites*; John Wiley & Sons, Ltd.: Hoboken, NJ, USA, 2013; pp. 11–107, ISBN 978-3-527-67422-0.
32. Chaabouni, E.; Gassara, F.; Brar, S.K. Biopolymers Synthesis and Application. In *Biotransformation of Waste Biomass into High Value Biochemicals*; Brar, S.K., Dhillon, G.S., Soccol, C.R., Eds.; Springer: New York, NY, USA, 2014; pp. 415–443, ISBN 978-1-4614-8005-1.
33. Prabhu, A.; Crapnell, R.D.; Eersels, K.; van Grinsven, B.; Kunhiraman, A.K.; Singla, P.; McClements, J.; Banks, C.E.; Novakovic, K.; Peeters, M. Reviewing the Use of Chitosan and Polydopamine for Electrochemical Sensing. *Curr. Opin. Electrochem.* **2022**, *32*, 100885. [CrossRef]
34. Sawant, S. Development of Biosensors from Biopolymer Composites. In *Biopolymer Composites in Electronics*; Elsevier: Amsterdam, The Netherlands, 2017; pp. 353–383.
35. Ramdzan, N.S.M.; Fen, Y.W.; Anas, N.A.A.; Omar, N.A.S.; Saleviter, S. Development of Biopolymer and Conducting Polymer-Based Optical Sensors for Heavy Metal Ion Detection. *Molecules* **2020**, *25*, 2548. [CrossRef]
36. Feng, K.; Wen, G. Absorbed Pb^{2+} and Cd^{2+} Ions in Water by Cross-Linked Starch Xanthate. *Int. J. Polym. Sci.* **2017**, *2017*, 6470306. [CrossRef]
37. Joly, N.; Ghemati, D.; Aliouche, D.; Martin, P. Interaction of Metal Ions with Mono-and Polysaccharides for Wastewater Treatment: A Review. *Nat. Prod. Chem. Res.* **2020**, *8*, 373.
38. Bashir, A.; Malik, L.A.; Ahad, S.; Manzoor, T.; Bhat, M.A.; Dar, G.; Pandith, A.H. Removal of Heavy Metal Ions from Aqueous System by Ion-Exchange and Biosorption Methods. *Environ. Chem. Lett.* **2019**, *17*, 729–754. [CrossRef]
39. Xu, D.; Zhou, B.; Yuan, R. Optimization of Coagulation-Flocculation Treatment of Wastewater Containing Zn (II) and Cr (VI). *IOP Publ.* **2019**, *227*, 052049–052055. [CrossRef]
40. Bolisetty, S.; Peydayesh, M.; Mezzenga, R. Sustainable Technologies for Water Purification from Heavy Metals: Review and Analysis. *Chem. Soc. Rev.* **2019**, *48*, 463–487. [CrossRef] [PubMed]
41. Zou, Y. Cu^{2+}, Cd^{2+}, and Pb^{2+} Ions Adsorption from Wastewater Using Polysaccharide Hydrogels Made of Oxidized Carboxymethyl Cellulose and Chitosan Grafted with Catechol Groups. *Iran. Polym. J.* **2024**, *33*, 57–66. [CrossRef]
42. Doyo, A.N.; Kumar, R.; Barakat, M.A. Recent Advances in Cellulose, Chitosan, and Alginate Based Biopolymeric Composites for Adsorption of Heavy Metals from Wastewater. *J. Taiwan Inst. Chem. Eng.* **2023**, *151*, 105095. [CrossRef]
43. Garg, S.; Goel, N. Encapsulation of Heavy Metal Ions via Adsorption Using Cellulose/ZnO Composite: First Principles Approach. *J. Mol. Graph. Model.* **2023**, *124*, 108566. [CrossRef] [PubMed]
44. Zhang, Z.; Chen, Y.; Wang, D.; Yu, D.; Wu, C. Lignin-Based Adsorbents for Heavy Metals. *Ind. Crops Prod.* **2023**, *193*, 116119. [CrossRef]
45. Naseer, A.; Jamshaid, A.; Hamid, A.; Muhammad, N.; Ghauri, M.; Iqbal, J.; Rafiq, S.; Khuram, S.; Shah, N.S. Lignin and Lignin Based Materials for the Removal of Heavy Metals from Waste Water-An Overview. *Z. Für Phys. Chem.* **2019**, *233*, 315–345. [CrossRef]
46. Santoso, S.P.; Kurniawan, A.; Angkawijaya, A.E.; Shuwanto, H.; Warmadewanthi, I.; Hsieh, C.-W.; Hsu, H.-Y.; Soetaredjo, F.E.; Ismadji, S.; Cheng, K.-C. Removal of Heavy Metals from Water by Macro-Mesoporous Calcium Alginate–Exfoliated Clay Composite Sponges. *Chem. Eng. J.* **2023**, *452*, 139261. [CrossRef]
47. Zhang, W.; Duo, H.; Li, S.; An, Y.; Chen, Z.; Liu, Z.; Ren, Y.; Wang, S.; Zhang, X.; Wang, X. An Overview of the Recent Advances in Functionalization Biomass Adsorbents for Toxic Metals Removal. *Colloid Interface Sci. Commun.* **2020**, *38*, 100308. [CrossRef]

48. Na, Y.; Lee, J.; Lee, S.H.; Kumar, P.; Kim, J.H.; Patel, R. Removal of Heavy Metals by Polysaccharide: A Review. *Polym. Plast. Technol. Mater.* **2020**, *59*, 1770–1790. [CrossRef]
49. Wu, S.; Kan, J.; Dai, X.; Shen, X.; Zhang, K.; Zhu, M. Ternary Carboxymethyl Chitosan-Hemicellulose-Nanosized TiO_2 Composite as Effective Adsorbent for Removal of Heavy Metal Contaminants from Water. *Fibers Polym.* **2017**, *18*, 22–32. [CrossRef]
50. Luo, X.; Yuan, J.; Liu, Y.; Liu, C.; Zhu, X.; Dai, X.; Ma, Z.; Wang, F. Improved Solid-Phase Synthesis of Phosphorylated Cellulose Microsphere Adsorbents for Highly Effective Pb^{2+} Removal from Water: Batch and Fixed-Bed Column Performance and Adsorption Mechanism. *ACS Sustain. Chem. Eng.* **2017**, *5*, 5108–5117. [CrossRef]
51. Luo, W.; Bai, Z.; Zhu, Y. Fast Removal of Co(II) from Aqueous Solution Using Porous Carboxymethyl Chitosan Beads and Its Adsorption Mechanism. *RSC Adv.* **2018**, *8*, 13370–13387. [CrossRef] [PubMed]
52. Kumar, R.; Sharma, R.K.; Singh, A.P. Grafting of Cellulose with N-Isopropylacrylamide and Glycidyl Methacrylate for Efficient Removal of Ni (II), Cu (II) and Pd (II) Ions from Aqueous Solution. *Sep. Purif. Technol.* **2019**, *219*, 249–259. [CrossRef]
53. Wang, J.; Liu, M.; Duan, C.; Sun, J.; Xu, Y. Preparation and Characterization of Cellulose-Based Adsorbent and Its Application in Heavy Metal Ions Removal. *Carbohydr. Polym.* **2019**, *206*, 837–843. [CrossRef]
54. Jiang, C.; Wang, X.; Wang, G.; Hao, C.; Li, X.; Li, T. Adsorption Performance of a Polysaccharide Composite Hydrogel Based on Crosslinked Glucan/Chitosan for Heavy Metal Ions. *Compos. Part B Eng.* **2019**, *169*, 45–54. [CrossRef]
55. Lin, Z.; Yang, Y.; Liang, Z.; Zeng, L.; Zhang, A. Preparation of Chitosan/Calcium Alginate/Bentonite Composite Hydrogel and Its Heavy Metal Ions Adsorption Properties. *Polymers* **2021**, *13*, 1891. [CrossRef]
56. Xu, X.; Ouyang, X.; Yang, L.-Y. Adsorption of Pb (II) from Aqueous Solutions Using Crosslinked Carboxylated Chitosan/Carboxylated Nanocellulose Hydrogel Beads. *J. Mol. Liq.* **2021**, *322*, 114523. [CrossRef]
57. Zhao, H.; Ouyang, X.-K.; Yang, L.-Y. Adsorption of Lead Ions from Aqueous Solutions by Porous Cellulose Nanofiber–Sodium Alginate Hydrogel Beads. *J. Mol. Liq.* **2021**, *324*, 115122. [CrossRef]
58. Mahmood-ul-Hassan, M.; Yasin, M.; Yousra, M.; Ahmad, R.; Sarwar, S. Kinetics, Isotherms, and Thermodynamic Studies of Lead, Chromium, and Cadmium Bio-Adsorption from Aqueous Solution onto *Picea smithiana* Sawdust. *Environ. Sci. Pollut. Res.* **2018**, *25*, 12570–12578. [CrossRef]
59. Zhang, S.; Arkin, K.; Zheng, Y.; Ma, J.; Bei, Y.; Liu, D.; Shang, Q. Preparation of a Composite Material Based on Self-Assembly of Biomass Carbon Dots and Sodium Alginate Hydrogel and Its Green, Efficient and Visual Adsorption Performance for Pb^{2+}. *J. Environ. Chem. Eng.* **2022**, *10*, 106921. [CrossRef]
60. Lian, Y.; Zhang, J.; Li, N.; Ping, Q. Preparation of Hemicellulose-Based Hydrogel and Its Application as an Adsorbent Towards Heavy Metal Ions. *BioResources* **2018**, *13*, 3208–3218. [CrossRef]
61. Qu, J.; Tian, X.; Jiang, Z.; Cao, B.; Akindolie, M.S.; Hu, Q.; Feng, C.; Feng, Y.; Meng, X.; Zhang, Y. Multi-Component Adsorption of Pb (II), Cd (II) and Ni (II) onto Microwave-Functionalized Cellulose: Kinetics, Isotherms, Thermodynamics, Mechanisms and Application for Electroplating Wastewater Purification. *J. Hazard. Mater.* **2020**, *387*, 121718. [CrossRef]
62. Choi, H.Y.; Bae, J.H.; Hasegawa, Y.; An, S.; Kim, I.S.; Lee, H.; Kim, M. Thiol-Functionalized Cellulose Nanofiber Membranes for the Effective Adsorption of Heavy Metal Ions in Water. *Carbohydr. Polym.* **2020**, *234*, 115881. [CrossRef] [PubMed]
63. Zhang, Y.; Ni, S.; Wang, X.; Zhang, W.; Lagerquist, L.; Qin, M.; Willför, S.; Xu, C.; Fatehi, P. Ultrafast Adsorption of Heavy Metal Ions onto Functionalized Lignin-Based Hybrid Magnetic Nanoparticles. *Chem. Eng. J.* **2019**, *372*, 82–91. [CrossRef]
64. Zhou, F.; Feng, X.; Yu, J.; Jiang, X. High Performance of 3D Porous Graphene/Lignin/Sodium Alginate Composite for Adsorption of Cd(II) and Pb(II). *Environ. Sci. Pollut. Res.* **2018**, *25*, 15651–15661. [CrossRef] [PubMed]
65. Malayoglu, U. Removal of Heavy Metals by Biopolymer (Chitosan)/Nanoclay Composites. *Sep. Sci. Technol.* **2018**, *53*, 2741–2749. [CrossRef]
66. Ijaz, I.; Bukhari, A.; Gilani, E.; Nazir, A.; Zain, H.; Bukhari, A.; Shaheen, A.; Hussain, S.; Imtiaz, A. Functionalization of Chitosan Biopolymer Using Two Dimensional Metal-Organic Frameworks and MXene for Rapid, Efficient, and Selective Removal of Lead (II) and Methyl Blue from Wastewater. *Process Biochem.* **2023**, *129*, 257–267. [CrossRef]
67. Khalil, T.E.; Abdel-Salam, A.H.; Mohamed, L.A.; El-Meligy, E.; El-Dissouky, A. Crosslinked Modified Chitosan Biopolymer for Enhanced Removal of Toxic Cr (VI) from Aqueous Solution. *Int. J. Biol. Macromol.* **2023**, *234*, 123719. [CrossRef] [PubMed]
68. Elgueta, E.; Becerra, Y.; Martínez, A.; Pereira, M.; Carrillo-Varela, I.; Sanhueza, F.; Nuñez, D.; Rivas, B.L. Adsorbents Derived from Xylan Hemicellulose with Removal Properties of Pollutant Metals. *Chin. J. Polym. Sci.* **2023**, *41*, 874–886. [CrossRef]
69. Radotić, K.; Djikanović, D.; Radosavljević, J.S.; Jović-Jovičić, N.; Mojović, Z. Comparative Study of Lignocellulosic Biomass and Its Components as Electrode Modifiers for Detection of Lead and Copper Ions. *J. Electroanal. Chem.* **2020**, *862*, 114010. [CrossRef]
70. Chen, Y.; Zhang, N.; Chen, X. Structurally Modified Polysaccharides: Physicochemical Properties, Biological Activities, Structure–Activity Relationship, and Applications. *J. Agric. Food Chem.* **2024**, *72*, 3259–3276. [CrossRef]
71. Zhao, D.; Zhu, Y.; Cheng, W.; Chen, W.; Wu, Y.; Yu, H. Cellulose-based Flexible Functional Materials for Emerging Intelligent Electronics. *Adv. Mater.* **2021**, *33*, 2000619. [CrossRef] [PubMed]
72. Swingler, S.; Gupta, A.; Gibson, H.; Kowalczuk, M.; Heaselgrave, W.; Radecka, I. Recent Advances and Applications of Bacterial Cellulose in Biomedicine. *Polymers* **2021**, *13*, 412. [CrossRef]

73. Ning, J.; Luo, X.; Wang, F.; Huang, S.; Wang, J.; Liu, D.; Liu, D.; Chen, D.; Wei, J.; Liu, Y. Synergetic Sensing Effect of Sodium Carboxymethyl Cellulose and Bismuth on Cadmium Detection by Differential Pulse Anodic Stripping Voltammetry. *Sensors* **2019**, *19*, 5482. [CrossRef] [PubMed]
74. Qin, D.; Hu, X.; Dong, Y.; Mamat, X.; Li, Y.; Wågberg, T.; Hu, G. An Electrochemical Sensor Based on Green γ-AlOOH-Carbonated Bacterial Cellulose Hybrids for Simultaneous Determination Trace Levels of Cd (II) and Pb (II) in Drinking Water. *J. Electrochem. Soc.* **2018**, *165*, B328–B334. [CrossRef]
75. Zinoubi, K.; Majdoub, H.; Barhoumi, H.; Boufi, S.; Jaffrezic-Renault, N. Determination of Trace Heavy Metal Ions by Anodic Stripping Voltammetry Using Nanofibrillated Cellulose Modified Electrode. *J. Electroanal. Chem.* **2017**, *799*, 70–77. [CrossRef]
76. Taheri, M.; Ahour, F.; Keshipour, S. Sensitive and Selective Determination of Cu^{2+} at D-Penicillamine Functionalized Nano-Cellulose Modified Pencil Graphite Electrode. *J. Phys. Chem. Solids* **2018**, *117*, 180–187. [CrossRef]
77. Priya, T.; Dhanalakshmi, N.; Karthikeyan, V.; Thinakaran, N. Highly Selective Simultaneous Trace Determination of Cd^{2+} and Pb^{2+} Using Porous Graphene/Carboxymethyl Cellulose/Fondaparinux Nanocomposite Modified Electrode. *J. Electroanal. Chem.* **2019**, *833*, 543–551. [CrossRef]
78. Teodoro, K.B.; Migliorini, F.L.; Facure, M.H.; Correa, D.S. Conductive Electrospun Nanofibers Containing Cellulose Nanowhiskers and Reduced Graphene Oxide for the Electrochemical Detection of Mercury (II). *Carbohydr. Polym.* **2019**, *207*, 747–754. [CrossRef]
79. Padmalaya, G.; Sreeja, B.; Dinesh Kumar, P.; Radha, S.; Poornima, V.; Arivanandan, M.; Shrestha, S.; Uma, T. A Facile Synthesis of Cellulose Acetate Functionalized Zinc Oxide Nanocomposite for Electrochemical Sensing of Cadmium Ions. *J. Inorg. Organomet. Polym. Mater.* **2019**, *29*, 989–999. [CrossRef]
80. Abdelhamid, H.N.; Georgouvelas, D.; Edlund, U.; Mathew, A.P. CelloZIFPaper: Cellulose-ZIF Hybrid Paper for Heavy Metal Removal and Electrochemical Sensing. *Chem. Eng. J.* **2022**, *446*, 136614. [CrossRef]
81. Zhang, B.; Chen, J.; Zhu, H.; Yang, T.; Zou, M.; Zhang, M.; Du, M. Facile and Green Fabrication of Size-Controlled AuNPs/CNFs Hybrids for the Highly Sensitive Simultaneous Detection of Heavy Metal Ions. *Electrochim. Acta* **2016**, *196*, 422–430. [CrossRef]
82. Bressi, V.; Celesti, C.; Ferlazzo, A.; Len, T.; Moulaee, K.; Neri, G.; Luque, R.; Espro, C. Waste-Derived Carbon Nanodots for Fluorimetric and Simultaneous Electrochemical Detection of Heavy Metals in Water. *Environ. Sci. Nano* **2024**, *11*, 1245–1258. [CrossRef]
83. Sotolářová, J.; Vinter, Š.; Filip, J. Cellulose Derivatives Crosslinked by Citric Acid on Electrode Surface as a Heavy Metal Absorption/Sensing Matrix. *Colloids Surf. A Physicochem. Eng. Asp.* **2021**, *628*, 127242. [CrossRef]
84. Wang, Z.; Yang, H.; Zhu, Z. Study on the Blends of Silk Fibroin and Sodium Alginate: Hydrogen Bond Formation, Structure and Properties. *Polymer* **2019**, *163*, 144–153. [CrossRef]
85. Chen, J.; Zhang, M.; Liao, Q.; Wang, L.; Li, H.; Niu, X.; Liu, X.; Wang, K. Integrated Polysaccharides via Amidation for Sensitive Electrochemical Detection of Heavy Metal Ions. *J. Mater. Sci. Mater. Electron.* **2022**, *33*, 8140–8150. [CrossRef]
86. Chrouda, A. A Novel Electrochemical Sensor Based on Sodium Alginate-Decorated Single-Walled Carbon Nanotubes for the Direct Electrocatalysis of Heavy Metals Ions. *Polym. Adv. Technol.* **2023**, *34*, 1807–1816. [CrossRef]
87. Crini, G.; Badot, P.-M.; Roberts, G.A.; Guibal, E. *Chitine et Chitosane: Du Biopolymère à l'application*; Presses Universitaires de. Franche-Comté: Besançon, France, 2009; p. 209, ISBN 2-84867-249-8.
88. Jiang, Y.; Wu, J. Recent Development in Chitosan Nanocomposites for Surface-based Biosensor Applications. *Electrophoresis* **2019**, *40*, 2084–2097. [CrossRef]
89. Hwang, J.-H.; Wang, X.; Pathak, P.; Rex, M.M.; Cho, H.J.; Lee, W.H. Enhanced Electrochemical Detection of Multiheavy Metal Ions Using a Biopolymer-Coated Planar Carbon Electrode. *IEEE Trans. Instrum. Meas.* **2019**, *68*, 2387–2393. [CrossRef]
90. Hadnine, S.; Zighed, L.; Abbassi, H.; Rahmouni, S.; Zouaoui, E. Determination of Hg (II) by Thiourea Grafted Chitosan Modified Carbon Paste Electrode: Reversibility and Electrochemical Parameters Studies. *Anal. Bioanal. Electrochem.* **2019**, *11*, 1716–1734.
91. Fort, C.I.; Cotet, L.C.; Vulpoi, A.; Turdean, G.L.; Danciu, V.; Baia, L.; Popescu, I.C. Bismuth Doped Carbon Xerogel Nanocomposite Incorporated in Chitosan Matrix for Ultrasensitive Voltammetric Detection of Pb (II) and Cd (II). *Sens. Actuators B Chem.* **2015**, *220*, 712–719. [CrossRef]
92. Pathak, P.; Hwang, J.-H.; Li, R.H.T.; Rodriguez, K.L.; Rex, M.M.; Lee, W.H.; Cho, H.J. Flexible Copper-Biopolymer Nanocomposite Sensors for Trace Level Lead Detection in Water. *Sens. Actuators B Chem.* **2021**, *344*, 130263. [CrossRef]
93. Zhou, S.-F.; Han, X.-J.; Liu, Y.-Q. SWASV Performance toward Heavy Metal Ions Based on a High-Activity and Simple Magnetic Chitosan Sensing Nanomaterials. *J. Alloys Compd.* **2016**, *684*, 1–7. [CrossRef]
94. Shang, J.; Zhao, M.; Qu, H.; Li, H.; Gao, R.; Chen, S. New Application of Pn Junction in Electrochemical Detection: The Detection of Heavy Metal Ions. *J. Electroanal. Chem.* **2019**, *855*, 113624. [CrossRef]
95. Guo, Z.; Luo, X.; Li, Y.; Zhao, Q.-N.; Li, M.; Zhao, Y.; Sun, T.; Ma, C. Simultaneous Determination of Trace Cd (II), Pb (II) and Cu (II) by Differential Pulse Anodic Stripping Voltammetry Using a Reduced Graphene Oxide-Chitosan/Poly-l-Lysine Nanocomposite Modified Glassy Carbon Electrode. *J. Colloid Interface Sci.* **2017**, *490*, 11–22. [CrossRef]
96. Wei, P.; Zhu, Z.; Song, R.; Li, Z.; Chen, C. An Ion-Imprinted Sensor Based on Chitosan-Graphene Oxide Composite Polymer Modified Glassy Carbon Electrode for Environmental Sensing Application. *Electrochim. Acta* **2019**, *317*, 93–101. [CrossRef]

97. Yin, J.; Zhai, H.; Wang, Y.; Wang, B.; Chu, G.; Guo, Q.; Zhang, Y.; Sun, X.; Guo, Y.; Zhang, Y. COF/MWCNTs/CLS-Based Electrochemical Sensor for Simultaneous and Sensitive Detection of Multiple Heavy Metal Ions. *Food Anal. Methods* **2022**, *15*, 3244–3256. [CrossRef]
98. Xu, T.; Dai, H.; Jin, Y. Electrochemical Sensing of Lead (II) by Differential Pulse Voltammetry Using Conductive Polypyrrole Nanoparticles. *Microchim. Acta* **2020**, *187*, 1–7. [CrossRef] [PubMed]
99. Singh, V.K.; Kushwaha, C.S.; Shukla, S. Potentiometric Detection of Copper Ion Using Chitin Grafted Polyaniline Electrode. *Int. J. Biol. Macromol.* **2020**, *147*, 250–257. [CrossRef] [PubMed]
100. Liu, Y.; Deng, Y.; Li, T.; Chen, Z.; Chen, H.; Li, S.; Liu, H. Aptamer-Based Electrochemical Biosensor for Mercury Ions Detection Using AuNPs-Modified Glass Carbon Electrode. *J. Biomed. Nanotechnol.* **2018**, *14*, 2156–2161. [CrossRef]
101. Liu, Y.; Lai, Y.; Yang, G.; Tang, C.; Deng, Y.; Li, S.; Wang, Z. Cd-Aptamer Electrochemical Biosensor Based on AuNPs/CS Modified Glass Carbon Electrode. *J. Biomed. Nanotechnol.* **2017**, *13*, 1253–1259. [CrossRef]
102. Mo, Z.; Liu, H.; Hu, R.; Gou, H.; Li, Z.; Guo, R. Amino-Functionalized Graphene/Chitosan Composite as an Enhanced Sensing Platform for Highly Selective Detection of Cu^{2+}. *Ionics* **2018**, *24*, 1505–1513. [CrossRef]
103. Wu, S.; Li, K.; Dai, X.; Zhang, Z.; Ding, F.; Li, S. An Ultrasensitive Electrochemical Platform Based on Imprinted Chitosan/Gold Nanoparticles/Graphene Nanocomposite for Sensing Cadmium (II) Ions. *Microchem. J.* **2020**, *155*, 104710. [CrossRef]
104. Wong, A.; Ferreira, P.A.; Santos, A.M.; Cincotto, F.H.; Silva, R.A.B.; Sotomayor, M.D.P.T. A New Electrochemical Sensor Based on Eco-Friendly Chemistry for the Simultaneous Determination of Toxic Trace Elements. *Microchem. J.* **2020**, *158*, 105292. [CrossRef]
105. Guo, C.; Wang, C.; Sun, H.; Dai, D.; Gao, H. A Simple Electrochemical Sensor Based on rGO/MoS_2/CS Modified GCE for Highly Sensitive Detection of Pb(Ii) in Tobacco Leaves. *RSC Adv.* **2021**, *11*, 29590–29597. [CrossRef]
106. Boultif, W.; Dehchar, C.; Belhocine, Y.; Zouaoui, E.; Rahali, S.; Zouari, S.E.; Sbei, N.; Seydou, M. Chitosan and Metal Oxide Functionalized Chitosan as Efficient Sensors for Lead (II) Detection in Wastewater. *Separations* **2023**, *10*, 479. [CrossRef]
107. Bouraoui, S.; Zazoua, A.; Braiek, M.; Jaffrezic-Renault, N. A New Sensitive and Selective Sensor for Heavy Metal Ions Based on Tannin Extracted from the Skin of *Punica granatum* L. *Int. J. Environ. Anal. Chem.* **2016**, *96*, 739–751. [CrossRef]
108. Zazoua, A.; Khedimallah, N.; Jaffrezic-Renault, N. Electrochemical Determination of Cadmium, Lead, and Nickel Using a Polyphenol–Polyvinyl Chloride—Boron-Doped Diamond Electrode. *Anal. Lett.* **2018**, *51*, 336–347. [CrossRef]
109. Suherman, A.L.; Kuss, S.; Tanner, E.E.L.; Young, N.P.; Compton, R.G. Electrochemical Hg^{2+} Detection at Tannic Acid-Gold Nanoparticle Modified Electrodes by Square Wave Voltammetry. *Analyst* **2018**, *143*, 2035–2041. [CrossRef]
110. Gonçalves, S.S.L.; Rudnitskaya, A.; Sales, A.J.M.; Costa, L.M.C.; Evtuguin, D.V. Nanocomposite Polymeric Materials Based on Eucalyptus Lignoboost® Kraft Lignin for Liquid Sensing Applications. *Materials* **2020**, *13*, 1637. [CrossRef] [PubMed]
111. Mahfoud, H.; Morakchi, K.; Hamel, A.; Bendjama, A.; Saifi, H.; Belghiche, R. Electrochemical Characterization of Modified Platinum Electrode by Using Lignin from Stone Olive as Ionophore. *J. Iran. Chem. Soc.* **2022**, *19*, 313–318. [CrossRef]
112. Bao, Q.-X.; Liu, Y.; Liang, Y.-Q.; Weerasooriya, R.; Li, H.; Wu, Y.-C.; Chen, X. Tea Polyphenols Mediated Zero-Valent Iron/Reduced Graphene Oxide Nanocomposites for Electrochemical Determination of Hg^{2+}. *J. Electroanal. Chem.* **2022**, *917*, 116428. [CrossRef]
113. Vicentini, F.C.; Silva, L.R.G.; Stefano, J.S.; Lima, A.R.F.; Prakash, J.; Bonacin, J.A.; Janegitz, B.C. Starch-Based Electrochemical Sensors and Biosensors: A Review. *Biomed. Mater. Devices* **2022**, *1*, 319–338. [CrossRef]
114. Alves, G.M.; da Silva, J.L.; Stradiotto, N.R. A Novel Citrus Pectin-Modified Carbon Paste Electrochemical Sensor Used for Copper Determination in Biofuel. *Measurement* **2021**, *169*, 108356. [CrossRef]
115. Arulraj, A.D.; Devasenathipathy, R.; Chen, S.-M.; Vasantha, V.S.; Wang, S.-F. Femtomolar Detection of Mercuric Ions Using Polypyrrole, Pectin and Graphene Nanocomposites Modified Electrode. *J. Colloid Interface Sci.* **2016**, *483*, 268–274. [CrossRef]
116. El Hamdouni, Y.; El Hajjaji, S.; Szabo, T.; Trif, L.; Felhősi, I.; Abbi, K.; Labjar, N.; Harmouche, L.; Shaban, A. Biomass Valorization of Walnut Shell into Biochar as a Resource for Electrochemical Simultaneous Detection of Heavy Metal Ions in Water and Soil Samples: Preparation, Characterization, and Applications. *Arab. J. Chem.* **2022**, *15*, 104252. [CrossRef]
117. de Oliveira Farias, E.A.; dos Santos, M.C.; de Araujo Dionísio, N.; Quelemes, P.V.; de Leite, J.R.S.A.; Eaton, P.; da Silva, D.A.; Eiras, C. Layer-by-Layer Films Based on Biopolymers Extracted from Red Seaweeds and Polyaniline for Applications in Electrochemical Sensors of Chromium VI. *Mater. Sci. Eng. B* **2015**, *200*, 9–21. [CrossRef]
118. Hwang, J.-H.; Fox, D.; Stanberry, J.; Anagnostopoulos, V.; Zhai, L.; Lee, W.H. Direct Mercury Detection in Landfill Leachate Using a Novel AuNP-Biopolymer Carbon Screen-Printed Electrode Sensor. *Micromachines* **2021**, *12*, 649. [CrossRef] [PubMed]
119. Mondal, B.; Banerjee, S.; Samanta, S.K.; Senapati, S.; Tripathy, T. Highly Selective and Sensitive Electrochemical Sensing of Trace Zn^{2+} Ions, by Grafted Tricholoma Mushroom Polysaccharide/Ag Composite Nanoparticles in Aqueous Medium. *Appl. Organomet. Chem.* **2021**, *35*, e6171. [CrossRef]
120. Silva, I.B.; de Araújo, D.M.; Vocciante, M.; Ferro, S.; Martínez-Huitle, C.A.; Dos Santos, E.V. Electrochemical Determination of Lead Using A Composite Sensor Obtained from Low-Cost Green Materials:Graphite/Cork. *Appl. Sci.* **2021**, *11*, 2355. [CrossRef]
121. Palisoc, S.T.; Vitto, R.I.M.; Noel, M.G.; Palisoc, K.T.; Natividad, M.T. Highly Sensitive Determination of Heavy Metals in Water Prior to and after Remediation Using Citrofortunella Microcarpa. *Sci. Rep.* **2021**, *11*, 1394. [CrossRef]

122. Qin, X.; Tang, D.; Zhang, Y.; Cheng, Y.; He, F.; Su, Z.; Jiang, H. An Electrochemical Sensor for Simultaneous Stripping Determination of Cd(II) and Pb(II) Based on Gold Nanoparticles Functionalized β-Cyclodextrin-Graphene Hybrids. *Int. J. Electrochem. Sci.* **2020**, *15*, 1517–1528. [CrossRef]
123. Elamin, M.B.; Chrouda, A.; Ali, S.M.A.; Alhaidari, L.M.; Jabli, M.; Alrouqi, R.M.; Renault, N.J. Electrochemical Sensor Based on Gum Arabic Nanoparticles for Rapid and In-Situ Detection of Different Heavy Metals in Real Samples. *Heliyon* **2024**, *10*, 4. [CrossRef]

chemosensors

MDPI

Review

A Review on Analytical Techniques for Quantitative Detection of Biogenic Amines in Aquatic Products

Zixin Chen [1], Jing Xie [1,2,3,4,*] and Jun Mei [1,2,3,4,*]

1 College of Food Science & Technology, Shanghai Ocean University, Shanghai 201306, China; m240401141@st.shou.edu.cn
2 Shanghai Professional Technology Service Platform on Cold Chain Equipment Performance and Energy Saving Evaluation, Shanghai Ocean University, Shanghai 201306, China
3 National Experimental Teaching Demonstration Center for Food Science and Engineering, Shanghai Ocean University, Shanghai 201306, China
4 Shanghai Engineering Research Center of Aquatic Product Processing & Preservation, Shanghai Ocean University, Shanghai 201306, China
* Correspondence: jxie@shou.edu.cn (J.X.); jmei@shou.edu.cn (J.M.)

Abstract: Aquatic products contain a large amount of protein, which can promote the production of a variety of biogenic amines through the function of microorganisms. Biogenic amines are a broad category of organic substances that contain nitrogen and have a low molecular weight. The presence of biogenic amines can cause the deterioration and excessive accumulation of aquatic products, which can cause damage to human health. Therefore, it is essential to discover a fast, convenient, and easy to operate method for the determination of biogenic amines in aquatic products. In this paper, the function and research significance of biogenic amines are analyzed from the aspects of their formation, toxicological properties, harm to the human body, and control methods. Several common direct detection techniques and indirect techniques for biogenic amines are briefly introduced especially sensors. This review provides references for efficient detection in the future.

Keywords: biogenic amines; aquatic products; detection methods; chemo-sensors

1. Introduction

Aquatic products contain a large amount of protein. During the storage and transportation of aquatic products, microorganisms can decompose the protein to form amino acids. However, there are some potential safety issues with aquatic products, which may be major sources of heavy metals, persistent organic pollutants, parasites, microorganisms, and certain natural toxins [1]. In addition, during the drying process, lipids (triglycerides and phospholipids) in aquatic products are broken down by lipase to produce free fatty acids, which undergo additional oxidation to create a variety of aromatic compounds, including alcohols, ketones, and fatty aldehydes [2]. Free amino acids undergo decarboxylation reactions to produce biogenic amines. Biogenic amines are a class of compounds with low molecular weight and containing nitrogen. Basic details and chemical structures of a number of common biogenic amines are represented in Table 1. They have certain biological activity, which is widely found in diverse foods, including cheese, wine, meat, and aquatic products [3]. Trace biogenic amines are essential active ingredients in living organisms and have important physiological functions in living cells. They can promote the growth of organisms, monitor the production of nucleic acids and proteins, eliminate free radicals, and so on. However, if humans consume a great number of biogenic amines from aquatic products, or biogenic amines build up to significant quantities within the human body, they probably cause harm to human health, resulting in respiratory system issues, vomiting, headaches, cramping in the abdomen, and other adverse physiological reactions [4]. Normally, several enzymes in the human gut, such as diamine oxidase (DAO), monoamine oxidase (MAO), and polyamine oxidase (PAO), can degrade biogenic amines, thus avoiding excessive accumulation [5]. Among biogenic amines, histamine has the strongest toxicity, as it can bind to receptors on the cell membrane to produce toxicity. Tyramine is also highly toxic, and when ingested in excess, toxic phenomena such as migraines and high blood pressure can occur.

In both fermented and non-fermented products, biogenic amines are frequently found, such as cheese containing 5–4500 mg kg^{-1}. There are 2400–5000 mg kg^{-1} biogenic amines in fish and beef liver, which contain biogenic amines of 340 mg kg^{-1} [6]. For unfermented foods, biogenic amines can be used as a biomarker to analyze the decomposition of chemical components in food, as well as indicators of spoilage in certain foods. There is a detection index called the biogenic amine index (BAI), which can determine the character of seafood products and make the results have a certain degree of scientific and measurable validity. Its calculation formula is:

$$\begin{aligned} BAI = (&mg\ kg^{-1}\ histamine + mg\ kg^{-1}\ putrescine \\ &+mg\ kg^{-1}\ cadaverine)/(1 \\ &+mg\ kg^{-1}\ spermine + mg\ kg^{-1} spermidine) \end{aligned}$$

It is considered that there is some quality loss in the product when the BAI exceeds 10 [7].

All amines from different foods in a meal should be added up to determine the entire quantity of biogenic amines consumed rather than considering a single food separately. At the same time, when consuming different foods, the cumulative effects of different amines should also be considered. Therefore, many countries have strict intake standards for biogenic amines. Timely detection of excessive biogenic amines in aquatic products can effectively guarantee that they are safe to consume and have a good flavor [8]. Therefore, the development of a quick and precise detection technique to identify the categories and concentrations of biogenic amines has progressively drawn attention from researchers. There are several indirect detection methods, which mainly involve detecting biogenic amines by detecting the presence of amine-producing bacteria. In addition, chromatography, immunological recognition, enzymatic reaction, pH variation, fluorometry, biosensors, chemo-sensors, and optical chemo-sensor systems are used as the direct detection methods. Among them, sensors such as chemo-sensors have become popular in recent years for being fast, simple, and cost-effective. Although chromatography is widely used in practical applications, its high equipment cost and strict requirements for operators limit its application. Therefore, in recent years, sensors, especially chemical sensors, have become popular. Researchers can design and choose appropriate technologies according to different purposes, such as using pH sensors when only determining the presence or absence of biogenic amines. This method is fast, easy to operate, and easy to observe. If qualitative and quantitative detection of biogenic amines is required, nanomaterials can be considered. Due to the wide range of choices and the great application prospects of chemical sensors, continuous improvement of chemical sensor technology is a future trend for the efficient detection of biogenic amines.

The purpose of this review is to provide theoretical support for the efficient detection of biogenic amines in the future by introducing the formation, classification, hazards, and inhibition measures of biogenic amines, and by focusing on the detection methods.

Table 1. Information of main biogenic amines.

Biogenic Amine	Relative Molecular Mass	Classification	Precursor	Chemical Structures	Reference
Tryptamine	160.22	Heterocyclic Amine	Tryptophan	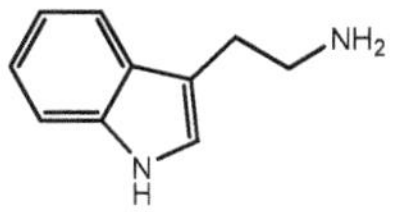	[9]
Histamine	111.15	Heterocyclic Amine	Histidine	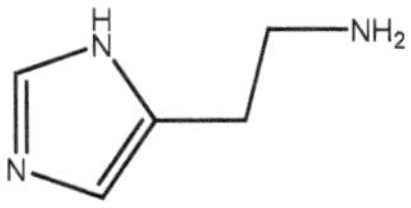	[10]
Tyramine	137.18	Aromatic Amine	Tyrosine	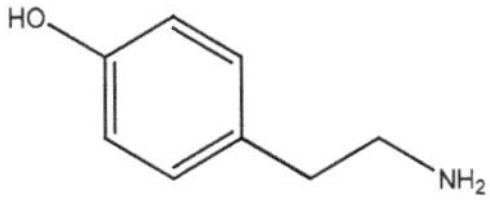	[11]
β-Phenylethylamine	121.18	Aromatic Amine	Phenylalanine	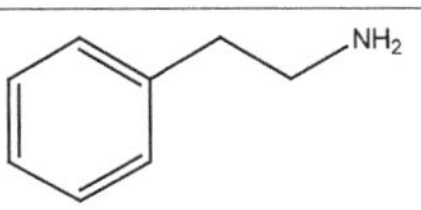	[12]
Spermine	202.34	Aliphatic Amine	Arginine Ornithine	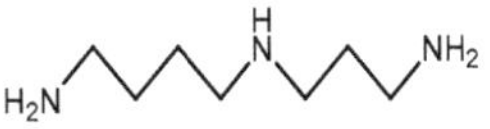	[13]
Spermidine	145.25	Aliphatic Amine	Arginine Ornithine	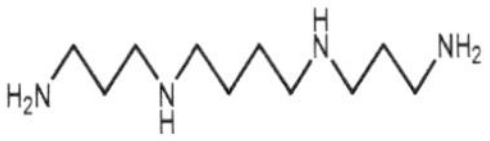	[14]
Cadaverine	102.18	Aliphatic Amine	Lysine	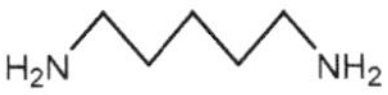	[15]

2. Biogenic Amines in Aquatic Products

2.1. Classification and Sources of Biogenic Amines

There are several different classification methods for biogenic amines due to the differences in the structure of precursor amino acids, the quantity of amino acids, and the source of biogenic amines.

According to the structure of precursor amino acids, there are three types of biogenic amines, heterocyclic, aromatic, and aliphatic. Heterocyclic compounds include serotonin and histamine. Aliphatic compounds include agmatine, spermidine, putrescine, spermine, and cadaverine. Aromatic compounds include β-phenylethylamine and tyramine. Some aromatic amines, such as serotonin and tyramine, have vasoconstrictive functions, while others, such as histamine and 5-hydroxytryptamine, have vasodilatory functions.

The second classification method relies on the quantity of amino acids. Biogenic amines can be separated into monoamines, like tyramine, histamine, and serotonin; diamines, such as cadaverine and putrescine; and polyamines, including agmatine, spermine, and spermidine.

According to the source, there are two types of biogenic amines: endogenous amines and exogenous amines [16]. Tyramine and histamine play a role in hormone transmission. Dopamine and serotonin act as psychoactive mediators in the central nervous system, and they have certain functions.

Under low-temperature conditions, there is a noticeable number of histamines in marine fish. Cadaverine, histamine, and putrescine are among the various biogenic amines that are present in various aquatic products, including sardines, mackerel, tuna, and herring. There are still many amines in raw fish and its products, the content of which needs to be determined according to whether the fish is fresh or not [17]. Meat and meat products contain abundant proteins and amino acids. During storage, proteins undergo hydrolysis to form peptides. Peptides are not always stable. They then further degrade into oligopeptides and even free amino acids. Under the function of microorganisms, biogenic amines like spermidine, cadaverine, spermine, and histamine are generated [18]. The biogenic amines in dairy products mainly include histamine, tyramine, cadaverine, putrescine, etc., mainly through protein degradation and microbial action in dairy products [19].

2.2. Formation Mechanism and Influence Factors

Due to the action of microorganisms such as proteases, peptidases, and amino acid decarboxylases in aquatic products, proteins are broken down into amino acids, which then undergo decarboxylation reactions to generate biogenic amines. Figure 1 shows the specific procedure. However, some aquatic products do not contain amino acid decarboxylases. In this case, aldehydes and ketones undergo amination reactions with amino groups to generate biogenic amines [20]. In most cases, biogenic amines are formed through decarboxylation reactions under the action of amino acid decarboxylases. Substrate amino acids are exchanged through membrane anti-transporters in extracellular media, and then biogenic amines are synthesized in the cytoplasm. For example, if the exchanged substrate amino acid is tryptophan, serotonin will be synthesized in the cytoplasm [21]. Figure 2 shows the main formation process of biogenic amines. In general, though there are few exceptions, such as putrescine being comprised of arginine and cadaverine being comprised of lysine, precursor amino acid names typically match those of biogenic amines. For example, tyrosine is the source of tyramine, while histidine is the source of histamine.

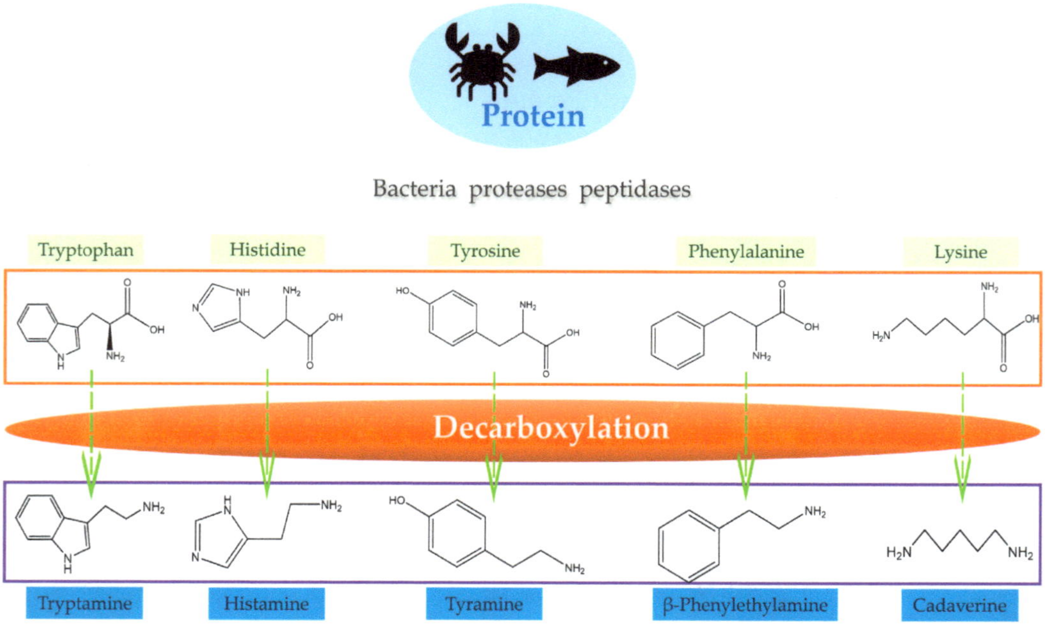

Figure 1. The process of protein degradation into biogenic amines.

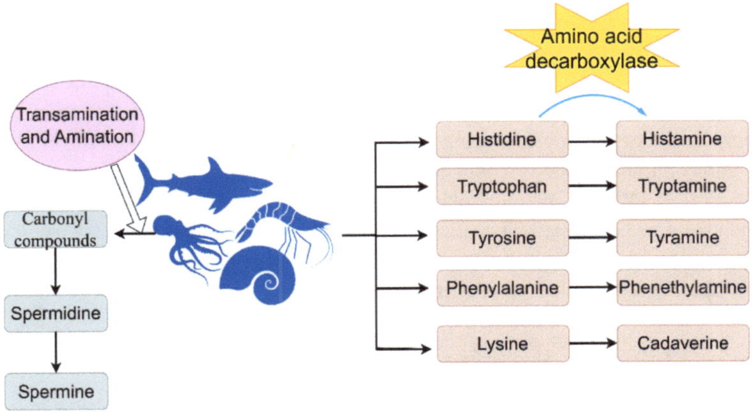

Figure 2. The biogenic amines formation (by Figdraw 2.0).

Some internal and external factors affect the generation of biogenic amines, such as pH, temperature, oxygen supply, and water activity. At the same time, if there are inadequate hygienic conditions for processing and storing food, aquatic products are prone to microbial contamination and the production of biogenic amines. When hygiene conditions are poor, there are various microorganisms in the environment that can rapidly grow under suitable conditions. They may also interact with each other to accelerate the production of biogenic amines. Under temperature conditions, microbial growth, and enzyme activity were inhibited with the decrease in temperature, and the generation of biogenic amines was effectively reduced. When the temperature is too high, the bacteria that produce biogenic amines can be killed, which greatly inhibits the generation of biogenic amines [22]. The optimal temperature range is 20–37 °C [23]. For pH, biogenic amines are more easily produced under acidic conditions. The main reason is that the optimal pH of amino acid decarboxylase is 4.0–5.5. Therefore, under acidic conditions, the content of amino acid decarboxylase gradually increases, causing biogenic amines like tyramine, histamine, and putrescine to significantly increase in content [24]. Oxygen supply also has a great impact on the biosynthesis of biogenic amines. Various bacteria produce different amounts of biogenic amines under different oxygen supply conditions. For example, the amount of putrescine produced by Enterobacter cloacae significantly decreases under anaerobic conditions, while the amount of putrescine synthesized by Klebsiella pneumoniae is less, but the synthesis amount of putrescine has significantly increased under anaerobic conditions [25]. It is worth noting that these influencing factors do not exist alone but work together to promote or inhibit the production of biogenic amines. At the same time, biogenic amines are thermally stable, which means that if the raw material itself contains biogenic amines, they are difficult to remove when products are being heated up, such as pasteurization and cooking. Therefore, biogenic amines are easily absorbed by the human body, posing a health hazard.

2.3. Hazard of Biogenic Amines

The global demand for aquatic products is gradually increasing, but a large amount of waste may be generated during the processing of aquatic products [26]. Excessive intake or accumulation of biogenic amines in the human body can produce a variety of diseases or health problems. They can cause negative physiological responses, like abdominal cramping, headaches, palpitations, vomiting, respiratory system disorders, and other symptoms of poisoning.

2.3.1. Excessive Intake and Accumulation of Biogenic Amines

Normally, biogenic amines intake from aquatic products can be rapidly broken down through amine oxidase or binding, but if certain populations are allergic to biogenic amines or take drugs containing monoamine inhibitors, the normal decomposition process of biogenic amines can be disrupted, leading to their continuous accumulation in the human body [25]. For example, drinking alcohol or taking enzyme drugs and antidepressants that inhibit histamine metabolism are more likely to cause histamine poisoning in humans [19]. When only histamine is ingested if consumed in small amounts, it may not cause harm at lower levels, but sometimes the body may ingest multiple biogenic amines simultaneously. Interactions occur between different biogenic amines like cadaverine and putrescine, which can suppress the activity of histamine oxidase, thus increasing histamine content and enhancing the toxicity of food [19,27,28].

After ingesting biogenic amines, they may accumulate continuously in the body. When biogenic amines accumulate to a certain concentration that exceeds the body's metabolic capacity, it can lead to biogenic amines poisoning. Histamine is the most toxic and can make blood vessels dilate, resulting in an obvious decrease in blood pressure. Next is tyramine, which can promote vasoconstriction. It can induce norepinephrine release and promote adverse reactions of histamine to increase blood pressure [29]. It is worth noting that various biogenic amines, combined with nitrogen, can produce carcinogens such as nitrite and enhance the poisonousness of tyramine and histamine [30]. For fish and other aquatic products, such as tuna, sardines, mackerel, salmon, etc., bacteria-rich muscle histidine in fish can multiply under appropriate temperatures, and the muscle histidine can be converted into histamine [31].

2.3.2. Poisoning of Biogenic Amines

Histamine poisoning, also known as scombroid fish poisoning, has the strongest toxic effect [31]. The main symptoms of poisoning include facial, neck, and upper arm flushing, urticaria, gastrointestinal symptoms, headache, and difficulty swallowing [32]. The incubation period of histamine poisoning is relatively short, usually 20–30 min, and the severity of symptoms is manifested as low or moderate [33]. Due to the fact that the symptoms of histamine poisoning are sometimes similar to allergy symptoms, histamine poisoning can be determined by measuring plasma histamine levels or whether high histamine foods have been consumed [34]. According to literature reports, the number of histamine poisoning cases caused by consuming tuna has been increasing year by year from 2014 to 2017 [33].

Tyramine poisoning, also known as cheese reaction, is characterized by elevated blood pressure, palpitations, and headaches, and it can occur 30 min after ingestion of food and several hours later [35]. Due to the potential interaction between monoamine oxidase inhibitors (MAOI) and tyramine toxicity, it is necessary to pay attention to whether the population is taking MAOI-related drugs [36]. Tyramine plays an important role in the gastrointestinal tract, and an increase in tyramine levels in the gastrointestinal tract may induce the release of inflammatory prostaglandins, leading to pro-inflammatory outcomes [37].

2.4. Control Methods for Biogenic Amines Excessive Accumulation in Aquatic Products

The methods for controlling excessive accumulation of biogenic amines are mainly through two methods: one is to avoid new biogenic amines appearing, and the other is to degrade the synthesized biogenic amines. Figure 3 shows the main control methods.

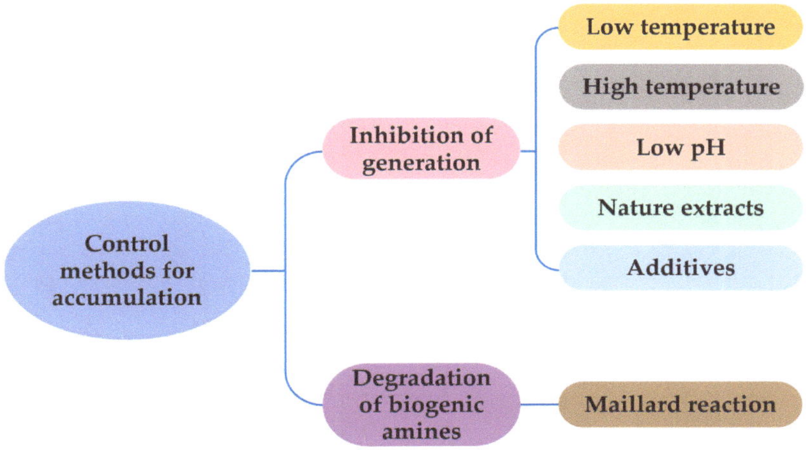

Figure 3. The main control methods for excessive accumulation of biogenic amines.

To inhibit the production of biogenic amines, three methods can be adopted: the first is to control the breakdown of amino acids, the second is to inhibit the propagation of microorganisms like amine-producing bacteria, and the third is to reduce the activity of amino acid decarboxylase.

For the propagation of producing amines bacteria and the activity of decarboxylase, one significant influencing factor is temperature, as both low and high temperatures can have significant impacts on decarboxylase and bacteria. At low temperatures, the enzyme bioactivity and growth of amine-producing bacteria decrease significantly. When ultra-low temperature conditions are reached, 5% to 30% of the water in the microbial cytoplasm begins to freeze, causing the concentration of cytoplasm to gradually increase [38]. When the temperature rises to 60 °C, the growth of amine-producing bacteria can also be inhibited [39]. WANG et al. [40] used brine immersion freezing (BIF) to treat tuna during the processing of canned tuna. The study found that yields of most bioactive substances were low at different stages of processing. Gardini et al. [41] found that low pH is also an effective method to inhibit the production of biogenic amines, and the generation amount increased with the increase in pH.

For canned aquatic products, various kinds of additives such as sodium chloride, sucrose, glucose, NaCl, glycine, lactic acid, citric acid, and sorbic acid were used to avoid the generation of biogenic amines. Food additives mainly inhibit the production of biogenic amines by suppressing the biological activity of amine-producing bacteria [42]. Jae-Hyung et al. [43] used seven different food additives, and the results showed that the glycine treatment group had the most significant decrease in the content of putrescine, cadaverine, and histamine.

Natural extracts such as cinnamon oil extract [44] can be added appropriately to effectively control the production of biogenic amines. In addition, Li et al. [45] found that natural proanthocyanidins have a significant inhibitory effect on putrescine, cadaverine, and tyramine, and this inhibitory mechanism is mainly achieved by affecting the undesirable microbial community and inhibiting microbial activity.

If aquatic products have been processed into canned products, it is difficult to directly remove the synthesized biogenic amines by using traditional refrigeration methods. Therefore, WANG et al. [40] studied the Maillard reaction of glucose with histamine by using fluorescence intensity and UV–VIS spectroscopy. Research has shown that the histamine content in canned tuna is significantly reduced, and the toxicity of Maillard reaction products is also significantly decreased.

2.5. Maximum Residual Limits of Biogenic Amines in Water Bodies

To ensure food safety, biogenic amine detection and management are essential. The safety standard for histamine in aquatic products varies from country to country. The US Food and Drug Administration (FDA) has defined a guidance level of histamine, and the limit of tyramine and β-phenylethylamine in aquatic products is 100–800 and 30 mg/kg [46], respectively. The EU regulates the healthy level of histamine for certain fish species at 100 mg/kg [46]. Table 2 represents the content of various biogenic amines in common aquatic products.

Table 2. Biogenic amine content of aquatic products (mg/kg).

Aquatic Products	Histamine	Cadaverine	Putrescine	Dopamine	Serotonin	Reference
Belt fish	2.6	24.2	15.9			[47]
Octopus	3.2	25.5	18.3			[47]
Common mackerel	1.9	1.4	0.4	<0.03		[48]
Common mullet	1.7	1.7	0.4	<0.03		[48]
Grass carp	2.51	0.90	1.32			[49]
Swimming crab	2.1	10.6	17.3	<0.1	0.1	[50]
Common sea squirt	3.4	18.7	12.5	<0.1	1.6	[50]
Chum salmon	1.4	<0.1	1.8	5.0	<0.1	[50]
Japanese scallop	<0.1	2.5	2.9	<0.1	<0.1	[50]
Silver pomfret	<0.1	<0.1	<0.1	<0.1	<0.1	[50]
Mackerel	2.3	4.8	0.9	1.6	1.2	[51]
Tuna	0.1	0.4	0.5	1.2	0.6	[51]

3. Sample Pre-Treatment Technology

Sample collection, sample pre-processing, analysis and detection, data processing, and reporting results are the four main steps of a comprehensive sample analysis process. The statistical results show that sample pre-treatment in these four steps takes up a considerable amount of time, some even accounting for 70% or more of the entire process. Therefore, in recent years, research on sample pre-treatment methods and techniques has attracted the attention of analysts. The application of appropriate sample pretreatment technology can effectively improve the accuracy, precision, sensitivity, selectivity, and analysis speed of the analytical method, reduce or eliminate matrix interference, and is also conducive to the enrichment of target compounds. During the pre-treatment process, the reaction characteristics of the sample should also be considered. For aquatic products, because of the abundance of fats, proteins, and other substances they contain, selecting appropriate extractants is also crucial. They can dissolve biogenic amines and precipitate proteins. In recent years, as technology and materials continue to advance, sample pre-treatment technology has also been constantly updated and improved to be more accurate and effective for various sample analyses. Here are five sample pre-treatment techniques: QuEChERS (quick, easy, cheap, effective, rugged, safe) [52], solid-phase extraction (SPE) [53], liquid–liquid extraction (LLE) [54], dispersive liquid–liquid microextraction (DLLME) [55], solid-phase microextraction (SPME) [56]. Each of the five technologies has its own characteristics; for example, LLE uses a large volume of solvents that may further exacerbate environmental problems, while SPME does not require solvents during the extraction process [57]. Table 3 shows more characteristics of each pre-treatment technology.

Table 3. Advantages and disadvantages of different sample pre-treatment technology.

Sample Pre-Treatment Technology	Advantages	Disadvantages	Reference
Liquid–liquid extraction (LLE)	Minimal damage to the analyte; Easy to operate	Time consuming; Low extraction ability; High consumption of organic solvent	[58]
Solid-phase extraction (SPE)	Reduced analysis steps; Easy automation; Using no organic solvents	Time-consuming; Relatively expensive	[59]
Solid-phase microextraction (SPME)	Fast, universal; Solvent-less separation	Fibers used may be broken; Coating can be stripped off; Needle can be bent	[60]
Dispersive liquid–liquid microextraction (DLLME)	Easy to operate; Fast; High preconcentration factor; Environmentally friendly	High consumption of solvents; Partition coefficient decrease	[61]
QuEChERS	Easy to operate; Fast; High cost-effectiveness; Less equipment required; Relatively small amounts of solvents	Limited scope of application; Not very suitable for traditional fermented meat products	[62]

3.1. Liquid–Liquid Extraction

LLE is extensively utilized in the fields of environmental, food, and biological analysis due to its simple equipment and operation [63,64]. When using the LLE method, salt-assisted LLE is often considered, as it does not need to be used with immiscible and toxic organic solvents, nor does it require severe mechanical oscillation [65]. Liu et al. [54] detected eight biogenic amines in wine using modified LLE; the limit of detection (LOD) and quantification (LOQ) were 0.001–0.050 mg/L and 0.005–0.167 mg/L, respectively. What's more, the detection time is effectively shortened, the amount of organic reagents is reduced, the cost has been effectively controlled, and the operation is simple and fast, with strong practicality.

3.2. Solid-Phase Extraction

SPE can be divided into the following categories: ion exchange SPE, reverse phase SPE, normal phase SPE, and mixed-mode SPE. The most appropriate method can be selected according to the characteristics of the seafood to be tested and the type and characteristics of different biogenic amines. For example, the interaction force in an aqueous phase sample is mainly van der Waals forces, and thus, reverse phase SPE can be used. The main advantages of SPE include a high recovery rate, reduced analysis steps, shortened analysis time, easy automation, compatibility with chromatographic analysis, and reduced use of organic solvents [66]. Sagratini et al. [53] determined eight biogenic amines, including spermine, cadaverine, spermidine, and so on, in fish; the LOD and LOQ were 0.02–0.25 mg/kg and 0.07–0.75 mg/kg.

3.3. Solid-Phase Microextraction

SPME is a relatively new and easily automated technology used for extracting analytes from gas, liquid, and solid matrices [56]. SPME overcomes the disadvantages of traditional sample pre-treatment techniques. It can integrate sampling, extraction, concentration, and injection, greatly accelerating the rate of analysis and detection. Its significant technological advantages are extensively utilized in fields including food, pharmaceutical industry, and environmental analysis. Headspace SPME (HS-SPME) is extensively used for the preparation and analysis of complex samples. This technique has low matrix interference clear spectra and can protect fibers from irreversible damage, which is caused by non-volatile coexisting compounds present in complex matrices [40]. Chen et al. [67] designed a functionalized mesoporous silica-coated SPE Arrow system to determine six biogenic amines, and the results showed that the LOD and LOQ were 1.1–26.8 $\mu g\ L^{-1}$ and 3.5–89.3 $\mu g\ L^{-1}$, respectively. HS-SPME is also applied to extract and determine the contents of putrescine, histamine, and tyramine in canned aquatic products. Figure 4 shows the application of SPME in recent years.

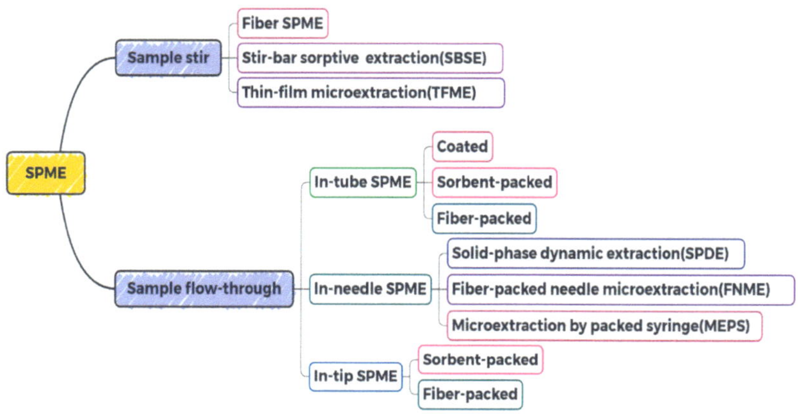

Figure 4. The application of SPME technology (by Xmind 24.01.14361).

3.4. Dispersive Liquid–Liquid Microextraction

DLLME is environmentally friendly, fast, simple, and easy. Figure 5 shows the basic process of applying the DLLME method, with red wine as the sample. Zhang et al. [55] used $CHCl_3$ as the extractant, and the dispersant was methanol. The results showed that the linear relationship performs well. The LOD and LOQ were at a low level, which was 1.77 and 5.33 $\mu g\ kg^{-1}$, respectively.

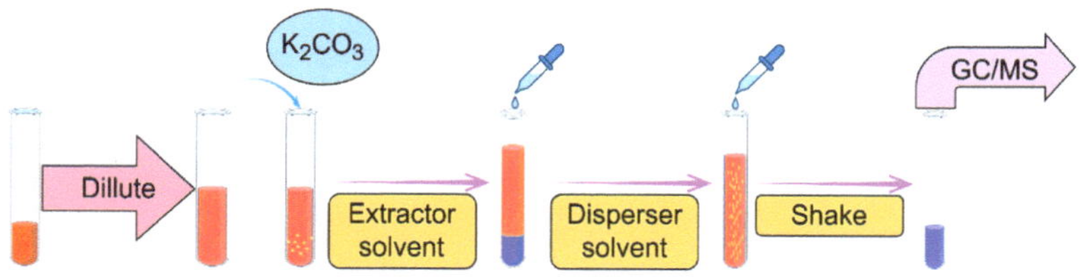

Figure 5. The process of the DLLME method (by Figdraw 2.0).

3.5. QuEChERS

QuEChERS is a widely used sample pre-treatment technique, which is essentially a sample pretreatment method formed by a combination of oscillation extraction, LLE for preliminary purification, and matrix dispersion SPE for purification. Compared with traditional methods (LLE, SPE), the QuEChERS method has many advantages, such as simple and fast operation, high cost-effectiveness, less equipment required, use of inert materials and relatively small amounts of solvents, etc. [62]. Guo et al. [52] researched the pollution characteristics of seven biogenic amines in eight types of canned sea fish samples. The study used carbon sphere QuEChERS mixed dispersion SPE coupled with high-performance liquid chromatography (HPLC) to analyze and determine the samples. The experimental data indicated that the experiment had a high recovery rate (92.3–97.7%), LOD, and LOQ of seven biogenic amines were 7.2–10.8 mg/kg and 24–36 mg/kg, respectively. Therefore, with this technique, biogenic amines in canned fish can be accurately detected.

4. Detection Techniques of Biogenic Amines

With the advancement of technology, there are diverse methods for detecting biogenic amines, including direct and indirect detection methods. The indirect detection methods do not directly identify biogenic amines but rather measure the activity of amine-producing bacteria. This type of method is extremely unstable and susceptible to various factors, such as the environment. On the contrary, direct detection methods yield more accurate results and can classify different biogenic amines with higher credibility. This review mainly introduces several specific methods for detecting biogenic amines. Figure 6 shows the classification of several detection methods in this review.

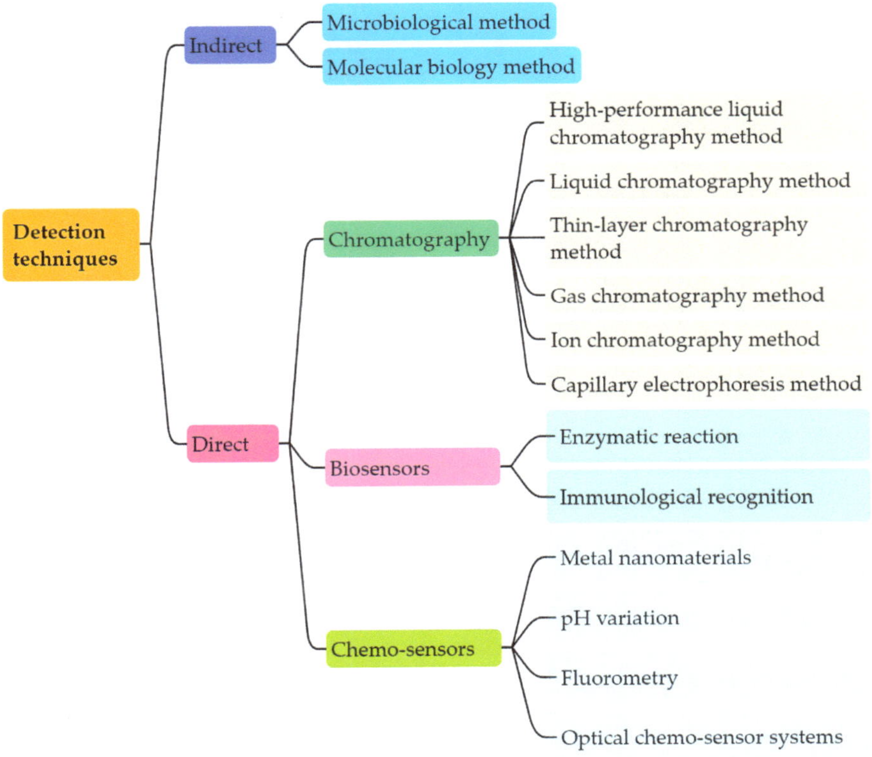

Figure 6. Classification of detection methods (by Xmind 24.01.14361).

4.1. Indirect Detection Technique of Biological Amines

The type of biogenic amines in aquatic products can be judged indirectly by detecting the amount and type of bacteria that can produce amines, including microbiological and molecular biology methods. Compared with the direct detection technology of biogenic amines, indirect detection technology is fast and simple, but its accuracy and specificity are poor. In addition, finding amine-producing bacteria does not always mean that a biogenic amine in aquatic products is present, and even if it is, it is unclear how much. The generation of biogenic amines is also influenced by environmental factors.

4.1.1. Microbiological Method

Proteins in aquatic products are broken down by microorganisms, such as proteases and peptidases, to form amino acids and other chemical substances. Free amino acids undergo decarboxylation reactions to produce biogenic amines. Therefore, indirect detection technology can determine biogenic amines by detecting the categories and quantities of microorganisms present in aquatic products. If amine-producing bacteria can grow in food, then it is highly likely that biogenic amines will be detected. When biogenic amines degrade, they can restrain the reproduction of harmful bacteria, degrade nitrites, and provide a good taste [68]. In aquatic products, the main amine-producing bacteria are Hafnia alvei, Klebsiella variicola, Proteus vulgaris, Morganella psychrotolerans, Morganella morganii, Pantoea agglomerans, Enterobacter aerogenes, Photobacterium phosphoreum, Acinetobacter baumannii, which are all Gram-negative contaminants [21]. Generally, selective culture media are used to identify amine-producing bacteria, and then alkaline biogenic amines are stained with the acid–base indicator bromocresol violet to screen for amine-producing bacteria [69]. However, there may be some alkaline metabolites [70] in the medium, which are produced by the complex metabolic processes of microorganisms. They can affect the identification results and cause false positives, so it is necessary to adjust the composition of the culture medium according to the specific type of biogenic amines. Therefore, although microbiological methods can detect biogenic amines, they have significant limitations and are susceptible to external interference.

4.1.2. Molecular Biology Method

Compared with traditional methods, molecular biology methods are rapid, scientific, and reliable, and no culture is required. Before biogenic amines are produced, it can predict whether a food will produce biogenic amines [71]. Multiple PCR technology has become increasingly popular in recent years, and it can simultaneously and rapidly detect multiple amine-producing bacteria [72]. In raw fish products, histamine can be produced because Gram-negative bacteria are present in the gut. The histamine in tuna and mackerel is produced by the decarboxylation of histidine decarboxylase (HDC), which exists in muscle tissue during the breakdown process [71]. Therefore, it is essential to efficiently detect bacteria that can produce histidine in order to prevent microbial invasion and reproduction and high-level histamine production during the storage and processing of aquatic products [71]. Takahashi et al. [73] designed a technique by PCR for rapid determination of bacteria that can generate histamine and is Gram-negative. What's more, they used single-strand conformation polymorphism (SSCP) technology to analyze the amplification products of the HDC gene for identification. The method collected 37 strains that can produce histamine and 470 strains that cannot produce histamine from fish and determined their histamine formation content using paper chromatography. Strains of P. phosphoreum, Proteus vulgaris, E. aerogenes, Enterobacter amnigenus, M. morganii, R. planticola, Hafnia alvei, P. damselae were positive by detecting by PCR, while the 470 strains that cannot produce histamine did not produce any amplification products. Table 4 presents some primer-related information used in the PCR assay.

Table 4. Primers used in the PCR assay.

Primer	Target Gene	Sequence	Amplicon Size (bp)
PUT1-F	ornithine decarboxylase	TWYMAYGCNGAYAARACNTAYYYTGT	1440
PUT1-R	ornithine decarboxylase	ACRCANAGNACNCCNGGNGGRTANGG	1440
HIS1-F	histidine decarboxylase	GGNATNGTNWSNTAYGAYMGNGCNGA	372
HIS2-R	histidine decarboxylase	TANGGNSANCCDATCATYTTRTGNCC	531
TDC-F	tyrosine decarboxylase	TGGYTNGTNCCNCARACNAARCAYTA	825
TDC-R	tyrosine decarboxylase	ACRTARTCNACCATRTTRAARTCNGG	825

4.2. Direct Detection Technique of Biological Amines

4.2.1. Chromatography

Chromatography can be used to determine the amounts of biogenic amines present. The following six common chromatographic detection techniques are introduced. They are high-performance liquid chromatography (HPLC), liquid chromatography (LC), ion chromatography (IC), capillary electrophoresis (CE), thin-layer chromatography (TLC), and gas chromatography (GC).

High-Performance Liquid Chromatography Method

The method most frequently employed for quantitative analysis of biogenic amines is HPLC, which can detect biogenic amines sensitively and obtain scientific and reliable data. Each component in a mixture can be identified, separated, and quantified using this method. An HPLC–MS/MS method was established by Nalazek-Rudnicka et al. [74] to identify biogenic amines in alcoholic beverages (beer and wine). It was derivatized with tosyl chloride. The technique had high sensitivity and good reproducibility. In this manner, the majority of biogenic amines can be found. Fu et al. [75] identified eight biogenic amines in aquatic products using HPLC. The findings demonstrated that there was a good linear relationship ($r^2 > 0.999$) among phenylethylamine, tryptamine, spermidine, histamine, putrescine, and cadaverine. The maximum LOD value for eight biogenic amines is 0.021 mg kg^{-1}, and the minimum value is 0.007 mg kg^{-1}. The LOQ value range of eight biogenic amines is 0.024–0.069 mg kg^{-1}. The spiked recovery rate was basically between 68% and 123%, indicating that this method can be considered when detecting biogenic amines in multiple aquatic products at once. During the operation of HPLC, due to the lack of suitable chromophores for most biogenic amines, derivatization with reagents such as dansyl chloride (Dns-Cl) and o-phthalaldehyde (OPA) is necessary before the detection of fluorescence or ultraviolet. However, the derivatization process of the current approach is time-consuming and laborious, and the price of Dns-Cl is relatively high [76,77].

Liquid Chromatography Method

The LC method is a commonly used method for detecting biogenic amines, second only to the HPLC method, and it also has high accuracy, sensitivity, and selectivity [78]. The mechanism of separation of LC is grounded in the different partition coefficients of all of the mixtures in the fixed phase and the mobile phase. LC has three categories, including liquid–solid chromatography, liquid–liquid chromatography, and bonded phase chromatography, which are mainly different from stationary phases. In addition, because of the different types of stationary phases, LC is classified into column chromatography, paper chromatography, and thin-layer chromatography. LC with pre- or post-column is mainly applied to biogenic amine separation and quantification [79]. Veciana-Nogues et al. [80] established a post-column derivatization LC method for biogenic amines detection in fish and its products. The method regulated the column and post-column apparatus for reactions under the condition of room temperature. The experiment chose 1 mL/min as the mobile rate of flow, and 0.5 mL/min was used as the derivatization reagent rate of flow. The findings demonstrated that the range of linear of various biogenic amines was 0.25–8.00 mg/L ($r^2 > 0.992$), and the recovery rate was between 92% and 103%, indicating that the method has certain accuracy and reproducibility.

The LC–MS method combines liquid chromatography with mass spectrometry. The benefit of using LC–MS is that it does not require derivatization, but it has high instrument costs and strict requirements for operators. Kosma et al. [81] determined β-phenylethylamine, cadaverine, putrescine, histamine, tyramine, and serotonin in trout samples frozen for 15 days. The experimental data indicated that on the 15th day, the concentration of serotonin, histamine, putrescine, and cadaverine was higher at 76.530 mg kg^{-1}, 85.530 mg kg^{-1}, 25.210 mg kg^{-1}, and 15.975 mg kg^{-1}, respectively, while β-phenylethylamine and tyramine had lower content, at 3.230 mg kg^{-1} and 0.165 mg kg^{-1}, respectively. There is a commercially available derivative reagent, 2,4,6-triethyl-3,5-dimethyl pyrylium trifluoromethane sulfonate (Py-Tag), which can be applied to aquatic products to detect biogenic amines. The significant advantages of Py-Tag include improved sensitivity, short reaction time, and minimal odor [82]. However, the drawback is the narrow range of biogenic amines that can be detected [83]. Py-Tag can selectively react rapidly with primary amine groups on carbon chains containing two or more carbon atoms under alkaline conditions [84]. Figure 7 shows the derivative products of histamine and Py-Tag after derivatization. The experiment showed that the spiked concentration of the sample was from 88% to 104%, and the relative standard deviation was less than 6.1%. The detection of specific biogenic amines can be accomplished with this technique.

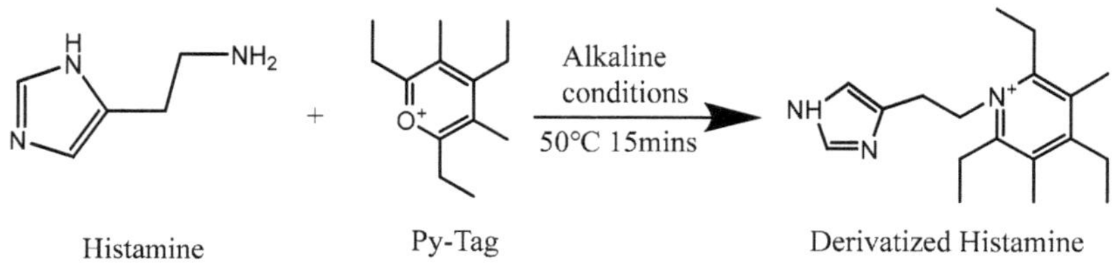

Figure 7. Derivative products of histamine and Py-Tag.

Thin-Layer Chromatography Method

TLC plays a great role in quickly separating and qualitatively analyzing small amounts of substances. Aladhadh et al. [85] determined several biogenic amines (spermine, cadaverine, spermidine, tyramine, histamine, and putrescine) in fish from retail stores by TLC method; the experience showed that the content of putrescine (17.28 mg/kg) and cadaverine (10.26 mg/kg) in frozen shrimp was high. Sardines in spicy tomato sauce contained less total biogenic amines, which is about 3.19 mg/kg. Spermidine, spermine, and tyramine were not detected in Jon West salmon. According to the research findings, different aquatic products have varying amounts of biogenic amines. Valls et al. [86] used five different layer solvents, including (a) a mixed solution of ethanol and ammonia, (b) a mixed solution of methanol and ammonia, (c) a mixed solution of chloroform and n-butyl acetate, (d) a mixed solution of chloroform, methanol, and ammonia, and (e) a mixed solution of acetate and ammonia. The separation result of acetone: ammonia solvent, the proportion is 95:5, was the best. Estimating the amount of certain biogenic amines in a sample can be done by comparing its Rf, shape, size, and color. The concentration range that TLC can estimate in this experiment was: the cadaverine content in salted and dried fish was 5–40 mg%, the tyramine content was 10–20 mg%, and the cadaverine, serotonin, and histamine contents in canned fish was 10–20 mg%, 5–10 mg%, and 10–60 mg%, respectively. Therefore, the TLC method can qualitatively and quantitatively analyze biogenic amines in mixtures.

Gas Chromatography Method

By using the various physical characteristics of substances, such as their adsorption capacity, affinity, solubility, and blocking effect, GC is a technique for separating and analyzing different elements in a mixture. Badrul et al. [87] used a GC-flame ionization detector (GC-FID) to detect heptylamine, tyramine, histamine, spermidine and cadaverine in fish, and confirmed the structure of biogenic amines using MS. It can be inferred by experiment that the LODs range of the five biogenic amines were 1.2–2.9 μg/mL, and the LOQs range were 3.98–9.65 μg/mL. High histamine concentrations (5.96 μg/mL) were detected in mackerel, while tyramine was the most detected in this study. In addition, the experience also showed that biogenic amines in fish did not accumulate all the time because of the presence of salt, and the process was effectively inhibited. At the same time, it had a certain preservative effect. Shalaby [88] found that sodium can restrict the accumulation of biogenic amines, and 2% sodium hexametaphosphate can delay the production of histamine. Mah and Hwang [43] revealed that adding salt to vitamin products can lower quantities of biogenic amines. Bonilla et al. [89] studied the "cold on column" GC method for analyzing cadaverine and putrescine, which did not require derivatization treatment. Prepare the tested biogenic amine into a standard mixture and inject it into the GC system 14 times, keeping the chromatographic conditions consistent throughout the experiment. According to the chromatogram, it was found that putrescine was eluted first, which took 6.073 min. Then heptylamine was eluted at 6.638 min, and finally, cadaverine was eluted at 7.031 min. In addition, the experiment had good reproducibility and quantitative analysis results.

Ion Chromatography Method

The principle of IC is to separate the anions and cations present in food at the same time through ion exchange and then carry out qualitative and quantitative analysis. For example, a low-capacity cation exchange resin is poured into the separation column, and an eluent solution of hydrochloric acid is used to analyze cations. At low pH values, all analytes are ionic, making this method especially appropriate for the polar amine analysis [90,91]. Kocar et al. [92] combined IC with MS to detect histamine in aquatic products and separated it using a cation exchange column. This method did not require additional derivatization operations, only pure water ultrasound for 5 min and vortex for 25 min for extraction. Then, by comparing the results with the HPLC detection results, researchers finally conducted a correlation analysis between the two. The experimental results indicated that the histamine content in fresh anchovy (sample 1) detected by IC–MS/MS was 4.51 ± 0.67 mg/kg. In 15% saline-treated anchovy (sample 2), it was 2.59 ± 0.98 mg/kg. In Danish fermented herring (sample 3), it was 11.25 ± 0.49 mg/kg. In Norwegian smoked salmon (sample 4), it was 1.67 ± 0.09 mg/kg. Using HPLC to detect histamine, the contents from sample 1 to sample 4 were 3.45 ± 0.02, 2.42 ± 0.03, 8.98 ± 0.36, and 1.81 ± 0.06 mg/kg, respectively. In addition, according to the correlation analysis, significant similarities were found in 56% of the results ($p > 0.05$). However, it was found that the correlation between IC–MS/MS and HPLC was poor when detecting other biogenic amines, and further research is needed.

Capillary Electrophoresis Method

CE is a novel form of technology for liquid-phase separation that uses capillary tubes as separation channels and requires an electric field powered by high-voltage direct current to provide power, ensuring the normal operation of the instrument. CE is used for detecting biogenic amines, with simple sample preparation and easy separation but low sensitivity. Therefore, a method combining CE with magnetic solid phase extraction (MSPE) was designed to improve detection sensitivity [93]. At the same time, a new type of MSPE adsorbent was used in the experiment, and Pt–Co–MWCNTs–COOH was created by combining the new magnetic field material Pt–Co with multi-walled carbon nanotubes (MWCNTs), where –COOH can provide more biogenic amine recognition sites for the adsorbent. The results demonstrated a strong linear relationship between peak area and biogenic amine concentration. The intra-day and inter-day precision of peak area was 1.3–9.0% and 2.2–9.6%, respectively. For migration time, the intra-day precision was 0.2–0.8%, while the inter-day precision was 0.7–1.4%, indicating that the accuracy of the MSPE–CE method was effectively improved. Similarly, molecular imprinting solid-phase extraction (MISPE) technology is combined with CE to detect histamine in food [94]. This method prepared a highly selective molecularly imprinted polymer (MIP) as an adsorbent, which has specific recognition sites. The results showed that the LOD and LOQ were 0.087 μg/L and 0.29 μg/L, with good repeatability. These experiments fully consider the limitations of the CE method and combine it with other techniques to improve the shortcomings of the technology itself, simplify sample pretreatment, and thus detect biogenic amines more sensitively and accurately.

4.2.2. Biosensors

A biosensor comprises molecular recognition elements, signal conversion parts, and processors [95]. The working mechanism of a biosensor is to first identify the target analyte and then generate a signal, which is then transformed into signals electrically by the signal conversion part. Certain physical or chemical changes can be caused by the primary functional components, such as microorganisms, enzymes, nucleic acids, and antibodies. In most cases, they can achieve a selective recognition function. The component that converts biological activity signals into electrical signals is a chemical or physical transducer. The output of biosensors is usually magnetic, mechanical, electrical, optical, or thermal signals while also considering whether the detection system is compatible with the sensor platform [96].

Enzymatic Reaction

The principle of using enzyme biosensors to detect biogenic amines is the assimilation of the biosensing electrode near the enzyme. Enzymes have two forms of action: producing electroactive substances or consuming electroactive reactants. In addition, enzyme biosensors can be separated into two kinds: inhibitory sensors and substrate sensors. Substrate biosensors usually assess target substrates and their enzyme reactions, while inhibitor biosensors typically evaluate the reducing activity of substances or enzymes [95,97,98]. Enzyme-based chemiluminescent biosensors have the advantages of speed, wide linear range, ease to operate, low LOD, and no need for monochromatic light [99]. Obervic-Miklikanin and Valzacchi developed two luminescent biosensors based on DAO and putrescine oxidase. Based on the findings, the linear range of the two biosensors was 1–2 mg/L. The LOD of putrescine oxidase biosensors was 0.8 mg/L, and the LOD of DAO biosensors was 1.3 mg/L [100]. Metal nanoparticles (NPs), including gold, platinum, molybdenum, and silver, as well as carbon nanoparticle materials, are known as nanoenzymes. They were widely used in the progress of nanoenzyme-based biosensors for detecting pollutants in food [101]. Kuo et al. [102] developed a sensor according to Ag/Au NPs. Spermine can be detected in urine samples using the sensor, and it can exhibit peroxidase-like and oxidase-like catalytic activity. The findings of the experiment showed that the Ag–Au/AgCl nanosensor exhibited highly efficient catalytic activity, with a linear range of 2.6 nM–8.0 μM and LOD of 0.87 nM. Figure 8 illustrates the basic principle of Ag/Au NPs synthesis.

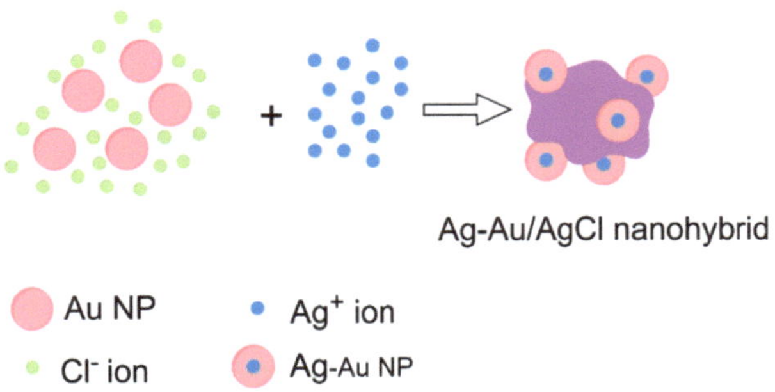

Figure 8. The basic principle of Ag/Au NPs synthesis (by Figdraw 2.0).

Sanz-Vicente et al. [103] designed an enzyme colorimetric analysis system to detect biogenic amines in tuna samples. The system uses tyramine oxidase (TAO) as the molecular recognition part and can simultaneously detect histamine and tyramine under pH = 8 conditions. Tyramine could be detected within 30 s, while histamine detection took about 4 min. In addition, the system was also connected to smartphones and did not require specialized training during use. It consumed fewer reagents and was a portable and green detection method.

Immunological Recognition

The principle of immune recognition is to use biogenic amines as antigens and utilize biological components of recognition such as antibodies [104], nucleic acid aptamers [105], molecularly imprinted polymer (MIP) [106], etc., to bind with antigens for the detection of biogenic amines content. Because of its simple structure, histamine cannot stimulate the production of specific antibodies and usually requires derivatization. In recent years, MIPs have been widely used as biological recognition components for detecting biogenic amines due to their stability, robustness, and specific recognition ability. Venkatesh et al. [107] demonstrated a flexible histamine sensing device that can be used to detect histamine in aqueous media, and its mechanism of action was based on impedance spectroscopy and MIP. What's more, they developed a portable smartphone that was a semi-quantitative histamine sensing device in various aqueous solutions and seafood.

Research has shown that many antibodies against histamine derivatives have been prepared. However, the reaction time for preparing antibodies is relatively long, and side reactions may occur during the experimental process. These issues need to be improved. Xu et al. [108] used enzyme-linked immunosorbent assay (ELISA) to conjugate histamine with fetal bovine ovalbumin or serum albumin as antigen and then injected the conjugate into the subcutaneous tissue of mice. Indirect competitive enzyme-linked immunosorbent assay (ic-ELISA) was used to detect the titer of the antiserum. The experiment could establish a standard curve to determine drug remnants, but the disadvantage was that it took a long time to carry out the whole detection [109]. The research results showed that the IC_{50} value was 1.2 μ g/mL, indicating that the antibody could be used for histamine detection. The LOD (IC_{10} value) was 89.0 ng/mL, and the range of linear was 100.0 ng/mL to 10.0 μg/mL.

If antibodies are used as biological recognition elements to form an immunosensor, the specificity of the sensor is strong due to its strong antigen–antibody reaction binding ability. Shkodra et al. [110] developed a novel immunosensor for histamine detection, which is according to single-walled carbon nanotubes (SWCNTs). After oxygen plasma treatment, histamine is competitively reacted with horseradish peroxidase (HRP)-coupled histamine and antihistamine antibodies. The results indicated that the detection range of histamine using this method was 0.5–50 ng/mL, and the method had high specificity and sensitivity.

4.2.3. Chemo-Sensors

Electrodes and chemical modification of the electrodes are necessary using chemical sensors to detect biogenic amines [111]. Platinum, gold, carbon, and silicon are frequently employed to identify biogenic amines in food and beverage samples [112]. For example, carbon nanotubes (CNTs) have a wide range of applications because of their high chemical and thermal stability [113]. Chemical sensors mainly consider electrochemical sensors, which are fast, simple, and cost-effective. The receptors of electrochemical sensors can be divided into chemical and biological categories; that is, the receptors are chemically or biologically modified, and then the receptors react with the analyte, generating electronic signals from an individual or a collection of analytes to obtain relevant data [112]. There are various methods for modifying receptors to generate electrical signals, such as current analysis, impedance analysis, and potentiometric analysis [114]. The current analysis method determines the concentration of the component by measuring the current generated by the measured component. The potential analysis method includes an electrode that is used to work and a reference electrode, which determines the concentration of the measured component by measuring the potential difference between the two. The impedance method determines the impedance from the analyte, including resistance and reactance.

Nanomaterials

In recent years, metal nanomaterials have become increasingly popular for testing and analysis of food safety. These materials possess distinct optical, electrical, physical, and chemical characteristics; additionally, their size, shape, structure, and surface characteristics can be altered [115]. The specific identification of biogenic amines is a common application for gold nanoparticles, nanorods, and nanoclusters. Du et al. [116] used a colorimetric chemical sensor array according to gold nanoparticles to detect the biogenic amine content produced while the raw fish was deteriorating (tuna). In the experiment, three carboxylate derivatives were used, including 11-mercaptodecanoic acid (S1), 4-mercaptobenzoic acid (S2), and 6-mercaptohexanoic acid (S3), to functionalize AuNPs. AuNPs functionalized with longer alkyl chains of 11-mercaptodecanoic acid can detect high concentrations of analytes [117]. When AuNPs came into contact with biogenic amines due to cross-reactivity interactions, aggregation-induced ultraviolet-visible (UV–VIS) spectral changes resulted in significant color changes in the solution. This experiment prepared two types of AuNPs (IS–AuNPs and DS–AuNPs), where IS–AuNPs were prepared by mixing Na_3Ct (0.65 mmol, 2 mL) with $HAuCl_4$ (0.25 mmol, 98 mL), while DS–AuNPs were prepared by mixing Na_3Ct (0.65 mmol, 99 mL) with $HAuCl_4$ (0.25 mmol, 1 mL). The experimental results showed that after surface functionalization with S1, S2, and S3, a slight spectral shift was observed in the extinction spectrum of IS–AuNP and its deep red color could be used for colorimetric sensors. The concentration of histamine gradually increased over time, while there was little change in spermidine and spermine concentrations. Through this method, biogenic amines can be qualitatively and quantitatively analyzed from mixtures and can also be used to detect freshness.

Due to the different aggregation behaviors of target biogenic amines, Abbasi-Moayed et al. [118] utilized AuNP and AgNP to create unique plasma patterns for each biogenic amines to detect and distinguish four biogenic amines, including spermine, spermidine, histamine, and serotonin. Due to the different compositions of AuNP and AgNP, there were significant differences in the color changes produced when exposed to different biogenic amines. Four biogenic amines were classified using principal component analysis–linear discrimination analysis (PCA–LDA). Furthermore, a colorimetric sensor array was designed to accurately distinguish between individual biogenic amines and their mixtures. The experimental results indicated that spermine and spermidine induced rapid aggregation of AuNPs, but they showed significant differences in the aggregation level of AgNPs, which could be used to distinguish spermine and spermidine. Serotonin and histamine hardly caused aggregation of AgNPs, while AuNPs exhibited significantly different aggregation, which could be distinguished by serotonin and histamine. From a color perspective, AgNP has turned from yellow to orange, and AuNP has turned from red to purple. Therefore, this method can distinguish biogenic amines intuitively, quickly, and simply due to the obvious color changes.

Cao et al. [119] developed a nanosystem for ratiometric fluorescence according to upconversion nanoparticles (UCNPs) for efficient detection of histamine in aquatic products. It acted exclusively on histamine by using diazonium ions as a selective chromogenic agent. A combination of azo reagents produced diazonium ions. During this process, UCNPs went through signal transduction. UCNPs have high chemical stability, non-spontaneous fluorescence, and great capacity to penetrate light, and can be used as fluorescent markers in assays [120]. This experiment selected different concentrations of histamine as samples, namely 0, 5, 10, 15, 20, 25, 50, 75, 100, 125, 150, 175, and 200 mg/L, and then added them to Na_2CO_3 and UCNPs solutions, followed by the addition of mixed azo reagents. Finally, the detection of colorimetric and upconversion fluorescence was achieved at room temperature. The experimental results indicated that in the separated emission and absorption spectra within the mixed nanosystem, the two primary fluorescence peaks of UCNP were located at 548 and 664 nm. If histamine was further added, a fresh absorption peak emerged at 548 nm and kept growing until it crossed over with the emission peak of upconversion fluorescence. Therefore, the luminescence intensity ratio I_{548}/I_{664} can be applied to ascertain the content of histamine.

pH Sensors

Detecting biogenic amines through pH sensors is a direct, convenient, and easy to observe method. Biogenic amines contain nitrogen elements and have a small molecular weight; they are mostly alkaline. Therefore, pH indicators such as anthocyanins, curcumin, bromophenol blue, bromocresol green, methyl red, etc., can effectively detect biogenic amines. When biogenic amines are present in aquatic products, color changes may appear, and a pH sensor can clearly show this change. Although this method is convenient for observation, it cannot accurately measure the content of biogenic amines and can only provide semi-quantitative information. Usually, the sensitivity is relatively low. Siripongdera et al. [121] used pH-sensitive infectious materials with a pH range of 5.2–6.8 as sensing elements to establish a colorimetric and LDI–MS dual detection platform for screening and quantitative detection of biogenic amines. This method selected bromocresol purple as the pH indicator to make a colorimetric sensor. The initial color of the sensor was yellow, and if it came into contact with alkaline biogenic amines, the color turned purple. The experimental results showed that after 30 min, the sensor for detecting cadaverine underwent a color change. At 8 h, the sensor turned purple instead of yellow when it detected putrescine. Zhong et al. [122] studied a colorimetric sensor array for detecting biogenic amines, which was made of a composite of pH-sensitive infectious materials and nanomaterials. The study showed that due to the existence of functional groups that were acidic on the exterior of nanomaterials, it was easy to combine with alkaline biogenic amines. The concentration of amine vapor generated by the nanoporous structure of nanomaterials/dye composites or substrates, a good linear detection range, and a detection limit were obtained. In addition, the reaction time was effectively shortened. Ding et al. [123] introduced cellulose into polyvinyl alcohol (PVA) and developed a pH sensor for detecting biogenic amines in spoilage shrimp. The color changed from yellow to brown, indicating the strong operability of the sensor. Therefore, using pH sensors to detect biogenic amines has great application prospects, and it can be considered to combine it with other materials for qualitative and quantitative analysis.

Fluorometry

Roth first proposed the use of OPA and reduced agents such as 2-mercaptoethanol (2-ME) to detect primary amino compounds [124]. However, traditional fluorescence detection equipment is expensive, takes a long time to analyze, has low sensitivity, and cannot qualitatively and quantitatively determine the total amount of biogenic amines in food. Therefore, Hasanova et al. [125] designed a fluorescent DTE AuNP/OPA (DTE: 1,4-dithioerythritol) method based on NPs in order to identify biogenic amines. The principle is that under alkaline conditions, one thiol group of DTE is covalently bound to AuNPs, while the other group of –SH is available and participates in the indole reaction between OPA and primary amines. The results showed that the emission spectra of histamine, 2-phenylethylamine, serotonin, and tyramine under 340 nm excitation exhibited a good linear relationship. The LOD range was between 4.20 and 27.1 nM, and this method effectively detected the total biogenic amine content with high operational feasibility. Peat et al. [126] combined a reverse-phase HPLC system with fluorescence to detect the levels of trypsin, 5-hydroxyindoleacetic acid (5-HIAA), 5-hydroxytryptamine (5-HT), dopamine, and norepinephrine in the rat brain. The research indicated that the optimal settings for simultaneously measuring these five substances were a wavelength of excitation of 290nm and a wavelength of emission of 330nm. Norepinephrine had the highest recovery rate (98%), followed by 5-HT, and 5-HIAA had the lowest recovery rate (90%). In addition, through this experiment, the 5-HT content was 1.2 ± 0.13 ($n = 6$) ng/mg wet tissue, the concentrations of dopamine and 5-HIAA were 7.9 ± 0.68 (n = 6) and 1.3 ± 0.13 (n = 6) ng/mg wet tissue, respectively.

A fluorescent probe CMA–Cl derived from coumarin derivatives was designed and synthesized to detect biogenic primary diamines such as cadaverine and putrescine [127]. Among them, diethylaminocoumarin is a multifunctional fluorescent group. It has some significant advantages, such as more fluorescence quantum, good light stability, and a simple synthesis process. Its visible light range absorption and fluorescence spectra made it useful for visual observation and biogenic amine detection. The detection principle of this fluorescent probe is due to the fact that primary diamines have two groups of amino acids, which can be specifically recognized by aldehyde and chloroquine groups on CMA–Cl and then undergo reactions involving nucleophilic substitution and condensation, causing significant changes in fluorescence intensity. The experimental results showed that the addition of cadaverine at 475 nm exhibited strong blue fluorescence, while the fluorescence intensity varied with the addition of other biogenic amines, indicating a certain selectivity for different biogenic amines. Based on this, the experiment also prepared CMA–Cl loaded test strips to track the content of biogenic primary diamines during fish spoilage. As the exposure time of fish samples to air increases, the degree of spoilage gradually increases, and the biogenic amines concentration gradually increases. The color of the test paper changed from yellow to white, which could achieve convenient and rapid detection of biogenic amines.

In addition, multi-functional molecular assemblies can be used to develop chemosensor. Among them, porphyrins can be used as colorimetric and fluorescent chemo-sensor due to their multiple binding sites and unique photophysical properties. Guo et al. [128] introduced a ditopic porphyrin-based chemo-sensor for detecting histamine, which was prepared from tetraphenylporphyrin (TPP) by adding a second binding site during the β–pyrrole functionalization strategy. This sensor had two receptor sites; one was carboxylic acid, and the other was metal zinc ion, which had a strong affinity for histamine and high binding constants. By using sensors to separately identify histamine, histidine, and nicotine, and according to the roughly linear correlation between each component's concentration and the emission peak ratio, it can be found that histamine was the most sensitive for identification.

Optical Chemo-Sensor Systems

Optical sensors mainly rely on the measurement of absorption rate, while fluorescent sensors combine with specific recognition elements to quantitatively analyze the intensity of fluorescence signals [129]. The absorption ability of biogenic amines in the visible light range is weak because they lack conjugated aromatic π–electron systems and do not have chemical structures that can be used for optical detection [130]. It is usually difficult to directly detect biogenic amines through optical sensors. Therefore, in order to obtain ideal detection performance and make it suitable for optical analysis, it is essential to use chromophores or fluorophore to derive bioamines and convert them into corresponding derivatives [131]. Optical sensors are appropriate for in vivo measurements and remote sensing, even at distances greater than kilometers. A portable sensor system or dipstick sensor has been designed based on various probes, such as reflectometry, luminescence, photometry, surface-enhanced Raman spectroscopy, or total internal reflection ellipsometry (SERS). In addition, compared to photometry and reflectometry, luminescence is more sensitive. It is mainly because luminescence is not affected by excitation light interference during the detection process [132]. Raman signals that are normally weak can increase by multiple orders of magnitude using SERS, aiding in the detection of chemical and biochemical substances [133].

The composition of a reflectometric sensor is simple, consisting of a light source, a filter, and a detector. Among them, the filter was used to select the detection wavelength. Biogenic amines sensing can be read out using a reflectometer and analyzed by using the standard of the International Commission on Illumination (CIE) system [134]. Embedding NIR dyes reactive with biogenic amines into electrospun nanofiber mats to form a reflectometric dipstick sensor and preparing electrospun nanofibers through a straightforward, conventional electrospinning process, which also contains S0378 cyanine dye absorbed at 800 nm [130]. Biogenic amines can undergo a color change by binding with dyes, from green to blue, and dipstick can be used to detect total amine content (TAC). During the experiment, as biogenic amines concentration rose, the blue color gradually deepened. The concentration started from 0.2 mM, and the blue change was most pronounced. Quantitative analysis of biogenic amines revealed that shrimp aged at room temperature were taken as the research object. The solution of biogenic amine was added to a dipstick, and the reflectance of the test paper was measured. Finally, a graph was plotted relative to biogenic amine concentration. The histamine concentration on the 0th, 1st, and 6th day of aging were 7.54 ± 0.96, 12.8 ± 0.8, and 21.7 ± 3.2 μ mol/g, respectively (n = 4).

Combining photometry with CE for indirect detection of biogenic amines [135]. One notable benefit of this approach is that it eliminates the need for derivative processing, saving a lot of time and energy. The experiment indicated that amines can be determined within the range of 0.05–1 μg mL^{-1}, and the recovery rates of several representative biogenic amines are between 90–110%, demonstrating long-term stability and reproducibility.

In the luminescence method, the application of ion covalent organic frameworks (iCOFs) was considered. These represented a novel class of porous material that was made up of ionic and covalent bonds with significant chemical stability, adsorption, and selectivity. A study has designed an iCOF chemo-sensor, which was formed by condensing triamino-guanidine hydrochloride salt (TGH • Cl) and phenanthroline-2,9-dicarbaldehyde (PD) [136]. The iCOF was abbreviated as TGH^+ • PD. Figure 9 shows its chemical structure and condensation method.

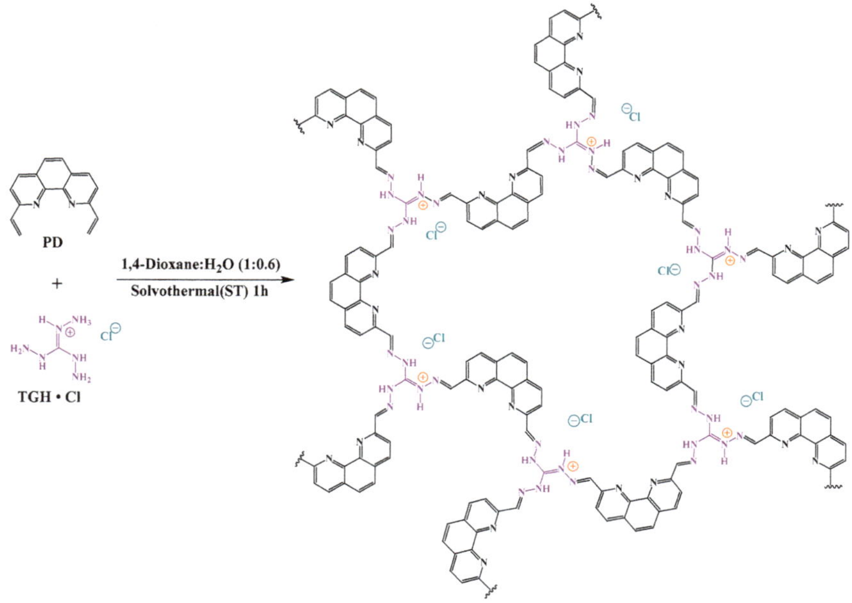

Figure 9. Chemical structure and condensation method.

TGH^+ • PD was easily dispersed in water and served as an electron donor, transferring electrons from phenanthroline to the electron acceptor guanidinium unit, forming intramolecular charge transfer (ICT), which results in a color change (orange). When it bound to the analyte, the fluorescence color changed [136]. The iCOF structure was characterized by a helical fiber morphology [136], which was attributed to the presence of water molecules. They were mainly located near the guanidine unit. In the experiment, the iCOF was treated with heat, and it was found that the helical structure was destroyed. If it came into contact with water molecules again, its morphology could be restored. In order to verify the effectiveness of TGH^+ • PD in detecting biogenic amines, fresh chicken meat was stored in a sealed beaker at 4 °C. The fluorescence intensity was not significant within two days, mainly due to the low amounts of biogenic amines produced under these conditions. Then, the sealed beaker was transferred to room temperature, and the fluorescence intensity significantly increased, indicating that the iCOF could effectively detect biogenic amines and act as an observing signal for spoilage. In addition, in order to investigate the practicality and convenience of TGH^+ • PD, its aqueous dispersion was applied to filter paper to prepare a test strip, which was then placed on top of spoiled chicken. As the amine vapor evaporated, the color of the detection strip changed from orange to yellow-green. Interestingly, if the yellow-green test strip was moved to fresh air, its color would change back to the initial orange. This experiment successfully validated the practicality of TGH^+ • PD and discovered a convenient, easy, and low-cost method for detecting biogenic amines.

5. Conclusions and Future Perspective

Aquatic products are rich in fat and protein. Under suitable conditions, microorganisms can grow and reproduce, inducing the generation of substantial quantities of biogenic amines, leading to the spoilage of aquatic products, and excessive human intake can also cause harm. Therefore, it is crucial to determine the types of biogenic amines and their concentrations in aquatic products. Microbiological and molecular biology methods can be used for the initial detection of biogenic amines due to their inability to be quantitatively analyzed. Chromatography such as HPLC, LC, and GC is widely used and the most common method, but sometimes requires high equipment and operators. Sensors, especially chemo-sensors, are widely developed for their speed, simplicity, and cost-effectiveness. Although nanomaterials have good detection performance for chemical sensors, they have certain specificity for different biogenic amines due to their different aggregation behaviors. The color change caused by the pH sensor through acid–base reaction makes the detection results easy to observe, but this method alone cannot be quantitatively analyzed and has low sensitivity. Similarly, fluorescence analysis has low sensitivity and cannot qualitatively and quantitatively detect total biogenic amines in aquatic products. Therefore, new technologies such as fluorescent probes have been developed to improve these drawbacks. This review summarized various detection methods for biogenic amines, all of which have certain drawbacks that need improvement. This review provides theoretical support for more efficient detection of biogenic amines in the future and making contributions to preserving human health and making sure aquatic products are safe to consume.

Author Contributions: Conceptualization, Z.C.; methodology Z.C.; software, Z.C.; validation, Z.C.; formal analysis, Z.C.; investigation, Z.C.; resources, J.M.; data curation, Z.C.; writing—original draft preparation, Z.C.; writing—review and editing, J.M. and J.X.; visualization, J.M. and J.X.; supervision, J.M. and J.X.; project administration, J.M. and J.X.; funding acquisition, J.X. All authors have read and agreed to the published version of the manuscript.

Funding: This research was supported by National Key Research and Development Program of China (2023YFD2401402) and Agriculture Research System of China (CARS-47).

Institutional Review Board Statement: Not applicable.

Informed Consent Statement: Not applicable.

Data Availability Statement: The data presented in this study are available in article. Data available in a publicly accessible repository.

Conflicts of Interest: The authors declare no conflicts of interest.

References

1. GarridoGamarro, E.; Svanevik, C.S.; Lundebye, A.-K.; Sanden, M.; D'Agostino, E.; Kjellevold, M.; Pincus, L.; Pucher, J. Challenges in the implementation of food safety and quality assurance systems in small-scale fisheries. *Food Qual. Saf.* **2023**, *7*, fyad007. [CrossRef]
2. Wang, S.Y.; Jian, C.; Hu, M.Y.; Zhao, L.; Sun, H.H.; Liu, Q.; Cao, R.; Xue, Y. Lipid changes and volatile compounds formation in different processing stages of dry-cured Spanish mackerel. *Food Qual. Saf.* **2024**, *8*, fyae026. [CrossRef]
3. Doeun, D.; Davaatseren, M.; Chung, M.S. Biogenic amines in foods. *Food Sci. Biotechnol.* **2017**, *26*, 1463–1474. [CrossRef] [PubMed]
4. Ding, T.; Li, Y. Biogenic amines are important indices for characterizing the freshness and hygienic quality of aquatic products: A review. *Lwt* **2024**, *194*, 115793. [CrossRef]
5. Ruiz-Capillas, C.; Herrero, A.M. Impact of Biogenic Amines on Food Quality and Safety. *Foods* **2019**, *8*, 62. [CrossRef]
6. Krízek, M.; Pelikánová, T. Determination of seven biogenic amines in foods by micellar electrokinetic capillary chromatography. *J. Chromatogr. A* **1998**, *815*, 243–250. [CrossRef]

7. Sarkadi, L.S. Amino acids and biogenic amines as food quality factors. *Pure Appl. Chem.* **2019**, *91*, 289–300. [CrossRef]
8. Li, T.; Wang, R.; Wang, P. The Development of an Ultra-Performance Liquid Chromatography-Tandem Mass Spectrometry Method for Biogenic Amines in Fish Samples. *Molecules* **2023**, *28*, 184. [CrossRef] [PubMed]
9. Hao, D.; Kaijun, X. Modified QuEChERS combined with ultra high performance liquid chromatography tandem mass spectrometry to determine seven biogenic amines in Chinese traditional condiment soy sauce. *Food Chem.* **2017**, *229*, 502–508. [CrossRef]
10. Nuo, D.; Yuting, C.; Wenhui, L.; Changxin, L.; Chunxia, L.; Zhouping, W.; Shijia, W. Ratiometric SERS aptasensing for simultaneous quantitative detection of histamine and tyramine in fishes. *Talanta* **2023**, *265*, 124891. [CrossRef]
11. Yifrach, Y.; Rahimi, R.; Baraban, J.H.; Bar, I. Ionization energies and ionization-induced structural changes in 2-phenylethylamine and its monohydrate. *J. Chem. Phys.* **2023**, *158*, 114305. [CrossRef]
12. Ziaee, E.; Shareghi, B.; Farhadian, S. A comparative study of structural and dynamical properties of bovine serum albumin in the presence of spermine. *J. Mol. Liq.* **2021**, *332*, 115853. [CrossRef]
13. Eslami-Farsani, R.; Farhadian, S.; Shareghi, B.; Asgharzadeh, S. Structural change of myoglobin structure after binding with spermidine. *J. Mol. Liq.* **2022**, *352*, 118691. [CrossRef]
14. Moradi, S.; Shareghi, B.; Saboury, A.A.; Farhadian, S. The influence of Cadaverine on the structure, stability, and activity of acid phosphatase. *J. Mol. Struct.* **2022**, *1247*, 131372. [CrossRef]
15. Wojcik, W.; Lukasiewicz-Mierzejewska, M.; Damaziak, K.; Bien, D. Biogenic Amines in Poultry Meat and Poultry Products: Formation, Appearance, and Methods of Reduction. *Animals* **2022**, *12*, 1577. [CrossRef] [PubMed]
16. Santos, M.H.S. Biogenic amines: Their importance in foods. *Int. J. Food Microbiol.* **1996**, *29*, 213–231. [CrossRef] [PubMed]
17. Schirone, M.; Esposito, L.; D'Onofrio, F.; Visciano, P.; Martuscelli, M.; Mastrocola, D.; Paparella, A. Biogenic Amines in Meat and Meat Products: A Review of the Science and Future Perspectives. *Foods* **2022**, *11*, 788. [CrossRef]
18. Stratton, J.E.; Hutkins, R.W.; Taylor, S.L. Biogenic Amines in Cheese and other Fermented Foods: A Review. *J. Food Prot.* **1991**, *54*, 460–470. [CrossRef] [PubMed]
19. Del Rio, B.; Fernandez, M.; Redruello, B.; Ladero, V.; Alvarez, M.A. New insights into the toxicological effects of dietary biogenic amines. *Food Chem.* **2024**, *435*, 137558. [CrossRef] [PubMed]
20. Naila, A.; Flint, S.; Fletcher, G.; Bremer, P.; Meerdink, G. Control of Biogenic Amines in Food-Existing and Emerging Approaches. *J. Food Sci.* **2010**, *75*, R139–R150. [CrossRef]
21. Maijala, R.L.; Eerola, S.H.; Aho, M.A.; Hirn, J.A. The effect of GDL-induced pH decrease on the formation of biogenic amines in meat. *J. Food Prot.* **1993**, *56*, 125–129. [CrossRef] [PubMed]
22. Karovicová, J.; Kohajdová, Z. Biogenic amines in food. *Chem. Pap.* **2005**, *59*, 70–79. [CrossRef]
23. Halasz, A.; Barath, A.; Simon-Sarkadi, L.; Holzapfel, W. Biogenic amines and their production by microorganisms in food. *Trends Food Sci. Technol.* **1994**, *5*, 42–49. [CrossRef]
24. Conz, A.; Davoli, E.; Franchi, C.; Diomede, L. Seafood loss prevention and waste reduction. *Food Qual. Saf.* **2024**, *8*, fyae017. [CrossRef]
25. HernandezJover, T.; IzquierdoPulido, M.; VecianaNogues, M.T.; MarineFont, A.; VidalCarou, M.C. Biogenic amine and polyamine contents in meat and meat products. *J. Agric. Food. Chem.* **1997**, *45*, 2098–2102. [CrossRef]
26. Emborg, J.; Dalgaard, P. Formation of histamine and biogenic amines in cold-smoked tuna: An investigation of psychrotolerant bacteria from samples implicated in cases of histamine fish poisoning. *J. Food Prot.* **2006**, *69*, 897–906. [CrossRef] [PubMed]
27. Bodmer, S.; Imark, C.; Kneubühl, M. Biogenic amines in foods: Histamine and food processing. *Inflamm. Res.* **1999**, *48*, 296–300. [CrossRef] [PubMed]
28. Qiaoqiao, L.; Ruoyu, S.; Pengfei, G.; Yutong, L.; Wei, C.; Chengtao, W. Biogenic amines in Huangjiu (Chinese rice wine): Formation, hazard, detection, and reduction. *LWT—Food Sci. Technol.* **2022**, *168*, 113952. [CrossRef]
29. Saha Turna, N.; Chung, R.; McIntyre, L. A review of biogenic amines in fermented foods: Occurrence and health effects. *Heliyon* **2024**, *10*, e24501. [CrossRef] [PubMed]
30. Barbieri, F.; Montanari, C.; Gardini, F.; Tabanelli, G. Biogenic Amine Production by Lactic Acid Bacteria: A Review. *Foods* **2019**, *8*, 17. [CrossRef] [PubMed]
31. Comas-Baste, O.; Sanchez-Perez, S.; Veciana-Nogues, M.T.; Latorre-Moratalla, M.; Vidal-Carou, M.d.C. Histamine Intolerance: The Current State of the Art. *Biomolecules* **2020**, *10*, 1181. [CrossRef] [PubMed]
32. Ladero, V.; Calles-Enriquez, M.; Fernández, M.; Alvarez, M.J.C.N.A.; Science, F. Toxicological effects of dietary biogenic amines. *Curr. Nutr. Food Sci.* **2010**, *6*, 145–156. [CrossRef]
33. Bruno, M.D.-P.; Flavia, B.C.; Maria, B.A.G. Health concerns associated with biogenic amines in food and interaction with amine oxidase drugs. *Curr. Opin. Food Sci.* **2023**, *54*, 101090. [CrossRef]
34. Marcobal, A.; De Las Rivas, B.; Maria Landete, J.; Tabera, L.; Munoz, R. Tyramine and Phenylethylamine Biosynthesis by Food Bacteria. *Crit. Rev. Food Sci. Nutr.* **2012**, *52*, 448–467. [CrossRef] [PubMed]

35. Pretorius, L.; Smith, C. *Aspalathus linearis* (Rooibos) and Agmatine May Act Synergistically to Beneficially Modulate Intestinal Tight Junction Integrity and Inflammatory Profile. *Pharmaceuticals* **2022**, *15*, 1097. [CrossRef]
36. Dong, S.L.; Niu, Y.B.; Wei, H.M.; Lin, Y.M.; Lu, X.; Yamashita, T.; Yu, K.F.; Takaki, K.; Yuan, C.H. Effect of super-chilling storage on maintenance of quality and freshness of the Pacific oyster (Crassostrea gigas). *Food Qual. Saf.* **2023**, *7*, fyad008. [CrossRef]
37. Bjornsdottir-Butler, K.; Bencsath, F.A.; McCarthy, S.; Benner, R.A., Jr. Heat Resistance of Histidine Decarboxylase from Gram-Negative Histamine-Producing Bacteria in Seafood. *J. Food Prot.* **2017**, *80*, 1273–1279. [CrossRef] [PubMed]
38. Wang, J.; Qu, Y.; Liu, Z.; Zhou, H. Formation, Analytical Methods, Change Tendency, and Control Strategies of Biogenic Amines in Canned Aquatic Products: A Systematic Review. *J. Food Prot.* **2021**, *84*, 2020–2036. [CrossRef]
39. Gardini, F.; Martuscelli, M.; Caruso, M.C.; Galgano, F.; Crudele, M.A.; Favati, F.; Guerzoni, M.E.; Suzzi, G. Effects of pH, temperature and NaCl concentration on the growth kinetics, proteolytic activity and biogenic amine production of *Enterococcus faecalis*. *Int. J. Food Microbiol.* **2001**, *64*, 105–117. [CrossRef] [PubMed]
40. Wu, S.; Niu, Y.; Wang, J.; Dao, X.; Lin, Y.; Chen, J. The Influence of Different Levels of Sodium Chloride, Sodium Nitrite, and Glucose on Biogenic Amines and Microbial Communities in Fermented Goat Meat Sausage. *Foods* **2024**, *13*, 817. [CrossRef] [PubMed]
41. Jae-Hyung, M.; Han-Joon, H. Effects of food additives on biogenic amine formation in myeolchi-jeot, a salted and fermented anchovy (Engraulis japonicus). *Food Chem.* **2009**, *114*, 168–173. [CrossRef]
42. Shulgin, Y.P.; Lazhentseva, L.Y.; Shulgina, L.V.; Kalenik, T.K.; Matveeva, V.A.; Piekoszewski, W. Quality Improvement of Canned Fish with the Use of Cinnamon Oil Extract. *Int. J. Food Eng.* **2017**, *13*. [CrossRef]
43. Li, J.; Jiang, K.; Yang, H.; Zhang, X.; Huang, H.; Ye, X.; Zhi, Z. Proanthocyanidins from Chinese Bayberry (Myrica rubra Sieb. et Zucc.) Leaves Effectively Inhibit the Formation of Biogenic Amines in the Brewing Soy Sauce. *Agriculture* **2023**, *13*, 2100. [CrossRef]
44. Zhang, X.; Fang, C.; Huang, D.; Yang, G.; Tang, Y.; Shi, Y.; Kong, C.; Cao, P.; Cai, Y. Determination of 8 biogenic amines in aquatic products and their derived products by high-performance liquid chromatography-tandem mass spectrometry without derivatization. *Food Chem.* **2021**, *361*, 130044. [CrossRef] [PubMed]
45. Hu, Y.; Huang, Z.; Li, J.; Yang, H. Concentrations of biogenic amines in fish, squid and octopus and their changes during storage. *Food Chem.* **2012**, *135*, 2604–2611. [CrossRef] [PubMed]
46. Young Mi, K.; Min Joo, K.; Sun Young, P.; Min Soo, H.; Jin-Soo, K. Survey and exposure assessment of biogenic amines in fish species commonly consumed in Korea. *J. Food Prot.* **2019**, *82*, 151–158. [CrossRef]
47. Zhai, H.; Yang, X.; Li, L.; Xia, G.; Cen, J.; Huang, H.; Hao, S. Biogenic amines in commercial fish and fish products sold in southern China. *Food Control* **2012**, *25*, 303–308. [CrossRef]
48. Min-Ki, K.; Jae-Hyung, M.; Han-Joon, H. Biogenic amine formation and bacterial contribution in fish, squid and shellfish. *Food Chem.* **2009**, *116*, 87–95. [CrossRef]
49. Jin Seok, M.; Yujin, K.; Keum Il, J.; Kyung-Ju, C.; Seung-Joon, Y.; Gun-Mook, Y.; So-Young, K.; Nam Soo, H. Analysis of biogenic amines in fermented fish products consumed in Korea. *Food Sci. Biotechnol.* **2010**, *19*, 1689–1692. [CrossRef]
50. Guo, X.; Dai, Z.; Zhang, W. Pollution, Exposure and Risk of Biogenic Amines in Canned Sea Fish: Classification of Analytical Methods Based on Carbon Spheres QuEChERS Extraction Combined with HPLC. *Molecules* **2022**, *27*, 6243. [CrossRef] [PubMed]
51. Sagratini, G.; Fernandez-Franzon, M.; De Berardinis, F.; Font, G.; Vittori, S.; Manes, J. Simultaneous determination of eight underivatised biogenic amines in fish by solid phase extraction and liquid chromatography-tandem mass spectrometry. *Food Chem.* **2012**, *132*, 537–543. [CrossRef] [PubMed]
52. Liu, Y.; Han, F.; Liu, Y.; Wang, W. Determination of Biogenic Amines in Wine Using Modified Liquid-Liquid Extraction with High Performance Liquid Chromatography-Fluorescence Detector. *Food Anal. Methods* **2020**, *13*, 911–922. [CrossRef]
53. Zhang, S.; Li, Z.; Qi, Y.; Yu, P.; Zhao, Q. A Routine and Sensitive Quantification of 2-Acetyl-1-Pyrroline in Shrimp by DSPE-DLLME Coupled to HPLC-UV. *Food Anal. Methods* **2022**, *15*, 2479–2486. [CrossRef]
54. Merkle, S.; Kleeberg, K.; Fritsche, J. Recent Developments and Applications of Solid Phase Microextraction (SPME) in Food and Environmental Analysis—A Review. *Chromatography* **2015**, *2*, 293–381. [CrossRef]
55. Nasiri, M.; Ahmadzadeh, H.; Amiri, A. Sample preparation and extraction methods for pesticides in aquatic environments: A review. *TrAC Trends Anal. Chem.* **2020**, *123*, 115772. [CrossRef]
56. Yu-Jia, Z.; Yuan, Z.; Yu, Z.; Guo-Hui, L.; Wen-Zhen, Y.; Xue-Song, F. A review of pretreatment and analytical methods of biogenic amines in food and biological samples since 2010. *J. Chromatogr. A* **2019**, *1605*, 360361. [CrossRef]
57. Luis Ordonez, J.; Maria Troncoso, A.; Garcia-Parrilla, M.C.; Maria Callejon, R. Recent trends in the determination of biogenic amines in fermented beverages—A review. *Anal. Chim. Acta* **2016**, *939*, 10–25. [CrossRef] [PubMed]
58. Otles, S.; Kartal, C. Solid-Phase Extraction (SPE): Principles and Applications in Food Samples. *Acta Sci. Pol. Technol. Aliment.* **2016**, *15*, 5–15. [CrossRef] [PubMed]
59. Jayasinghe, G.D.T.M.; Jinadasa, B.K.K.K.; Pawel, P.; Aydi, A. Critical review on microextraction techniques used in determination of histamine in food samples. *Discov. Food* **2022**, *2*, 8. [CrossRef]

60. Mohammed, G.I.; Bashammakh, A.S.; Alsibaai, A.A.; Alwael, H.; El-Shahawi, M.S. A critical overview on the chemistry, clean-up and recent advances in analysis of biogenic amines in foodstuffs. *TrAC Trends Anal. Chem.* **2016**, *78*, 84–94. [CrossRef]
61. Santana-Mayor, A.; Rodríguez-Ramos, R.; Herrera-Herrera, A.V.; Socas-Rodríguez, B.; Rodríguez-Delgado, M.A. Updated overview of QuEChERS applications in food, environmental and biological analysis (2020–2023). *TrAC Trends Anal. Chem.* **2023**, *169*, 117375. [CrossRef]
62. Yuan, W.; Lijie, X.; Ruifeng, L.; Xianyi, L.; Fei, Z.; Shiling, L. Modified QuEChERS combined with UPLC-MS/MS to determine eight biogenic amines in Xinjiang smoked horsemeat sausages. *Food Sci. Technol.* **2022**, *42*, e93521. [CrossRef]
63. Heydarzadeh, M.; Heydari, R. Determination of 2, 4-dichlorophenoxyacetic acid in environmental and food samples using salt-assisted liquid-liquid extraction coupled with micro-channel and high-performance liquid chromatography. *Sep. Sci. Plus* **2022**, *5*, 305–313. [CrossRef]
64. Ismaili, A.; Heydari, R.; Rezaeepour, R. Monitoring the oleuropein content of olive leaves and fruits using ultrasound-and salt-assisted liquid-liquid extraction optimized by response surface methodology and high-performance liquid chromatography. *J. Sep. Sci.* **2016**, *39*, 405–411. [CrossRef] [PubMed]
65. Jiang, H.; Yang, S.; Tian, H.; Sun, B. Research progress in the use of liquid-liquid extraction for food flavour analysis. *Trends Food Sci. Technol.* **2023**, *132*, 138–149. [CrossRef]
66. Chen, M.; Lan, H.; Pan, D.; Zhang, T. Hydrophobic Mesoporous Silica-Coated Solid-Phase Microextraction Arrow System for the Determination of Six Biogenic Amines in Pork and Fish. *Foods* **2023**, *12*, 578. [CrossRef] [PubMed]
67. Li, Y.; Yu, Z.; Zhu, Y.; Cao, Z. Selection of nitrite-degrading and biogenic amine-degrading strains and its involved genes. *Food Qual. Saf.* **2020**, *4*, 225–235. [CrossRef]
68. Wakinaka, T.; Iwata, S.; Takeishi, Y.; Watanabe, J.; Mogi, Y.; Tsukioka, Y.; Shibata, Y. Isolation of halophilic lactic acid bacteria possessing aspartate decarboxylase and application to fish sauce fermentation starter. *Int. J. Food Microbiol.* **2019**, *292*, 137–143. [CrossRef]
69. LopezSabater, E.I.; RodriguezJerez, J.J.; HernandezHerrero, M.; MoraVentura, M.T. Incidence of histamine-forming bacteria and histamine content in scombroid fish species from retail markets in the Barcelona area. *Int. J. Food Microbiol.* **1996**, *28*, 411–418. [CrossRef]
70. Landete, J.M.; de las Rivas, B.; Marcobal, A.; Muñoz, R. Molecular methods for the detection of biogenic amine-producing bacteria on foods. *Int. J. Food Microbiol.* **2007**, *117*, 258–269. [CrossRef]
71. Bozic, J.T.; Butinar, L.; Marusic, M.B.; Korte, D.; Vodopivec, B.M. Determination of biogenic amines formation by autochthonous lactic acid bacteria from 'Refosk' grapes using different analytical methods. *Lwt-Food Sci. Technol.* **2022**, *156*, 112908. [CrossRef]
72. Takahashi, H.; Kimura, B.; Yoshikawa, M.; Fujii, T. Cloning and sequencing of the histidine decarboxylase genes of gram-negative, histamine-producing bacteria and their application in detection and identification of these organisms in fish. *Appl. Environ. Microbiol.* **2003**, *69*, 2568–2579. [CrossRef] [PubMed]
73. Nalazek-Rudnicka, K.; Wasik, A. Development and validation of an LC-MS/MS method for the determination of biogenic amines in wines and beers. *Monatsh Chem.* **2017**, *148*, 1685–1696. [CrossRef] [PubMed]
74. Fu, Q.; Zheng, H.; Han, X.; Cao, L.; Sui, J. Development of a highly sensitive HPLC method for the simultaneous determination of eight biogenic amines in aquatic products. *Acta Chromatogr.* **2021**, *33*, 378–386. [CrossRef]
75. Jiang, W.; Xu, Y.; Li, C.; Dong, X.; Wang, D. Biogenic amines in commercially produced Yulu, a Chinese fermented fish sauce. *Food Addit. Contam. Part B* **2014**, *7*, 25–29. [CrossRef] [PubMed]
76. Li, G.; Dong, L.; Wang, A.; Wang, W.; Hu, N.; You, J. Simultaneous determination of biogenic amines and estrogens in foodstuff by an improved HPLC method combining with fluorescence labeling. *LWT—Food Sci. Technol.* **2014**, *55*, 355–361. [CrossRef]
77. Abdurrahman Munir, M.; Haji Badri, K. The importance of derivatizing reagent in chromatography applications for biogenic amine detection in food and beverages. *J. Anal. Methods Chem.* **2020**, *2020*, 5814389. [CrossRef]
78. Bomke, S.; Seiwert, B.; Dudek, L.; Effkemann, S.; Karst, U. Determination of biogenic amines in food samples using derivatization followed by liquid chromatography/mass spectrometry. *Anal. Bioanal. Chem.* **2009**, *393*, 247–256. [CrossRef] [PubMed]
79. Veciana-Nogues, M.T.; Hernandez-Jover, T.; Marine-Font, A.; Vedal-Carou, M.D.C. Liquid chromatographic method for determination of biogenic amines in fish and fish products. *J. AOAC Int.* **1995**, *78*, 1045–1050. [CrossRef] [PubMed]
80. Kosma, I.; Badeka, A. Determination of six underivatized biogenic amines by LC-MS/MS and study of biogenic amine production during trout (Salmo trutta) storage in ice. *Food Addit. Contam. Part A Chem. Anal. Control Expo. Risk Assess.* **2021**, *38*, 476–487. [CrossRef]
81. Koo, P.-L.; Lim, G.-K. A review on analytical techniques for quantitative detection of histamine in fish products. *Microchem. J.* **2023**, *189*, 108499. [CrossRef]
82. Shiono, K.; Tsutsumi, T.; Nabeshi, H.; Ikeda, A.; Yokoyama, J.; Akiyama, H. Simple and rapid determination of biogenic amines in fish and fish products by liquid chromatography-tandem mass spectrometry using 2,4,6-triethyl-3,5-dimethyl pyrylium trifluoromethanesulfonate as a derivatization reagent. *J. Chromatogr. A* **2021**, *1643*, 462046. [CrossRef] [PubMed]

83. Tatsuta, Y.; Tanaka, Y.; Ikeda, A.; Matsukawa, S.; Katano, H.; Taira, S. Nanoparticle-Assisted Laser Desorption/Ionization Mass Spectrometry (Nano-PALDI MS) with Py-Tag for the Analysis of Small Molecules. *Mass Spectrom.* **2017**, *6*, S0069. [CrossRef] [PubMed]
84. Aladhadh, M.; Nasser Binjawhar, D.; Abd El-Kader Ebrahim, H.N.E.; Radhi, K.S.; Almatrafi, M.; Fayad, E.; Al-Saman, M.A.; Elsanhoty, R.M. Investigation of Biogenic Amine Levels and Microbiological Activity as Quality Markers in Some Dairy and Fish Products in Food Markets in the Kingdom of Saudi Arabia. *ACS Omega* **2024**, *9*, 19193–19202. [CrossRef] [PubMed]
85. Valls, J.E.; Bello, R.A.; Kodaira, M.S. Semiquantitative analysis by thin-layer chromatography (TLC) of biogenic amines in dried, salted and canned fish products. *J. Food Qual.* **2002**, *25*, 165–176. [CrossRef]
86. Badrul, H.A.; Inayatullah, A.; Munir, M.A. Fish Analysis Containing Biogenic Amines Using Gas Chromatography Equipped With Flame Ionization And Mass Spectrometer Detectors. *Sci. Technol. Indones.* **2021**, *6*. [CrossRef]
87. Shalaby, A.R. Significance of biogenic amines to food safety and human health. *Food Res. Int.* **1996**, *29*, 675–690. [CrossRef]
88. Bonilla, M.; Enriquez, L.G.; McNair, H.M. Use of cold on-column injection for the analysis of putrescine and cadaverine by gas chromatography. *J. Chromatogr. Sci.* **1997**, *35*, 53–56. [CrossRef]
89. Scavnicar, A.; Rogelj, I.; Kocar, D.; Kose, S.; Pompe, M. Determination of Biogenic Amines in Cheese by Ion Chromatography with Tandem Mass Spectrometry Detection. *J. AOAC Int.* **2018**, *101*, 1542–1547. [CrossRef] [PubMed]
90. Kocar, D.; Kose, S.; Tufan, B.; Scavnicar, A.; Pompe, M. Determination of Biogenic Amines in Fresh Fish and Processed Fish Products Using IC-MS/MS. *Foods* **2021**, *10*, 1746. [CrossRef] [PubMed]
91. Kocar, D.; Köse, S.; Koral, S.; Tufan, B.; Scavnicar, A.; Pompe, M. Analysis of Biogenic Amines Using Immunoassays, HPLC, and a Newly Developed IC-MS/MS Technique in Fish Products-A Comparative Study. *Molecules* **2021**, *26*, 6156. [CrossRef]
92. Fan, Y.; Yu, R.; Waterhouse, G.I.N.; Wang, R.; Sun, Y.; Xu, Z. Development of a capillary electrophoresis method based on magnetic solid-phase extraction for simultaneous and sensitive detection of eight biogenic amines in foods. *J. Sci. Food Agric.* **2024**, *104*, 3256–3264. [CrossRef]
93. Fan, Y.; Yu, R.; Chen, Y.; Sun, Y.; Waterhouse, G.I.N.; Xu, Z. A Capillary Electrophoresis Method Based on Molecularly Imprinted Solid-Phase Extraction for Selective and Sensitive Detection of Histamine in Foods. *Molecules* **2022**, *27*, 6987. [CrossRef] [PubMed]
94. Verma, N.; Hooda, V.; Gahlaut, A.; Gothwal, A.; Hooda, V. Enzymatic biosensors for the quantification of biogenic amines: A literature update. *Crit. Rev. Biotechnol.* **2020**, *40*, 1–14. [CrossRef]
95. Vasconcelos, H.; Coelho, L.C.C.; Matias, A.; Saraiva, C.; Jorge, P.A.S.; de Almeida, J.M.M.M. Biosensors for Biogenic Amines: A Review. *Biosensors* **2021**, *11*, 82. [CrossRef] [PubMed]
96. Singh, S.; Kumar, V.; Dhanjal, D.S.; Datta, S.; Prasad, R.; Singh, J. Biological biosensors for monitoring and diagnosis. *Microb. Biotechnol.* **2020**, 317–335. [CrossRef]
97. Lange, J.; Wittmann, C. Enzyme sensor array for the determination of biogenic amines in food samples. *Anal. Bioanal. Chem.* **2002**, *372*, 276–283. [CrossRef]
98. Iranifam, M. Analytical applications of chemiluminescence systems assisted by carbon nanostructures. *TrAC-Trends Anal. Chem.* **2016**, *80*, 387–415. [CrossRef]
99. Omanovic-Miklicanin, E.; Valzacchi, S. Development of new chemiluminescence biosensors for determination of biogenic amines in meat. *Food Chem.* **2017**, *235*, 98–103. [CrossRef] [PubMed]
100. Ahangari, H.; Kurbanoglu, S.; Ehsani, A.; Uslu, B. Latest trends for biogenic amines detection in foods: Enzymatic biosensors and nanozymes applications. *Trends Food Sci. Technol.* **2021**, *112*, 75–87. [CrossRef]
101. Kuo, P.-C.; Lien, C.-W.; Mao, J.-Y.; Unnikrishnan, B.; Chang, H.-T.; Lin, H.-J.; Huang, C.-C. Detection of urinary spermine by using silver-gold/silver chloride nanozymes. *Anal. Chim. Acta* **2018**, *1009*, 89–97. [CrossRef] [PubMed]
102. Sanz-Vicente, I.; Rivero, I.; Marcuello, L.; Montano, M.P.; de Marcos, S.; Galban, J. Portable colorimetric enzymatic disposable biosensor for histamine and simultaneous histamine/tyramine determination using a smartphone. *Anal. Bioanal. Chem.* **2023**, *415*, 1777–1786. [CrossRef]
103. Givanoudi, S.; Heyndrickx, M.; Depuydt, T.; Khorshid, M.; Robbens, J.; Wagner, P. A Review on Bio- and Chemosensors for the Detection of Biogenic Amines in Food Safety Applications: The Status in 2022. *Sensors* **2023**, *23*, 613. [CrossRef] [PubMed]
104. Hasanzadeh, M.; Shadjou, N.; de la Guardia, M. Aptamer-based assay of biomolecules: Recent advances in electro-analytical approach. *TrAC Trends Anal. Chem.* **2017**, *89*, 119–132. [CrossRef]
105. Rotariu, L.; Lagarde, F.; Jaffrezic-Renault, N.; Bala, C. Electrochemical biosensors for fast detection of food contaminants trends and perspective. *TrAC Trends Anal. Chem.* **2016**, *79*, 80–87. [CrossRef]
106. Venkatesh, S.; Yeung, C.C.; Li, T.; Lau, S.C.; Sun, Q.J.; Li, L.Y.; Li, J.H.; Lam, M.H.W.; Roy, V.A.L. Portable molecularly imprinted polymer-based platform for detection of histamine in aqueous solutions. *J. Hazard. Mater.* **2021**, *410*, 124609. [CrossRef]
107. Xu, L.; Zhou, J.; Eremin, S.; Dias, A.C.P.; Zhang, X. Development of ELISA and chemiluminescence enzyme immunoassay for quantification of histamine in drug products and food samples. *Anal. Bioanal. Chem.* **2020**, *412*, 4739–4747. [CrossRef]
108. Jiaxu, X.; Hongfei, Y.; Liangni, Q.; Jixiang, L.; Long, L.; Xiaohui, F.; Dapeng, P. Rapid detection of fluoroquinolone residues in aquatic products based on a gold-labeled microwell immunochromatographic assay. *Food Qual. Saf.* **2022**, *6*, fyac033. [CrossRef]

109. Shkodra, B.; Abera, B.D.; Cantarella, G.; Douaki, A.; Avancini, E.; Petti, L.; Lugli, P. Flexible and Printed Electrochemical Immunosensor Coated with Oxygen Plasma Treated SWCNTs for Histamine Detection. *Biosens.* **2020**, *10*, 35. [CrossRef] [PubMed]
110. Degefu, H.; Amare, M.; Tessema, M.; Admassie, S. Lignin modified glassy carbon electrode for the electrochemical determination of histamine in human urine and wine samples. *Electrochim. Acta* **2014**, *121*, 307–314. [CrossRef]
111. Munir, M.A.; Badri, K.H.; Heng, L.Y.; Inayatullah, A.; Badrul, H.A. A Modest Approach of Electrochemical Sensor to Determine Biogenic Amines in Food and Beverages. *JSI* **2020**, *1*, 162–173. [CrossRef]
112. Heng, L.Y.; Badri, K.H.; Munir, M.A. Biogenic Amines Detection by Chromatography and Sensor Methods: A Comparative Review. *Sci. Technol. Indones.* **2020**, *5*. [CrossRef]
113. Justino, C.I.; Freitas, A.C.; Pereira, R.; Duarte, A.C.; Santos, T.A.R. Recent developments in recognition elements for chemical sensors and biosensors. *TrAC Trends Anal. Chem.* **2015**, *68*, 2–17. [CrossRef]
114. Dervisevic, M.; Dervisevic, E.; Şenel, M. Recent progress in nanomaterial-based electrochemical and optical sensors for hypoxanthine and xanthine. A review. *Microchim. Acta* **2019**, *186*, 749. [CrossRef] [PubMed]
115. Du, L.; Lao, Y.; Sasaki, Y.; Lyu, X.; Gao, P.; Wu, S.; Minami, T.; Liu, Y. Freshness monitoring of raw fish by detecting biogenic amines using a gold nanoparticle-based colorimetric sensor array. *RSC Adv.* **2022**, *12*, 6803–6810. [CrossRef] [PubMed]
116. Prasad, B.; Stoeva, S.I.; Sorensen, C.M.; Klabunde, K.J. Digestive ripening of thiolated gold nanoparticles: The effect of alkyl chain length. *Langmuir* **2002**, *18*, 7515–7520. [CrossRef]
117. Abbasi-Moayed, S.; Orouji, A.; Hormozi-Nezhad, M.R. Multiplex Detection of Biogenic Amines for Meat Freshness Monitoring Using Nanoplasmonic Colorimetric Sensor Array. *Biosensors* **2023**, *13*, 803. [CrossRef] [PubMed]
118. Cao, Y.; Wang, X.; Feng, T.; Li, Z.; Xue, C.; Xu, J. Ratiometric fluorescent nanosystem based on upconversion nanoparticles for histamine determination in seafood. *Food Chem.* **2022**, *390*, 133194. [CrossRef] [PubMed]
119. Rong, Y.; Hassan, M.M.; Ouyang, Q.; Chen, Q. Lanthanide ion (Ln^{3+})-based upconversion sensor for quantification of food contaminants: A review. *Compr. Rev. Food Sci. Food Saf.* **2021**, *20*, 3531–3578. [CrossRef]
120. Siripongpreda, T.; Siralertmukul, K.; Rodthongkum, N. Colorimetric sensor and LDI-MS detection of biogenic amines in food spoilage based on porous PLA and graphene oxide. *Food Chem.* **2020**, *329*, 127165. [CrossRef]
121. Zhong, X.H.; Huo, D.Q.; Fa, H.B.; Luo, X.G.; Wang, Y.; Zhao, Y.N.; Hou, C.J. Rapid and ultrasensitive detection of biogenic amines with colorimetric sensor array. *Sens. Actuators B* **2018**, *274*, 464–471. [CrossRef]
122. Ding, L.; Li, X.; Hu, L.C.; Zhang, Y.C.; Jiang, Y.; Mao, Z.P.; Xu, H.; Wang, B.J.; Feng, X.L.; Sui, X.F. A naked-eye detection polyvinyl alcohol/cellulose-based pH sensor for intelligent packaging. *Carbohydr. Polym.* **2020**, *233*, 115859. [CrossRef]
123. Roth, M. Fluorescence reaction for amino acids. *Anal. Chem.* **1971**, *43*, 880–882. [CrossRef]
124. Hasanova, N.; Çelik, S.E.; Apak, R. Dithioerythritol functionalized gold nanoparticles—based fluorometric sensing of biogenic amines in food samples. *J. Food Compos. Anal.* **2022**, *114*, 104837. [CrossRef]
125. Peat, M.A.; Gibb, J.W. High-performance liquid chromatographic determination of indoleamines, dopamine, and norepinephrine in rat brain with fluorometric detection. *Anal. Biochem.* **1983**, *128*, 275–280. [CrossRef]
126. Zhu, B.; Jiang, L.; Chen, T.; Bao, G.-M.; Zeng, L.; Hu, X.; Yuan, H.-Q. A colorimetric and fluorescence lighting-up probe for the determination of biogenic primary diamine during the spoilage of fish. *Dyes Pigm.* **2021**, *186*, 108963. [CrossRef]
127. Guo, Q.-N.; Li, Z.-Y.; Chan, W.-H.; Lau, K.-C.; Crossley, M.J. Appending zinc tetraphenylporphyrin with an amine receptor at β-pyrrolic carbon for designing a selective histamine chemosensor. *Supramol. Chem.* **2010**, *22*, 122–129. [CrossRef]
128. Sun, F.; Zhang, J.; Yang, Q.; Wu, W. Quantum dot biosensor combined with antibody and aptamer for tracing food-borne pathogens. *Food Qual. Saf.* **2021**, *5*, fyab019. [CrossRef]
129. Mobarez, S.N.; Wongkaew, N.; Simsek, M.; Baeumner, A.J.; Duerkop, A. Dipsticks with Reflectometric Readout of an NIR Dye for Determination of Biogenic Amines. *Chemosensors* **2020**, *8*, 99. [CrossRef]
130. Plotka-Wasylka, J.M.; Morrison, C.; Biziuk, M.; Namiesnik, J. Chemical Derivatization Processes Applied to Amine Determination in Samples of Different Matrix Composition. *Chem. Rev.* **2015**, *115*, 4693–4718. [CrossRef]
131. Danchuk, A.I.; Komova, N.S.; Mobarez, S.N.; Doronin, S.Y.; Burmistrova, N.A.; Markin, A.V.; Duerkop, A. Optical sensors for determination of biogenic amines in food. *Anal. Bioanal. Chem.* **2020**, *412*, 4023–4036. [CrossRef]
132. Zhang, Q.; Han, J.J.; Chen, Y.H.; Jia, Z.Q.; Pan, X.H.; Rani, K.K.; Zhou, J.Z.; Jiao, T.H.; Chen, Q.M.; Wu, D.Y. Rapid fabrication of large-area and uniform surface-enhanced Raman spectroscopy substrate of Au nano-hemisphere array and its application in the detection of Malachite Green in tilapia. *Food Qual. Saf.* **2023**, *7*, fyac061. [CrossRef]
133. Schaude, C.; Meindl, C.; Froehlich, E.; Attard, J.; Mohr, G.J. Developing a sensor layer for the optical detection of amines during food spoilage. *Talanta* **2017**, *170*, 481–487. [CrossRef]
134. Arce, L.; Rios, A.; Valcarcel, M. Selective and rapid determination of biogenic amines by capillary zone electrophoresis. *Chromatographia* **1997**, *46*, 170–176. [CrossRef]
135. Das, G.; Garai, B.; Prakasam, T.; Benyettou, F.; Varghese, S.; Sharma, S.K.; Gandara, F.; Pasricha, R.; Baias, M.; Jagannathan, R.; et al. Fluorescence turn on amine detection in a cationic covalent organic framework. *Nat. Commun.* **2022**, *13*, 3904. [CrossRef]

136. Nandi, S.; Mandal, S.; Sanmartin Matalobos, J.; Sahana, A.; Das, D. Interaction of water with a benzimidazole derivative: Fluorescence and colorimetric recognition of trace level water involving intramolecular charge transfer process. *J. Mol. Recognit.* **2016**, *29*, 5–9. [CrossRef]

chemosensors

MDPI

Review

Origami-Inspired Biosensors: Exploring Diverse Applications and Techniques for Shape-Changing Sensor Platforms

Shikha Patil [1,†], Shariq Suleman [1,†], Nigar Anzar [1], Jagriti Narang [1,*], Roberto Pilloton [2,*], Suna Timur [3], Emine Guler Celik [4], Chandra S. Pundir [5] and Sudheesh K. Shukla [6,7]

1 Department of Biotechnology, School of Chemical and Life Sciences, Jamia Hamdard, New Delhi 110062, India; shikhapatil29@gmail.com (S.P.); shariqsuleman07@gmail.com (S.S.); nigarsheikh111@gmail.com (N.A.)
2 Institute of Crystallography, National Research Council (CNR-IC), 00015 Rome, Italy
3 Department of Biochemistry, Faculty of Science, Ege University, 35100 Izmir, Turkey; suna.timur@ege.edu.tr
4 Department of Bioengineering, Faculty of Engineering, Ege University, 35100 Izmir, Turkey; emine.guler.celik@ege.edu.tr or gulercelik.emine@gmail.com
5 Department of Biochemistry, Maharshi Dayanand University, Rohtak 124001, India; pundircs@rediffmail.com
6 Centre for Nanoscience and Nano Bioelectronics, School of Chemical Engineering and Physical Sciences, Lovely Professional University, Phagwara 144411, Punjab, India; sudheeshkshukla010@gmail.com
7 Department of Chemical Science, University of Johannesburg (Doornfontein Campus), Johannesburg 2008, South Africa
* Correspondence: jags_biotech@yahoo.co.in (J.N.); roberto.pilloton@cnr.it (R.P.)
† These authors contributed equally to this work.

Abstract: Biosensors are widely used across industries such as healthcare, food safety, and environmental monitoring, offering high stability and sensitivity compared to conventional methods. Recently, origami—the art of folding 2D structures into 3D forms—has emerged as a valuable approach in biosensor development, enabling the creation of shape-changing devices. These origami-based biosensors are particularly useful in precision medicine, rapid diagnostics, and resource-limited settings, offering affordable, highly precise, and portable solutions with diverse applications. Paper and biological substrates like DNA have been integrated with origami techniques to develop biosensors with enhanced functionality. The incorporation of aptamer origami into both paper and DNA biosensors further increases sensitivity and specificity for target detection. The concept of paper-based origami biosensors originated from using paper as a platform for biological assays, leading to significant advancements in design and functionality. These devices employ folding techniques to create channels and wells for manipulating samples and detecting target molecules through reactions with specific reagents. Similarly, DNA origami, introduced in 2006, has revolutionized biosensors by enabling the creation of precise molecular systems with tunable properties. Paper-based and DNA origami biosensors have immense potential to transform biosensing technologies in healthcare, food safety, and environmental monitoring. This review explores diverse origami-based biosensor techniques and their applications, including the role of aptamer origami in paper and DNA biosensors.

Keywords: origami; oPAD; DNA origami; aptamer

1. Introduction

Origami, the ancient Japanese art of folding two-dimensional paper into intricate three-dimensional structures, has found a transformative role in biosensing. Originally a creative art form, the principles of origami have been adapted by scientists to develop dynamic, shape-changing structures with vast potential for biosensor applications [1]. These innovative biosensors, often called origami-based biosensors, are used for the detection of a variety of analytes like glucose, viruses, and pesticides, leveraging their unique structural properties to enhance sensitivity and functionality [2]. DNA origami, an extension of this technique, has also emerged as a powerful tool in biomolecular sensing, providing new opportunities for precise and reliable detection [3]. These innovative biosensors can detect analytes like glucose, viruses, and pesticides with remarkable sensitivity, achieving detection limits as low as 8.86 pM for specific targets, far surpassing traditional biosensors, which often lack such adaptability and precision. The programmability of DNA origami enables the creation of complex structures that amplify signals, significantly improving performance in challenging environments [4,5].

The development of origami-based biosensors offers numerous advantages over traditional sensing technologies, particularly in resource-limited settings such as rural areas, where access to sophisticated diagnostic tools is restricted [6]. These biosensors are cost-effective, portable, easy to manufacture, and scalable, making them ideal for point-of-care (POC) diagnostics, environmental monitoring, and food safety. In particular, the integration of origami techniques into paper-based analytical devices (PADs) has allowed researchers to create flexible, three-dimensional structures capable of performing complex multi-step assays, such as immunoassays, in a simplified and efficient manner [7]. This approach enhances assay specificity and sensitivity while reducing operational steps and assay time, addressing the need for rapid and low-cost detection methods [8].

In addition to paper-based substrates, biological materials such as DNA are increasingly being used to create origami biosensors. DNA origami, a rapidly advancing area of nanotechnology, holds immense promise for applications ranging from disease diagnosis to drug discovery and environmental monitoring [9]. DNA offers several key advantages, including high stability, predictability, programmability, and ease of synthesis. These have driven the development of increasingly complex DNA-based biosensors capable of multiplex detection and target specificity [4]. DNA origami-based biosensors are particularly noted for their ability to distinguish between specific and non-specific interactions, offering high sensitivity and precision [10]. Moreover, the large-scale production of DNA origami structures is cost-effective, making them an attractive option for biomedical applications, especially when compared to other treatments like antisense oligonucleotides [3]. The combination of DNA origami with other biosensing technologies marks a promising direction for advancing sensor capabilities. For example, integrating DNA origami with paper-based systems results in hybrid biosensors that harness the strengths of each technology. DNA origami, functionalized with aptamers or other biomolecular probes, can serve as concrete sensing elements within paper substrates. This integration could develop low-cost devices capable of multiplex detection with improved sensitivity and specificity [11,12]. Table 1 provides a comparative overview of paper-based and DNA origami-based biosensors, highlighting the distinct advantages of each.

Another significant advancement in biosensing is the incorporation of aptamers—short, engineered DNA or RNA strands that selectively bind to specific target molecules—into origami structures. Aptamer origami enhances biosensor performance by increasing the surface area for target capture, thereby improving binding affinity and detection sensitivity. In paper-based biosensors, aptamer origami is integrated into the paper substrate, where target molecules bind to the aptamer, leading to a detectable signal, such as a color change [13]. Similarly, aptamers are folded into complex three-dimensional structures in DNA origami biosensors, further enhancing the device's specificity and sensitivity [14].

This review will explore the use of origami techniques in the development of biosensing devices, with a focus on the different materials employed—such as paper, DNA, and aptamers—and the unique advantages they bring to biosensor design and application.

Table 1. Comparison of paper-based and DNA-based origami biosensors and aptamer origami biosensors.

	Paper Origami Biosensors	DNA Origami Biosensors	Aptamer Origami Biosensor
Material Composition	Cellulose-based paper	DNA strands	Single stranded oligonucleotides (DNA/RNA)
Fabrication Techniques	Cutting, folding, and assembling 3D structures with paper	DNA origami technique (scaffold DNA and staple strands for folding)	Aptamer-based folding (using aptamers for target binding and folding)
Detection Mechanisms	Colorimetric, electrochemical, fluorescence-based	Fluorescence, FRET, SPR, electrochemical	Fluorescence, FRET, SPR, electrochemical
Target Analytes	Pathogens, environmental toxins, small molecules	Proteins, nucleic acids, metal ions	Small molecules, proteins, ions, pathogens
Sensitivity	Moderate, depending on design and readout method	High sensitivity due to precise molecular design	Moderate to high, depending on aptamer specificity
Applications	POC diagnostics, Food safety, environmental monitoring	Medical diagnostics, drug delivery, nanoscale sensing	Medical diagnostics, biosensing, therapeutic monitoring
Advantages	Cost-effective, simple, disposable, portable	High precision, customizable structures	High specificity, versatility in target binding
Limitations	Lower sensitivity compared to DNA origami	Complex fabrication, higher cost	Limited by aptamer selection and stability

2. Paper-Based Origami Biosensors

Paper-based origami biosensors are built upon using paper as a platform for biological assays. The origin of these biosensors can be traced back to 2007, when the Whiteside group introduced the first paper-based biosensor for glucose and protein detection in artificial urine samples [15]. Since then, researchers have expanded on this idea by incorporating advanced sensing technologies such as microfluidics and nanomaterials into these devices [16]. In 2011, Liu and Crooks advanced the field by developing PADs that used origami folding techniques to create three-dimensional microfluidic channels. This breakthrough allowed for detecting various biomolecules, including proteins and DNA [17,18].

Paper-based origami biosensors have since been applied to various fields, such as environmental analysis, food safety, and clinical diagnostics. These biosensors use paper folding in specific ways to form channels and wells, which hold and manipulate biological samples. The samples are treated with reagents that react with target molecules, producing measurable signals detectable by a sensor [19]. Paper, as a substrate, offers many advantages for fabricating electroanalytical devices due to its wide availability, flexibility, high creasability, and eco-friendly disposal through burning. Its rough surface also provides a large area for the physical adsorption of biomolecules and reagents [8].

Paper-based origami biosensors can be classified based on the number of folds used in their construction.

2.1. Types of Paper Based Origami Biosensor

2.1.1. Single Folding

In single-folding biosensors, the device is created by folding the paper once [Figure 1a]. Liang et al. designed a biosensor by folding a paper strip lengthwise to form two tabs: a base tab and a cover tab. This simple folding method eliminated electroactive interference from other substances, improving detection specificity [20]. Similarly, Li et al. developed a single-fold glucose biosensor with a detection and enzyme immobilization zone separated by a single crease. Folding the paper brought these zones together for glucose detection, having an LOD of 0.05 mM and a linear range of 1 to 12 mM [21].

In another experiment, Li et al. used this method to design an immunosensing device to detect prostate antigen. They created a 3D sensor by folding two wax pads, one consisting of the electrodes and the other consisting of working electrodes. The detection process involved electrochemical enzymatic redox cycling. The device is characterized by an LOD of 0.0012 ng/mL and a linear range of 0.005–100 ng/mL. Using Au nanoparticles and electrodeposited MnO nanowires increased the working electrode's surface area, enhancing sensitivity [22].

While single folding offers simplicity and cost advantages, its functionality may be limited for assays requiring more complex fluidic control or structural features.

2.1.2. Double Folding

Double-folding biosensors involve folding the paper twice, creating multiple layers [Figure 1b]. Sun et al. created an origami μPAD for glycoprotein detection, which included a detection pad, a channel pad, and a washing pad. By folding the channel pad, the washing buffer was directed to the washing pad through a semi-hydrophilic zone, preventing sample contamination and enabling accurate detection. This device demonstrated a linear range of 1–107 pg/L and an LOD of 0.87 pg/mL [23].

Compared to single folding, double folding enhances fluidic control and reduces contamination risks, making it suitable for multi-step assays. However, it requires more intricate fabrication and precise folding alignment. This added complexity makes double folding a bridge between single folding's simplicity and the advanced functionalities of multiple folding

2.1.3. Multiple Folding

Multiple-folding biosensors, such as the one developed by Ding et al. for detecting organophosphorous pesticides, involve the use of three or more folded pads [Figure 1c]. Their biosensor featured a central detection pad surrounded by folding tabs, allowing for sequential folding to perform bioassays manually. The device achieved a linear range of 0.1–1 nM and an LOD of 0.06 nM. This multi-pad approach eliminated the need for separate reservoirs and facilitated efficient miniaturized analysis [24]. Additionally, Sun et al. developed a multiple-fold immunosensor to detect analytes like human chorionic gonadotropin (HCG), prostate-specific antigen (PSA), and carcinoembryonic antigen. This sensor utilized zinc oxide nanorods and reduced graphene oxide to enhance electron transmission and incorporated a screen-printed electrode array on paper sample zones for the precise and sensitive detection of multiple analytes [25].

While multiple folding facilitates miniaturization and multiplexing, its complexity poses reproducibility and user handling challenges. Nevertheless, the integration of advanced nanomaterials in these designs enhances sensitivity, making them suitable for high-precision applications

2.1.4. POP Up

Inspired by pop-up greeting cards, Wang et al. created a pop-up ePAD for detecting β-hydroxybutyrate [Figure 1d]. This device uses a reversible mechanical valve to control fluid connectivity by applying pressure to switch between "on" and "off" states. The sensor demonstrated a linear range of 0.1–6.0 mM and an LOD of 0.3 mM [26]. In another example, Srisomwat et al. designed a pop-up DNA biosensor for detecting label-free hepatitis B virus DNA. Using a cellulose paper substrate, they immobilized a DNA probe, allowing for hybridization detection of the target DNA with minimized contamination risk. This pop-up design also featured fluidic control, allowing for easy reconfiguration and rapid, low-cost detection without the need for complex labeling procedures [27].

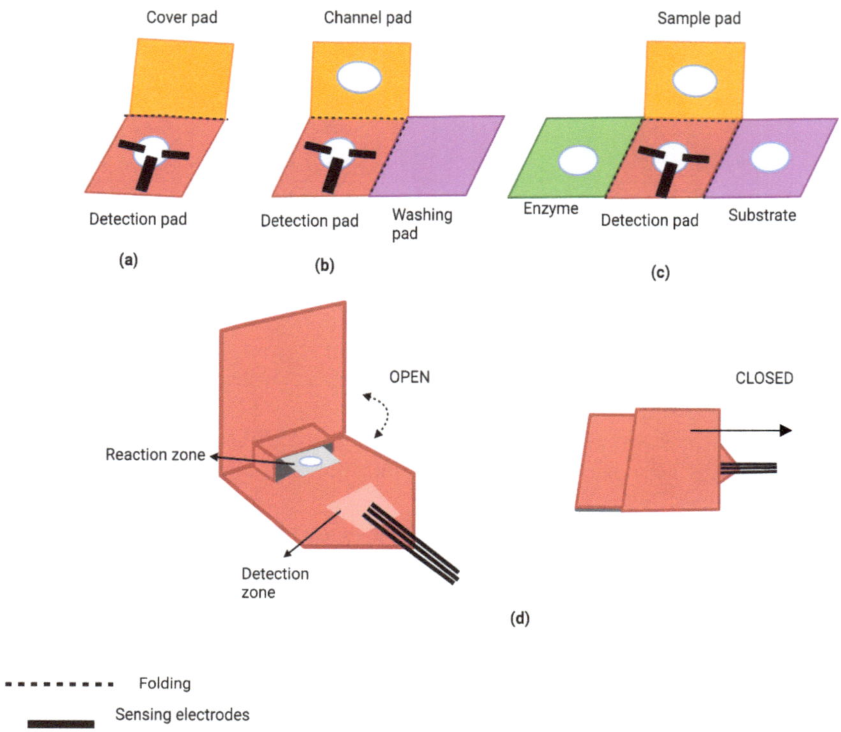

Figure 1. The general structure of paper-based origami biosensors: (**a**) single folding; (**b**) double folding; (**c**) multiple folding, which provides various pads for the substrate and enzyme, making the detection process suitable in miniaturized devices; (**d**) pop-up, in which the structure provides a reversible, mechanical connectivity of system where upon closing the pad, the reaction zone nears the detection zone and the analysis of the analyte takes place (redrawn from [26]).

2.2. *Applications of Paper Origami in Biosensing*

2.2.1. Nucleic Acid Detection

Nucleic acid testing is a critical technique in molecular diagnostics used to identify pathogens responsible for diseases due to their nucleic acid content. Detecting nucleic acids is crucial in POC applications, where paper-based origami biosensors show great promise. For example, Yu et al. developed a three-dimensional paper platform for electrochemical DNA detection, utilizing screen-printed electrodes coated with graphene and gold nanoparticles to immobilize captured DNA. When target single-stranded DNA (ssDNA) was present, the capture probe hybridized with it, triggering a reaction with an electroactive amplification label [24]. Scida et al. demonstrated a similar approach for ssDNA detection using fluorescence on an origami paper analytical device (oPAD). This method involved the hybridization of ssDNA and the subsequent detection of a quencher-labeled ssDNA displaced from a fluorophore-labeled ssDNA. The versatility of oPAD was further showcased by incorporating logical operations like OR and AND gates into the system [27].

2.2.2. Proteins Detection

Boonkaew et al. introduced a label-free electrochemical immunosensor on an origami PAD (oPAD) to detect C-reactive protein (CRP). They designed a specific oPAD pattern that allowed for the integration of multiple electrode modification steps into a single device. Using electrochemical impedance spectroscopy (EIS), the sensor measured changes in charge transfer between the electrode and the redox couple $[Fe(CN)_6]^{3-/4-}$, enabling CRP detection. This device demonstrated high sensitivity, stability, and selectivity for CRP detection, with no hindrance from common proteins such as bilirubin, BSA, or myoglobin. CRP levels were successfully measured in human serum samples, proving the potential usage of this biosensor in clinical diagnostics [28].

2.2.3. Virus Detection

Paper-based origami biosensors are highly suitable for the POC diagnosis of viral diseases. Various oPADs have been developed to detect viruses such as hepatitis B, HIV, and SARS-CoV-2. For example, Chen et al. developed a 3D oPAD for detecting human immunodeficiency virus (HIV). The 3D-tPAD featured components like strips, detection pads, indication pads, and absorbent pads, with specific features such as hydrophilic channels and hydrophobic zones created via wax printing. The device also incorporated a timer function to control the ELISA procedure by adding a washing buffer at timed intervals. The HIV detection signal was triggered by a color change on the indication pad, allowing for the easy visualization of results [29].

Following the COVID-19 pandemic, rapid diagnostic devices gained significant attention. Yakoha et al. designed a 3D electrochemical paper-based biosensor for detecting SARS-CoV-2 antibodies in human serum. The 3D origami device comprised three layers: a working pad, a counter pad, and a closing pad. Detection occurred when immunoglobulins from the serum formed a complex with the immobilized SARS-CoV-2 spike protein on the counter pad. This immunocomplex formation triggered a redox reaction ($[Fe(CN)_6]^{3-/4-}$), which was monitored using square-wave voltammetry (SWV) [30]. Figure 2 illustrates the device components and detection procedure of this COVID-19 biosensor. Upon folding, the immunoglobulins bind to the spike protein on the counter pad, enabling the detection of SARS-CoV-2 antibodies via SWV.

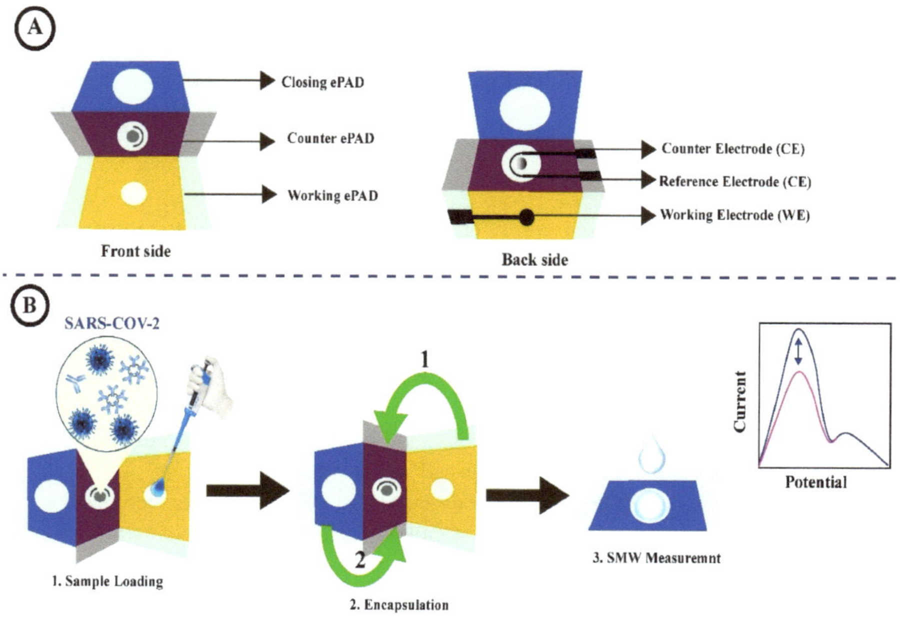

Figure 2. Schematic illustration of the (**A**) device components (front and back side) and (**B**) detection procedure of the COVID-19 ePAD; the sample is loaded on a working pad, and upon folding, the immunoglobulins bind with the deposited spike protein of SARS-CoV-2 on the counter pad. This immunocomplex formation leads to the detection of SARS-CoV-2 in human sera by means of SWV measurement.

2.2.4. Detection of Heavy Metals

Heavy metals are significant environmental pollutants that threaten human health [31,32]. Current methods for water analysis, such as spectrophotometry and traditional ELISA, are often expensive, time-consuming, and require highly trained personnel and sophisticated equipment [33–35]. As a more accessible alternative, oPADs have been developed to detect heavy metals. Heavy metal ions like Pb^{2+}, Hg^{2+}, Cd^{2+}, Cu^{2+} and Zn^{2+} are common environmental contaminants. A microfluidic paper sensor, developed by Martín-Yerga et al., enabled both the electrochemical and colorimetric detection of these ions. This sensor used screen-printed electrodes on a polyester film substrate to detect Cd^{2+} and Pb^{2+} levels. At the same time, colorimetric analysis was employed to detect the presence of other metal ions such as Fe^{2+}, Cu^{2+}, Ni^{2+}, and Cr^{2} [36]. Xiao et al. designed a 3D origami paper biosensing system for detecting silver ions using a portable, highly sensitive glucose meter. This biosensor used a nanoporous membrane embedded with reagents, where silver nanoparticles grew in situ to block pores and amplify detection signals. This device successfully detected Ag^{+} in various water samples, such as tap, drinking, pond, and soil water [37].

2.2.5. Agriculture and Food Safety

Pesticides are widely utilized on a global scale to increase food production and meet the demands of the growing world population. The constant use of pesticides has, however, resulted in food, soil, and water pollution, which is a significant problem [38,39]. To address this issue, Arduini and their colleagues developed an oPAD for the detection of various classes of pesticides by combining different enzyme-inhibition biosensors. By determining the ability to inhibit the enzymes butyrylcholinesterase, alkaline phosphatase, and tyrosinase displayed by the pesticides paraoxon, 2,4-dichlorophenoxyacetic acid, and atrazine, respectively, the detection was performed [40].

The presence of foodborne pathogens in food poses a prominent risk to public health [41]. These pathogens are living organisms like bacteria, viruses, and other microorganisms that can lead to foodborne illnesses when consumed. Foodborne illnesses can be categorized into two types: foodborne infections, caused by ingesting live pathogens that multiply in the digestive system, and foodborne intoxications, resulting from toxins produced by pathogens in the food [42]. oPADs have been effective in detecting various foodborne bacteria, including *E. coli*, *E. faecalis*, *L. monocytogenes*, *S. aureus*, and *S. typhimurium* [43,44]. The genetic material extracted from bacteria or viruses is usually minimal in quantity. It is crucial to amplify the extracted genetic material to detect a low number of pathogens in food analysis to achieve a reliable LOD [45]. He et al. demonstrated a method for detecting *S. typhimurium* using an amplification-based nucleic acid test (NAT) and an origami paper device. The origami paper device consisted of layers for drawing the sample solution, for DNA extraction, and for loop-mediated isothermal amplification (LAMP) and electrochemical sensing. The detection was performed via DPV once the LAMP reaction was achieved on the sensor. This method detected *S. typhimurium* at very low levels, reaching 5 CFU/mL and 2 CFU/mL in milk samples and drinking water, respectively [46].

An overview of the applications of different types of origami paper-based biosensors is shown in Table 2.

Table 2. Summary of types of origami paper-based biosensors.

Biosensor Type	Target	Sensing Substrate	Linear Range	LOD	Ref.
Single folding	Glucose	Glucose preloaded on paper	0–24 mM	-	[20]
	Glucose	Glucose oxidase + ferrocenecarboxylic acid	1–12 mM	0.05 mM	[21]
	Prostate protein antigen	Carbon nanosperes-glucose oxidase-monoclonal antibody label	0.005–100 ng/mL	0.0012 ng/mL	[22]
	ssDNA	AuNPs/GS modified SPWPE	0.0008–500 pM	0.2 fM	[47]
	Cd^{2+}, Ni^{2+}, Pb^{2+}, Fe^{2+}, Cu^{2+} and Cr^{2+}	Bi and potassium ferricyanide	0.25–7.5 ng	0.25 ng	[36]
Double folding	Glycoproteins	SiO_2@Au/dsDNA/CeO_2 nanocomposite	1–10^7 pg/mL	0.87 pg/mL	[23]
	ssDNA	fluorophore-labeled ssDNA	-	<5 nM	[48]
	SARS-CoV-2 antibodies	spike protein receptor-binding domain (SP RBD) of SARS-CoV-2	-	1 ng/ml	[30]
Multiple folding	Organophosphorus pesticides	Inhibition of Butyrylcholinesterase, with butyrylcholine-sensitive membrane	0.1 and 1.0 nM	0.06 nM	[24]
	(a) HCG (b) PSA(c) carcinoembryonic antigen	Reduced graphene oxide/Ag@BSA/2° antibody as signal label.	(a) 0.002–120 mIU/mL (b) 0.001–110 pg/mL (c) 0.001–100 pg/mL	(a) 0.0007 mIU/mL (b) 0.35 pg/mL (c) 0.33 pg/mL	[25]
	HIV p24	anti-HIV-1 p24	0.03 ng/mL to 3 ng/mL	0.01 ng/mL	[29]
	(i) paraoxon, (ii) 2,4-dichlorophenoxyacetic acid (iii) atrazine	(i) butyrylcholinesterase, (ii) alkaline phosphatase, (iii) tyrosinase	(i) Upto 20 ppb (ii) Upto 600 ppb (iii) 10–100 PPB	(i) 2 ppb (ii) 50 ppb (iii) -	[39]
Pop up	β-hydroxybutyrate	3-hydrozybutyrate dehydrogenase	0.1–6.0 mM	0.3 mM	[26]

3. DNA Origami

In 2006, Paul W.K. Rothemund introduced the DNA origami technique, where numerous small single-stranded DNAs (ssDNAs) were used to fold a long ssDNA into desired shapes [49]. This technique involves folding a long ssDNA with smaller complementary DNA strands called "staple strands", followed by heat-annealing in a buffer to create the origami structure [Figure 3a]. This method builds upon earlier work that demonstrated the potential of DNA as a material for constructing stable, self-assembling structures. Initial studies focused on creating DNA junctions and branched molecules, which showed that DNA could be engineered to form stable, predictable shapes [50]. These early innovations paved the way for more advanced DNA-based designs, such as DNA origami. DNA origami has found diverse applications across fields such as nanotechnology and medicine. It is employed in molecular surface patterning, nanoparticle positioning, nanorobotics, targeted drug delivery, molecular recognition, and biosensing [51–54]. Due to its affinity and interactions with other nucleic acids, DNA origami has been used in biosensing platforms. Biosensing through DNA origami can be categorized into binding-based biosensors and nanopores [55].

3.1. Types of DNA Origami Biosensor

3.1.1. Binding-Based Biosensors

Binding-based DNA origami biosensor detection is based on molecular interactions (nucleic acid–nucleic acid, nucleic acid–protein, etc.). In nucleic acid–nucleic acid interactions, the sensing occurs by anchoring the probe DNA with a complementary target nucleic acid sequence. DNA–DNA interactions and RNA–DNA interactions lead to the formation of ds hybrid nucleic acid, which can be visualized by means of atomic force microscopy (AFM). If the target nucleic acid sequence is not complementary with the probe DNA, it remains single-stranded and therefore cannot be seen in AFM [56]. The DNA tile is another nanoscale structure used in biosensing. It consists of scaffold DNA, which is a long single-stranded DNA that serves as the backbone, folded into a specific shape; helper DNA, a short strand that binds to the scaffold, stabilizing and shaping the structure; and index DNA, which aids in self-assembly and precise alignment [57]. Yan et al. developed a label-free RNA hybridization assay in which they utilized DNA origami to create a water-soluble nucleic acid probe "tile" [Figure 3b(2)]. They used the rectangle-shaped design to form origami tiles with different DNA probe sequences complementary to three genes—Rag-1, β-actin, and c-myc. When the RNA solution was applied to the tile, the protruding probe hybridized with target RNA and formed a V-shaped structure which was then sensed with AFM [58]. This was the first experiment in which a DNA origami structure was used in a biosensor [55]. DNA origami has also been used in protein biomarker detection. In 2011, Komiyama et al. created a "DNA origami plier", which acts as a nano-sized pinching device [Figure 3b(1)]. The opening and closing of this nanomechanical DNA origami plier occur selectively based on the specific target molecule. The shape transition was then visualized in AFM. The researchers detected streptavidin using a biotinylated-DNA origami plier [59].

3.1.2. Nanopores

Nanopores are widely used in biosensing applications. The sensing is based on the principle that the nanopores connect two electrolyte solutions reservoirs, and when the voltage is applied, the flow of current through the pore is measured. The single target molecule blocks the nanopore, which affects the current flow, and therefore, the target's presence can be determined [60]. The advancement in nanopore-based sequencing technologies in recent years has made nanopore-based sensing devices more competent. The nanopores can be classified into biological nanopores and solid-state nanopores. The former are developed by inserting natural proteins into lipid bilayer [61], whereas the latter are artificial nanopores created by drilling pores in synthetic silicon-based membranes using concentrated electron or ion beams [62]. DNA origami has been applied to nanopores for producing hybrid nanopores. This can be achieved in two different ways—(1) by trapping a DNA origami structure at the mouth of a solid state nanopore and (2) by means of the insertion of a DNA origami structure, coated with hydrophobic moieties, into a lipid bilayer [Figure 3b(4)] [63]. Hybrid nanopores are achieved by capturing DNA origami within a solid-state nanopore, taking inspiration from Hall et al.'s approach in 2010, where they guided the protein nanopore, alpha-hemolysin, into a solid-state nanopore to create a hybrid architecture [64]. This technique combines the benefits of precisely tailored nanoconstructs and a more durable substrate compared to a lipid bilayer. Another method of utilizing DNA nanostructures in nanopore sensing involves inserting a structure into a lipid bilayer, mimicking the behavior of membrane proteins in cellular membranes that regulate molecule and ion transport. The hydrophilic nature of DNA's charged phosphate backbone necessitates the incorporation of hydrophobic chemical groups in the DNA nanostructure to overcome the substantial energy cost associated with creating a pore in the lipid bilayer [63].

DNA origami nanopores can act as biosensors for detecting various biomolecules, including ssDNA, dsDNA, and proteins [65–67]. Furthermore, they have advantages over traditional nanopores. Their characteristics can be modified, expanding their applications as single-molecule detectors due to their stability, reversibility, tailored size, and chemical modifications [68].

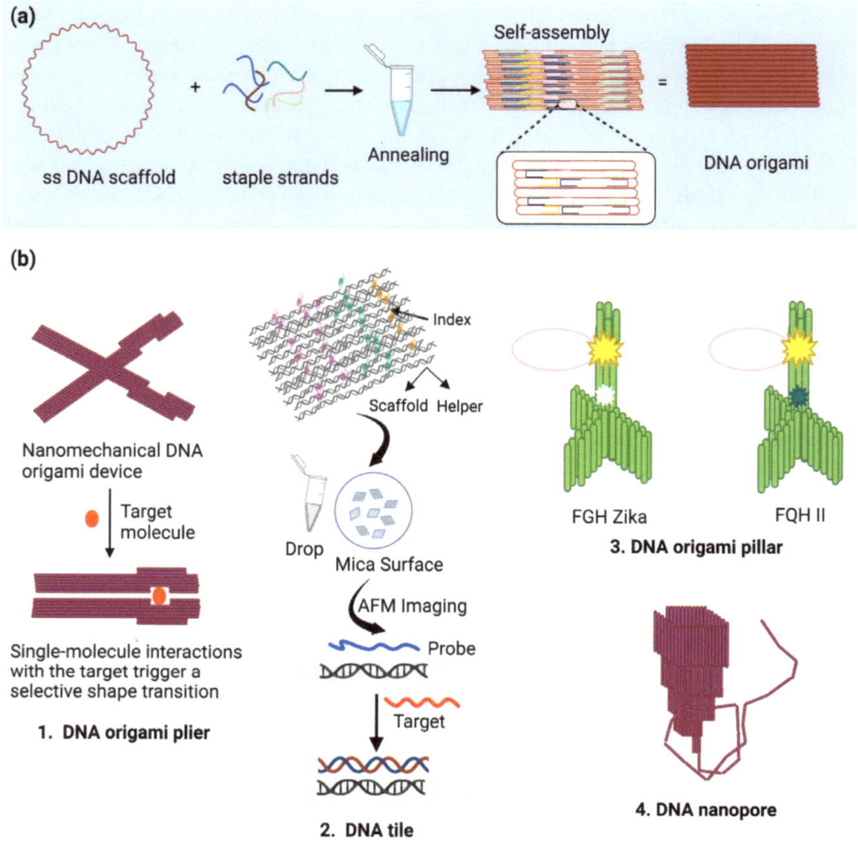

Figure 3. Synthesis and utilization of DNA origami in developing various structures. (**a**) The synthesis process begins with designing a lengthy ssDNA scaffold, usually derived from a bacteriophage genome. Complementary short DNA strands, called staple strands, are then created and combined with the scaffold in a controlled reaction. Through precise base-pairing interactions between the staples and the scaffold, a sophisticated computer algorithm guides the formation of the DNA origami structure. The staples effectively pull the scaffold into specific configurations, resulting in the final nanostructure. (**b**) Different structures: (**1**) DNA origami plier: opening and closing triggered by the target [59]; (**2**) DNA tile: consisting of scaffold, helper, and index DNA [58]; (**3**) DNA origami pillar [69]; (**4**) DNA nanopore [65].

3.2. Applications of DNA Origami in Biosensing

3.2.1. Nucleic Acid/SNP Detection

SNPs can be detected using a nucleic acid origami platform. Label-free SNP detection has been achieved in homogenous solutions using DNA origami chips and toehold-mediated strand-displacement reactions. These origami chips contain ssDNA-captured probes aligned with biotinylated and partially complementary reporter probes. Streptavidin acts as a marker and appears as a white bulge under AFM. When a fully complementary strand binds to the capture probe, the reporter probe is displaced, causing streptavidin's characteristics to vanish. This is not the case when there is even a single nucleotide mismatch in the sequence [70,71].

Subramanian et al. demonstrated the potential of DNA nanotechnology to detect single nucleotide polymorphisms (SNPs) through a unimolecular approach [72]. This technique involved combining atomic force microscopy (AFM) with DNA origami patterns to create a visual representation of the target nucleotide in the probe sequence. The origami design included graphical symbols for all four nucleotides, with the symbol representing the test nucleotide disappearing upon probe sequence addition. SNP detection relied on the kinetic process of branch migration, which had previously been successful in solution-state multiplex SNP analysis [73]. This isothermal method ensured unidirectional branch migration from the toehold region to the opposite end. The system also incorporated a photocleavable linker that could be broken upon irradiation, allowing the signal-producing component to be released by the probe strand. AFM images were analyzed by computer to provide a direct readout of the probe nucleotide. The system was also able to detect heterozygous diploid genomes using pairs of probes. Despite being immobilized on the origami scaffold, the strand exchange process was not hindered.

Viruses are composed of nucleic acids. To detect virus-related nucleic acids, DNA origami can be employed. Ochmann et al. developed a detection method to identify Zika-specific artificial DNA and RNA using optical antennas created by DNA origami. The DNA origami antenna consists of a pillar [Figure 3b(3)] with a silver nanoparticle on top, an adjacent fluorescence-quenching hairpin, and a fluorescent dye integrated at the base of the origami. By introducing specific Zika DNA/RNA, the hairpin opens, resulting in fluorescence recovery, while the silver nanoparticles enhance the fluorescence intensities [69].

Williamson et al. present a novel strategy that utilizes DNA origami technology to amplify electrochemical signals generated from DNA hybridization (Figure 4). Their approach employs a sandwich assay to enhance charge transfer resistance (RCT), significantly improving the LOD by two orders of magnitude compared to conventional label-free electrochemical DNA (e-DNA) biosensors. This sensor demonstrates a linear range between 10 pM and 1 nM for target, eliminating the need for probe labeling [5].

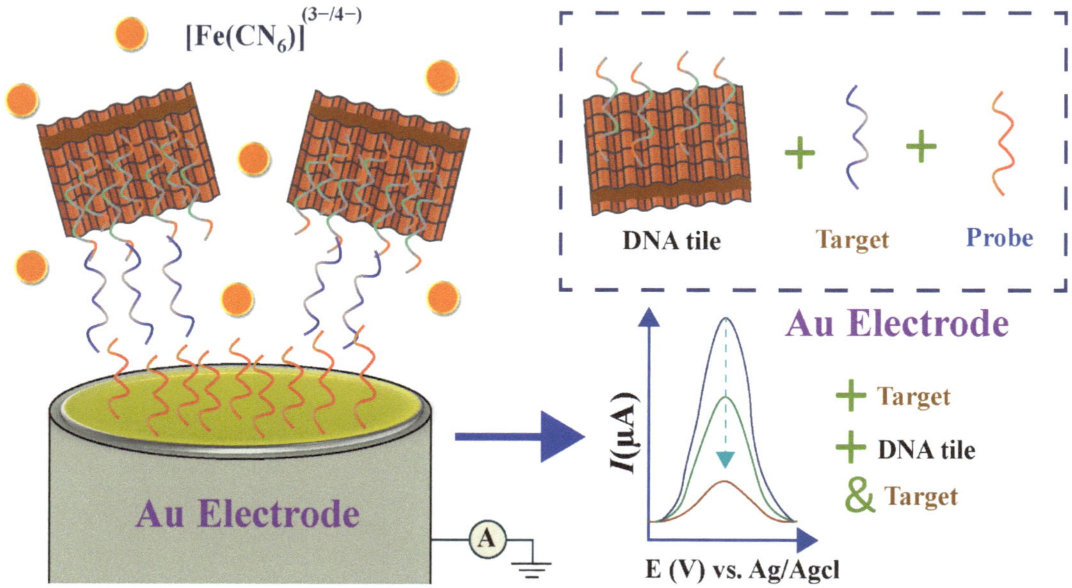

Figure 4. Signal amplification in the biosensor facilitated by DNA origami tiles. The DNA origami (brown) incorporates capture strands that bind to the target strands, forming a complex that subsequently attaches to the single-stranded DNA probe-functionalized electrode (FE), comprising probes and a polycrystalline gold electrode (PGE). This interaction modulates the distribution of redox species.

3.2.2. Protein Detection

Raveendran et al. developed a biosensor platform for quantitative single-molecule detection by means of a nanopore-based readout using DNA origami. A hollow rectangular DNA sheet was functionalized with a target-specific aptamer for human CRP at its center. This design enabled differentiation between DNA origami structures in the presence and in the absence of a target protein by analyzing the peak shape, amplitude, and dwell time during nanopore translocation [74]. Yan et al. developed an ELISA with magnetic beads and rolling circle amplification (RCA)-based DNA belts that is sensitive and selective for the detection of PSA. RCA produces DNA nanostructures that are then folded into DNA belts with biotin-coated staples to amplify the signal. Then, magnetic bead ELISA for PSA detection uses high-order nanostructures. By utilizing DNA origami's precise flexibility with RCA, this method has great selectivity [75].

3.2.3. pH Detection

DNA origami has also been used in pH sensing. Kumuya and colleagues devised a single-molecule pH sensor utilizing AFM imaging in response to the pH-responsive conformational changes of a nanomechanical DNA origami plier. The DNA origami nanoconstruct consists of two levers that are 170 nm long and 20 nm wide connected by a holliday-juction fulcrum, with each lever containing nine pairs of C-rich 12-mer sequences (i-binder). Under acidic conditions, when the construct is introduced with a short DNA sequence called an i-motif, it interacts with the i-binder, forming a quadruplex which results in changes in the shape of the DNA plier from an open form to a closed form. The shape transition was visualized through atomic force microscopy imaging [76]. Zhang et al. developed a DNA origami nanocaliper which changes its conformation depending upon the surrounding pH. The origami nanocaliper consists of pH-responsive triplex DNA between two arms. The shape transition of the caliper can be determined by TEM, in which the DNA nanostructure shows a large hinge angle at acidic pH, whereas in basic conditions, it shows a small hinge angle [77].

3.2.4. Enzyme Activity

Tintore and colleagues developed a DNA origami platform for analyzing the enzymatic activity of human O6-alkylguanine-DNA alkyltransferase (hAGT). This is a protein responsible for the repair of O6-methyl guanine, providing resistance to chemotherapeutic agents, and is therefore considered a relevant prognosis marker of cancer. Using DNA quadruplex and α-thrombin protein, the researchers developed a biosensing platform for detection of the enzymatic activity of hAGT. The detection is based upon the conformational change of the DNA quadruplex upon binding with the α-thrombin protein. The interaction was visualized under AFM imaging [78].

3.2.5. Chemical Reactions

Voigt et al. used DNA origami for single-molecule analysis of chemical reactions. In 2010, the authors reported the use of origami structures as an addressable support to achieve and visualize the cleavage and formation of individual chemical bonds. They were able to demonstrate a bond-cleavage reaction, where DNA origami with biotinylated staple strands was used. The addition of streptavidin led to bright spots. The biotinylated strands were incorporated with three linkers, type A, type B and type C. 1,4-dithiothreitol and singlet oxygen photosensitized by eosin were used for the cleavage of linkers B and C, respectively. The reactions were monitored by AFM based on the disappearance of streptavidin. Similarly, the authors demonstrated bond-forming reactions and photochemical reactions in same study [77].

An overview of the applications of DNA origami biosensors is shown in Table 3.

Table 3. Summary table of the applications of DNA origami biosensors.

Applications	Target	Sensing Component	Detection/Visualization Technique	Efficiency/ LOD	Ref.
Nucleic acid detection	Rag-1, c-myc and β-actin	DNA origami tile having complementary probe	Atomic Force Microscopy	~1000 molecules	[58]
SNP detection	SM (single-base mismatch) DNA	-	"toehold"-mediated strand-displacement reaction/Atomic Force Microscopy	-	[71]
Protein detection	Streptavidin	Biotinylated DNA plier	Atomic Force Microscopy	2 molecules	[59]
	Prostate-specific antigen (PSA)	RCA based DNA belts	Magnetic bead-based ELISA/AFM	50 aM	[75]
	C-reactive protein (CRP)	CRP-specific aptamer	AFM	3 nM	[74]
pH detection	HEPES buffer	DNA origami plier	AFM	-	[76]
	pH buffer	DNA nanocaliper	Transmission electron microscope	-	[79]
Enzyme activity	human O6-alkylguanine-DNA alkyltransferase (hAGT)	DNA quadruplex	AFM	-	[78]

4. Aptamers in Biosensors

Aptamers are short, single-stranded oligonucleotides that fold into distinct three-dimensional structures, allowing them to bind to targets with high specificity and affinity. These targets include small molecules, inorganic compounds, proteins, and entire cells. Aptamers are constructed through an in vitro process called the Systematic Evolution of Ligands by Exponential Enrichment (SELEX) and have been employed for precise detection, inhibition, and characterization of various targets [80].

Researchers have been working to offer simple, quick, and analytical systems with high sensitivity and specificity in order to overcome the drawbacks of conventional analytical methods, such as their high cost and protracted detection processes. Due to their high sensitivity, simplicity, and strong affinity for their targets, aptamers have been able to significantly advance this field. Aptamers are a useful tool in biosensors due to their simplicity of labeling and modification, excellent chemical and thermal stability compared to antibodies, and other factors [14].

While both RNA/DNA aptamers and DNA origami utilize the unique properties of nucleic acids, they serve distinct roles in biotechnology. Aptamers enhance biosensor functionality through specific target recognition, while DNA origami provides structural frameworks that can support various biomolecular applications. Understanding these differences is crucial for leveraging their respective strengths in developing advanced diagnostic tools and therapeutic strategies. Aptamer-based biosensors primarily focus on the molecular recognition and detection aspects, whereas DNA origami biosensors emphasize creating programmable, nanoscale platforms for signal transduction, molecular interactions, or multi-target detection. The integration of these two approaches often results in hybrid systems that amplify functionality and efficiency in sensing or therapeutic applications [81,82].

Aptamers have been incorporated with both oPAD and DNA origami biosensors. The paper-based sensors typically take advantage of the strand transfer generated by aptamer target binding. The aptamers change their shape in the presence of the target, displacing the partially complementary strands. To produce a detectable signal in reaction to the strand shift, enzymes or nanoparticles can be utilized. For instance, the target-specific strand shift could set off an enzyme reaction that results in a color change or electron migration, or it could disassemble AuNP-tagged ssDNAs that, when they amass on the paper, create a colorimetric signal [83]. Aptamers present a significant opportunity for facile integration with custom-designed DNA origami structures, enabling them to acquire practical functionalities. These modified aptamers have been employed in diverse research areas, encompassing (i) immobilizing target molecules through aptamers, as exemplified by nanoarrays and biosensor applications; (ii) inducing conformational changes in DNA nanostructures by utilizing aptamers, with the intended outcomes being either biosensor advancements or molecular computing capabilities; and (iii) leveraging aptamers for the targeted delivery of drugs to specific (cancer) cells [84].

4.1. Aptamer in Paper Biosensors

Zang et al. developed a paper-based biosensor for adenosine detection using an aptamer-based approach. This system leveraged toehold-mediated strand displacement (TMSD), a method in which an input strand is replaced by a specific output strand. TMSD amplification, in combination with a bead-linked aptamer assembly, enabled adenosine detection. In this setup, the adenosine target caused the release of the bead-linked strand, which initiated a hybridization chain reaction (HCR) that captured streptavidin conjugated to glucose oxidase (GOx). The GOx then catalyzed glucose oxidation, producing hydrogen peroxide (H2O2). This, in turn, reacted with potassium permanganate (KMnO4) embedded in the paper, causing a color change from purple to colorless [85]. Similarly, an in-field electrochemical sensing of adenosine was achieved using a paper device activated by TMSD. The device consisted of a carbon electrode and $[Fe(CN)6]^{3-}$, along with a bead-linked aptamer/GOx-tagged strand assembly on the other side. Upon adding a solution containing adenosine targets to the device, the targets diffused to the beads. The adenosine triggered TMSD through the aptamers linked to the beads, leading to the conversion of $[Fe(CN)6]^{3-}$ to $[Fe(CN)6]^{4-}$ by the GOx-tagged strands. As a result, a capacitor connected to the paper became charged, and upon discharge, a short but amplified current flow was generated. This paper device effectively charged the capacitor only when the target was present, thereby converting a biomolecular signal into an electronic one, akin to a biobattery [86].

Additionally, researchers developed a 3D microfluidic origami nano-aptasensor for the rapid and precise electrochemical detection of the peanut allergen Ara h1. This microfluidic chip featured dual detection sites and utilized aptamer-functionalized black phosphorus nanosheets (BPNSs) to enhance signal sensitivity. The sensor's performance was optimized by analyzing aptamer concentration, self-assembly duration, and aptamer–antigen interactions [87].

4.2. Aptamers in DNA Origami Biosensors

Godonoga and colleagues developed a DNA origami biosensor integrated with aptamers designed specifically to target the malarial biomarker plasmodium falciparum lactate dehydrogenase (PfLDH). This design utilized rectangular DNA origami functionalized with aptamers that demonstrated precise recognition of PfLDH, as confirmed by AFM. Remarkably, the bound PfLDH retained its enzymatic activity, and high-speed AFM provided insights into the dynamic interactions between the protein and the aptamers. This study highlights the potential of incorporating DNA aptamers into supramolecular DNA frameworks for malaria biomarker detection, paving the way for advanced nanotechnology-driven diagnostic tools for malaria detection [88].

Wagenknecht et al. introduced a novel system utilizing split aptamers integrated into a DNA origami tweezer, enabling dual fluorescence signal outputs. The split aptamers, functionalized with donor and acceptor fluorophores, exhibit FRET when positioned within 10 nm of each other. In the absence of ATP, the aptamers remain apart, leading to green fluorescence (indicating the "open" state of the DNA origami with no FRET signal). Upon ATP binding, the aptamers converge, shifting the fluorescence from green to red (signifying the "closed" state of the DNA origami with an active FRET signal). This platform not only provides fluorescence-based detection but also offers topographical insights when combined with AFM, establishing itself as an innovative bimodal sensor platform [89].

5. Challenges in Practical Applications of Origami Biosensor

Paper-based and DNA origami biosensors offer innovative, low-cost solutions for various biosensing applications, yet both face significant challenges that limit their broader adoption, particularly in high-precision fields like healthcare.

Paper-based sensors benefit from the porous nature of paper for reagent absorption but are highly susceptible to environmental factors like temperature and humidity, leading to inconsistent assay outcomes. Cross-contamination between assay regions and insufficient detection limits further hinder their reliability, particularly in sensitive medical diagnostics [90]. DNA origami biosensors, known for their precision in molecular recognition, struggle with high fabrication costs and complexity, involving the synthesis of long DNA strands and intricate assembly processes. Large-scale production remains impractical, and advanced detection methods, such as atomic force microscopy or fluorescence, add to the cost and complexity, making them unsuitable for routine or POC use. Both approaches also face issues with environmental stability, as fluctuations in temperature and pH can compromise performance [91].

The integration of origami designs with microfabrication technologies introduces further challenges. Rigid components used for sensing and computation are incompatible with the flexible nature of origami structures, increasing system complexity and reducing efficiency [92]. Modular designs in DNA origami sensors offer flexibility but require tailored solutions for each application, consuming significant time and resources. Performance issues, such as low signal gain and analyte-specific modifications, complicate broader use. Additionally, limitations in existing readout mechanisms, which are often costly and time-intensive, restrict their practicality for rapid testing [93]. Addressing these challenges requires innovations in materials, fabrication, and detection techniques to enhance the functionality, reliability, and scalability of origami biosensors across diverse applications [94,95].

6. Conclusions and Outlook

The utilization of origami folding techniques in the development of paper biosensors and DNA biosensors has revolutionized the field of biosensor technology. Origami-inspired designs have allowed for the creation of biosensors that are low-cost, portable, and easy to use, making them accessible to a wider range of users, including those in low-resource settings. The use of origami in biosensor technology has been particularly advantageous in the development of paper-based biosensors. By using origami to create microfluidic channels, it is possible to create complex fluidic networks in a compact and easily transportable format. Additionally, the use of origami has allowed for the creation of paper biosensors that can detect a wide range of analytes, including glucose, cholesterol, and various pathogens. DNA biosensors have also benefitted from the use of origami. By incorporating DNA strands into origami structures, it is possible to create biosensors that are highly specific and sensitive to particular DNA sequences. This has applications in medical diagnostics, environmental monitoring, and forensic science. Origami folding techniques have also been used to create biosensors that are integrated with electronic components, allowing for real-time data analysis and the wireless transmission of results. This has the potential to greatly improve the efficiency and accuracy of biosensing, making it possible to rapidly detect and respond to threats such as infectious diseases. Despite the many advantages of origami-inspired biosensors, there are still challenges that need to be addressed. For example, the creation of complex origami structures requires precision fabrication techniques that are not yet widely available. Additionally, the integration of electronic components into origami structures can be challenging, requiring specialized expertise in both engineering and biology.

In conclusion, the use of origami folding techniques in paper biosensors and DNA biosensors has opened up new avenues for the development of low-cost, portable, and highly specific biosensors. The potential applications of these biosensors are vast, ranging from medical diagnostics to environmental monitoring to national security. As research in this field continues to advance, we can expect to see even more exciting developments in the near future.

Author Contributions: Conceptualization, S.P., S.S. and N.A.; methodology, S.P., S.S. and N.A.; software, S.P.; validation, J.N., R.P. and S.T.; formal analysis, J.N. and R.P.; investigation, J.N., R.P., S.T., E.G.C., C.S.P. and S.K.S.; resources, S.P., S.S., and N.A.,; data curation, S.P., S.S. and N.A.; writing—original draft preparation, S.P., S.S. and N.A.; writing—review and editing, S.P., S.S. and N.A.; visualization, J.N., R.P., S.T., E.G.C., C.S.P. and S.K.S.; supervision, J.N. and R.P.; project administration, J.N.; funding acquisition, J.N. All authors have read and agreed to the published version of the manuscript.

Funding: The Department of Biotechnology provided funding for this study under grant number BT/PR31594/MED/32/738/2020. J.N and Dr. E.G.C. also acknowledge the TUBITAK for 2221-Fellowships for visiting scientist and Scientists on Sabbatical Leave support.

Institutional Review Board Statement: Not applicable.

Informed Consent Statement: Not applicable.

Data Availability Statement: Not applicable.

Conflicts of Interest: The authors declare no conflicts of interest.

References

1. Chen, Y.; Peng, R.; You, Z. Origami of Thick Panels. *Science (1979)* **2015**, *349*, 396–400. [CrossRef] [PubMed]

2. Colozza, N.; Caratelli, V.; Moscone, D.; Arduini, F. Origami Paper-Based Electrochemical (Bio)Sensors: State of the Art and Perspective. *Biosensors* **2021**, *11*, 328. [CrossRef] [PubMed]
3. Loretan, M.; Domljanovic, I.; Lakatos, M.; Rüegg, C.; Acuna, G.P. DNA Origami as Emerging Technology for the Engineering of Fluorescent and Plasmonic-Based Biosensors. *Materials* **2020**, *13*, 2185. [CrossRef] [PubMed]
4. Wang, S.; Zhou, Z.; Ma, N.; Yang, S.; Li, K.; Teng, C.; Ke, Y.; Tian, Y. Dna Origami-Enabled Biosensors. *Sensors* **2020**, *20*, 6899. [CrossRef]
5. Williamson, P.; Piskunen, P.; Ijäs, H.; Butterworth, A.; Linko, V.; Corrigan, D.K. Signal Amplification in Electrochemical DNA Biosensors Using Target-Capturing DNA Origami Tiles. *ACS Sens.* **2023**, *8*, 1471–1480. [CrossRef] [PubMed]
6. Singh, A.T.; Lantigua, D.; Meka, A.; Taing, S.; Pandher, M.; Camci-Unal, G. Paper-Based Sensors: Emerging Themes and Applications. *Sensors* **2018**, *18*, 2838. [CrossRef] [PubMed]
7. Lazzarini, E.; Pace, A.; Trozzi, I.; Zangheri, M.; Guardigli, M.; Calabria, D.; Mirasoli, M. An Origami Paper-Based Biosensor for Allergen Detection by Chemiluminescence Immunoassay on Magnetic Microbeads. *Biosensors* **2022**, *12*, 825. [CrossRef] [PubMed]
8. Sahraei, N.; Mazloum-Ardakani, M.; Hoseynidokht, F. Electrochemical Paper-Based Biosensors for Point-of-Care Diagnostics: Detection Methods and Applications. *J. Electrochem. Sci. Eng.* **2022**, *12*, 399–419. [CrossRef]
9. Huang, Y.; Nguyen, M.K.; Natarajan, A.K.; Nguyen, V.H.; Kuzyk, A. A DNA Origami-Based Chiral Plasmonic Sensing Device. *ACS Appl. Mater. Interfaces* **2018**, *10*, 44221–44225. [CrossRef] [PubMed]
10. Chandrasekaran, A.R.; Punnoose, J.A.; Zhou, L.; Dey, P.; Dey, B.K.; Halvorsen, K. DNA Nanotechnology Approaches for MicroRNA Detection and Diagnosis. *Nucleic Acids Res.* **2019**, *47*, 10489–10505. [CrossRef] [PubMed]
11. Gao, X.; Feng, L.; Deng, R.; Wang, B.; He, Y.; Zhang, L.; Luo, D.; Chen, M.; Chang, K. Bottom-up DNA Nanostructure-Based Paper as Point-of-Care Diagnostic: From Method to Device. *Interdiscip. Med.* **2024**, *2*, e20230033. [CrossRef]
12. Lee, N.E.; Hong, J.H.; Lee, S.; Yoo, Y.K.; Kim, K.H.; Park, J.S.; Kim, C.; Yoon, J.; Yoon, D.S.; Lee, J.H. Integration of an Aptamer-Based Signal-On Probe and a Paper-Based Origami Preconcentrator for Small Molecule Biomarkers Detection. *BioChip J.* **2023**, *17*, 439–446. [CrossRef]
13. Wu, W.; Zhang, J.; Zheng, M.; Zhong, Y.; Yang, J.; Zhao, Y.; Wu, W.; Ye, W.; Wen, J.; Wang, Q.; et al. An Aptamer-Based Biosensor for Colorimetric Detection of Escherichia Coli O157:H7. *PLoS ONE* **2012**, *7*, e48999. [CrossRef] [PubMed]
14. Sameiyan, E.; Bagheri, E.; Ramezani, M.; Alibolandi, M.; Abnous, K.; Taghdisi, S.M. DNA Origami-Based Aptasensors. *Biosens. Bioelectron.* **2019**, *143*, 111662. [CrossRef] [PubMed]
15. Martinez, A.W.; Phillips, S.T.; Butte, M.J.; Whitesides, G.M. Patterned Paper as a Platform for Inexpensive, Low-Volume, Portable Bioassays. *Angew. Chem. Int. Ed.* **2007**, *46*, 1318–1320. [CrossRef] [PubMed]
16. Ge, X.; Asiri, A.M.; Du, D.; Wen, W.; Wang, S.; Lin, Y. Nanomaterial-Enhanced Paper-Based Biosensors. *TrAC Trends Anal. Chem.* **2014**, *58*, 31–39. [CrossRef]
17. Liu, H.; Crooks, R.M. Three-Dimensional Paper Microfluidic Devices Assembled Using the Principles of Origami. *J. Am. Chem. Soc.* **2011**, *133*, 17564–17566. [CrossRef] [PubMed]
18. Liu, H.; Xiang, Y.; Lu, Y.; Crooks, R.M. Aptamer-Based Origami Paper Analytical Device for Electrochemical Detection of Adenosine. *Angew. Chem. Int. Ed.* **2012**, *51*, 6925–6928. [CrossRef] [PubMed]
19. Kuswandi, B.; Hidayat, M.A.; Noviana, E. Paper-Based Sensors for Rapid Important Biomarkers Detection. *Biosens. Bioelectron. X* **2022**, *12*, 100246. [CrossRef]
20. Liang, B.; Zhu, Q.; Fang, L.; Cao, Q.; Liang, X.; Ye, X. An Origami Paper Device for Complete Elimination of Interferents in Enzymatic Electrochemical Biosensors. *Electrochem. Commun.* **2017**, *82*, 43–46. [CrossRef]
21. Li, W.; Qian, D.; Wang, Q.; Li, Y.; Bao, N.; Gu, H.; Yu, C. Fully-Drawn Origami Paper Analytical Device for Electrochemical Detection of Glucose. *Sens. Actuators B Chem.* **2016**, *231*, 230–238. [CrossRef]
22. Li, L.; Xu, J.; Zheng, X.; Ma, C.; Song, X.; Ge, S.; Yu, J.; Yan, M. Growth of Gold-Manganese Oxide Nanostructures on a 3D Origami Device for Glucose-Oxidase Label Based Electrochemical Immunosensor. *Biosens. Bioelectron.* **2014**, *61*, 76–82. [CrossRef]
23. Sun, X.; Jian, Y.; Wang, H.; Ge, S.; Yan, M.; Yu, J. Ultrasensitive Microfluidic Paper-Based Electrochemical Biosensor Based on Molecularly Imprinted Film and Boronate Affinity Sandwich Assay for Glycoprotein Detection. *ACS Appl. Mater. Interfaces* **2019**, *11*, 16198–16206. [CrossRef] [PubMed]
24. Ding, J.; Li, B.; Chen, L.; Qin, W. A Three-Dimensional Origami Paper-Based Device for Potentiometric Biosensing. *Angew. Chem. Int. Ed.* **2016**, *55*, 13033–13037. [CrossRef] [PubMed]
25. Sun, G.; Zhang, L.; Zhang, Y.; Yang, H.; Ma, C.; Ge, S.; Yan, M.; Yu, J.; Song, X. Multiplexed Enzyme-Free Electrochemical Immunosensor Based on ZnO Nanorods Modified Reduced Graphene Oxide-Paper Electrode and Silver Deposition-Induced Signal Amplification Strategy. *Biosens. Bioelectron.* **2015**, *71*, 30–36. [CrossRef] [PubMed]
26. Wang, C.C.; Hennek, J.W.; Ainla, A.; Kumar, A.A.; Lan, W.J.; Im, J.; Smith, B.S.; Zhao, M.; Whitesides, G.M. A Paper-Based Pop-up Electrochemical Device for Analysis of Beta-Hydroxybutyrate. *Anal. Chem.* **2016**, *88*, 6326–6333. [CrossRef]
27. Srisomwat, C.; Teengam, P.; Chuaypen, N.; Tangkijvanich, P.; Vilaivan, T.; Chailapakul, O. Pop-up Paper Electrochemical Device for Label-Free Hepatitis B Virus DNA Detection. *Sens. Actuators B Chem.* **2020**, *316*, 128077. [CrossRef]

28. Boonkaew, S.; Chaiyo, S.; Jampasa, S.; Rengpipat, S.; Siangproh, W.; Chailapakul, O. An Origami Paper-Based Electrochemical Immunoassay for the C-Reactive Protein Using a Screen-Printed Carbon Electrode Modified with Graphene and Gold Nanoparticles. *Microchim. Acta* **2019**, *186*, 153. [CrossRef] [PubMed]
29. Chen, C.A.; Yuan, H.; Chen, C.W.; Chien, Y.S.; Sheng, W.H.; Chen, C.F. An Electricity- And Instrument-Free Infectious Disease Sensor Based on a 3D Origami Paper-Based Analytical Device. *Lab Chip* **2021**, *21*, 1908–1915. [CrossRef]
30. Yakoh, A.; Pimpitak, U.; Rengpipat, S.; Hirankarn, N.; Chailapakul, O.; Chaiyo, S. Paper-Based Electrochemical Biosensor for Diagnosing COVID-19: Detection of SARS-CoV-2 Antibodies and Antigen. *Biosens. Bioelectron.* **2021**, *176*, 112912. [CrossRef]
31. Wang, Z.; Luo, P.; Zha, X.; Xu, C.; Kang, S.; Zhou, M.; Nover, D.; Wang, Y. Overview Assessment of Risk Evaluation and Treatment Technologies for Heavy Metal Pollution of Water and Soil. *J. Clean. Prod.* **2022**, *379*, 134043. [CrossRef]
32. Asim, M.; Nageswara Rao, K. Assessment of Heavy Metal Pollution in Yamuna River, Delhi-NCR, Using Heavy Metal Pollution Index and GIS. *Environ. Monit. Assess* **2021**, *193*, 103. [CrossRef] [PubMed]
33. Malikula, R.S.; Kaonga, C.C.; Mapoma, H.W.T.; Chiipa, P.; Thulu, F.G.D. Heavy Metals and Nutrients Loads in Water, Soil, and Crops Irrigated with Effluent from WWTPs in Blantyre City, Malawi. *Water* **2022**, *14*, 121. [CrossRef]
34. Xu, L.; Suo, X.-y.; Zhang, Q.; Li, X.-p.; Chen, C.; Zhang, X.Y. ELISA and Chemiluminescent Enzyme Immunoassay for Sensitive and Specific Determination of Lead (II) in Water, Food and Feed Samples. *Foods* **2020**, *9*, 305. [CrossRef]
35. Fu, X.; Chen, E.; Ma, B.; Xu, Y.; Hao, P.; Zhang, M.; Ye, Z.; Yu, X.; Li, C.; Ji, Q. Establishment of an Indirect Competitive Enzyme-Linked Immunosorbent Method for the Detection of Heavy Metal Cadmium in Food Packaging Materials. *Foods* **2021**, *10*, 413. [CrossRef] [PubMed]
36. Rattanarat, P.; Dungchai, W.; Cate, D.; Volckens, J.; Chailapakul, O.; Henry, C.S. Multilayer Paper-Based Device for Colorimetric and Electrochemical Quantification of Metals. *Anal. Chem.* **2014**, *86*, 3555–3562. [CrossRef]
37. Xiao, W.; Gao, Y.; Zhang, Y.; Li, J.; Liu, Z.; Nie, J.; Li, J. Enhanced 3D Paper-Based Devices with a Personal Glucose Meter for Highly Sensitive and Portable Biosensing of Silver Ion. *Biosens. Bioelectron.* **2019**, *137*, 154–160. [CrossRef] [PubMed]
38. Soliman Sabra, F.; El-Deeb Mehana, E.-S. Pesticides Toxicity in Fish with Particular Reference to Insecticides. *Asian J. Agric. Food Sci.* **2015**, *3*, 1.
39. Aktar, W.; Sengupta, D.; Chowdhury, A. Impact of Pesticides Use in Agriculture: Their Benefits and Hazards. *Interdiscip. Toxicol.* **2009**, *2*, 1–12. [CrossRef] [PubMed]
40. Arduini, F.; Cinti, S.; Caratelli, V.; Amendola, L.; Palleschi, G.; Moscone, D. Origami Multiple Paper-Based Electrochemical Biosensors for Pesticide Detection. *Biosens. Bioelectron.* **2019**, *126*, 346–354. [CrossRef]
41. Jabeen, N.; Shahzad, K. Studies on Identification of the Food Born Fungal Pathogens and Their Pathogenic Effects on Human Health. *Acta Sci. Agric.* **2019**, *3*, 186–191. [CrossRef]
42. Khiyami, M.; Al-Faris, N.; Busaeed, B.; Sher, H. Food Borne Pathogen Contamination in Minimally Processed Vegetable Salads in Riyadh, Saudi Arabia. *J. Med. Plant Res.* **2011**, *5*, 444–451.
43. Wang, K.; Lin, X.; Zhang, M.; Li, Y.; Luo, C.; Wu, J. Review of Electrochemical Biosensors for Food Safety Detection. *Biosensors* **2022**, *12*, 959. [CrossRef] [PubMed]
44. Ivanišević, I.; Milardović, S.; Kassal, P. Recent Advances in (Bio)Chemical Sensors for Food Safety and Quality Based on Silver Nanomaterials. *Food Technol. Biotechnol.* **2021**, *59*, 216–237. [CrossRef] [PubMed]
45. Kuswandi, B.; Hidayat, M.A.; Noviana, E. Paper-Based Electrochemical Biosensors for Food Safety Analysis. *Biosensors* **2022**, *12*, 1088. [CrossRef] [PubMed]
46. He, T.; Li, J.; Liu, L.; Ge, S.; Yan, M.; Liu, H.; Yu, J. Origami-Based "Book" Shaped Three-Dimensional Electrochemical Paper Microdevice for Sample-to-Answer Detection of Pathogens. *RSC Adv.* **2020**, *10*, 25808–25816. [CrossRef]
47. Lu, J.; Ge, S.; Ge, L.; Yan, M.; Yu, J. Electrochemical DNA Sensor Based on Three-Dimensional Folding Paper Device for Specific and Sensitive Point-of-Care Testing. *Electrochim. Acta* **2012**, *80*, 334–341. [CrossRef]
48. Scida, K.; Li, B.; Ellington, A.D.; Crooks, R.M. DNA Detection Using Origami Paper Analytical Devices. *Anal. Chem.* **2013**, *85*, 9713–9720. [CrossRef] [PubMed]
49. Rothemund, P.W.K. Folding DNA to Create Nanoscale Shapes and Patterns. *Nature* **2006**, *440*, 297–302. [CrossRef]
50. Seeman, N.C. DNA in a Material World. *Nature* **2003**, *421*, 427–431. [CrossRef]
51. Zadegan, R.M.; Norton, M.L. Structural DNA Nanotechnology: From Design to Applications. *Int. J. Mol. Sci.* **2012**, *13*, 7149–7162. [CrossRef]
52. Ramm, B.; Khmelinskaia, A.; Franquelim, H.G.; Schwille, P. Patterning DNA Origami on Membranes Through Protein Self-Organization. In *Natural Computing Series*; Springer: Singapore, 2023; Volume Part F821.
53. Hartl, C.; Frank, K.; Amenitsch, H.; Fischer, S.; Liedl, T.; Nickel, B. Position Accuracy of Gold Nanoparticles on DNA Origami Structures Studied with Small-Angle X-Ray Scattering. *Nano Lett.* **2018**, *18*, 2609–2615. [CrossRef] [PubMed]
54. Dietz, H. Toward Applications for DNA Nanotechnology—More Bricks To Build With. *ChemBioChem* **2016**, *17*, 1046–1047. [CrossRef] [PubMed]
55. Wang, P.; Meyer, T.A.; Pan, V.; Dutta, P.K.; Ke, Y. The Beauty and Utility of DNA Origami. *Chem* **2017**, *2*, 359–382. [CrossRef]

56. Chandrasekaran, A.R.; Anderson, N.; Kizer, M.; Halvorsen, K.; Wang, X. Beyond the Fold: Emerging Biological Applications of DNA Origami. *ChemBioChem* **2016**, *17*, 1081–1089. [CrossRef]
57. Ke, Y.; Nangreave, J.; Yan, H.; Lindsay, S.; Liu, Y. Developing DNA Tiles for Oligonucleotide Hybridization Assay with Higher Accuracy and Efficiency. *Chem. Commun.* **2008**, *43*, 5622–5624. [CrossRef] [PubMed]
58. Ke, Y.; Lindsay, S.; Chang, Y.; Liu, Y.; Yan, H. Self-Assembled Water-Soluble Nucleic Acid Probe Tiles for Label-Free RNA Hybridization Assays. *Science (1979)* **2008**, *319*, 180–183. [CrossRef] [PubMed]
59. Kuzuya, A.; Sakai, Y.; Yamazaki, T.; Xu, Y.; Komiyama, M. Nanomechanical DNA Origami "single-Molecule Beacons" Directly Imaged by Atomic Force Microscopy. *Nat. Commun.* **2011**, *2*, 449. [CrossRef]
60. Hernández-Ainsa, S.; Keyser, U.F. DNA Origami Nanopores: Developments, Challenges and Perspectives. *Nanoscale* **2014**, *6*, 14121–14132. [CrossRef] [PubMed]
61. Kasianowicz, J.J. Nanometer-Scale Pores: Potential Applications for Analyte Detection and DNA Characterization. *Dis. Markers* **2002**, *18*, 185–191. [CrossRef]
62. Storm, A.J.; Chen, J.H.; Ling, X.S.; Zandbergen, H.W.; Dekker, C. Fabrication of Solid-State Nanopores with Single-Nanometre Precision. *Nat. Mater.* **2003**, *2*, 537–540. [CrossRef] [PubMed]
63. Bell, N.A.W.; Keyser, U.F. Nanopores Formed by DNA Origami: A Review. *FEBS Lett.* **2014**, *588*, 3564–3570. [CrossRef] [PubMed]
64. Hall, A.R.; Scott, A.; Rotem, D.; Mehta, K.K.; Bayley, H.; Dekker, C. Hybrid Pore Formation by Directed Insertion of α-Haemolysin into Solid-State Nanopores. *Nat. Nanotechnol.* **2010**, *5*, 874–877. [CrossRef]
65. Bell, N.A.W.; Engst, C.R.; Ablay, M.; Divitini, G.; Ducati, C.; Liedl, T.; Keyser, U.F. DNA Origami Nanopores. *Nano Lett.* **2012**, *12*, 512–517. [CrossRef]
66. Wei, R.; Martin, T.G.; Rant, U.; Dietz, H. DNA Origami Gatekeepers for Solid-State Nanopores. *Angew. Chem. Int. Ed.* **2012**, *51*, 4864–4867. [CrossRef] [PubMed]
67. Hernández-Ainsa, S.; Bell, N.A.W.; Thacker, V.V.; Göpfrich, K.; Misiunas, K.; Fuentes-Perez, M.E.; Moreno-Herrero, F.; Keyser, U.F. DNA Origami Nanopores for Controlling DNA Translocation. *ACS Nano* **2013**, *7*, 6024–6030. [CrossRef] [PubMed]
68. Hernández-Ainsa, S.; Keyser, U.F. DNA Origami Nanopores: An Emerging Tool in Biomedicine. *Nanomedicine* **2013**, *8*, 1551–1554. [CrossRef] [PubMed]
69. Ochmann, S.E.; Vietz, C.; Trofymchuk, K.; Acuna, G.P.; Lalkens, B.; Tinnefeld, P. Optical Nanoantenna for Single Molecule-Based Detection of Zika Virus Nucleic Acids without Molecular Multiplication. *Anal. Chem.* **2017**, *89*, 13000–13007. [CrossRef] [PubMed]
70. Zhang, Z.; Wang, Y.; Fan, C.; Li, C.; Li, Y.; Qian, L.; Fu, Y.; Shi, Y.; Hu, J.; He, L. Asymmetric DNA Origami for Spatially Addressable and Index-Free Solution-Phase DNA Chips. *Adv. Mater.* **2010**, *22*, 2672–2675. [CrossRef]
71. Zhang, Z.; Zeng, D.; Ma, H.; Feng, G.; Hu, J.; He, L.; Li, C.; Fan, C. A DNA-Origami Chip Platform for Label-Free SNP Genotyping Using Toehold-Mediated Strand Displacement. *Small* **2010**, *6*, 1854–1858. [CrossRef] [PubMed]
72. Subramanian, H.K.K.; Chakraborty, B.; Sha, R.; Seeman, N.C. The Label-Free Unambiguous Detection and Symbolic Display of Single Nucleotide Polymorphisms on DNA Origami. *Nano Lett.* **2011**, *11*, 910–913. [CrossRef]
73. Panyutin, I.G.; Hsieh, P. The Kinetics of Spontaneous DNA Branch Migration. *Proc. Natl. Acad. Sci. USA* **1994**, *91*, 2021–2025. [CrossRef] [PubMed]
74. Raveendran, M.; Lee, A.J.; Sharma, R.; Wälti, C.; Actis, P. Rational Design of DNA Nanostructures for Single Molecule Biosensing. *Nat. Commun.* **2020**, *11*, 4384. [CrossRef] [PubMed]
75. Yan, J.; Hu, C.; Wang, P.; Liu, R.; Zuo, X.; Liu, X.; Song, S.; Fan, C.; He, D.; Sun, G. Novel Rolling Circle Amplification and DNA Origami-Based DNA Belt-Involved Signal Amplification Assay for Highly Sensitive Detection of Prostate-Specific Antigen (PSA). *ACS Appl. Mater. Interfaces* **2014**, *6*, 20372–20377. [CrossRef]
76. Kuzuya, A.; Watanabe, R.; Yamanaka, Y.; Tamaki, T.; Kaino, M.; Ohya, Y. Nanomechanical DNA Origami PH Sensors. *Sensors* **2014**, *14*, 19329–19335. [CrossRef] [PubMed]
77. Voigt, N.V.; Tørring, T.; Rotaru, A.; Jacobsen, M.F.; Ravnsbæk, J.B.; Subramani, R.; Mamdouh, W.; Kjems, J.; Mokhir, A.; Besenbacher, F.; et al. Single-Molecule Chemical Reactions on DNA Origami. *Nat. Nanotechnol.* **2010**, *5*, 200–203. [CrossRef]
78. Tintoré, M.; Gállego, I.; Manning, B.; Eritja, R.; Fàbrega, C. DNA Origami as a DNA Repair Nanosensor at the Single-Molecule Level. *Angew. Chem. Int. Ed.* **2013**, *52*, 7747–7750. [CrossRef]
79. Zhang, X.; Pan, L.; Guo, R.; Zhang, Y.; Li, F.; Li, M.; Li, J.; Shi, J.; Qu, F.; Zuo, X.; et al. DNA Origami Nanocalipers for PH Sensing at the Nanoscale. *Chem. Commun.* **2022**, *58*, 3673–3676. [CrossRef]
80. Adachi, T.; Nakamura, Y. Aptamers: A Review of Their Chemical Properties and Modifications for Therapeutic Application. *Molecules* **2019**, *24*, 4229. [CrossRef]
81. Sequeira-Antunes, B.; Ferreira, H.A. Nucleic Acid Aptamer-Based Biosensors: A Review. *Biomedicines* **2023**, *11*, 3201. [CrossRef] [PubMed]
82. Lee, H.; Xie, T.; Kang, B.; Yu, X.; Schaffter, S.W.; Schulman, R. Plug-and-Play Protein Biosensors Using Aptamer-Regulated in Vitro Transcription. *Nat. Commun.* **2024**, *15*, 7973. [CrossRef] [PubMed]

83. Yoo, H.; Jo, H.; Oh, S.S. Detection and beyond: Challenges and Advances in Aptamer-Based Biosensors. *Mater. Adv.* **2020**, *1*, 2663–2687. [CrossRef]
84. Sakai, Y.; Islam, M.S.; Adamiak, M.; Shiu, S.C.C.; Tanner, J.A.; Heddle, J.G. DNA Aptamers for the Functionalisation of DNA Origami Nanostructures. *Genes* **2018**, *9*, 571. [CrossRef]
85. Zhang, Y.; Gao, D.; Fan, J.; Nie, J.; Le, S.; Zhu, W.; Yang, J.; Li, J. Naked-Eye Quantitative Aptamer-Based Assay on Paper Device. *Biosens. Bioelectron.* **2016**, *78*, 538–546. [CrossRef] [PubMed]
86. Wang, L.; Ma, W.; Chen, W.; Liu, L.; Ma, W.; Zhu, Y.; Xu, L.; Kuang, H.; Xu, C. An Aptamer-Based Chromatographic Strip Assay for Sensitive Toxin Semi-Quantitative Detection. *Biosens. Bioelectron.* **2011**, *26*, 3059–3062. [CrossRef] [PubMed]
87. Jiang, H.; Guo, Q.; Zhang, C.; Sun, Z.; Weng, X. Microfluidic Origami Nano-Aptasensor for Peanut Allergen Ara H1 Detection. *Food Chem.* **2021**, *365*, 130511. [CrossRef]
88. Godonoga, M.; Lin, T.Y.; Oshima, A.; Sumitomo, K.; Tang, M.S.L.; Cheung, Y.W.; Kinghorn, A.B.; Dirkzwager, R.M.; Zhou, C.; Kuzuya, A.; et al. A DNA Aptamer Recognising a Malaria Protein Biomarker Can Function as Part of a DNA Origami Assembly. *Sci. Rep.* **2016**, *6*, 21266. [CrossRef] [PubMed]
89. Walter, H.K.; Bauer, J.; Steinmeyer, J.; Kuzuya, A.; Niemeyer, C.M.; Wagenknecht, H.A. DNA Origami Traffic Lights with a Split Aptamer Sensor for a Bicolor Fluorescence Readout. *Nano Lett.* **2017**, *17*, 2467–2472. [CrossRef]
90. Hosseini, S.; Vázquez-Villegas, P.; Martínez-Chapa, S.O. Paper and Fiber-Based Bio-Diagnostic Platforms: Current Challenges and Future Needs. *Appl. Sci.* **2017**, *7*, 863. [CrossRef]
91. Linko, V.; Keller, A. Stability of DNA Origami Nanostructures in Physiological Media: The Role of Molecular Interactions. *Small* **2023**, *19*, e2301935. [CrossRef]
92. Yan, W.; Li, S.; Deguchi, M.; Zheng, Z.; Rus, D.; Mehta, A. Origami-Based Integration of Robots That Sense, Decide, and Respond. *Nat. Commun.* **2023**, *14*, 1553. [CrossRef] [PubMed]
93. Jeon, B.; Guareschi, M.M.; Stewart, J.M.; Wu, E.; Gopinath, A.; Arroyo-Currás, N.; Dauphin-Ducharme, P.; Plaxco, K.W.; Lukeman, P.S.; Rothemund, P.W.K. Modular DNA Origami-Based Electrochemical Detection of DNA and Proteins. *arXiv* **2023**, arXiv:2312.06554.
94. Chang, K.; Zhao, Y.; Wang, M.; Xu, Z.; Zhu, L.; Xu, L.; Wang, Q. Advances in Metal-Organic Framework-Plasmonic Metal Composites Based SERS Platforms: Engineering Strategies in Chemical Sensing, Practical Applications and Future Perspectives in Food Safety. *Chem. Eng. J.* **2023**, *459*, 141539. [CrossRef]
95. Wang, Q.; Chang, K.; Yang, Q.; Wu, W. Semiconductor-Based Surface-Enhanced Raman Scattering Sensing Platforms: State of the Art, Applications and Prospects in Food Safety. *Trends Food Sci. Technol.* **2024**, *147*, 104460. [CrossRef]

chemosensors

MDPI

Review

Multi-Template Molecularly Imprinted Polymeric Electrochemical Biosensors

Meltem Agar [1,2], Maisem Laabei [3,4], Hannah S. Leese [1,5] and Pedro Estrela [1,2,*]

1 Centre for Bioengineering & Biomedical Technologies (CBio), University of Bath, Bath BA2 7AY, UK; ma2680@bath.ac.uk (M.A.); hsl25@bath.ac.uk (H.S.L.)
2 Department of Electronic and Electrical Engineering, University of Bath, Bath BA2 7AY, UK
3 Department of Life Sciences, University of Bath, Bath BA2 7AY, UK; maisem.laabei@bristol.ac.uk
4 School of Cellular and Molecular Medicine, University of Bristol, Bristol BS8 1TD, UK
5 Department of Chemical Engineering, University of Bath, Bath BA2 7AY, UK
* Correspondence: p.estrela@bath.ac.uk

Abstract: Dual- or multi-template molecularly imprinted polymers have been an attractive research field for many years as they allow simultaneous detection of more than one target with high selectivity and sensitivity by creating template-specific recognition sites for multiple targets on the same functional monomer. Dual/multi-template molecular imprinting techniques have been applied to identify, extract, and detect many targets, from heavy metal ions to viruses, by different methods, such as high-performance liquid chromatography (HPLC), liquid chromatography–mass spectrometry (LC-MS), and piezoelectric, optical, and electrochemical methods. This article focuses on electrochemical sensors based on dual/multi-template molecularly imprinted polymers detecting a wide range of targets by electrochemical methods. Furthermore, this work highlights the use of these sensors for point-of-care applications, their commercialization and their integration with microfluidic systems.

Keywords: molecularly imprinted polymer; multi-template; electrochemical sensor

1. Introduction

There is a pressing worldwide need to detect a wide range of substances that affect human health, food safety, water quality and the environment; for example, human biomarkers, drugs, bacteria, heavy metal ions, pesticides, etc. [1–5]. The detection method, therefore, should be cheap, rapid, reliable, have high selectivity and specificity and not require intense people-power. In simplistic terms, biosensors are analytical devices consisting of a transducer and a bioreceptor (target recognition molecule). Ideally, they are easy to use, fast responding, have high selectivity toward the target and do not require sample preparation beforehand. Molecules such as antibodies, aptamers, peptides, deoxyribonucleic acids and enzymes are used as bioreceptors in biosensors [6]. Although the combination of natural receptors with label-free transducers allows for the successful implementation of a plethora of sensor devices, natural biological receptors also have inherent drawbacks: their chemical and physical stability and shelf-life are limited, especially antibodies and enzymes. Additionally, their compatibility with most transducer surfaces is limited, necessitating the design of adequate linker layers.

Some of the disadvantages of natural receptors can be overcome by employing so-called antibody mimetics: robust, artificial receptors that are able to bind their targets with an affinity comparable to their natural counterparts. Molecularly imprinted polymers

(MIPs) have great potential to be robust artificial receptors. The history of molecular imprinting dates back to the 1930s, when Polyakov synthesized silica gel in the presence of aromatic hydrocarbons. By the 1970s, researchers began using different templates for imprinting silica gel. In 1970 and 1972, organic polymers replaced silica gels, and non-covalent imprinting was introduced by Mosbach, marking significant advancements in the field [7,8].

MIPs offer high specificity, stability, cost-effectiveness, and reusability, while also being budget-friendly, simple to utilize, highly selective, and sensitive to targets. On the other hand, they have limitations such as template leakage, slow binding kinetics, cross-reactivity and lower affinity.

The synthesis of MIPs is straightforward and consists of three steps: (i) formation of the functional monomer and template; (ii) polymerization of the functional monomer–template complex with the cross-linker and initiator; and (iii) template removal to create three-dimensional cavities for specific recognition [9].

The interaction between a template and functional monomers that takes place in the first stage of MIP synthesis is crucial as it affects the physical properties and recognition of the MIP and the stability of the template–monomer complex [10]. Among these interactions, non-covalent interaction is the most preferred. In this approach, the template–monomer complex interacts via van der Waals forces, hydrogen bonding, π–π, dipole–dipole or ion–dipole interactions. They are weak interactions and offer some advantages, such as easy binding and template removal from the polymer, permitting a simplified process that eliminates the requirement for chemical derivatization of the template [7].

MIPs are commonly formed via free radical polymerization, which includes bulk, multi-step swelling, suspension, emulsion, seed, and precipitation polymerization. These polymerization methods suffer from low imprinting capacity, the need for a large amount of template, poor recognition and incomplete template removal [11]. In order to eliminate or ease these drawbacks, different MIP preparation techniques, such as the sol-gel process, surface and epitope imprinting and electropolymerization, have been adopted [12–14]. It is important to choose the most suitable polymerization technique according to the chemical and intrinsic properties of the template. For example, the sol-gel method allows MIP fabrication at room temperature and prevents thermal decomposition of the template, but at the same time, there is a risk of the template dissolving in the solvent. Likewise, while surface imprinting allows for high binding capacity, it requires the use of pure templates. The dimensions of the template are also important in determining the polymerization method to be chosen: polymerization methods used for small molecules might not be suitable for macromolecules such as bacteria and cells. If an appropriate method is not found, the template molecules might not be effectively removed from the polymer matrix or might not be properly imprinted.

These are very important parameters that affect the performance of the MIP. For example, functional monomers strongly interact with the target via functional groups of the target to form a template–functional monomer complex. If a suitable monomer is not chosen, a stable template–monomer complex cannot be achieved, leading to unsuccessful molecular recognition. In order to arrange the configuration of a functional monomer around the template to obtain a rigid polymeric matrix, cross-linkers are used. The amount of cross-linker has an influence on the mechanical stability of the polymeric matrix and recognition sites. The porogen and initiator are responsible for forming a porous structure, which enables the template to diffuse through an MIP and start polymerization thermally or photochemically [11,15].

MIPs allow multiplexed detection as long as they are imprinted with multi-targets (templates) under appropriate conditions. With multi-target MIPs (MT-MIPs), which are imprinted with more than one target, simultaneous detection of at least two targets can be achieved using less material, reducing the costs and time requirements. The MT-MIP preparation steps and different interactions between the templates and the functional monomer are shown in Figure 1. The preparation of MT-MIPs is similar to that of MIPs imprinted with a single template. The synthesis of MT-MIPs begins with the formation of complexes between the different templates and functional monomers through covalent or non-covalent interactions. This is followed by the simultaneous polymerization of the functional monomer–template complexes with a cross-linker and an initiator. In the final step, the templates are removed from the polymer to create three-dimensional cavities for specific recognition [16]. Various types of interactions are employed in the fabrication of MT-MIPs, as shown in Figure 1. Different polymerization methods, such as bulk polymerization, precipitation polymerization, emulsion polymerization, suspension polymerization, electropolymerization, and surface imprinting polymerization, can be used to fabricate MT-MIPs. As per single-template MIPs, each polymerization method has its own drawbacks and should be selected based on the properties of the templates.

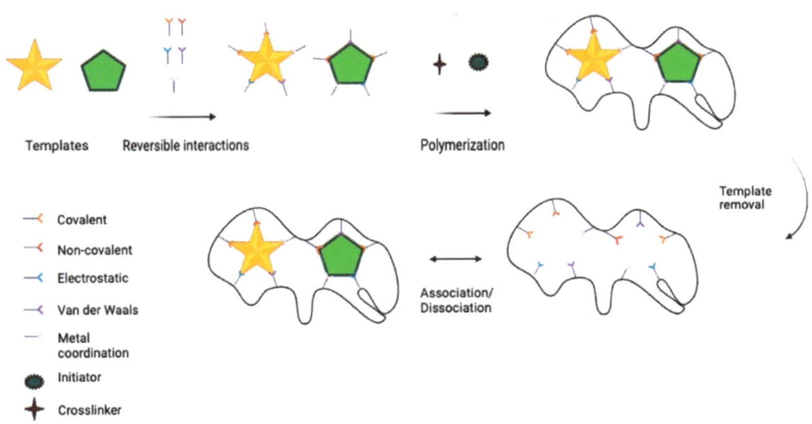

Figure 1. Preparation procedures for MT-MIPs and various interactions of templates (analyte) and MT-MIPs.

Since non-covalent interactions are advantageous—they allow for easier template removal, the creation of reusable recognition sites, and dynamic interactions—monomers that can form non-covalent bonds with templates are preferred. Examples include methacrylic acid (MAA) [17], acrylamide (AM) [18], 4-vinylpyridine (4-VP) [19], and 2-vinylpyridine (2-VP) [20]. The choice of cross-linker should take into account the interaction between the templates and the monomers; an inappropriate cross-linker can disrupt or break the bonds between them. For this reason, divinylbenzene (DVB) [21] and ethylene glycol dimethacrylate (EGDMA) [22] are generally used to support non-covalent interactions. For instance, Nurrokhimah et al. synthesized a molecularly imprinted polymer incorporated with graphene oxide and magnetite nanoparticles, which was used as a magnetic solid-phase extraction adsorbent for the simultaneous extraction and determination of cefoperazone, cephalexin, and cefazolin [23]. For the synthesis of MT-MIPs, Fe_3O_4@SiO_2-NH_2/GOx nanoparticles were first dispersed in acetonitrile with a specific amount of cefoperazone, cefazolin, and cephalexin as templates. The functional monomer MAA was added, and the mixture was sonicated for 15 min and then stirred for 12 h at room temperature. The solution was transferred to a three-neck flask, and EGDMA and AIBN were added as the cross-linker and initiator, respectively. Polymerization occurred under a nitrogen atmosphere at 60 °C for 24 h. Subsequently, the coated nanoparticles were washed with a mixture of methanol and acetic acid (8:2, v/v) to remove the template molecules, followed by a methanol rinse. The final nanocomposite adsorbent was dried under a vacuum. In this study, MAA was chosen as the functional monomer due to its carboxyl group, which can form strong hydrogen bonds and ionic interactions with the templates. EGDMA was used as the cross-linker because of its ability to create a rigid polymer network. EGDMA is ideal for ensuring that the polymer matrix remains stable and maintains its shape even after template removal and reusability, and it does not disrupt the hydrogen bonds between MAA and the templates. The bulk polymerization technique was used for polymer formation with this method, where AIBN (azobisisobutyronitrile) was employed as the initiator to start the polymerization process. A porogen (solvent mixture), typically acetonitrile, was used to help dissolve the monomer and ensure the formation of a uniform polymer matrix. The choice of these chemicals, coupled with the bulk polymerization method, provided an effective strategy for creating highly selective and reusable MT-MIPs for pharmaceutical applications.

While preparing MIPs, there are points to be taken into consideration regardless of whether it is a multi- or single-target MIP, including the selection and amount of monomer, cross-linker, porogen and initiator suitable for the target, the use of an appropriate polymerization method and the choice of effective washing solution [10,24]. Choosing templates with the same features is important in terms of the easy preparation of MT-MIPs and the templates showing the same interactions with other MIP components. If templates with different properties are selected, MT-MIPs are more difficult to prepare, and one target may not be imprinted as effectively as the other or may not be removed from the polymer matrix after washing. Therefore, while preparing MT-MIP with templates with different features, the properties of the different types of templates to be imprinted should be considered separately and the appropriate polymerization method and MIP components should be selected accordingly. In this context, templates used in molecular imprinting can be divided into four groups: ions, organic molecules, biomacromolecules and cells/viruses [25].

Similar to MIPs, imprinting three-dimensional biomolecules in MT-MIPs poses challenges due to their high molecular weights and sizes, particularly regarding template removal and low binding efficiency. To overcome these challenges, alternative imprinting strategies such as surface imprinting and epitope imprinting have been developed. Surface imprinting creates recognition sites at or near the surface of the MIP, allowing biomolecules to access the cavities more easily. This improves the binding efficiency and facilitates efficient template removal. On the other hand, epitope imprinting uses an epitope—a small, recognizable fragment or sequence of the biomolecule—as the template instead of the entire molecule. This strategy simplifies template removal and reduces the risk of incomplete elution or cavity deformation, further enhancing the efficiency and precision of the imprinting process [26,27].

The fact that MT-MIPs allow for the simultaneous detection of multiple templates is a significant advantage over MIPs; however, the detection performance of MT-MIPs also needs to be evaluated. In several studies, MT-MIPs demonstrated similar results when detecting templates both individually and as mixtures, maintaining consistent linear ranges and limits of detection (LODs) [28–30]. For instance, in the study conducted by Fatma et al., the MT-MIP for chlorambutil and dacarbazine achieved LODs of 0.037 ng/mL and 0.016 ng/mL in mixtures, and 0.035 ng/mL and 0.014 ng/mL individually [28]. In comparison, the LOD for dacarbazine obtained with the MIP developed by Prasad et al. was 0.02 ng/mL [31]. These results demonstrate that if the appropriate MIP components and methods are selected, MT-MIPs can detect templates with high selectivity and sensitivity.

Several techniques, such as fluorescence [32–34], quartz crystal microbalance (QCM) [35,36], chemiluminescence [37,38], high-performance liquid chromatography

(HPLC) [39], surface- enhanced Raman scattering (SERS) [40] and electrochemical methods [41,42], have been used in relation to MT-MIPs. Among them, electrochemical methods are regarded as a more efficient technique in terms of the detection of many different targets since these methods have advantages in their simple manipulation, cost-effectiveness, high sensitivity, easy sample preparation steps, simplicity and fast response [43,44]. In the same study conducted by Fatma et al., the performance of the electrochemical MT-MIP was compared with HPLC and UV methods, revealing that the limit of detection achieved with the electrochemical methods was significantly lower than that obtained with HPLC and UV [28]. This underscores the sensitivity of electrochemical methods compared to other detection techniques.

To date, MT-MIPs have been used to detect many different targets simultaneously. In this review, the detection of a variety of targets by electrochemical methods will be discussed according to their target classification. The performance of MT-MIPs in aqueous solutions will be evaluated. Recent progress in MT-MIP-based electrochemical sensors for point-of-care applications will be reviewed and their commercialization and integration with microfluidic systems will be assessed.

2. Detection of Targets by MT-MIP

2.1. Detection of Ions

Many different targets can be detected by molecularly imprinted polymer-based sensors and one of these targets is ions. Imprinted polymers prepared for the detection of ions can be called "ion-imprinted polymers" instead of molecularly imprinted polymers. While the target for molecularly imprinted polymers is molecules, for an ion-imprinted polymer, it is an ion [45]. Ion-imprinted polymers are attractive as they have high environmental stability, reusability and easy synthesis processes [46].

Some elements are essential for our health and nutrition and the proper function of our immune system, such as zinc and copper; however, their excessive intake can be harmful. On the other hand, certain elements, such as heavy metals and lanthanides, are extremely toxic at minute concentrations and if ingested or exposed to can cause serious health problems. Accordingly, detection of these elements is vital and they need to be detected in a highly sensitive and selective manner.

Prasad et al. demonstrated an electrochemical sensor to detect cadmium and copper, aiming to prevent the side effects of excessive exposure to or intake of these heavy metal contaminants. The sensor was fabricated using a biocompatible monomer (2-acrylamidoethyldihydrogen phosphate (AEDP)), a trapped ligand (L-histidine), a cross-linker (ethylene glycol dimetharylate (EGDMA)) and an initiator (2,2-azoisobutyronitrile (AIBN)) that were thermo-polymerized with template ions and embedded in a sol-gel matrix [47]. The inter-metallic effect between Cd(II) and Cu(II) was reduced by cavities created after ion removal because cavities allow strong and independent binding. Reducing the inter-metallic effect also significantly reduced the non-linear relationship between the peak current and ionic concentration. The recognition capability of the dual-ion-imprinted polymer was assessed by differential pulse anodic stripping voltammetry (DPASV). The sensor exhibited a limit of detection (LOD) of 0.053 and 0.035 ng/mL for Cd(II) and Cu(II) ions, respectively. The limit of detection for Cd(II) of the sensor produced is lower than the safe drinking water limit (3 μg/L) determined by the World Health Organization [48]. In addition, the produced sensor exhibited a lower LOD in terms of detecting Cu than previously reported Cu MIP sensors [49,50].

In another study by Prasad et al., screen-printed carbon electrodes (SPCE) were modified with COCl-modified magnetic iron oxide nanoparticles (NPs) by drop casting (Figure 2) [51]. Thermal polymerization with the functional monomer (but-2-enedioic acid bis-[(2-amino-ethyl)-amide]) was employed in the presence of template ions (cerium(IV) and gadolinium(III)), cross-linker, initiator and multiwalled carbon nanotubes (MWCNTs). HCl solution was used to remove ions from the polymeric matrix to create cavities. After simultaneous analysis of Ce(IV) and Gd(III) by DPASV, the LOD was obtained as 0.063 ng/mL for Ce(IV) and 0.182 ng/mL for Gd(III). The LOD for Ce(IV) is approximately 76 times lower than the one obtained by spectrophotometry [52]. The sensor was also tested with increasing concentrations of one ion while the concentration of the other ion was kept fixed in order to investigate the effect of one ion on the other one in terms of the redox behavior, and for both ions, linear calibration plots were obtained. This was an indication of the weak intermolecular effects between Cu(II) and Zn(II) ions.

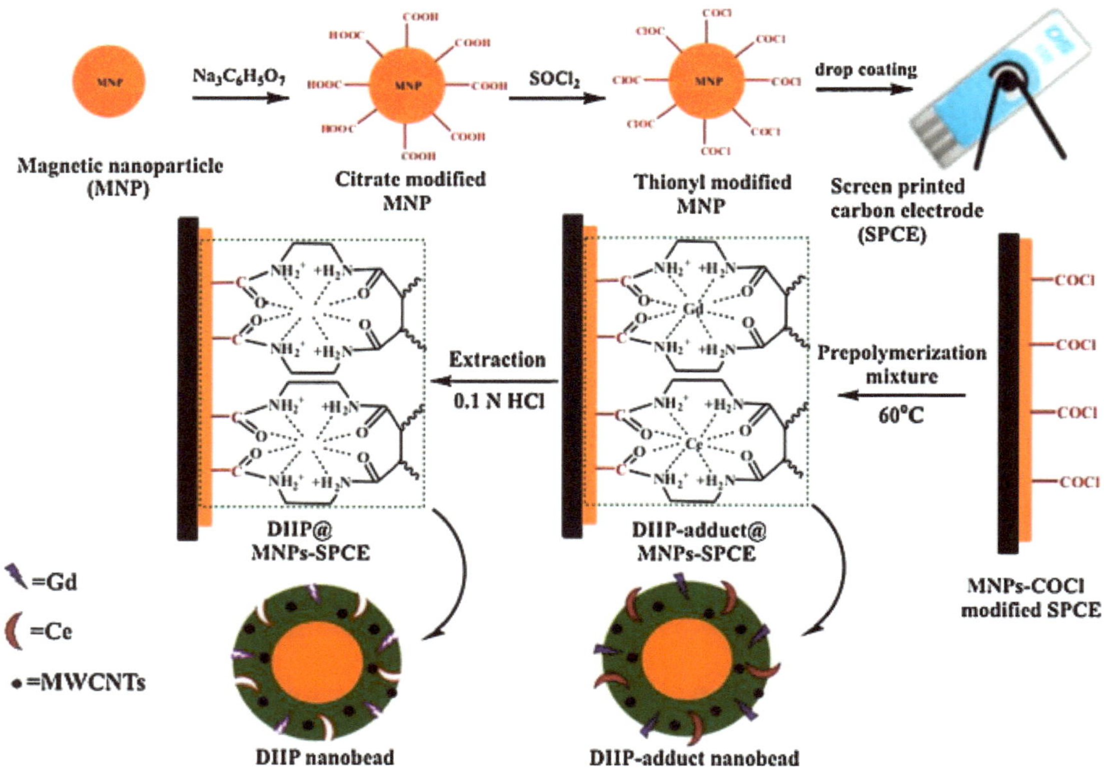

Figure 2. Fabrication of an ion-imprinted polymer-based screen-printed gold electrode to detect Ce(IV) and Gd (III). Reproduced with permission from [51].

Although copper and zinc are important elements for our body and immune system and have a critical effect on homeostasis and oxidative stress, they can be toxic at high concentrations [53,54]. Inductively coupled plasma mass spectrometry (ICP-MS) is considered the gold standard for trace element analysis since it has high specificity and sensitivity (ng/mL), but it has some drawbacks as it requires costly equipment and laboratory set-up, highly trained personnel and multiple high-purity gases [55]. Pencil graphite electrodes (PGEs) were used by Kumar et al. for simultaneous detection of copper and zinc [56]. In this study, important features of MWCNTs, such as high electroconductivity and good stability, were utilized and MWCNTs were mixed with bis-(2-acryloylamino-ethyl)-phosphinic acid (BAAP), Zn(II) and Cu(II), EGDMA and AIBN, which were used as the monomer, templates, cross-linker and initiator, respectively, to make the non-conducting MIP film conductive.

After thermal polymerization, the template ions were removed by an ethylenediaminetetraacetic acid (EDTA) solution. The DPASV was measured for different concentrations of both ions and 0.0159 μg/L and 0.0275 μg/L were obtained as the LOD in aqueous sample for Cu(II) and Zn(II), respectively. In order to evaluate the selectivity of the sensor, Fe^{+3}, Ca^{2+}, Mg^{2+}, nitrate, urea, ascorbic acid, and dopamine were used as interfering substances. It was observed that the produced sensor did not show any response to interfering substances. The proposed sensor for Cu(II) and Zn(II) detection may be an alternative to ICP-MS because it has an easy production process and provides as low detection limits as ICP-MS.

2.2. Detection of Biomarkers

The majority of biomarkers are biomacromolecules with large molecules with high molecular weights (1–100 kDa), such as proteins, enzymes, and nucleic acids. While the detection of biomacromolecules is very important in various aspects, their imprinting is difficult due to their large dimensions, complex structures, insolubility in organic solvents, slow mass transfer and structural flexibility in solution. These challenges can be overcome by using different imprinting methods, such as surface and epitope imprinting, using appropriate polymerization methods in which the MIP thickness can be controlled, such as electropolymerization, considering the large dimensions of the biomacromolecule, and using nanomaterials that reduce mass transfer resistance and have a large surface to volume ratio in MIPs [57–59].

The detection of small molecules such as hydrocortisone and testosterone is also vital in terms of early diagnosis, prognosis and treatment [60,61]. 8-hydroxy-20-deoxyguanosine (8-OHdG) and 3-nitrotyrosine (3-NT) are critical biomarkers: 8-OHdG is a biomarker of DNA damage and 3-NT is a biomarker of Alzheimer's and Parkinson's diseases. Nontawong et al. fabricated a dual-imprinted paper-based electrochemical sensor to detect 3-NT and 8-OhdG simultaneously [62]. Silica nanospheres modified with silver nanoparticles were used as the imprinting surface to improve the sensitivity and selectivity of the sensor because nanomaterials provide a larger surface/mass ratio and easily accessible recognition cavities (Figure 3a). Modified nanospheres were coated with L-cysteine via the thiol group and polymerized in the presence of 3-NT and guanosine (a dummy of 8-OHdG), *N*-isopropylacrylamide (NIPAM), N,N-(1,2 dihydroxyethylene) bis-acrylamide (DHEBA) and AIBN separately, followed by template removal with methanol/acetic acid solution to produce 3-NT- and 8-OhdG-based MIPs. In the paper-based sensor fabrication step, hydrophobic barrier layers were printed on filter paper to create three-dimensional circular reservoirs (Figure 3b). Four electrodes (two electrodes as working electrodes for 3-NT and 8-OHdG, reference and counter electrodes) were then fabricated and assembled on filter paper for electrochemical detection. In order to fabricate working electrodes, graphene ink was mixed with 3-NT- and 8-OHdG-based MIPs. The performance of the sensor was evaluated by square wave voltammetry (SWV). For detection, 3-NT and 8-OHdG showed well-defined oxidation peaks and the current responses increased with the increasing concentration of both templates. The LODs were determined as 2.7 nM for 3-NT and 13.8 nM for 8-OHdG—lower than in previous studies [63–65]—with wide linear dynamic ranges.

An electrochemical sensor for the simultaneous detection of carbohydrate antigen 72–4 (CA72-4) and carbohydrate antigen 19–9 (CA19-9) gastric cancer tumor markers was proposed by Luo et al. [66]. Detection of tumor markers was achieved via glycosyl imprinting and lectin-specific binding as a two-step detection. In the first step, the MIP was synthesized by electropolymerization of the characteristic glycopeptide STn and SLe^a found on the surface of CA72-4 and CA19-9, respectively, 2-aminophenylboronic acid and aminophenylthiophenol-modified nanogold. After elution to create cavities and readsorption for binding of CA72-4 and CA19-9, the secondary specific recognition of CA72-4 and CA19-9 was assessed. In the second step, SNA modified with cysteine (Cys) and AuNPs for CA72-4 and MAL modified with AuNPs and ferrocenecarboxylic acid (Fc) for CA19-9 were prepared and incubated to bind to the glycosyl groups of CA72-4 and CA19-9. Differential pulse voltammetry (DPV) was employed to evaluate the performance of Cys and Fc as redox probes. The MAL-Au-Fc probe showed excellent redox properties with well-defined redox peaks; on the other hand, the SNA-Au-Cys probe gave a sensitive oxidation peak but a weaker reduction peak. According to the CV and EIS results used to assess the sensor performance, the produced sensor recognized both tumor markers specifically in about 30 min, with 0.0041 U/mL and 0.0032 U/mL LODs for CA72-4 and CA19-9, respectively. These LOD values make the sensor a powerful candidate for CA72-4 and CA19-9 detection when compared to performance of other electrochemical sensors for the detection of both markers [67,68].

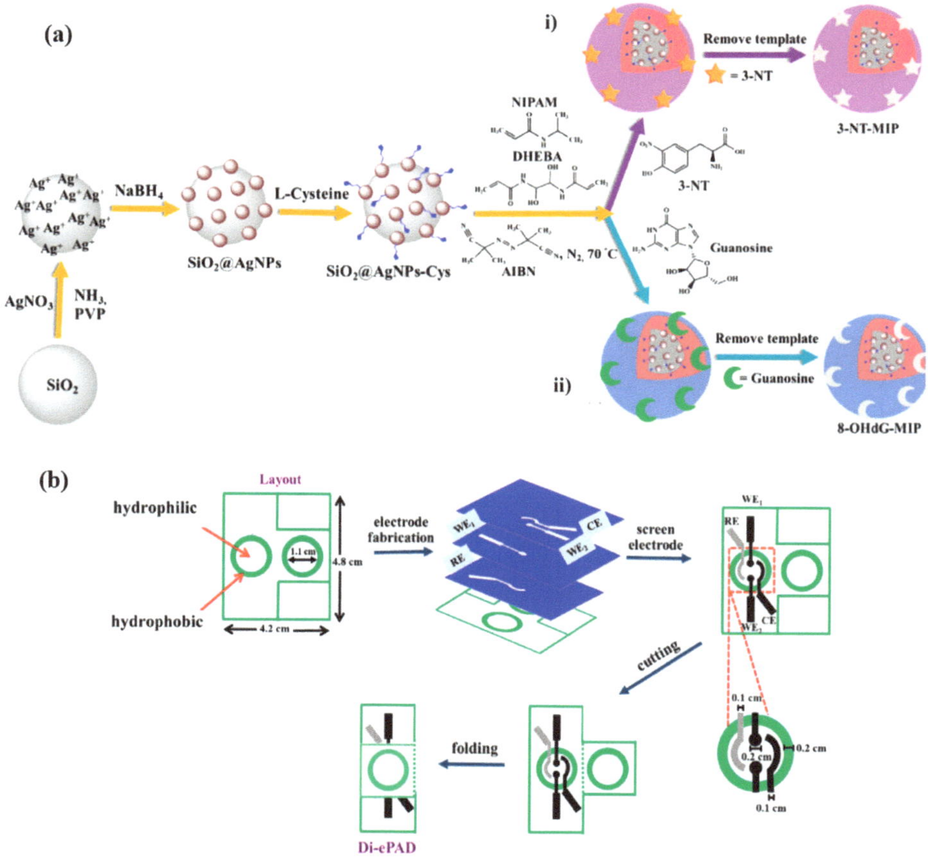

Figure 3. (**a**) Preparation of (**i**) 3-NT and (**ii**) 8-OHdG MIPs on SiO_2@AgNPs-Cys obtained by the modification of SiO_2 with $AgNO_3$, $NaBH_4$ and L-cysteine, respectively, before radical polymerization where 3-NT and guanosine were used as monomers. (**b**) Fabrication of the dual-imprinted paper-based electrochemical sensor by creating a hydrophobic reservoir on a filter paper to be used by voltametric cells by using Penguard enamel and constructing four electrodes by in-house screen printing and finally folding the spare reservoir on the electrodes to detect 3-NT and 8-OHdG. Reproduced with permission from [62].

Wang et al. produced an MIP-based electrochemical sensor to detect alpha-fetoprotein (AFP) and carcinoembryonic antigen (CEA), which are tumor markers for liver and bowel cancer in particular, respectively [69]. In this study, metallic labels were prepared by removing iron from recombinant ferritin to form apoferritin (r-Apo) and adding Cd^{2+} and Pb^{2+} and mixing with a graphene–Au composite. Finally, it was incubated with primary antibodies solution. Dual-template magnetic MIP (DT-MMIP) was prepared by polymerization of AFP and CEA and dopamine on Fe_3O_4 nanoparticles and removal of AFP and CEA by SDS solution. For electrochemical detection, DT-MMIP was incubated with AFP and CEA and dispersed into metallic label solution. The SWV results showed that the anodic peak currents of Cd^{2+} and Pb^{2+} increased with increasing concentrations of tumor markers. The LOD values were 0.3 and 0.35 pg/mL for AFP and CEA, respectively, which are at least ten times lower than in the study where AFP and CEA were detected simultaneously by an electrochemical assay [70].

Another study on the detection (one-by-one) of AFP and CEA by a dual-template molecularly imprinted polymer (DT-MIP) was conducted by Taheri et al. [71]. The sensor was established on a fluorine-doped tin oxide (FTO) electrode by electropolymerizing methyl orange (MO), AFP, CEA and pyrrole (Py) and removing AFP and CEA with NaOH. In the one-by-one detection method, DT-MIP was exposed to CEA until no more R_{ct} changes observed in the EIS. Thus, all the CEA-specific cavities were occupied by CEA and afterward DT-MIP was incubated with AFP many times until it gave a linear regression after EIS measurements. For the determination of CEA, DT-MIP was washed with NaOH to remove both templates and exposed to AFP for occupation of the AFP-specific cavities. Subsequently, CEA detection was carried out. The CV and EIS results confirmed that polypyrrole (PPy) and MO increased the conductivity as after the polymerization of them, the current increased in CV and the R_{ct} decreased in EIS. After incubation with AFP and CEA since the cavities were occupied by AFP and CEA, CV showed lower current as a result of bare electron transfer and EIS displayed higher impedance as a consequence of higher resistance of the double layer. DT-MIP had the detection limits of 1.6 pg/mL for CEA and 3.3 pg/mL for AFP. These are satisfactory results in comparison to the LODs obtained by electrochemical immunosensors [69,72,73].

Prostate-specific antigen (PSA) and myoglobin (Myo) are both proteins and biomarkers of prostate cancer. It is acknowledged that their high concentration in men's blood is an indicator of prostate cancer. Their detection is very important to diagnose the cancer at early stages. In accordance with this purpose, Karami et al. constructed an antibody molecularly imprinted polymer-based immunosensor to detect prostate-specific antigen and myoglobin markers [74]. Gold screen-printed electrodes (SPE) were modified with 3,3′-dithiodipropionicacid di(N-hydroxysuccinimide ester) (DSP) and PSA and Myo were attached to the modified electrode surface via covalent bonds. Subsequently, polymerization was carried out in the presence of acrylamide (AM) as a monomer, N,N-methylenebisacrylamide (NNMBA) as a cross-linker, and PSA and Myo as the templates. Oxalic acid (Oac) was selected as the elution solution to remove entrapped PSA and Myo from the polymeric matrix as it can break peptide bonds (Figure 4). For nanocomposite (NCP) synthesis, Fe_3O_4, MWCNTs, graphene oxide (GO) and PSA-specific antibody were used. EIS measurements were run at two different stages for detection of PSA and Myo. First, it was measured when the MIP was incubated with PSA and Myo. Second, it was measured when NCP was incubated with MIP, which was already incubated with PSA and Myo. This time, binding resulted from the interaction between PSA and the PSA-specific antibody. The R_{ct} difference between two EIS measurements was attributed to Myo binding. After the EIS results, it was confirmed that the MIP-based sensor is highly sensitive, with 5.4 pg/mL and 0.83 ng/mL LODs for PSA and Myo, respectively, well below the required clinical range [75]. Moreover, NCP is a proper sensing interface for PSA detection with high conductivity.

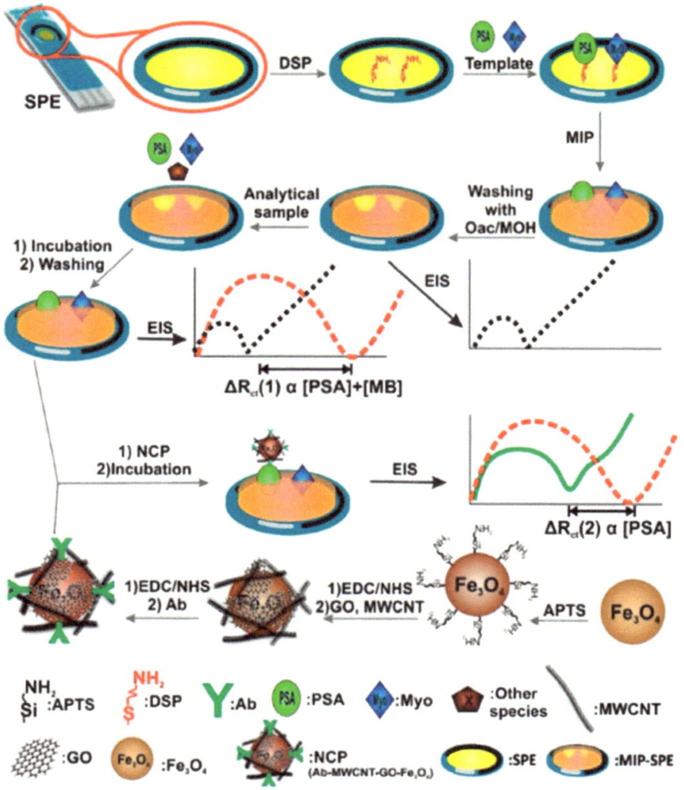

Figure 4. Schematic illustration of the process of MIP and NCP synthesis, along with the detection of PSA and Myo using EIS after incubating the sensor with PSA and Myo, and the NCP-PSA antibody, respectively. Reproduced with permission from [74].

Epidermal growth factor receptor (EGFR) and vascular endothelial growth factor (VEGF) are valuable cancer biomarkers that can provide important information for early cancer diagnosis. For simultaneous detection of these biomarkers, Johari-Ahar et al. developed a biosensor consisting of MIPs and antibody-conjugated nano-liposomes [76]. The MIPs were prepared in the same way and using the same chemicals as the MIP in the above article [74], except utilizing EGFR and VEGF as templates in this study. Antibody-conjugated nano-liposomes were designed by preparation of Cu(II)- and Cd(II)-loaded liposomes and conjugation of EGFR- and VEGF-specific antibodies with Cd(II)- and Cu(II)-loaded liposomes, respectively. Before evaluating the performance of the sensor, it was exposed to EGFR and VEGF and then incubated with antibody-conjugated nano-liposomes. EIS measurements showed that the created cavities were specific for EGFR and VEGF as the R_{ct} increased with the incubation of the biomarkers and the use of antibody-conjugated nano-liposomes amplified the electrochemical signal. The LODs were calculated to be 0.01 pg/mL for EGFR and 0.005 pg/mL for VEGF. The high sensitivity, selectivity and reproducibility of the proposed sensor make it a superior candidate among other electrochemical sensors produced for EGFR and VEGF detection [77–79].

Pandey et al. introduced a nanocube-shaped dual imprinted polymer-based electrochemical sensor for the detection of hemoglobin (Hb) and glycated hemoglobin (HbA1c), which are biomarkers of gestational diabetes mellitus [80]. In the sensor fabrication process, 3 amino-phenyl boronic acid (APBA), rhodamine b, HbA1c and Hb were electropolymerized on the carbon-paste-coated aluminum foil. During electropolymerization, APBA and rhodamine b were attached to each other via amide bonds; on the other hand, HbA1c and Hb were bound to a boronic acid moiety via a cis-diol bond of glucose and attached to a rhodamine b moiety via H-bonding with the presence of amino acid groups of Hb. HbA1c and Hb were extracted electrochemically. The sensor performance was analyzed both individually and simultaneously by DPV. In both individual measurements, the DPV responses increased linearly with an increase in the concentration of HbA1c and Hb. For simultaneous determination of HbA1c and Hb, DPV showed a regression linear curve for both biomarkers. Furthermore, well-defined separate peaks were obtained at their respective potentials, as determined during individual DPV measurements. The sensor demonstrated very low LODs (0.084 ng/mL for Hb and 0.095 ng/mL for HbA1c) as well as being very flexible, with the electrochemical response remaining unchanged despite being bent 450 times.

Immunoglobulins sometimes act as a biomarker and provide important information about health. Detection of the antibodies produced in the first and later stages of diseases is clinically important in terms of early diagnosis of the disease, determining its stage and identifying the treatments that need to be applied. Liu et al. proposed a dual molecularly imprinted polymer-based electrochemical sensor to detect IgG and IgM, where AuNPs, GO and MWCNTs were utilized to enhance the electrochemical signals and increase the stability of the signal probes [81]. Electropolymerization of Py was followed by template removal with acetic acid and SDS solution. The produced sensor had very low LODs, with 28.80 pg/mL for IgG and 0.58 pg/mL for IgM, and showed high selectivity toward a mixture of other substances, such as BSA, HGB, L-Trp and D-Tyr.

Overviews of the imprinted MT-MIP-based electrochemical sensors developed for the detection of ions and biomacromolecules are presented in Tables 1 and 2, respectively.

Table 1. Summary of ion-imprinted MT-MIP-based electrochemical sensors.

Template	MIP Components	Elution Solution	Electrochemical Method	Linear Range	LOD	Application	Ref.
Cd(II) Cu(II)	AEDP, L-histidine, EGDMA, AIBN	EDTA	DPASV	0.124–2.989 ng/mL 0.124–0.725 ng/mL	0.053 ng/mL 0.035 ng/mL	Human blood serum Cow's milk Lake water	[47]
Ce(IV) Gd(III)	But-2-enedioic acid bis-[(2-amino-ethyl)-amide], EGDMA AIBN	HCl	DPASV	0.27–5.35 ng/mL 0.75–9.45 ng/mL	0.063 ng/mL 0.182 ng/mL	Water Human serum	[51]
Cu(II) Zn(II)	BAAP, EGDMA, AIBN	EDTA	DPASV	0.098–23.80 µg/L	0.0159 µg/L 0.0275 µg/L	-	[56]

Table 2. Summary of biomacromolecule-imprinted MT-MIP-based electrochemical sensors.

Template	MIP Components	Elution Solution	Electrochemical Method	Linear Range	LOD	Application	Ref.
8-OHdG 3-NT	NIPAM, DHEBA, AIBN	Methanol/ acetic acid	SWV	0.05–500 μM 0.01–500 μM	0.0138 μM 0.0027 μM	Urine Serum	[62]
CA72-4 CA19-9	2-aminopheny-lboronic acid	Methanol/ acetic acid	DPV	0.005–100.0 U/mL	0.0041 U/mL 0.0032 U/mL	Serum	[66]
AFP CEA	Dopamine	SDS	SWV	0.001–5 ng/mL	0.3 pg/mL 0.35 pg/mL	Human serum	[69]
AFP CEA	Pyrrole	NaOH	EIS	$10–10^4$ pg/mL $5–10^4$ pg/mL	3.3 pg/mL 1.6 pg/mL	Human serum	[71]
PSA Myo	AM, NNMBA,	Oac	EIS	0.01–100 ng/mL 1–20,000 ng/mL	5.4 pg/mL 0.83 ng/mL	Serum Urine	[74]
EGFR VEGF	AM, NNMBA	Oac	PSA	0.05–50,000 pg/mL 0.01–7000 pg/mL	0.01 pg/mL 0.005 pg/mL	Serum	[76]
Hb HbA1c	APBA	PBS (overoxi-dation)	DPV	0.1–250 ng/mL 0.5–235 ng/mL	0.084 ng/mL 0.095 ng/mL	Blood	[80]
IgG IgM	Pyrrole	Acetic acid/SDS	DPV	0.05–500 ng/mL 0.001–100 ng/mL	0.0288 ng/mL 0.00058 ng/mL	Serum	[81]

2.3. Detection of Amino Acids

Amino acids are the building blocks of proteins and the most important organic molecules for organisms. They are found in two forms: levorotatory (L-) and dextrorotatory (D-) amino acids. Their detection is critical for many fields, including medicine, agriculture, and food, and also for tissue metabolism as they take part in many human body functions and sometimes act as biomarkers of different diseases.

A one-by-one detection method was adopted by Prasad et al. to detect D- and L-aspartic acid enantiomeric pairs by a dual-template molecularly imprinted polymer-based electrochemical sensor [82]. The surface "grafting from" approach was followed for sensor fabrication. After modification of a pencil graphite electrode (PGE) with AuNPs, free radical polymerization was conducted in the presence of N-acryloyl pyrrolidine-2,5-dione (NAPD, functional monomer), EGDMA (cross-linker), AIBN (initiator), D- and L-aspartic acid (templates) and MWCNTs, followed by template removal with NaOH and phosphate buffer. Although enantioselective analysis of D- and L-aspartic acid is challenging since they have same oxidation potential, the produced sensor managed to distinguish between them with 1.11 and 1.14 ng/mL LODs for D- and L-aspartic acid, respectively.

In another study to detect D-cysteine (D-Cys) and L-cysteine (L-Cys), Hou et al. used a magnetic glassy carbon electrode (MGCE), which was drop-coated with molybdenum disulfide-ionic liquid (MoS_2-IL) and electrodeposited with chitosan (CS) before drop-coating with MIPs, including methacrylic acid (MAA), acrylic amide (AM), N-isopropylacrylamide (NIPAM) as monomers, N,N methylenebis(acrylamide) (MBA) as cross-linker, D- and L-cysteine as templates and Fe_3O_4 NPs as the framework material [83] (Figure 5a). The templates were extracted with acetic acid and acetonitrile solution. Each step in the sensor fabrication was observed by CV and EIS. Electrochemical detection was carried out by DPV through a one-by-one detection method (vector method) as the oxidation potential of both templates overlaps. The DPV results revealed that the sensor was able to detect D- and L-cysteine by a one-by-one detection method, which allows the detection of one target after the sensor is saturated with the other target (Figure 5b). The LODs of

L-Cys and D-Cys were 0.7402 pg/mL and 0.6136 pg/mL, respectively. In comparison to the reported electrochemical chiral detection of L-Cys and D-Cys, the produced sensor showed higher sensitivity, which can be attributed to the outstanding electrical conductivity and large surface area of MoS_2-IL [84,85].

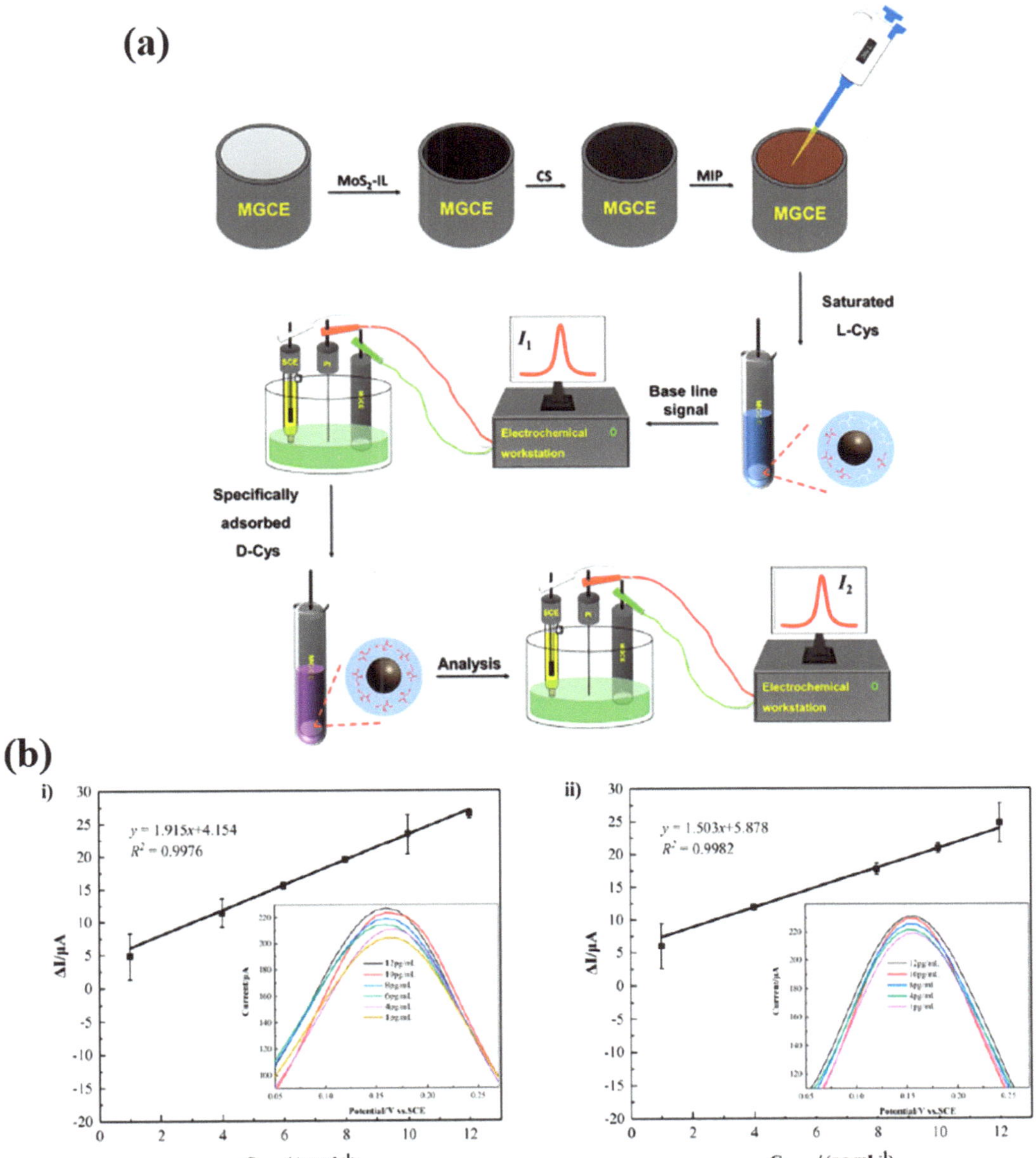

Figure 5. (**a**) Schematic illustration of the preparation of MIP/MoS_2-IL/CS/MGCE and the set-up for electrochemical enantioanalysis of D-Cys and L-Cys, and (**b**) the linear relationship between the current response and the L-Cys concentration (**i**) and D-Cys concentration (**ii**) (insets: DPV responses for L-Cys (**i**) and D-Cys (**ii**)). Reproduced with permission from [83].

2.4. Detection of Pharmaceutical Compounds

Pharmaceuticals are drugs used to treat diseases, reduce symptoms, or stop the progression of disease after its initial stages. While their use in low doses may cause the treatment to be ineffective, their use in high doses may be toxic or cause adverse side effects [86]. The effectiveness of pharmaceuticals depends on the dose used as well as the impurities of the pharmaceuticals [87]. Pharmaceuticals should be impurity-free as impurities may reduce the effectiveness of the drug. For all these reasons, the monitoring, detection and quantification of pharmaceuticals are important for patient health. Different analytical techniques, such as chromatographic, gravimetric and spectroscopic techniques, can be used for these purposes, but the advantages of MIPs over these methods make it a powerful technique and different pharmaceuticals have been detected by MIPs.

Chlorambucil (Chb) is used for cancer treatment and dacarbazine (Dac) is used for malignant melanoma, Hodgkin's lymphoma and soft tissue sarcoma. They both have similar side effects, and to avoid these, their dosage should be adjusted carefully, and this reveals the need for a sensor for their analysis and detection. By use of acryloylated tetraamine cobalt phthalocyanine (aTACoPC) as a crosslinking monomer, a dual imprinted polymer-based electrochemical sensor was fabricated on a reduced graphene oxide ceramic electrode (rGOCE) by Fatma et al. to detect Chb and Dac [28]. During the DT-MIP synthesis process, Chb, Dac, aTACoPC and AIBN were mixed to form a prepolymer mixture and spin-coated on an rGOCE, followed by free radical polymerization. Finally, the rGOCE was dipped in acetonitrile-methanol solution to retrieve Chb and Dac. The DPASV results showed that the sensor with a high imprinting factor could differentiate and detect both templates simultaneously and successively. The sensor had good stability as no deviation in current was observed over more than one month. Additionally, five electrodes produced under similar conditions gave identical responses by the DPASV measurements, indicating the reproducibility of the sensor.

Antipyrine (AnP) and ethionamide (ETH) are nonsteroidal anti-inflammatory drugs used for clinical applications to reduce pain and as an antibiotic used for tuberculosis treatment, respectively. Their overdose usage can result in multiple side effects. The sensor developed by Singh et al. detected AnP and ETH sensitively [88]. Reduced graphene oxide (RGO) was prepared and drop-coated on a glassy carbon electrode (GCE). A pre-polymerization solution was prepared with 3-thiophene acetic acid (3-TAA), AnP and ETH in phosphate-buffered saline (PBS) and electropolymerization was performed by CV. Afterwards, the MIP-modified GCE was eluted with methanol-acetic acid solution to remove AnP and ETH and create cavities complementary in size and shape to AnP and ETH. The MIP-based GCE sensor was evaluated using $K_3[Fe(CN)_6]$ as a redox probe by CV. Because 3-TAA has insulating properties, the current response decreased after electropolymerization, but with the removal of AnP and ETH, the current increased as cavities were created. The performance of the sensor in terms of the detection of AnP and ETH individually was assessed by DPV. The LODs were found to be 0.117 μM for AnP and 0.15 μM for ETH. When compared to other sensors produced for AnP and ETH detection, these low LODs can be attributed to the higher conductivity of RGO, which is used in electrochemical sensors to increase the sensitivity of target detection [89,90].

Sulfadiazine (SDZ) and acetaminophen (AP) were detected simultaneously by an electrochemical sensor as their excessive consumption is harmful. Sun et al. firstly modified GCE with a highly conductive graphene oxide@covalent organic framework composite (GO@COF) [91]. SDZ, AP, pyrrole and tetrabutyl ammonium perchlorate (TBAP) were electropolymerized in acetonitrile. Subsequently, polypyrrole was overoxidized in NaOH solution for template extraction. First, all the SDZ and AP were detected individually, with oxidation peaks at 0.36 V and 0.86 V for AP and SDZ, respectively. Following this, the sensor was incubated with AP and SDZ at the same time for simultaneous detection and two distinct oxidation peaks were observed at 0.36 V and 0.86 V. It was determined that the current response increased with increasing AP and SDZ concentrations and this revealed a strong linear relationship between the current and the analyte concentration. The sensor also demonstrated good selectivity, accuracy, and stability for AP and SDZ detection with a wide range of concentrations and low LODs.

2.5. Detection of Neurotransmitters

Neurotransmitters are endogenous chemicals called messengers of the body that amplify, transmit and convert signals in cells [92]. Neurotransmitters are of great importance for human health and any imbalance in the level of neurotransmitters or the absence of neurotransmitters leads to various neurological and mental diseases, such as Alzheimer's and Parkinson's diseases [93]. Therefore, their detection and concentration determination are very important for the treatment of diseases. Since different neurotransmitters have very similar redox potentials for *in vivo* detection, it is difficult to detect them simultaneously by electrochemical methods [94]. Despite having similar redox potentials, this issue can be tackled by using MIPs due to their target-specific cavities.

Dopamine (DA) and epinephrine (EP) were detected by a three-dimensional hybrid network consisting of a molecularly imprinted polymer and MWCNTs [95]. In this study, where poly(9-carbazoleacetic acid) was synthesized and used as a functional monomer for the first time, for the simultaneous detection of DA and EP, although DA and EP have the same molecular structure, EP was used as a pseudo-template for MIP preparation since DA is a little smaller than EP and DA-imprinted MIP cavities do not let EP enter the cavities, leading to low sensitivity. After modification of GCE with MWCNT 9-carbazoleacetic acid, EP was electropolymerized on the electrode, followed by NaOH washing and ethanol for EP extraction. The advantage of using 9-carbazoleacetic acid provided enough covalent interactions with both templates and MWCNTs, which created a high specific surface area and a high conductivity sensor, resulting in low LODs of 0.015 μM for DA and 0.023 μM for EP, with high selectivity and sensitivity.

Another study on the detection of DA and EP was conducted by Fatma et al. [96]. Firstly, graphene oxide/carbon black composite (GO/CB) was prepared. Acryloylated-GO/CB (aGO/CB) was then synthesized and used as a crosslinking monomer. After free radical polymerization of the crosslinking monomer, DA, EP and AIBN (initiator) on SPCE, triethylamine (TEA)-methanol solution removed DA and EP from the polymer matrix and a one monomer dual imprinted polymer (OMNiDIP) was created (Figure 6a). The effect of each modification on the detection of DA and EP was assessed by DPASV. According to the results, the GO/CB composite significantly improved the response of the sensor when compared to CB and GO separately, but it was not enough to differentiate both templates (Figure 6b). After employing the MIP, the GO/CB composite sensor managed to differentiate DA and EP and detect them with LODs of 0.028 ng/mL for DA and 0.017 ng/mL for EP.

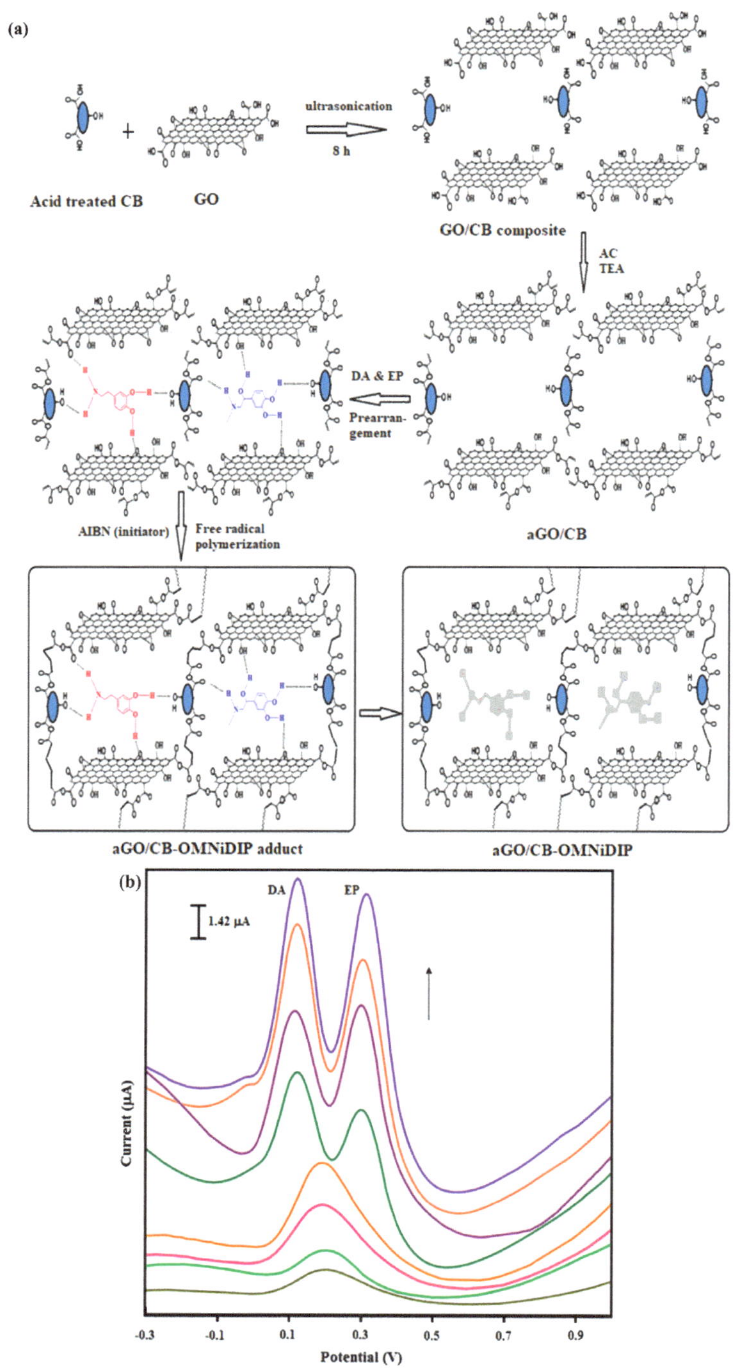

Figure 6. (**a**) Schematic protocol for the synthesis of aGO/CB-OMNiDIP, and (**b**) DPASV responses for DA and EP on different electrodes; from bottom to top: bare SPCE, CB/SPCE, GO/SPCE, GO/CB composite/SPCE, aCB-DIP/SPCE, aGO-DIP/SPCE, aGO/CB-DIP/SPCE and aGO/CB-OMNiDIP/SPCE. Reproduced with permission from [96].

2.6. Detection of Environmental Pollutants

Environmental pollutants, including chemicals, heavy metals, pesticides, herbicides, and plastics, are a threat to human health as they cause different pollutions and have adverse effects on the climate. This reveals the importance of their detection and analysis, both for global health and for the protection of the environment.

4-nitrophenol (4-NP) and hydroquinone (HQ) are both phenolic compounds that are dangerous environmental contaminants and pose a significant health threat due to their long-term aqueous stability. Thus, early detection prior to water contamination is crucial. A surface-imprinted polymeric film was fabricated on GCE for the detection of 4-NP and HQ by Singh et al. [97]. 4-amino thiophenol (4-ATP) and p-phenylenediamine (p-PD) with aromatic rings were selected as functional monomers because of their interaction with the template molecules via hydrophobic and π–π interactions. The functional monomers and templates were electropolymerized in an HCl-supporting electrolyte. The templates were extracted by immersing the electrodes in methanol/water solution. After individual detection of 4-NP and p-PD, the LODs were determined as 0.14 μM and 0.37 μM for HQ and 4-NP, respectively. For simultaneous detection, the DPV responses were recorded for different 4-NP and HQ concentrations, and this showed two oxidation peaks at around 0.1 V (HQ) and 0.9 V (4-NP) as they were obtained at individual detection measurements. This showed that there was no interference with the templates. Additionally, lower LODs were obtained for simultaneous detection, showing that the imprinted film managed to distinguish both templates well.

In another study, platinum nanoparticle (PtNP)-decorated amino-mesoporous silica nanoparticles (MSN-PtNPs) were used as supporting material for a dual-template molecularly imprinted polymer coating for the detection of paraquat (PQ) and glyphosate (GLY), both representatives of broad-spectrum herbicides that can damage aquatic organisms if released into water systems and can cause serious health issues for humans if allowed to accumulate *in vivo*. After polymerization of PQ and GLY with acrylic acid (AA) and N-vinyl-2-pyrrolidone (VP) as monomers, DHEBA as a cross-linker, potassium peroxydisulfate ($K_2S_2O_8$) as the initiator and removing the template by sonicating in water, the sensor was fabricated on a graphite electrode by manual screen-printing and modified with MIP-coated MSN-PtNPs, as shown in Figure 7. The simultaneous determination results showed that the sensor gave a linear response toward increasing concentrations of PQ and GLY; 3.1 nM and 4.0 nM were obtained as the LODs of PQ and GLY, respectively, with linear calibration curves in the range of 0.025–500 μM for both analytes by DPV [98]. These results meet the maximum contaminant levels of PQ (0.012 μM) and GLY (4.140 μM) in drinking water [99,100].

Rao et al. utilized nitrogen-doped carbon nanosheet frameworks (Fe-NCNFs) decorated with Fe to be coated with MIP for simultaneous detection of mebendazole (Meb) and catechol (CC), which are environmental pollutants [101]. As Fe nanoparticles increase electrocatalytical activity and carbon nanomaterials help nanoparticles to boost their electroactivity, by taking advantage of these features, the Fe-NCNFs had larger specific surface area and fast electron transport [102,103]. Fe-NCNFs were prepared via a chemical blowing process and GCE was modified with Fe-NCNF. Meb was imprinted on the modified GCE by electropolymerization in the presence of MAA and $LiClO_4$, followed by the removal of Meb with acetic acid/methanol solution. The sensor detected Meb and CC, with Meb recognized through the high binding affinity of the MIP and specific cavities, and CC detected through its adsorption and electrochemical oxidation by Fe-NCNFs. The sensor has a low limit of detection of 0.06 μM for Meb and 0.004 μM for CC.

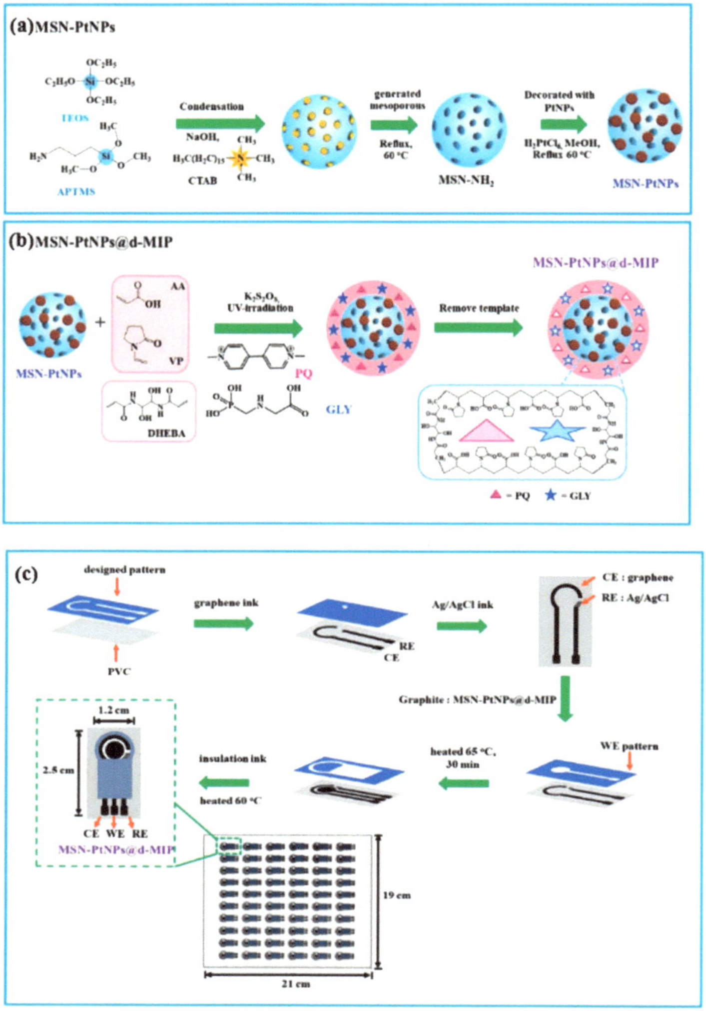

Figure 7. Schematic representation of synthesis of the (**a**) MSN-PtNPs and (**b**) dual imprinted MSN-PtNPs and (**c**) fabrication of the PQ and GLY dual-MIP sensor. Reproduced with permission from [98].

2.7. Detection of Cells and Viruses

Outbreaks and infections caused by bacteria and viruses have been a major concern for public health. Despite significant advancements in medical technology and treatments, as well as important developments in the field, the COVID-19 pandemic has starkly highlighted the devastating consequences of diseases caused by pathogens, which can lead to alarmingly high mortality rates. In terms of preventing diseases that bacteria and viruses cause, their early detection is of critical importance. Although many single-template MIP-based electrochemical sensors were fabricated for bacteria and virus detection [104–107], only a couple of multi-template MIP-based electrochemical sensors have been produced so far. Moakhar et al. developed a novel electrochemical sensor to detect two types of biomarkers: viral proteins from influenza A H1N1 and SARS-CoV-2, as well as specific antibodies (IgM and IgG) against SARS-CoV-2 [42]. This sensor was designed to analyze saliva samples for viral proteins and blood samples for antibodies, with the goal of facilitating the early detection and prevention of viral respiratory infections. In this study, three 1 µm sized gold nano/micro-sized island (NMI) electrodes, which comprise fluidic assays were electropolymerized with o-PD separately and built-in recognition sites, were created after removal with NaOH for the detection of viral particles in saliva and antibodies in blood (Figure 8c). The fluidic assay was used in an NFluidEX device, which has a multiplexed microfluidic delivery system, automated custom-made potentiostat and cartridge for sample collection (Figure 8d). NfluidEX was integrated with a smart phone via Wi-Fi and Bluetooth controllers for signal analyses and display of the results. NfluidEX showed a low limit of detection with high sensitivity and specificity and low cross-reactivity with the help of employing an NMI/MIP assay and using a proper monomer and finding high binding affinity regions between the monomer and the target proteins as a result of molecular-docking studies. The quantitative feature of the NFluidEX was evaluated by comparing it with real-time quantitative polymerase chain reaction (RT-qPCR), which is the gold standard for viruses. Patients clinically diagnosed with SARS-CoV-2 were found to be positive in both the saliva and blood tests using NFluidEX, and these results were consistent with those obtained through PCR and ELISA tests. This developed device can be used as a point-of-care device for early diagnosis to monitor and prevent the spread of viral infections due to its excellent features as it has multi-MIP detection system, allowing simultaneous detection of virus and antibodies within 11 min.

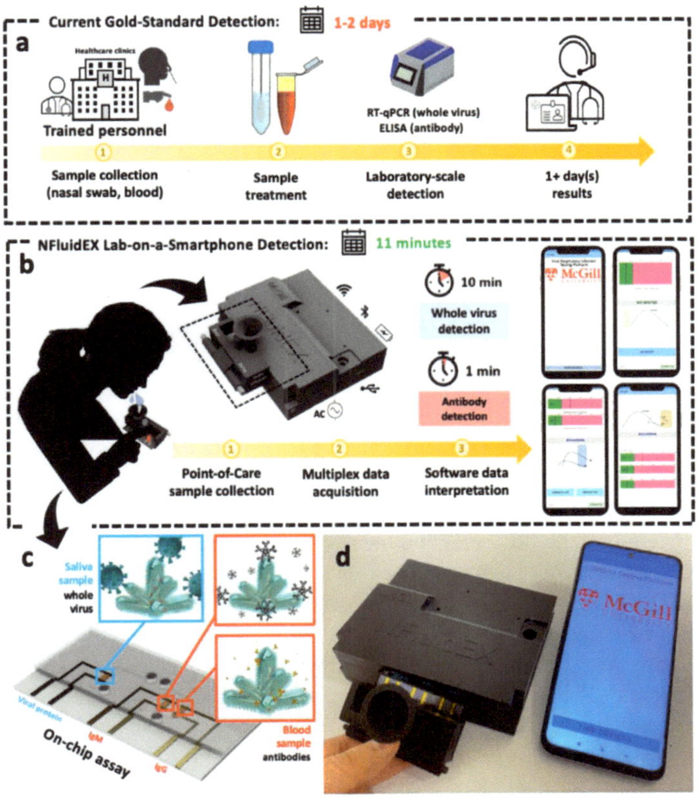

Figure 8. Schematic representation of the NfluidEX. (**a**) Current gold standard detection methods for diagnosis. (**b**) Steps of detection by NfluidEX. (**c**) On-chip assay for whole-virus detection in saliva samples and antibody detection in blood samples. (**d**) Real image of the NfluidEX device. Reproduced with permission from [42].

There are some challenges when imprinting whole bacteria and viruses because of their large dimensions when compared to small molecules such as nucleic acids, amino acids and proteins. For example, (i) a bulky, highly cross-linked polymer matrix may slow down the diffusion of microorganisms to the cavities as microorganisms have large dimensions; (ii) bacteria have many functional groups on their cell wall and this can make cavities hard to create and cause the heterogeneity of the binding affinity; (iii) by their nature, microorganisms can secrete various chemicals to adapt to the environment, which may cause the selectivity of the sensor to decrease; and (iv) template removal can be challenging [108,109]. These challenges can be overcome by employing different techniques and methods. For example, instead of using whole-cell imprinting, the surface components of microorganisms such as epitope and lipopolysaccaride can be imprinted, or in case of whole-cell imprinting, suitable and facile methods should be chosen [109].

When developing an MIP-based sensor for microorganism detection, due to the complex dimensions and size, the thickness of the polymer film is important and therefore the electropolymerization method, where the thickness of the MIP film can be easily controlled, is generally preferred. Moreover, electropolymerization is also advantageous as microorganisms are doped directly into the polymer matrix, which creates cavities with high affinity [110].

Since bacteria have many functional groups exposed on their surface, monomer selection is crucial for both the imprinting and the template removal processes. Dopamine [111], APBA [112] and pyrrole [113,114] are commonly used monomers. Dopamine has many functional groups, such as phenyl, amino, and hydroxyl groups, that can react with bacteria [115]. 3-aminophenylboronic acid (3-APBA) has a boronic acid group and it can specifically interact with cis-diol, which presents on the bacterial surface [104]. Pyrrole has excellent properties, including low nonspecific adsorption, good conductivity, superior stability, efficient polymerization at mild conditions and an N–H interaction that ensures high selectivity [116].

Although it is difficult to remove microorganisms from polymeric films, a variety of different useful methods are available. Acidic solutions and surfactants [117], enzyme treatment, overoxidation [118], multistep extraction procedures, including enzyme treatment, the use of surfactant and overoxidation [105,112] have been used for the removal of microorganisms.

Although the detection of microorganisms is more difficult than the detection of small molecules due to the reasons mentioned above, multiplexed detection can be achieved by using an appropriate monomer, eluent solution and imprinting method [109,119].

Escherichia coli (*E. coli*) O157:H7 and *Staphylococcus aureus* (*S. aureus*) are pathogenic bacteria, and they have caused many outbreaks that caused several illnesses [120–122]. Their detection is of great importance to prevent outbreaks and protect public health. A dual-bacteria-imprinted polymer (DBIP) sensor was reported by Xu et al. for *E. coli* O157:H7 and *S. aureus* detection [123]. In the DBIP preparation process, o-PD was electropolymerized on the GCE by CV in the presence of *E. coli* O157:H7 and *S. aureus*; subsequently, both bacteria were eluted by soaking the modified GCE in cetyltrimethylammonium bromide/acetic acid (CTAB/Hac) solution for 10 min. Quantitative detection of *E. coli* O157:H7 and *S. aureus* was performed separately by incubating modified GCE with both bacteria individually and measured using EIS. The LODs of the sensor were obtained as 9.4 CFU/mL for *E. coli* 0157:H7 and 9.5 CFU/mL for *S. aureus*. *E. coli* O6 and *S. hemolyticus* were used as interference bacteria to test the selectivity of the sensor and the highest EIS responses were observed for *E. coli* O157:H7 + *S. aureus* and a mixture of interference bacteria + *E. coli* O157:H7 + *S. aureus*, indicating that the sensor was not affected by closely related strains (interference bacteria). As the sensor has a short fabrication time (20 min), high selectivity and sensitivity, it can be a promising tool to monitor and detect multiple pathogenic bacteria simultaneously.

An overview of the imprinted MT-MIP-based electrochemical sensors developed for the detection of organic molecules and pathogens are presented in Tables 3 and 4, respectively. Other MT-MIP-based sensors for a range of analytes, not discussed in this review, are presented in Table 5.

Table 3. Summary of organic-molecule-imprinted MT-MIP-based electrochemical sensors.

Template	MIP Components	Elution Solution	Electrochemical Method	Linear Range	LOD	Application	Ref.
D-aspartic acid L-aspartic acid	NAPD, EGDMA, AIBN	NaOH/ Phosphate buffer	DPASV	3.89–66.23 ng/mL 3.99–66.12 ng/mL	1.11 ng/mL 1.14 ng/mL	CSF Blood serum Pharmaceutical samples	[82]
D-Cys L-Cys	MAA, AM, NIPAM, MBA	Acetic acid/ Acetonitrile	DPV	1–12 pg/mL	0.6136 pg/mL 0.7402 pg/mL	Fetal bovine serum	[83]
Chb Dac	aTACoPC, AIBN	Acetonitrile/ Methanol	DPASV	0.159–28.524 ng/mL 0.069–35.278 ng/mL	0.037 ng/mL 0.016 ng/mL	Blood serum Urine Pharmaceutical samples	[28]
AnP ETH	3-TAA	Methanol/ Acetic acid	DPV	0.05–0.6 μM 0.03–1.2 μM	0.117 μM 0.15 μM	Human blood serum	[88]
SDZ AP	Pyrrole, TBAP	NaOH (Overoxidation)	DPV	0.5–200 μM 0.05–20 μM	0.16 μM 0.032 μM	Pork Chicken	[91]
DA EP	9-carbazoleacetic acid	NaOH/ Ethanol	DPSV	0.04–70 μM	0.015 μM 0.023 μM	Rat plasma	[95]
DA EP	aGO/CB, AIBN	TEA/ Methanol	DPASV	0.12–4.578 ng/mL 0.075–1.188 ng/mL	0.028 ng/mL 0.017 ng/mL	Blood serum Urine Pharmaceutical samples	[96]
4-NP HQ	4-ATP, p-PD	Methanol/ Water	DPV	0.8–200 μM	0.37 μM 0.14 μM	Water (distilled, packaged, tap, river)	[97]
PQ GLY	AA, VP, DHEBA, $K_2S_2O_8$	Sonication in water	DPV	0.025–500 μM	0.0031 μM 0.004 μM	Water (reservoir, pond, wastewater)	[98]
Meb CC	MAA, $LiClO_4$	Methanol/ Acetic acid	DPV	0.01–1.5 μM 0.5–25 μM	0.004 μM 0.06 μM	Water (tap, river)	[101]

CSF: Cerebrospinal fluid.

Table 4. Summary of cell- and microorganism-imprinted MT-MIP-based electrochemical sensors.

Template	MIP Components	Elution Solution	Electrochemical Method	Linear Range	LOD	Application	Ref.
Viral particles IgG IgM	o-PD	NaOH	EIS	9.60×10^3–3.84×10^8 particles/mL 10^1–10^4 pg/μL 10^1–10^4 pg/μL	2091.6 particles/mL 3.63 pg/μL 2.79 pg/μL	Saliva Plasma Blood	[42]
E. coli O157:H7 *S. aureus*	o-PD	CTAB/HAc	EIS	-	9.4 CFU/mL 9.5 CFU/mL	Apple juice	[123]

Table 5. Additional MT-MIP-based sensors for the detection of different targets.

Template	MIP Components	Elution Solution	Electrochemical Method	Linear Range	LOD	Application	Ref.
NE UA	TAT, AIBN	TEA/ Methanol	DPASV	2.98–40.69 ng/mL 1.94–43.59 ng/mL	0.66 ng/mL 0.44 ng/mL	Blood serum Urine Pharmaceutical samples	[124]
HQ CC	Melamine	Ethanol/ Water	DPV	10–100 μM (for both)	3.1 μM 3.5 μM	River water	[125]
AA DA	TAT, EGDMA	ACN/ TEA	DPASV	8.28–77.92 ng/mL 0.10–5.24 ng/mL	2.21 ng/mL 0.22 ng/mL	CSF Blood serum Pharmaceutical samples	[29]
CA TPH	L-arginine	NaOH	DPV	0.01–1.0 μM 0.1–100.0 μM	1.3 nM 20.0 nM	Green tea Urine	[126]
UA Tyr	AMT	Ethanol	DPV	0.01 μM–100 μM 0.1 μM–400 μM	0.0032 μM 0.046 μM	Serum Urine	[127]
AA Tyr	m-DB, o-AP	Nitric acid	DPV	0.1–300 μM 0.01–180 μM	0.03 μM 0.003 μM	Human serum	[128]
CLB RAC	o-PD	NaOH (overoxidation)	CV	1 pM–8 nM (for both)	0.303 pM (for both)	Urine Raw pork CLB tablets	[129]
OX DZ	MAA, EGDMA, AIBN	Methanol/ Acetic acid	DPV	0.01–200 μM 0.05–150 μM	59 nM 21 nM	Urine Tablet	[130]
GLY GLU	EGDMA, TEA	Acetonitrile/ TEA	DPASV	3.98–176.23 ng/mL 0.54–3.96 ng/mL	0.35 ng/mL 0.19 ng/mL	Soil Human serum	[30]
Adrenaline UA	Dopamine, PBS	Methanol/ Acetic acid	OECTs	0.5 pM–10 μM 1 pM–1 mM	1 pM (for both)	Urine	[131]
CFZ AVI	o-PD, PBS	NaOH (overoxidation)	SWV	50–1000 μM 1–1000 μM	35 μM 0.5 μM	Human serum Rabbit	[132]
RIF INZ	Pyrrole	Methanol/ Water	AdSDPV	0.08–85 μM (for both)	0.287 nM 0.371 nM	Pharmaceutical samples Blood serum Urine	[133]

Table 5. *Cont.*

Template	MIP Components	Elution Solution	Electrochemical Method	Linear Range	LOD	Application	Ref.
DA Chlorpromazine	Nicotinamide	Methanol/ Acetic acid	DPV	0.05–8 μM/ 8–40 μM 0.005–2 μM	2.8 nM 0.25 nM	Human serum Urine Pharmaceutical sample	[41]
DA UA	o-PD, PBS	H_2SO_4 (overoxidation)	DPV	2.0–180 μM 5.0–160 μM	0.3 μM 0.4 μM	Bovine serum	[134]
DA Ade	AM	PBS (overoxidation)	DPV	0.6–200 μM 0.4–300 μM	0.12–0.37 μM 0.15–0.36 μM	Human serum	[135]
NPX MTH OMZ	MAA, EGDMA, AIBN	Acetic acid/ Ethanol	DPV	5.0 nM–100 μM 1.0 nM–130 μM 5.0 nM–100 μM	1.0 nM 0.7 nM 1.5 nM	Human plasma Urine Tap water Tablet	[136]

NE: Norepinephrine, UA: Uric acid, TAT: 2,4,6-trisacrylamido-1,3,5-triazine, Ery: Erythromycin, Cla: Clarithromycin, Azi: Azithromycin, mPD: m-phenylenediamine, AA: Ascorbic acid, CA: Catechin, TPH: Theophylline, G: Guanine, X: Xanthine, Tyr: Tyrosine, AMT: 2-amino-5-mercapto-1, 3, 4-thiadiazole, m-DB: m-dihydroxy benzene, o-AP: o-aminophenol, CLB: Clenbuterol hydrochloride, RAC: Ractopamine, OX: Oxazepam, DZ: Diazepam, GLU: Glufosinate, OECT: Organic electrochemical transistor, CFZ: Ceftazidime, AVI: Avibactam, RIF: Rifampicin, INZ: Isoniazid, CPZ: Chlorpromazine, Ade: Adenine, NPX: Naproxen, MTH: Methocarbamol, OMZ: Omeprazole.

3. Integration of Microfluidics and Commercialization

The detection of biomarkers, substances and pathogens that can affect public health and cause diseases is vital for early-stage detection and to make accurate diagnoses in a short time, which facilitates the initiation of an effective treatment regime. Current diagnostic tools have disadvantages, including the costs, requiring trained personnel, and the slow time to diagnosis, and are generally devices that are difficult to transport, preventing use in remote environments. Therefore, the need for effective point-of-care (POC) diagnostic tools is greatly increasing. POC diagnostics is a new strategy for real-time, rapid, accurate, and on-site detection at the patient's point of need, as depicted in Figure 9.

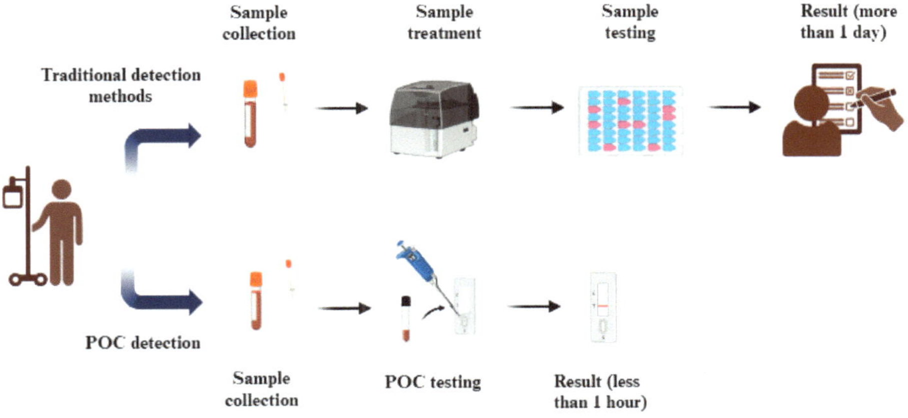

Figure 9. Schematic illustration of disease detection using traditional methods relying on centralized laboratories and POC testing approaches.

Microfluidic systems control and manipulate small amounts of liquids (typically μL to nL or lower) using microscale-level channels [137]. They enable smaller samples and reagents volumes, portability, precise reaction control, parallelization, high surface to volume ratio and spatio-temporal resolution [138]. MIPs with many advantages can be employed in the design of microfluidic systems for POC applications. Integration of MIPs with microfluidic devices allows an increase in sensitivity and selectivity. MIP-based microfluidic devices have been used for electrochemical detection of biomarkers [139,140], amino acids [141,142], hormones [143] and drugs [144,145].

Multiplexed detection is performed by three approaches: spatial separation of detection sites, regional separation or the use of different labels and biorecognition elements [146]. Microfluidic devices are suitable platforms for multiplexed detection because of the characteristic properties and design [147–149]. Microfluidics can have separate individual chambers for each analyte; thus, each analyte can only interact with its biorecognition element, reducing the possible cross-reactivity [150]. While complex and long processes are required for the detection of a single component and are more complicated for multiplexed detection, with microfluidic devices, the sample preparation, incubation and detection can be automated, significantly reducing complications and requiring less time [137].

Considering the benefits of microfluidics in terms of multiplexed detection, the integration of MIPs with microfluidics can lead to significant developments in the field of multiplexed detection by MIPs. Integrating MT-MIPs with microfluidic systems offers great potential for real-time analysis of target molecules in complex samples. To achieve this integration, the microfluidic device must be designed to accommodate MT-MIPs, often incorporating channels that allow for the continuous flow of sample solutions through a series of reaction zones. The MT-MIPs are typically loaded into the microfluidic channels by adsorbing them onto microbeads or directly onto the surfaces of the channels. Magnetic nanoparticles are often integrated for easy manipulation and to help remove excess template or interfere with non-specific binding [151,152]. Potential challenges for the integration of MT-MIPs within the microfluidic system are linked to the matrix interference, integration complexity and clogging of channels. To minimize the matrix effects, sample pre-treatments such as filtration and dilution can help remove large substances. Utilizing advances in droplet-based microfluidics can make it easier to control the particle size and distribution to control the integration complexity. Using hydrophilic materials can reduce the particle adhesion and optimizing the flow rate can prevent particle accumulation [152]; both methods can reduce the possibility of clogging.

The integration of MT-MIPs with microfluidic systems is also of great importance for the commercialization of MIPs. Several commercial MIP products are produced by companies such as MIP diagnostics (NanoMIPs), Sigma Aldrich (SupelMIP), Aspira Biosystems, Semorex, Affinisep and Biotage. Early commercialization of MIP products started for purification and separation applications. Biotage, Sigma Aldrich and Affinisep offer solid-phase extraction (SPE) cartridges for a broad range of applications, including healthcare, food safety and environmental analysis. Semorex and Aspira Biosystems synthesize MIPs on a large scale for detection purposes. Semorex produces MIPs for protein detection that can be further used for therapeutics for cancer [153]. MIPs synthesized by epitope imprinting are sold by Aspira Biosystems for microorganisms' detection [154]. Sixth Wave, an MIP-based nanotechnology company, has offered many successful MIP products for the extraction of cannabinoids, which are in the process of commercializing now, and for the detection of COVID-19 [155]. Sixth Wave has also produced MIPs for metal extraction and purification for mining applications.

However, there are bottlenecks in the commercialization of MIPs, with the main one being the production of high-affinity MIPs with a homogeneous size and shape on a large scale [153]. Failure to ensure homogeneity in terms of the size, shape and affinity reduces the reproducibility of MIPs, which has an undesirable effect on the commercialization of MIPs, but recent improvements in polymer science, methodology and imprinting technology [156–158] has paved the way to ameliorate bottlenecks in the way of commercialization of MT-MIPs. MT-MIPs often require expensive raw materials and complex synthesis methods, which can increase the production costs. To address this, researchers are exploring the use of cheaper monomers and solvents, optimizing the synthesis process to reduce waste, and improving the scalability of production. Additionally, integrating more cost-effective production techniques, such as microfluidic systems, can reduce costs by enabling precise and efficient polymerization processes and improve the stability and reliability for sensor applications. Ensuring the stability of MT-MIPs in various environmental conditions is crucial for their practical application, particularly in sensor technologies. One challenge is the potential degradation of the polymer under harsh conditions (e.g., high temperature or exposure to solvents). To improve the stability, researchers are focusing on enhancing the chemical robustness of the polymers through the selection of appropriate cross-linkers and functional monomers. Additionally, the development of composite materials, such as incorporating MT-MIPs with nanoparticles, can enhance both the mechanical strength and the stability of the sensor. In complex matrices, such as biological or environmental samples, the selectivity and sensitivity of MT-MIP sensors can be compromised due to interference from non-target substances. To mitigate this, the design of MT-MIPs with highly specific binding sites tailored for multiple targets is essential. Optimizing the polymerization process to ensure the formation of high-fidelity binding sites can help improve both selectivity and sensitivity. Moreover, integrating MT-MIPs with microfluidic platforms allows for better control over the interaction between the sensor and the sample, further enhancing the performance [10,25]. Furthermore, practically all the MIP products are currently singleplex MIPs; the production of commercially viable MT-MIPs still has a way to go.

4. Future Perspectives

Molecularly imprinted polymers utilized as artificial receptors have many advantages over natural receptors, making MIPs good recognition elements for sensing applications. The MIP production process is straightforward, and by taking the properties of the targets into consideration, MIPs can be employed for multiplexed detection, which allows the detection of more than one target simultaneously, with many benefits, including saving time and reagents. Electrochemical methods have been preferred to be used in the detection of multiple targets by MT-MIPs because of their significant properties, such as the high sensitivity, simplicity, and fast response. A broad range of targets from amino acids to viruses can be detected by MT-MIP-based electrochemical sensors with high sensitivity and selectivity.

MIPs are preferred over natural receptors because of their high environmental durability, low cost, long shelf life and significant robustness. Despite these advantages, MIPs have some drawbacks, such as the low binding efficiency, challenges in template removal, difficulty in imprinting large molecules, leakage of template, slow rebinding kinetics, cross-selectivity, and sometimes reduced sensitivity [159,160]. All these drawbacks can potentially be addressed by employing appropriate strategies. For example, to overcome the challenges associated with template removal and the imprinting of large molecules, both epitope imprinting [13] and surface imprinting [161] can be utilized. The low binding efficiency can be improved by using MIP nanoparticles, more flexible monomers, and nanomaterials. MIP nanoparticles can enhance the target accessibility, while more flexible polymers can adapt to slight conformational changes.

The recognition efficiency of MIPs can be further enhanced by employing surface imprinting, nanoparticles, microfluidic systems, and hybrid recognition strategies that incorporate highly specific aptamers with MIPs. Aptamers are nucleic acid sequences (single-stranded DNA or RNA) that can be recognized and bound to their target molecule. Aptamers offer great benefits, including being chemically stable, easily modified chemically and easily synthesized, which can increase the sensitivity and selectivity. Because of the unique properties of both aptamers and MIPs, they have been used as a hybrid recognition element for the detection of many substances [162–165]. MIPs are more stable against pH, temperature changes and organic solvents than aptamers and aptamers are more selective than MIPs. By combining MIPs and aptamers, the selectivity and sensitivity can be enhanced, and increased stability and high binding affinity can be obtained [159].

Template leakage is another common limitation of MIPs. To eliminate or alleviate this issue, dummy templates, structural analogues of the target molecules, can be used [166]. After polymerization, UV or plasma treatments can be applied to degrade residual templates. Buried binding sites within the polymer may slow the diffusion of target molecules. This limitation can be overcome by using surface imprinting and nanomaterials to create accessible binding sites, thereby increasing the surface area and enhancing the binding rates. Additionally, utilizing highly selective functional monomers that interact only with unique functional groups of the template, along with hybrid MIPs, can help reduce the effect of cross-reactivity.

In MT-MIPs, the analyte may sometimes contain multiple recognizable substances simultaneously. For example, if two templates have the same oxidation potentials, it can make the specific recognition of the templates challenging. In such cases, a "surface grafting" approach can be used to distinguish and detect specific targets [82]. For non-electroactive templates, introducing electroactive labels specific to each analyte can be another strategy for distinguishing multiple recognizable substances. Each label can produce a distinct, recognizable electrochemical signal.

So far, many MIPs and MT-MIPs have been produced for sensing applications targeting various analytes, including both electroactive and non-electroactive targets. Electroactive targets, such as inorganic ions, certain pharmaceuticals (including paracetamol and epinephrine), and environmental pollutants (such as phenol), have been detected using MIPs and MT-MIPs [167–169]. Non-electroactive targets, including proteins such as prostate-specific antigen (PSA), lipids, and bacteria, have also been detected by MIPs and MT-MIPs. For example, Tamboli et al. constructed a MOSFET device to detect PSA in human plasma by using a hybrid synthetic receptor consisting of an MIP and a PSA-specific aptamer [170]. In this study, the aptamer-coupled MIP was immobilized on a gold electrode, and the response generated as a result of binding was converted into an electrical signal by a field-effect transistor. The sensor performance was analyzed by exposing the sensor to different PSA concentrations and measuring the resulting voltage changes corresponding to those concentrations. In another study, Agar et al. developed an electrochemical sensor utilizing aptamers and MIPs as recognition elements for the multiplexed detection of *Escherichia coli* (*E. coli*) and *Staphylococcus aureus* (*S. aureus*) [171]. After preparing two different sensors—one for *E. coli* and the other for *S. aureus*—both sensors were transferred onto the same electrode array to conduct multiplexed detection of both bacteria. Non-Faradaic electrochemical impedance spectroscopy (EIS) measurements were employed to evaluate the sensor response.

The application of MT-MIPS and MIPs on complex matrices faces several challenges, such as matrix interference, cross-reactivity and limited accessibility. In terms of the matrix interference effect, non-target components in the sample matrix can occupy recognition sites or interfere with detection signals, reducing the specificity and sensitivity. Co-existing molecules structurally similar to templates may bind to the recognition sites and cause cross-reactivity. The complex nature of real samples can hinder target molecules from accessing recognition sites effectively, inducing limited accessibility. To overcome these challenges, several methods can be introduced. Designing MT-MIPS or MIPs with surface binding sites can improve the accessibility for target molecules and reduce non-specific binding. Sample pre-treatments such as filtration [172], centrifugation [173] or dilution can eliminate unwanted matrix components. Using hybrid materials such as magnetic nanoparticles or graphene oxide can enhance separation from complex samples and reduce interference. In the study conducted by Nurrokhimah et al., $Fe_3O_4@SiO_2$-based magnetic multi-template molecularly imprinted polymers (MT-MIPs) were developed for simultaneous detection of antibiotics (cephalexin, cefazolin, and cefoperazone) in milk [23]. The synthesis involved a composite material to improve the extraction efficiency and reduce the matrix interference. Pre-treatment processes, like centrifugation and filtration, were used to reduce milk's complex matrix interference, while washing steps optimized the removal of non-specific binding.

Considering the advantages provided by the design of microfluidic systems, their integration with MT-MIP-based electrochemical sensors for multiplexed detection is encouraging. Many companies that previously produced MIPs for purification and separation applications can produce MIPs that can be used for multiplexed detection by eliminating some of the problems that prevent MIPs from being produced on a large scale, and thus MT-MIPs may become available as POC diagnostic tools in the near future.

MIPs are very promising artificial receptors that can replace natural recognition elements. MT-MIP sensors provide the ability to measure different analytes on the same sample. The MIPs' capability of detecting a broad range of targets, incorporation with other recognition elements, integration of microfluidics and easy preparation process allow them to be used for multiplexed detection of different targets.

Author Contributions: Conceptualization, M.A.; investigation, M.A.; writing—original draft preparation, M.A.; writing—review and editing, M.L., H.S.L. and P.E.; supervision, M.L., H.S.L. and P.E. All authors have read and agreed to the published version of the manuscript.

Funding: M.A. was funded by the Ministry of National Education of Türkiye through their YLSY International Graduate Education Scholarship program.

Institutional Review Board Statement: Not applicable

Informed Consent Statement: Not applicable

Data Availability Statement: Not applicable

Conflicts of Interest: The authors declare no conflicts of interest.

References

1. Aydin, E.B.; Aydin, M.; Sezginturk, M.K. Biosensors in Drug Discovery and Drug Analysis. *Curr. Anal. Chem.* **2019**, *15*, 467–484. [CrossRef]
2. Abu, H.; Hossain, M.A.M.; Marlinda, A.; Al Mamun, M.; Simarani, K.; Johan, M.R. Nanomaterials Based Electrochemical Nucleic Acid Biosensors for Environmental Monitoring: A Review. *Appl. Surf. Sci. Adv.* **2021**, *4*, 100064. [CrossRef]
3. Chaudhry, G.E.S.; Akim, A.M.; Safdar, N.; Yasmin, A.; Begum, S.; Sung, Y.Y.; Sifzizul, T.; Muhammad, T. Cancer and Disease Diagnosis-Biosensor as Potential Diagnostic Tool for Biomarker Detection. *J. Adv. Pharm. Technol. Res.* **2022**, *13*, 243–247. [CrossRef] [PubMed]
4. Mi, F.; Hu, C.M.; Wang, Y.; Wang, L.; Peng, F.; Geng, P.F.; Guan, M. Recent Advancements in Microfluidic Chip Biosensor Detection of Foodborne Pathogenic Bacteria: A Review. *Anal. Bioanal. Chem.* **2022**, *414*, 2883–2902. [CrossRef] [PubMed]
5. Chen, Z.L.; Xie, M.J.; Zhao, F.G.; Han, S.Y. Application of Nanomaterial Modified Aptamer-Based Electrochemical Sensor in Detection of Heavy Metal Ions. *Foods* **2022**, *11*, 1404. [CrossRef] [PubMed]

6. Naresh, V.; Lee, N. A Review on Biosensors and Recent Development of Nanostructured Materials-Enabled Biosensors. *Sensors* **2021**, *21*, 1109. [CrossRef]
7. Sajini, T.; Mathew, B. A Brief Overview of Molecularly Imprinted Polymers: Highlighting Computational Design, Nano and Photo-Responsive Imprinting. *Talanta Open* **2021**, *4*, 20. [CrossRef]
8. Refaat, D.; Aggour, M.; Farghali, A.; Mahajan, R.; Wiklander, J.; Nicholls, I.; Piletsky, S. Strategies for Molecular Imprinting and the Evolution of MIP Nanoparticles as Plastic Antibodies-Synthesis and Applications. *Int. J. Mol. Sci.* **2019**, *20*, 6304. [CrossRef] [PubMed]
9. Wackerlig, J.; Lieberzeit, P.A. Molecularly Imprinted Polymer Nanoparticles in Chemical Sensing—Synthesis, Characterisation and Application. *Sens. Actuators B-Chem.* **2015**, *207*, 144–157. [CrossRef]
10. Hasanah, A.N.; Safitri, N.; Zulfa, A.; Neli, N.; Rahayu, D. Factors Affecting Preparation of Molecularly Imprinted Polymer and Methods on Finding Template-Monomer Interaction as the Key of Selective Properties of the Materials. *Molecules* **2021**, *26*, 5612. [CrossRef] [PubMed]
11. Chen, L.X.; Wang, X.Y.; Lu, W.H.; Wu, X.Q.; Li, J.H. Molecular Imprinting: Perspectives and Applications. *Chem. Soc. Rev.* **2016**, *45*, 2137–2211. [CrossRef]
12. Kodakat, K.; Kumar, K.G. Fabrication of a Selective and Sensitive Electro-synthesized Molecularly Imprinted Polymer-based Electrochemical Sensor for the Determination of Xanthine. *J. Appl. Electrochem.* **2023**, *53*, 2259–2272. [CrossRef]
13. Gupta, N.; Shah, K.; Singh, M. An Epitope-Imprinted Piezoelectric Diagnostic Tool for *Neisseria meningitidis* detection. *J. Mol. Recognit.* **2016**, *29*, 572–579. [CrossRef] [PubMed]
14. Wang, Y.L.; Gao, Y.L.; Wang, P.P.; Shang, H.; Pan, S.Y.; Li, X.J. Sol-gel Molecularly Imprinted Polymer for Selective Solid Phase Microextraction of Organophosphorous Pesticides. *Talanta* **2013**, *115*, 920–927. [CrossRef] [PubMed]
15. Lah, N.F.C.; Ahmad, A.L.; Low, S.C.; Zaulkiflee, N.D. Isotherm and Electrochemical Properties of Atrazine Sensing Using PVC/MIP: Effect of Porogenic Solvent Concentration Ratio. *Membranes* **2021**, *11*, 657. [CrossRef]
16. Wang, S.; Zhang, L.; Zeng, J.; Hu, X.; Wang, X.; Yu, L.; Wang, D.; Cheng, L.; Ahmed, R.; Romanovski, V.; et al. Multi-templates Molecularly Imprinted Polymers for Simultaneous Recognition of Multiple Targets: From Academy to Application. *Trac-Trends Anal. Chem.* **2023**, *166*, 117173. [CrossRef]
17. Nishimura, K.; Okamura, N.; Kimachi, T.; Haginaka, J. Evaluation of Molecularly Imprinted Polymers for Chlorpromazine and Bromopromazine Prepared by Multi-step Swelling and Polymerization Method-The Application for the Determination of Chlorpromazine and Its Metabolites in Rat Plasma by Column-switching LC. *J. Pharm. Biomed. Anal.* **2019**, *174*, 248–255. [CrossRef]
18. Sun, C.; Wang, J.; Huang, J.; Yao, D.; Wang, C.; Zhang, L.; Hou, S.; Chen, L.; Yuan, C. The Multi-Template Molecularly Imprinted Polymer Based on SBA-15 for Selective Separation and Determination of *Panax notoginseng* Saponins Simultaneously in Biological Samples. *Polymers* **2017**, *9*, 653. [CrossRef]
19. Ji, W.; Xie, H.; Zhou, J.; Wang, X.; Ma, X.; Huang, L. Water-compatible Molecularly Imprinted Polymers for Selective Solid Phase Extraction of Dencichine from the Aqueous Extract of *Panax notoginseng*. *J. Chromatogr. B-Anal. Technol. Biomed. Life Sci.* **2016**, *1008*, 225–233. [CrossRef] [PubMed]
20. Nkosi, S.; Mahlambi, P.; Chimuka, L. Synthesis, Characterisation and Optimisation of Bulk Molecularly Imprinted Polymers from Nonsteroidal Anti-inflammatory Drugs. *S. Afr. J. Chem.-Suid-Afr. Tydskr. Vir Chem.* **2022**, *76*, 56–64. [CrossRef]
21. Miura, C.; Funaya, N.; Matsunaga, H.; Haginaka, J. Monodisperse, Molecularly Imprinted Polymers for Creatinine by Modified Precipitation Polymerization and Their Applications to Creatinine Assays for Human Serum and Urine. *J. Pharm. Biomed. Anal.* **2013**, *85*, 288–294. [CrossRef]
22. Wu, X.; Shimizu, K. Development of Molecularly Imprinted Polymers as Tailored Templates for the Solid-state [2+2] photodimerization. *Biosens. Bioelectron.* **2009**, *25*, 640–646. [CrossRef]
23. Nurrokhimah, M.; Nurerk, P.; Kanatharana, P.; Bunkoed, O. A Nanosorbent Consisting of a Magnetic Molecularly Imprinted Polymer and Graphene Oxide for Multi-residue Analysis of Cephalosporins. *Microchim. Acta* **2019**, *186*, 822. [CrossRef] [PubMed]
24. Pratama, K.F.; Manik, M.E.R.; Rahayu, D.; Hasanah, A.N. Effect of the Molecularly Imprinted Polymer Component Ratio on Analytical Performance. *Chem. Pharm. Bull.* **2020**, *68*, 1013–1024. [CrossRef] [PubMed]
25. Murdaya, N.; Triadenda, A.L.; Rahayu, D.; Hasanah, A.N. A Review: Using Multiple Templates for Molecular Imprinted Polymer: Is It Good? *Polymers* **2022**, *14*, 4441. [CrossRef] [PubMed]
26. Xu, R.; Tian, J.; Guan, Y.; Zhang, Y. Peptide-Cross-Linked Protein-Imprinted Polymers: Easy Template Removal and Excellent Imprinting Effect. *CCS Chem.* **2019**, *1*, 544–552. [CrossRef]
27. Ge, Y.; Turner, A. Too Large to Fit? Recent Developments in Macromolecular Imprinting. *Trends Biotechnol.* **2008**, *26*, 218–224. [CrossRef]
28. Fatma, S.; Prasad, B.B.; Singh, K.; Singh, R.; Jaiswal, S. A Reduced Graphene Oxide Ceramic Electrode Modified with One MoNomer Doubly Imprinted Acryloylated Tetraamine Cobalt Phthalocyanine Polymer for the Simultaneous Analysis of Anticancerous Drugs. *Sens. Actuators. B Chem.* **2019**, *281*, 139–149. [CrossRef]

29. Bali Prasad, B.; Jauhari, D.; Prasad Tiwari, M. A Dual-template Imprinted Polymer-modified Carbon Ceramic Electrode for Ultra Trace Simultaneous Analysis of Ascorbic Acid and Dopamine. *Biosens. Bioelectron.* **2013**, *50*, 19–27. [CrossRef]
30. Prasad, B.B.; Jauhari, D.; Tiwari, M.P. Doubly Imprinted Polymer Nanofilm-modified Electrochemical Sensor for Ultra-trace Simultaneous Analysis of Glyphosate and Glufosinate. *Biosens. Bioelectron.* **2014**, *59*, 81–88. [CrossRef] [PubMed]
31. Prasad, B.; Pathak, P. Development of Surface Imprinted Nanospheres Using the Inverse Suspension Polymerization Method for Electrochemical Ultra Sensing of Dacarbazine. *Anal. Chim. Acta* **2017**, *974*, 75–86. [CrossRef]
32. Tang, K.L.; Chen, Y.; Wang, X.N.; Zhou, Q.; Lei, H.B.; Yang, Z.X.; Zhang, Z.H. Smartphone-integrated Tri-color Fluorescence Sensing Platform Based on Acid-sensitive Fluorescence Imprinted Polymers for Dual-mode Visual Intelligent Detection of Ibuprofen, Chloramphenicol and Florfenicol. *Anal. Chim. Acta* **2023**, *1260*, 341174. [CrossRef] [PubMed]
33. Zhu, L.; Mei, X.C.; Peng, Z.C.; Yang, J.; Li, Y.C. A Paper-based Microfluidic Sensor Array Combining Molecular Imprinting Technology and Carbon Quantum Dots for the Discrimination of Nitrophenol Isomers. *J. Hazard. Mater.* **2022**, *435*, 129012. [CrossRef]
34. Wang, L.Y.; Li, B.W.; Wang, J.A.; Qi, J.; Li, J.H.; Ma, J.P.; Chen, L.X. A Rotary Multi-positioned Cloth/Paper Hybrid Microfluidic Device for Simultaneous Fuorescence Sensing of Mercury and Lead Ions by Using Ion Imprinted Technologies. *J. Hazard. Mater.* **2022**, *428*, 128165. [CrossRef] [PubMed]
35. Feng, F.; Zheng, J.W.; Qin, P.; Han, T.; Zhao, D.Y. A Novel Quartz Crystal Microbalance Sensor Array Based on Molecular Imprinted Polymers for Simultaneous Detection of Clenbuterol and Its Metabolites. *Talanta* **2017**, *167*, 94–102. [CrossRef] [PubMed]
36. Liu, N.; Li, X.L.; Ma, X.H.; Ou, G.R.; Gao, Z.X. Rapid and Multiple Detections of Staphylococcal Enterotoxins by Two-dimensional Molecularly Imprinted Film-coated QCM Sensor. *Sens. Actuators B-Chem.* **2014**, *191*, 326–331. [CrossRef]
37. Cai, Y.; He, X.; Cui, P.L.; Liu, J.; Li, Z.B.; Jia, B.J.; Zhang, T.; Wang, J.P.; Yuan, W.Z. Preparation of a Chemiluminescence Sensor for Multi-detection of Benzimidazoles in Meat Based on Molecularly Imprinted Polymer. *Food Chem.* **2019**, *280*, 103–109. [CrossRef] [PubMed]
38. Zhang, T.; Liu, J.; Wang, J.P. Preparation of a Molecularly Imprinted Polymer Based Chemiluminescence Sensor for the Determination of Amantadine and Rimantadine in Meat. *Anal. Methods* **2018**, *10*, 5025–5031. [CrossRef]
39. Haginaka, J.; Tabo, H.; Matsunaga, H. Preparation of Molecularly Imprinted Polymers for Organophosphates and Their Application to the Recognition of Organophosphorus Compounds and Phosphopeptides. *Anal. Chim. Acta* **2012**, *748*, 1–8. [CrossRef]
40. Yan, M.M.; She, Y.X.; Cao, X.L.; Ma, J.; Chen, G.; Hong, S.H.; Shao, Y.; Abd El-Aty, A.M.; Wang, M.; Wang, J. A Molecularly Imprinted Polymer with Integrated Gold Nanoparticles for Surface Enhanced Raman Scattering Based Detection of the Triazine Herbicides, Prometryn and Simetryn. *Microchim. Acta* **2019**, *186*, 143. [CrossRef] [PubMed]
41. Lu, Z.; Li, Y.; Liu, T.; Wang, G.; Sun, M.; Jiang, Y.; He, H.; Wang, Y.; Zou, P.; Wang, X.; et al. A Dual-Template Imprinted Polymer Electrochemical Sensor Based on AuNPs and Nitrogen-doped Graphene Oxide Quantum Dots Coated on NiS_2/Biomass Carbon for Simultaneous Determination of Dopamine and Chlorpromazine. *Chem. Eng. J.* **2020**, *389*, 124417. [CrossRef]
42. Siavash Moakhar, R.; del Real Mata, C.; Jalali, M.; Shafique, H.; Sanati, A.; Vries, J.; Strauss, J.; AbdElFatah, T.; Ghasemi, F.; McLean, M.; et al. A Versatile Biomimic Nanotemplating Fluidic Assay for Multiplex Quantitative Monitoring of Viral Respiratory Infections and Immune Responses in Saliva and Blood. *Adv. Sci.* **2022**, *9*, 2204246. [CrossRef] [PubMed]
43. Wang, L.; Zhang, W. Molecularly Imprinted Polymer (MIP) Based Electrochemical Sensors and Their Recent Advances in Health Applications. *Sens. Actuators Rep.* **2023**, *5*, 100153. [CrossRef]
44. Ostojic, J.; Herenda, S.; Besic, Z.; Milos, M.; Galic, B. Advantages of an Electrochemical Method Compared to the Spectrophotometric Kinetic Study of Peroxidase Inhibition by Boroxine Derivative. *Molecules* **2017**, *22*, 1120. [CrossRef] [PubMed]
45. Kusumkar, V.V.; Galambos, M.; Viglasova, E.; Dano, M.; Smelkova, J. Ion-Imprinted Polymers: Synthesis, Characterization, and Adsorption of Radionuclides. *Materials* **2021**, *14*, 1083. [CrossRef] [PubMed]
46. Fu, J.Q.; Chen, L.X.; Li, J.H.; Zhang, Z. Current Status and Challenges of Ion Imprinting. *J. Mater. Chem. A* **2015**, *3*, 13598–13627. [CrossRef]
47. Bali Prasad, B.; Jauhari, D.; Verma, A. A Dual-Ion Imprinted Polymer Embedded in Sol–Gel Matrix for the Ultra Trace Simultaneous Analysis of Cadmium and Copper. *Talanta* **2014**, *120*, 398–407. [CrossRef] [PubMed]
48. Behbahani, M.; Barati, M.; Bojdi, M.K.; Pourali, A.R.; Bagheri, A.; Tapeh, N.A.G. A Nanosized Cadmium(II)-Imprinted Polymer for Use in Selective Trace Determination of Cadmium in Complex Matrices. *Microchim. Acta* **2013**, *180*, 1117–1125. [CrossRef]
49. Shamsipur, M.; Fasihi, J.; Khanchi, A.; Hassani, R.; Alizadeh, K.; Shamsipur, H. A Stoichiometric Imprinted Chelating Resin for Selective Recognition of Copper(II) Ions in Aqueous Media. *Anal. Chim. Acta* **2007**, *599*, 294–301. [CrossRef] [PubMed]
50. Birlik, E.; Ersöz, A.; Denizli, A.; Say, R. Preconcentration of Copper Using Double-Imprinted Polymer via Solid Phase Extraction. *Anal. Chim. Acta* **2006**, *565*, 145–151. [CrossRef]
51. Prasad, B.B.; Jauhari, D. Double-ion Imprinted Polymer @Magnetic Nanoparticles Modified Screen Printed Carbon Electrode for Simultaneous Analysis of Cerium and Gadolinium Ions. *Anal. Chim. Acta* **2015**, *875*, 83–91. [CrossRef] [PubMed]

52. Karim, M.M.; Lee, S.H.; Kim, Y.S.; Bae, H.S.; Hong, S.B. Fluorimetric Determination of Cerium(IV) with Ascorbic Acid. *J. Fluoresc.* **2006**, *16*, 17–22. [CrossRef] [PubMed]
53. Focarelli, F.; Giachino, A.; Waldron, K.J. Copper Microenvironments in the Human Body Define Patterns of Copper Adaptation in Pathogenic Bacteria. *PLoS Pathog.* **2022**, *18*, e1010617. [CrossRef] [PubMed]
54. Chasapis, C.T.; Loutsidou, A.C.; Spiliopoulou, C.A.; Stefanidou, M.E. Zinc and Human Health: An Update. *Arch. Toxicol.* **2012**, *86*, 521–534. [CrossRef] [PubMed]
55. Wilschefski, S.C.; Baxter, M.R. Inductively Coupled Plasma Mass Spectrometry: Introduction to Analytical Aspects. *Clin. Biochem. Rev.* **2019**, *40*, 115–133. [CrossRef]
56. Kumar, D.; Madhuri, R.; Prasad Tiwari, M.; Sinha, P.; Bali Prasad, B. Molecularly Imprinted Polymer-Modified Electrochemical Sensor for Simultaneous Determination of Copper and Zinc. *Adv. Mater. Lett.* **2011**, *2*, 294–297. [CrossRef]
57. Lv, Y.Q.; Tan, T.W.; Svec, F. Molecular Imprinting of Proteins in Polymers Attached to The Surface of Nanomaterials for Selective Recognition of Biomacromolecules. *Biotechnol. Adv.* **2013**, *31*, 1172–1186. [CrossRef] [PubMed]
58. Dinc, M.; Esen, C.; Mizaikoff, B. Recent Advances on Core-Shell Magnetic Molecularly Imprinted Polymers for Biomacromolecules. *Trac-Trends Anal. Chem.* **2019**, *114*, 202–217. [CrossRef]
59. Mazzotta, E.; Di Giulio, T.; Malitesta, C. Electrochemical Sensing of Macromolecules Based on Molecularly Imprinted Polymers: Challenges, Successful Strategies, and Opportunities. *Anal. Bioanal. Chem.* **2022**, *414*, 5165–5200. [CrossRef]
60. El-Schich, Z.; Zhang, Y.; Feith, M.; Beyer, S.; Sternbæk, L.; Ohlsson, L.; Stollenwerk, M.; Wingren, A.G. Molecularly Imprinted Polymers in Biological Applications. *Biotechniques* **2020**, *69*, 406–419. [CrossRef] [PubMed]
61. Song, Q.M.; Wang, B.W.; Lv, Y.Q. Molecularly imprinted monoliths: Recent Advances in the Selective Recognition of Biomacromolecules Related Biomarkers. *J. Sep. Sci.* **2022**, *45*, 1469–1481. [CrossRef]
62. Nontawong, N.; Ngaosri, P.; Chunta, S.; Jarujamrus, P.; Nacapricha, D.; Lieberzeit, P.A.; Amatatongchai, M. Smart Sensor for Assessment of Oxidative/Nitrative Stress Biomarkers Using A Dual-Imprinted Electrochemical Paper-Based Analytical Device. *Anal. Chim. Acta* **2022**, *1191*, 339363. [CrossRef] [PubMed]
63. Martins, G.V.; Tavares, A.P.M.; Fortunato, E.; Sales, M.G.F. Paper-Based Sensing Device for Electrochemical Detection of Oxidative Stress Biomarker 8-Hydroxy-2′-deoxyguanosine (8-OHdG) in Point-of-Care. *Sci. Rep.* **2017**, *7*, 14558. [CrossRef]
64. Wang, S.Q.; Sun, G.H.; Chen, Z.G.; Liang, Y.W.; Zhou, Q.; Pan, Y.F.; Zhai, H.Y. Constructing a Novel Composite of Molecularly Imprinted Polymer-Coated AuNPs Electrochemical Sensor for the Determination of 3-Nitrotyrosine. *Electrochim. Acta* **2018**, *259*, 893–902. [CrossRef]
65. Jia, L.P.; Wang, H.S. Electrochemical Reduction Synthesis of Graphene/Nafion Nanocomposite Film and Its Performance on the Detection of 8-Hydroxy-2′-Deoxyguanosine in the Presence of Uric Acid. *J. Electroanal. Chem.* **2013**, *705*, 37–43. [CrossRef]
66. Luo, K.; Zhao, C.; Luo, Y.; Pan, C.; Li, J. Electrochemical Sensor for the Simultaneous Detection of CA72-4 And CA19-9 Tumor Markers Using Dual Recognition via Glycosyl Imprinting and Lectin-Specific Binding for Accurate Diagnosis of Gastric Cancer. *Biosens. Bioelectron.* **2022**, *216*, 114672. [CrossRef] [PubMed]
67. Hong, G.L.; Chen, R.T.; Xu, L.Y.; Lu, X.; Yang, Z.Q.; Zhou, G.B.; Li, L.; Chen, W.; Peng, H.P. One-pot Ultrasonic Synthesis of Multifunctional Au Nanoparticle-Ferrocene-WS_2 Nanosheet Composite for the Construction of an Electrochemical Biosensing Platform. *Anal. Chim. Acta* **2020**, *1099*, 52–59. [CrossRef] [PubMed]
68. Wang, R.; Feng, J.J.; Liu, W.D.; Jiang, L.Y.; Wang, A.J. A Novel Label-Free Electrochemical Immunosensor Based on the Enhanced Catalytic Currents of Oxygen Reduction by AuAg Hollow Nanocrystals for Detecting Carbohydrate Antigen 199. *Biosens. Bioelectron.* **2017**, *96*, 152–158. [CrossRef]
69. Wang, D.; Gan, N.; Zhang, H.; Li, T.; Qiao, L.; Cao, Y.; Su, X.; Jiang, S. Simultaneous Electrochemical Immunoassay Using Graphene–Au Grafted Recombinant Apoferritin-Encoded Metallic Labels As Signal Tags and Dual-Template Magnetic Molecular Imprinted Polymer As Capture Probes. *Biosens. Bioelectron.* **2015**, *65*, 78–82. [CrossRef] [PubMed]
70. Kong, F.Y.; Xu, B.Y.; Xu, J.J.; Chen, H.Y. Simultaneous Electrochemical Immunoassay Using Cds/DNA and Pbs/DNA Nanochains As Labels. *Biosens. Bioelectron.* **2013**, *39*, 177–182. [CrossRef] [PubMed]
71. Taheri, N.; Khoshsafar, H.; Ghanei, M.; Ghazvini, A.; Bagheri, H. Dual-template Rectangular Nanotube Molecularly Imprinted Polypyrrole for Label-Free Impedimetric Sensing of AFP and CEA As Lung Cancer Biomarkers. *Talanta* **2022**, *239*, 123146. [CrossRef]
72. Zhao, X.Q.; Wang, J.; Chen, H.; Xu, H.; Bai, L.J.; Wang, W.X.; Yang, H.W.; Wei, D.L.; Yuan, B.Q. A Multiple Signal Amplification Based on PEI and rGO Nanocomposite for Simultaneous Multiple Electrochemical Immunoassay. *Sens. Actuators B-Chem.* **2019**, *301*, 127071. [CrossRef]
73. Li, L.H.; Wei, Y.; Zhang, S.P.; Chen, X.S.; Shao, T.L.; Feng, D.X. Electrochemical Immunosensor Based on Metal Ions Functionalized CNSs@Au NPs Nanocomposites As Signal Amplifier for Simultaneous Detection of Triple Tumor Markers. *J. Electroanal. Chem.* **2021**, *880*, 114882. [CrossRef]

74. Karami, P.; Bagheri, H.; Johari-Ahar, M.; Khoshsafar, H.; Arduini, F.; Afkhami, A. Dual-modality Impedimetric Immunosensor for Early Detection of Prostate-Specific Antigen and Myoglobin Markers Based on Antibody-Molecularly Imprinted Polymer. *Talanta* **2019**, *202*, 111–122. [CrossRef]
75. Merriel, S.W.D.; Pocock, L.; Gilbert, E.; Creavin, S.; Walter, F.M.; Spencer, A.; Hamilton, W. Systematic Review and Meta-Analysis of the Diagnostic Accuracy of Prostate-Specific Antigen (PSA) for the Detection of Prostate Cancer in Symptomatic Patients. *BMC Med.* **2022**, *20*, 54. [CrossRef] [PubMed]
76. Johari-Ahar, M.; Karami, P.; Ghanei, M.; Afkhami, A.; Bagheri, H. Development of a Molecularly Imprinted Polymer Tailored on Disposable Screen-Printed Electrodes for Dual Detection of EGFR and VEGF Using Nano-Liposomal Amplification Strategy. *Biosens. Bioelectron.* **2018**, *107*, 26–33. [CrossRef]
77. Li, R.B.; Huang, H.M.; Huang, L.Z.; Lin, Z.Y.; Guo, L.H.; Qiu, B.; Chen, G.N. Electrochemical Biosensor for Epidermal Growth Factor Receptor Detection with Peptide Ligand. *Electrochim. Acta* **2013**, *109*, 233–237. [CrossRef]
78. Omidfar, K.; Darzianiazizi, M.; Ahmadi, A.; Daneshpour, M.; Shirazi, H. A High Sensitive Electrochemical Nanoimmunosensor Based on Fe_3O_4/TMC/Au Nanocomposite and PT-Modified Electrode for the Detection of Cancer Biomarker Epidermal Growth Factor Receptor. *Sens. Actuators B-Chem.* **2015**, *220*, 1311–1319. [CrossRef]
79. Nonaka, Y.; Abe, K.; Ikebukuro, K. Electrochemical Detection of Vascular Endothelial Growth Factor with Aptamer Sandwich. *Electrochemistry* **2012**, *80*, 363–366. [CrossRef]
80. Pandey, I.; Tiwari, J.D. A Novel Dual Imprinted Conducting Nanocubes Based Flexible Sensor for Simultaneous Detection of Hemoglobin and Glycated Haemoglobin in Gestational Diabetes Mellitus Patients. *Sens. Actuators. B Chem.* **2019**, *285*, 470–478. [CrossRef]
81. Liu, Z.; Yin, Z.-Z.; Zheng, G.; Zhang, H.; Zhou, M.; Li, S.; Kong, Y. Dual-template Molecularly Imprinted Electrochemical Biosensor for IgG-IgM Combined Assay Based on a Dual-Signal Strategy. *Bioelectrochemistry* **2022**, *148*, 108267. [CrossRef] [PubMed]
82. Prasad, B.B.; Jaiswal, S.; Singh, K. Ultra-trace Analysis of D-And L-Aspartic Acid Applying One-By-One Approach on a Dual Imprinted Electrochemical Sensor. *Sens. Actuators. B Chem.* **2017**, *240*, 631–639. [CrossRef]
83. Hou, H.; Tang, S.; Wang, W.; Liu, M.; Liang, A.; Sun, L.; Luo, A. Electrochemical Enantioanalysis of D-and L-Cysteine with a Dual-Template Molecularly Imprinted Sensor. *J. Electrochem. Soc.* **2022**, *169*, 037506. [CrossRef]
84. Zaidi, S.A. Facile and Efficient Electrochemical Enantiomer Recognition of Phenylalanine Using Β-Cyclodextrin Immobilized on Reduced Graphene Oxide. *Biosens. Bioelectron.* **2017**, *94*, 714–718. [CrossRef]
85. Yang, X.; Niu, X.H.; Mo, Z.L.; Wang, J.; Shuai, C.; Pan, Z.; Liu, Z.Y.; Liu, N.J.; Guo, R.B. 3D Nitrogen and Sulfur Co -Doped Graphene/Integrated Polysaccharides for Electrochemical Recognition Tryptophan Enantiomers. *J. Electrochem. Soc.* **2019**, *166*, B1053–B1062. [CrossRef]
86. Afsharara, H.; Asadian, E.; Mosta, B.; Banan, K.; Bigdeli, S.A.; Hatamabadi, D.; Keshavarz, A.; Hussain, C.M.; Kecili, R.; Ghorbani-Bidkorpeh, F. Molecularly Imprinted Polymer-Modified Carbon Paste Electrodes (MIP-CPE): A Review on Sensitive Electrochemical Sensors for Pharmaceutical Determinations. *Trac-Trends Anal. Chem.* **2023**, *160*, 116949. [CrossRef]
87. Ramanavicius, S.; Samukaite-Bubniene, U.; Ratautaite, V.; Bechelany, M.; Ramanavicius, A. Electrochemical Molecularly Imprinted Polymer Based Sensors for Pharmaceutical and Biomedical Applications (Review). *J. Pharm. Biomed. Anal.* **2022**, *215*, 114739. [CrossRef]
88. Singh, R.; Singh, M. Design of Imprinting Matrix for Dual Template Sensing via Electropolymerized Polythiophene Films. *J. Mol. Recognit.* **2022**, *35*, e2962. [CrossRef]
89. Mulik, B.B.; Dhumal, S.T.; Sapner, V.S.; Rehman, N.; Dixit, P.P.; Sathe, B.R. Graphene Oxide-Based Electrochemical Activation of Ethionamide Towards Enhanced Biological Activity. *Rsc Adv.* **2019**, *9*, 35463–35472. [CrossRef] [PubMed]
90. Kushwaha, A.; Singh, S.; Gupta, N.; Singh, A.K.; Singh, M. Synthesis and Characterization of Antipyrine-Imprinted Polymers and Their Application for Sustained Release. *Polym. Bull.* **2018**, *75*, 5235–5252. [CrossRef]
91. Sun, Y.; He, J.; Waterhouse, G.I.N.; Xu, L.; Zhang, H.; Qiao, X.; Xu, Z. A Selective Molecularly Imprinted Electrochemical Sensor With GO@COF Signal Amplification for the Simultaneous Determination of Sulfadiazine and Acetaminophen. *Sens. Actuators. B Chem.* **2019**, *300*, 126993. [CrossRef]
92. Teleanu, R.I.; Niculescu, A.G.; Roza, E.; Vladâcenco, O.; Grumezescu, A.M.; Teleanu, D.M. Neurotransmitters-Key Factors in Neurological and Neurodegenerative Disorders of the Central Nervous System. *Int. J. Mol. Sci.* **2022**, *23*, 5954. [CrossRef] [PubMed]
93. Si, B.; Song, E. Recent Advances in the Detection of Neurotransmitters. *Chemosensors* **2018**, *6*, 1. [CrossRef]
94. Si, B.; Song, E. Molecularly Imprinted Polymers for the Selective Detection of Multi-Analyte Neurotransmitters. *Microelectron. Eng.* **2018**, *187–188*, 58–65. [CrossRef]
95. Liu, W.; Cui, F.; Li, H.; Wang, S.; Zhuo, B. Three-dimensional Hybrid Networks of Molecularly Imprinted Poly(9-Carbazoleacetic Acid) and MWCNTs for Simultaneous Voltammetric Determination of Dopamine and Epinephrine in Plasma Sample. *Sens. Actuators. B Chem.* **2020**, *323*, 128669. [CrossRef]

96. Fatma, S.; Prasad, B.B.; Jaiswal, S.; Singh, R.; Singh, K. Electrochemical Simultaneous Analysis of Dopamine and Epinephrine Using Double Imprinted One Monomer Acryloylated Graphene Oxide-Carbon Black Composite Polymer. *Biosens. Bioelectron.* **2019**, *135*, 36–44. [CrossRef] [PubMed]
97. Singh, R.; Singh, M. Highly Selective and Specific Monitoring of Pollutants Using Dual Template Imprinted MIP Sensor. *J. Electroanal. Chem.* **2022**, *926*, 116939. [CrossRef]
98. Thimoonnee, S.; Somnet, K.; Ngaosri, P.; Chairam, S.; Karuwan, C.; Kamsong, W.; Tuantranont, A.; Amatatongchai, M. Fast, Sensitive and Selective Simultaneous Determination of Paraquat and Glyphosate Herbicides in Water Samples Using a Compact Electrochemical Sensor. *Anal. Methods* **2022**, *14*, 820–833. [CrossRef] [PubMed]
99. Núñez, O.; Moyano, E.; Puignou, L.; Galceran, M.T. Sample Stacking with Matrix Removal for the Determination of Paraquat, Diquat and Difenzoquat in Water by Capillary Electrophoresis. *J. Chromatogr. A* **2001**, *912*, 353–361. [CrossRef] [PubMed]
100. Guo, J.J.; Zhang, Y.; Luo, Y.L.; Shen, F.; Sun, C.Y. Efficient Fluorescence Resonance Energy Transfer Between Oppositely Charged CdTe Quantum Dots and Gold Nanoparticles for Turn-on Fluorescence Detection of Glyphosate. *Talanta* **2014**, *125*, 385–392. [CrossRef]
101. Rao, H.; Liu, X.; Ding, F.; Wan, Y.; Zhao, X.; Liang, R.; Zou, P.; Wang, Y.; Wang, X.; Zhao, Q. Nitrogen-doped Carbon Nanosheet Frameworks Decorated with Fe and Molecularly Imprinted Polymer for Simultaneous Detection of Mebendazole and Catechol. *Chem. Eng. J.* **2018**, *338*, 478–487. [CrossRef]
102. Ahmed, J.; Ahamad, T.; AlShehri, S.M. Iron-Nickel Nanoparticles as Bifunctional Catalysts in Water Electrolysis. *Chemelectrochem* **2017**, *4*, 1222–1226. [CrossRef]
103. Yang, C.; Denno, M.E.; Pyakurel, P.; Venton, B.J. Recent Trends in Carbon Nanomaterial-Based Electrochemical Sensors for Biomolecules: A Review. *Anal. Chim. Acta* **2015**, *887*, 17–37. [CrossRef] [PubMed]
104. Golabi, M.; Kuralay, F.; Jager, E.W.H.; Beni, V.; Turner, A.P.F. Electrochemical Bacterial Detection Using Poly(3-Aminophenylboronic Acid)-Based Imprinted Polymer. *Biosens. Bioelectron.* **2017**, *93*, 87–93. [CrossRef] [PubMed]
105. Tokonami, S.; Nakadoi, Y.; Takahashi, M.; Ikemizu, M.; Kadoma, T.; Saimatsu, K.; Dung, L.Q.; Shiigi, H.; Nagaoka, T. Label-Free and Selective Bacteria Detection Using a Film with Transferred Bacterial Configuration. *Anal. Chem.* **2013**, *85*, 4925–4929. [CrossRef] [PubMed]
106. Ayankojo, A.G.; Boroznjak, R.; Reut, J.; Öpik, A.; Syritski, V. Molecularly Imprinted Polymer Based Electrochemical Sensor for Quantitative Detection of SARS-CoV-2 Spike Protein. *Sens. Actuators B-Chem.* **2022**, *353*, 131160. [CrossRef] [PubMed]
107. Tancharoen, C.; Sukjee, W.; Thepparit, C.; Jaimipuk, T.; Auewarakul, P.; Thitithanyanont, A.; Sangma, C. Electrochemical Biosensor Based on Surface Imprinting for Zika Virus Detection in Serum. *ACS Sens.* **2019**, *4*, 69–75. [CrossRef] [PubMed]
108. Amorim, M.S.; Sales, M.G.F.; Frasco, M.F. Recent Advances in Virus Imprinted Polymers. *Biosens. Bioelectron. X* **2022**, *10*, 100131. [CrossRef]
109. Dar, K.K.; Shao, S.; Tan, T.; Lv, Y. Molecularly Imprinted Polymers for the Selective Recognition of Microorganisms. *Biotechnol. Adv.* **2020**, *45*, 107640. [CrossRef]
110. Crapnell, R.D.; Hudson, A.; Foster, C.W.; Eersels, K.; van Grinsven, B.; Cleij, T.J.; Banks, C.E.; Peeters, M. Recent Advances in Electrosynthesized Molecularly Imprinted Polymer Sensing Platforms for Bioanalyte Detection. *Sensors* **2019**, *19*, 1204. [CrossRef] [PubMed]
111. Chen, S.; Chen, X.; Zhang, L.; Gao, J.; Ma, Q. Electrochemiluminescence Detection of Escherichia coli O157: H7 Based on a Novel Polydopamine Surface Imprinted Polymer Biosensor. *ACS Appl. Mater. Interfaces* **2017**, *9*, 5430–5436. [CrossRef] [PubMed]
112. Yasmeen, N.; Etienne, M.; Sharma, P.S.; El-Kirat-Chatel, S.; Helú, M.B.; Kutner, W. Molecularly Imprinted Polymer As a Synthetic Receptor Mimic for Capacitive Impedimetric Selective Recognition of *Escherichia coli* K-12. *Anal. Chim. Acta* **2021**, *1188*, 339177. [CrossRef] [PubMed]
113. Shan, X.L.; Yamauchi, T.; Shiigi, H.; Nagaoka, T. Binding Constant of the Cell-shaped Cavity Formed on a Polymer for Escherichia Coli O157. *Anal. Sci.* **2018**, *34*, 483–486. [CrossRef] [PubMed]
114. Wu, J.K.; Wang, R.N.; Lu, Y.F.; Jia, M.; Yan, J.; Bian, X.J. Facile Preparation of a Bacteria Imprinted Artificial Receptor for Highly Selective Bacterial Recognition and Label-Free Impedimetric Detection. *Anal. Chem.* **2019**, *91*, 1027–1033. [CrossRef]
115. Bezdekova, J.; Hutarova, J.; Tomeckova, K.; Vaculovicova, M. Isolation and Detection of Bacteria Using Magnetic Molecularly Imprinted Polymers. In Proceedings of the 25th International Phd Students Conference (Mendelnet 2018), Brno, Czechia, 7–8 November 2018; pp. 484–488.
116. Yasmeen, N.; Etienne, M.; Sharma, P.S.; Kutner, W. Artificial Receptors for Electrochemical Sensing of Bacteria. *Curr. Opin. Electrochem.* **2023**, *39*, 101291. [CrossRef]
117. Roushani, M.; Sarabaegi, M.; Rostamzad, A. Novel Electrochemical Sensor Based on Polydopamine Molecularly Imprinted Polymer for Sensitive and Selective Detection of *Acinetobacter baumannii*. *J. Iran. Chem. Soc.* **2020**, *17*, 2407–2413. [CrossRef]
118. Buensuceso, C.E.; Tiu, B.D.B.; Lee, L.P.; Sabido, P.M.G.; Nuesca, G.M.; Caldona, E.B.; del Mundo, F.R.; Advincula, R.C. Electropolymerized-molecularly Imprinted Polymers (E-MIPS) As Sensing Elements for the Detection of Dengue Infection. *Anal. Bioanal. Chem.* **2022**, *414*, 1347–1357. [CrossRef]

119. Idil, N.; Mattiasson, B. Imprinting of Microorganisms for Biosensor Applications. *Sensors* **2017**, *17*, 708. [CrossRef]
120. Le, H.H.T.; Dalsgaard, A.; Andersen, P.S.; Nguyen, H.M.; Ta, Y.T.; Nguyen, T.T. Large-Scale *Staphylococcus aureus* Foodborne Disease Poisoning Outbreak among Primary School Children. *Microbiol. Res.* **2021**, *12*, 43–52. [CrossRef]
121. Samadpour, M.; Stewart, J.; Steingart, K.; Addy, C.; Louderback, J.; McGinn, M.; Ellington, J.; Newman, T. Laboratory Investigation of an *E. coli* O157:H7 Outbreak Associated with Swimming in Battle Ground Lake, Vancouver, Washington. *J. Environ. Health* **2002**, *64*, 16–20, 25, 26.
122. Osborn, B.; Hatfield, J.; Lanier, W.; Wagner, J.; Oakeson, K.; Casey, R.; Bullough, J.; Kache, P.; Miko, S.; Kunz, J.; et al. Shiga Toxin-Producing Escherichia coli O157:H7 Illness Outbreak Associated with Untreated, Pressurized, Municipal Irrigation Water—Utah, 2023. *MMWR Morb. Mortal. Wkly. Rep.* **2024**, *73*, 411–416. [CrossRef] [PubMed]
123. Xu, X.L.; Lin, X.H.; Wang, L.L.; Ma, Y.X.; Sun, T.; Bian, X.J. A Novel Dual Bacteria-Imprinted Polymer Sensor for Highly Selective and Rapid Detection of Pathogenic Bacteria. *Biosensors* **2023**, *13*, 868. [CrossRef] [PubMed]
124. Prasad, B.B.; Fatma, S. One MoNomer Doubly Imprinted Dendrimer Nanofilm Modified Pencil Graphite Electrode for Simultaneous Electrochemical Determination of Norepinephrine and Uric Acid. *Electrochim. Acta* **2017**, *232*, 474–483. [CrossRef]
125. Hu, C.; Huang, H.; Sun, H.; Yan, Y.; Xu, F.; Liao, J. Simultaneous Analysis of Catechol and Hydroquinone by Polymelamine/CNT with Dual-Template Molecular Imprinting Technology. *Polymer* **2022**, *242*, 124593. [CrossRef]
126. Lu, Z.; Du, X.; Sun, M.; Zhang, Y.; Li, Y.; Wang, X.; Wang, Y.; Du, H.; Yin, H.; Rao, H. Novel Dual-Template Molecular Imprinted Electrochemical Sensor for Simultaneous Detection of CA And TPH Based on Peanut Twin-Like $NiFe_2O_4/CoFe_2O_4$/NCDs Nanospheres: Fabrication, Application and DFT Theoretical Study. *Biosens. Bioelectron.* **2021**, *190*, 113408. [CrossRef] [PubMed]
127. Zheng, W.; Zhao, M.; Liu, W.; Yu, S.; Niu, L.; Li, G.; Li, H.; Liu, W. Electrochemical Sensor Based on Molecularly Imprinted Polymer/Reduced Graphene Oxide Composite for Simultaneous Determination of Uric Acid and Tyrosine. *J. Electroanal. Chem.* **2018**, *813*, 75–82. [CrossRef]
128. Karazan, Z.M.; Roushani, M. Electrochemical Sensor Based on Molecularly Imprinted Copolymer for Selective and Simultaneous Determination of Ascorbic Acid and Tyrosine. *Anal. Bioanal. Chem. Res.* **2023**, *10*, 269–278. [CrossRef]
129. Li, X.; Li, Y.; Yu, P.; Tong, Y.; Ye, B.-C. A High Sensitivity Electrochemical Sensor Based on a Dual-Template Molecularly Imprinted Polymer for Simultaneous Determination of Clenbuterol Hydrochloride and Ractopamine. *Analyst* **2021**, *146*, 6323–6332. [CrossRef] [PubMed]
130. Vahidifar, M.; Es'haghi, Z. Magnetic Nanoparticle-Reinforced Dual-Template Molecularly Imprinted Polymer for the Simultaneous Determination of Oxazepam and Diazepam Using an Electrochemical Approach. *J. Anal. Chem.* **2022**, *77*, 625–639. [CrossRef]
131. Hao, P.; Zhu, R.; Tao, Y.; Jiang, W.; Liu, X.; Tan, Y.; Wang, Y.; Wang, D. Dual-Analyte Sensing with a Molecularly Imprinted Polymer Based on Enhancement-Mode Organic Electrochemical Transistors. *ACS Appl. Mater. Interfaces* **2023**, *15*, 30567–30579. [CrossRef] [PubMed]
132. Wang, X.; Liu, Y.; Liu, J.; Qu, J.; Huang, J.; Tan, R.; Yu, Y.; Wu, J.; Yang, J.; Li, Y.; et al. A Bifunctional Electrochemical Sensor for Simultaneous Determination of Electroactive and Non-Electroactive Analytes: A Universal Yet Very Effective Platform Serving Therapeutic Drug Monitoring. *Biosens. Bioelectron.* **2022**, *208*, 114233. [CrossRef]
133. Rawool, C.R.; Srivastava, A.K. A Dual Template Imprinted Polymer Modified Electrochemical Sensor Based on Cu Metal Organic Framework/Mesoporous Carbon for Highly Sensitive and Selective Recognition of Rifampicin and Isoniazid. *Sens. Actuators. B Chem.* **2019**, *288*, 493–506. [CrossRef]
134. Li, N.; Nan, C.; Mei, X.; Sun, Y.; Feng, H.; Li, Y. Electrochemical Sensor Based on Dual-Template Molecularly Imprinted Polymer and Nanoporous Gold Leaf Modified Electrode for Simultaneous Determination of Dopamine and Uric Acid. *Mikrochim. Acta* **2020**, *187*, 496. [CrossRef] [PubMed]
135. Zhang, T.; Xuan, X.; Li, M.; Li, C.; Li, P.; Li, H. Molecularly Imprinted Ni-Polyacrylamide-Based Electrochemical Sensor for the Simultaneous Detection of Dopamine and Adenine. *Anal. Chim. Acta* **2022**, *1202*, 339689. [CrossRef]
136. Vahidifar, M.; Es'haghi, Z.; Oghaz, N.M.; Mohammadi, A.A.; Kazemi, M.S. Multi-template Molecularly Imprinted Polymer Hybrid Nanoparticles for Selective Analysis of Nonsteroidal Anti-Inflammatory Drugs and Analgesics in Biological and Pharmaceutical Samples. *Environ. Sci. Pollut. Res. Int.* **2022**, *29*, 47416–47435. [CrossRef]
137. Whitesides, G.M. The Origins and the Future of Microfluidics. *Nature* **2006**, *442*, 368–373. [CrossRef]
138. Regmi, S.; Poudel, C.; Adhikari, R.; Luo, K.Q. Applications of Microfluidics and Organ-on-a-Chip in Cancer Research. *Biosensors* **2022**, *12*, 459. [CrossRef] [PubMed]
139. Qi, J.; Li, B.W.; Zhou, N.; Wang, X.Y.; Deng, D.M.; Luo, L.Q.; Chen, L.X. The Strategy of Antibody-Free Biomarker Analysis by In-Situ Synthesized Molecularly Imprinted Polymers on Movable Valve Paper-Based Device. *Biosens. Bioelectron.* **2019**, *142*, 111533. [CrossRef] [PubMed]
140. Sharma, P.S.; Iskierko, Z.; Noworyta, K.; Cieplak, M.; Borowicz, P.; Lisowski, W.; D'Souza, F.; Kutner, W. Synthesis and Application of a "Plastic Antibody" in Electrochemical Microfluidic Platform for Oxytocin Determination. *Biosens. Bioelectron.* **2018**, *100*, 251–258. [CrossRef]

141. Kong, Q.K.; Wang, Y.H.; Zhang, L.N.; Xu, C.X.; Yu, J.H. Highly Sensitive Microfluidic Paper-based Photoelectrochemical Sensing Platform Based on Reversible Photo-Oxidation Products and Morphology Preferable Multi-plate ZnO Nanoflowers. *Biosens. Bioelectron.* **2018**, *110*, 58–64. [CrossRef] [PubMed]
142. Ge, L.; Wang, S.M.; Yu, J.H.; Li, N.Q.; Ge, S.G.; Yan, M. Molecularly Imprinted Polymer Grafted Porous Au-Paper Electrode for an Microfluidic Electro-Analytical Origami Device. *Adv. Funct. Mater.* **2013**, *23*, 3115–3123. [CrossRef]
143. Kellens, E.; Bove, H.; Vandenryt, T.; Lambrichts, J.; Dekens, J.; Drijkoningen, S.; D'Haen, J.; De Ceuninck, W.; Thoelen, R.; Junkers, T.; et al. Micro-patterned Molecularly Imprinted Polymer Structures on Functionalized Diamond-coated Substrates for Testosterone Detection. *Biosens. Bioelectron.* **2018**, *118*, 58–65. [CrossRef] [PubMed]
144. Liu, J.; Zhang, Y.; Jiang, M.; Tian, L.P.; Sun, S.G.; Zhao, N.; Zhao, F.L.; Li, Y.C. Electrochemical Microfluidic Chip Based on Molecular Imprinting Technique Applied for Therapeutic Drug Monitoring. *Biosens. Bioelectron.* **2017**, *91*, 714–720. [CrossRef]
145. Weng, C.H.; Yeh, W.M.; Ho, K.C.; Lee, G.B. A Microfluidic System Utilizing Molecularly Imprinted Polymer Films for Amperometric Detection of Morphine. *Sens. Actuators B-Chem.* **2007**, *121*, 576–582. [CrossRef]
146. Dincer, C.; Bruch, R.; Kling, A.; Dittrich, P.S.; Urban, G.A. Multiplexed Point-of-Care Testing—xPOCT. *Trends Biotechnol.* **2017**, *35*, 728–742. [CrossRef]
147. Fava, E.L.; Silva, T.A.; do Prado, T.M.; de Moraes, F.C.; Faria, R.C.; Fatibello, O. Electrochemical Paper-based Microfluidic Device for High Throughput Multiplexed Analysis. *Talanta* **2019**, *203*, 280–286. [CrossRef] [PubMed]
148. Somvanshi, S.B.; Ulloa, A.M.; Zhao, M.; Liang, Q.Y.; Barui, A.K.; Lucas, A.; Jadhav, K.M.; Allebach, J.P.; Stanciu, L.A. Microfluidic Paper-based Aptasensor Devices for Multiplexed Detection of Pathogenic Bacteria. *Biosens. Bioelectron.* **2022**, *207*, 114214. [CrossRef] [PubMed]
149. Glatz, R.T.; Ates, H.C.; Mohsenin, H.; Weber, W.; Dincer, C. Designing Electrochemical Microfluidic Multiplexed Biosensors for On-Site Applications. *Anal. Bioanal. Chem.* **2022**, *414*, 6531–6540. [CrossRef] [PubMed]
150. Volpetti, F.; Garcia-Cordero, J.; Maerkl, S.J. A Microfluidic Platform for High-Throughput Multiplexed Protein Quantitation. *PLoS ONE* **2015**, *10*, e0117744. [CrossRef] [PubMed]
151. Pérez-Alvarez, M.; Arroyo-Manzanares, N.; Campillo, N.; Viñas, P. Magnetic Molecularly Imprinted Polymers for Selective Extraction of Aflatoxins from Feeds. *Toxins* **2024**, *16*, 120. [CrossRef]
152. Orbay, S.; Sanyal, A. Molecularly Imprinted Polymeric Particles Created Using Droplet-Based Microfluidics: Preparation and Applications. *Micromachines* **2023**, *14*, 763. [CrossRef]
153. Lowdon, J.W.; Diliën, H.; Singla, P.; Peeters, M.; Cleij, T.J.; van Grinsven, B.; Eersels, K. MIPs for Commercial Application in Low-Cost Sensors and Assays—An Overview of the Current Status Quo. *Sens. Actuators B-Chem.* **2020**, *325*, 128973. [CrossRef]
154. Turner, N.W.; Jeans, C.W.; Brain, K.R.; Allender, C.J.; Hlady, V.; Britt, D.W. From 3D to 2D: A Review of the Molecular Imprinting of Proteins. *Biotechnol. Prog.* **2006**, *22*, 1474–1489. [CrossRef]
155. Dixit, C.K.; Bhakta, S.; Reza, K.K.; Kaushik, A. Exploring Molecularly Imprinted Polymers As Artificial Antibodies for Efficient Diagnostics and Commercialization: A Critical Overview. *Hybrid Adv.* **2022**, *1*, 100001. [CrossRef]
156. Baldoneschi, V.; Palladino, P.; Banchini, M.; Minunni, M.; Scarano, S. Norepinephrine as New Functional Monomer for Molecular Imprinting: An Applicative Study for the Optical Sensing of Cardiac Biomarkers. *Biosens. Bioelectron.* **2020**, *157*, 112161. [CrossRef]
157. Garcia-Mutio, D.; Gómez-Caballero, A.; Gotiandia, A.; Larrauri, I.; Goicolea, M.; Barrio, R. Controlled Grafting of Molecularly Imprinted Films on Gold Microelectrodes Using a Self-Assembled Thiol Iniferter. *Electrochim. Acta* **2018**, *279*, 57–65. [CrossRef]
158. Perez-Puyana, V.; Wieringa, P.; Guerrero, A.; Romero, A.; Moroni, L. (Macro)Molecular Imprinting of Proteins on PCL Electrospun Scaffolds. *ACS Appl. Mater. InterfacES* **2021**, *13*, 29293–29302. [CrossRef]
159. Ali, G.K.; Omer, K.M. Molecular Imprinted Polymer Combined with Aptamer (MIP-Aptamer) As a Hybrid Dual Recognition Element for Bio(Chemical) Sensing Applications. Review. *Talanta* **2022**, *236*, 122878. [CrossRef] [PubMed]
160. Liu, Y.X.; Dykstra, G. Recent Progress on Electrochemical (Bio)Sensors Based on Aptamer-Molecularly Imprinted Polymer Dual Recognition. *Sens. Actuators Rep.* **2022**, *4*, 100112. [CrossRef]
161. Phonklam, K.; Wannapob, R.; Sriwimol, W.; Thavarungkul, P.; Phairatana, T. A Novel Molecularly Imprinted Polymer PMB/MWCNTs Sensor for Highly-Sensitive Cardiac Troponin T Detection. *Sens. Actuators B-Chem.* **2020**, *308*, 127630. [CrossRef]
162. Rad, A.O.; Azadbakht, A. An Aptamer Embedded in a Molecularly Imprinted Polymer for Impedimetric Determination of Tetracycline. *Microchim. Acta* **2019**, *186*, 56. [CrossRef]
163. Mahmoud, A.M.; Alkahtani, S.A.; Alyami, B.A.; El-Wekil, M.M. Dual-recognition Molecularly Imprinted Aptasensor Based on Gold Nanoparticles Decorated Carboxylated Carbon Nanotubes for Highly Selective and Sensitive Determination of Histamine in Different Matrices. *Anal. Chim. Acta* **2020**, *1133*, 58–65. [CrossRef] [PubMed]
164. Li, S.H.; Ma, X.H.; Pang, C.H.; Tian, H.; Xu, Z.; Yang, Y.; Lv, D.Z.; Ge, H.L. Fluorometric Aptasensor for Cadmium(II) by Using an Aptamer-Imprinted Polymer As the Recognition Element. *Microchim. Acta* **2019**, *186*, 823. [CrossRef]
165. Shen, M.M.; Kan, X.W. Aptamer and Molecularly Imprinted Polymer: Synergistic Recognition and Sensing of Dopamine. *Electrochim. Acta* **2021**, *367*, 137433. [CrossRef]

166. Yuan, X.; Yuan, Y.; Gao, X.; Xiong, Z.; Zhao, L. Magnetic Dummy-template Molecularly Imprinted Polymers Based on Multi-Walled Carbon Nanotubes for Simultaneous Selective Extraction and Analysis of Phenoxy Carboxylic Acid Herbicides in Cereals. *Food Chem.* **2020**, *333*, 127540. [CrossRef] [PubMed]
167. Wang, X.; Luo, J.; Yi, C.; Liu, X. Paracetamol Sensor Based on Molecular Imprinting by Photosensitive Polymers. *Electroanalysis* **2013**, *25*, 1907–1916. [CrossRef]
168. Tadi, K.; Motghare, R.; Ganesh, V. Electrochemical Detection of Epinephrine Using a Biomimic Made Up of Hemin Modified Molecularly Imprinted Microspheres. *RSC Adv.* **2015**, *5*, 99115–99124. [CrossRef]
169. Abu-Alsoud, G.; Bottaro, C. Porous Thin-film Molecularly Imprinted Polymer Device for Simultaneous Determination of Phenol, Alkylphenol and Chlorophenol Compounds in Water. *Talanta* **2021**, *223*, 121727. [CrossRef] [PubMed]
170. Tamboli, V.; Bhalla, N.; Jolly, P.; Bowen, C.; Taylor, J.; Bowen, J.; Allender, C.; Estrela, P. Hybrid Synthetic Receptors on MOSFET Devices for Detection of Prostate Specific Antigen in Human Plasma. *Anal. Chem.* **2016**, *88*, 11486–11490. [CrossRef]
171. Agar, M.; Laabei, M.; Leese, H.S.; Estrela, P. Aptamer-Molecularly Imprinted Polymer Sensors for the Detection of Bacteria in Water. *Biosens. Bioelectron.* 2024, *in press*. [CrossRef]
172. Gros, M.; Pizzolato, T.; Petrovic, M.; de Alda, M.; Barceló, D. Trace Level Determination of B-Blockers in Waste Waters by Highly Selective Molecularly Imprinted Polymers Extraction Followed by Liquid Chromatography-Quadrupole-Linear Ion Trap Mass Spectrometry. *J. Chromatogr. A* **2008**, *1189*, 374–384. [CrossRef] [PubMed]
173. Yang, H.; Zhou, W.; Guo, X.; Chen, F.; Zhao, H.; Lin, L.; Wang, X. Molecularly Imprinted Polymer As SPE Sorbent for Selective Extraction of Melamine in Dairy Products. *Talanta* **2009**, *80*, 821–825. [CrossRef]

chemosensors

MDPI

Review

Current and Future Diagnostics for Hepatitis C Virus Infection

Hussein Zilouchian [1,2,†], Omair Faqah [1,3,†], Md Alamgir Kabir [1,3], Dennis Gross [2], Rachel Pan [2], Shane Shaifman [2], Muhammad Awais Younas [4], Muhammad Abdul Haseeb [1], Emmanuel Thomas [5] and Waseem Asghar [1,3,6,*]

[1] Asghar-Lab, Micro and Nanotechnology in Medicine, College of Engineering and Computer Science, Boca Raton, FL 33431, USA; ofaqah2022@fau.edu (O.F.); mkabir2016@fau.edu (M.A.K.); mhaseeb2019@fau.edu (M.A.H.)
[2] College of Medicine, University of Central Florida, Orlando, FL 32827, USA
[3] Department of Electrical Engineering and Computer Science, Florida Atlantic University, Boca Raton, FL 33431, USA
[4] Manchester Royal Infirmary, Manchester University NHS Foundation Trust, Manchester M13 9WL, UK
[5] Department of Pathology and Laboratory Medicine, University of Miami School of Medicine, Miami, FL 33136, USA
[6] Department of Biomedical Engineering (Affiliate Appointment), Florida Atlantic University, Boca Raton, FL 33431, USA
* Correspondence: wasghar@fau.edu
† These authors contributed equally to this work.

Abstract: Hepatitis C virus (HCV), a member of the Flaviviridae family, is an RNA virus enclosed in an envelope that infects approximately 50 million people worldwide. Despite its significant burden on public health, no vaccine is currently available, and many individuals remain unaware of their infection due to the often asymptomatic nature of the disease. Early detection of HCV is critical for initiating curative treatments, which can prevent long-term complications such as cirrhosis, liver cancer, and decompensated liver disease. However, conventional diagnostic approaches available, such as enzyme immunoassays (EIAs) and polymerase chain reaction (PCR)-based methods, are often costly, time-intensive, and challenging to be implemented in resource-limited settings. This review provides an overview of HCV disease and the structural components of the virus, illustrating how different diagnostic methods target various parts of the viral structure. It examines current diagnostic tests and assays, highlighting their mechanisms, applications, and limitations, which necessitates the development of improved detection methods. Additionally, the paper explores emerging technologies in HCV detection that could offer affordable, accessible, and easy-to-use diagnostic solutions, particularly for deployment in low-resource and point-of-care settings. These advancements have the potential to contribute significantly to achieving the World Health Organization's (WHO) target of eliminating HCV as a public threat by 2030.

Keywords: hepatitis C; point-of-care (POC); molecular testing; HCV diagnostics; microfluidics; PCR

1. Introduction

The hepatitis C virus (HCV) is an enveloped RNA virus belonging to the Flaviviridae family [1]. The virus is transmitted parenterally through multiple routes, including sharing needles and syringes, nosocomial transmission, and blood transfusions [2,3]. Men who engage in sexual activity with other men face an elevated risk of contracting the disease, especially those infected with HIV [2]. Moreover, the transmission of HCV can occur vertically from the mother to the child during pregnancy [4]. HCV was first discovered in 1989 when Choo et al. found complementary DNA that was constructed from a patient who received a diagnosis of non-A, non-B viral hepatitis (NANBH) [5,6]. Prior to this discovery, the primary mode of viral transmission was the transfusion of contaminated blood products. Kuo et al. later created the first specific assay to detect HCV from circulating HCV antibodies [6]. At the time of the discovery of HCV, it constituted up to 90 percent of transfusion-associated hepatitis cases [6].

HCV prevalence is estimated to be around 50 million people [7]. The HCV virus has six genotypes: HCV 1, 2, 3, 4, 5, and 6 [8]. The most widespread genotype is 1, accounting for 59.7% of global infections [9]. Furthermore, genotypes 3, 2, and 4 comprise 25.7%, 8.6%, and 3.8% of HCV cases worldwide, respectively [9]. HCV genotypes 1 and 3 are the most common worldwide; however, genotypes 4 and 5 are more common in lower-income countries [9]. As per WHO, the Eastern Mediterranean region exhibits the highest prevalence globally, while the Americas have the lowest prevalence (Figure 1) [7]. WHO specifies the main hurdles in these developing countries as limited decentralization of testing, lack of local production of in vitro diagnostics (IVDs), and the inability to sustain the cost associated with expensive tests and employ human resources to process them [7]. A total of 1.3 million deaths were attributed to viral hepatitis in 2022, which was the second leading cause of death in communicable diseases after COVID-19 [7]. The majority of deaths were caused by hepatitis B (HBV-83%) and HCV (17%) [7]. The WHO estimates that out of the 36.7 million people with HIV, an estimated 2.3 million individuals, ranging from 1.3 to 4.4 million people, are co-infected with HCV [10]. This is primarily due to the shared transmission routes, such as injection drug use and unprotected sexual contact.

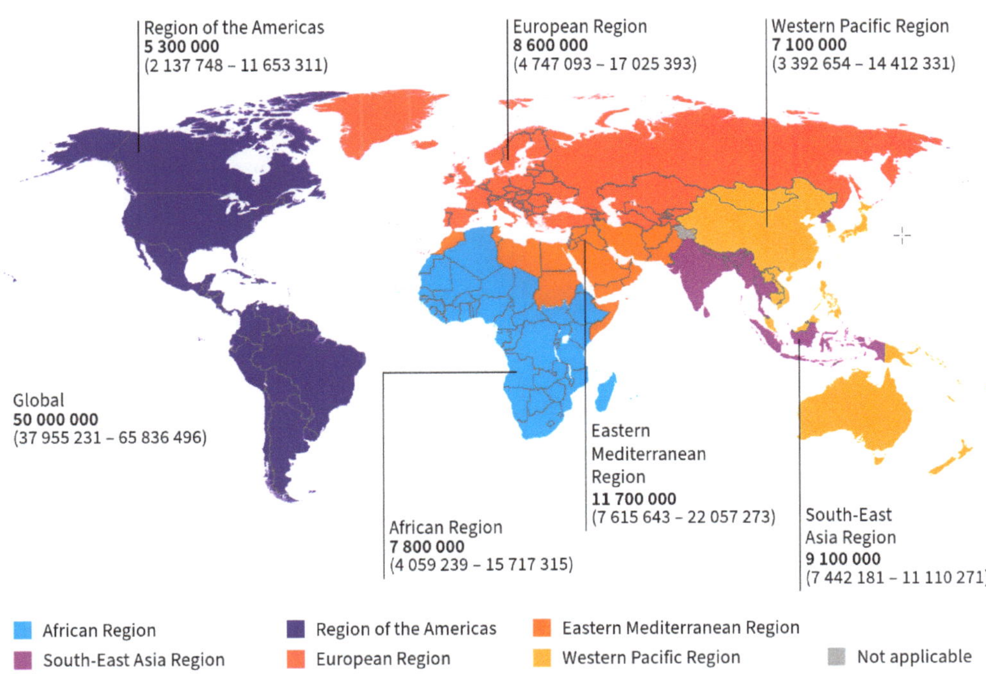

Figure 1. The world map shows the prevalence of chronic HCV globally in 2022. While HCV is prevalent throughout the world, the Eastern Mediterranean region exhibits the highest prevalence [7].

HCV can cause either acute or chronic hepatitis [11,12]. Acute HCV presents similarly to other acute hepatitis viruses clinically, with symptoms encompassing malaise, nausea, jaundice, right-upper-quadrant pain (RUQ), and bilirubinuria [12]. The average HCV incubation period is 14–84 days [3]. A small percentage of acute HCV infections become fulminant hepatitis, also known as acute liver failure [13]. Acute HCV infections lead to chronic HCV infections in 75–85% of the infected people [11]. Patients with chronic hepatitis frequently experience a long-term, asymptomatic course. However, the infection can progress to hepatic failure and hepatocellular carcinoma [11].

Since no vaccine currently exists for HCV, effective treatment depends upon early diagnosis and antiviral medication. Direct-acting antivirals (DAAs) for HCV are oral medications taken over an 8–12-week period and have been shown to significantly improve cure rates to achieve a sustained virologic response (SVR) in over 90% of patients, indicating no detectable levels of the virus [14]. Effective DAA regimens are specific to the HCV genotype, highlighting the importance of diagnostics in determining the appropriate therapy [15]. Therefore, addressing WHO's aim to eliminate HCV by 2030 requires developing robust diagnostics that allow healthcare professionals to identify undiagnosed patients so they can be linked to appropriate care [7,16].

Current guidelines of the Centers for Disease Control and Prevention (CDC) for HCV testing recommend first performing an HCV antibody (Ab) test. If nonreactive, no further testing is required. If the patient is Ab positive, reflex testing should be undertaken using an HCV RNA assay [17]. If HCV RNA is detected in a patient along with an anti-HCV-positive result, a diagnosis of chronic HCV infection is made, and the patient should be linked to care for assessment of liver disease and subsequent initiation of antiviral therapy [17]. However, it is difficult to differentiate between a prior resolved infection (spontaneous viral clearance) and a case of obtaining a false-positive anti-HCV test result along with a negative HCV RNA test. Additional testing should be pursued in these patients [17]. HCV testing is currently limited in large parts of the world, especially economically disadvantaged regions. Point-of-care (POC) technology is paramount to minimizing these disparities in care, and it may lower the cost associated with traditional testing that leverages reflex HCV RNA in patients who are HCV Ab-positive. This review will focus on current conventional technologies and future technologies that can be expanded to POC settings. To meet WHO's goal of eliminating HCV by 2030, advancements in diagnostic approaches are essential to enable early and accurate detection, facilitate prompt treatment initiation, and overcome challenges related to diverse HCV genotypes and viral strains [18].

2. Genome and Virion Structure

HCV is classified as an enveloped, positive-sense, single-stranded RNA (ssRNA). Upon entering hepatocytes, the virus facilitates the direct translation of its structural and non-structural proteins. Its genome is approximately 9.6 kb long. The virus includes a 5′ noncoding region (NCR), a site of internal ribosomal entry (IRES), an open reading frame for about 3000 base pairs, and a 3′ NCR. Internal ribosome entry is a crucial process for viral protein synthesis, highlighting the importance of the 5′ NCR in viral replication [19]. This makes the 5′ NCR region a highly conserved one in the HCV genome and, therefore, a critical target for diagnostic assays that target the viral RNA [20]. HCV RNA can be detected within 2 weeks of exposure, preceding antibody development [21]. For self-resolving cases, the RNA levels show a drop after 6 months [22]. Many assays utilize the quantitative measurement of the HCV RNA to detect active infection and monitor treatment efficiency. The initially transcribed polyprotein is modified co-translationally and post-translationally with the help of protease present in the host cell to produce ten mature proteins. Three mature proteins are structural, and seven are nonstructural among the ten mature proteins produced. Residing at the 5′ end of the open reading frame (ORF), the structural proteins of the virus consist of a core nucleocapsid protein (C) as well as two envelope glycoproteins

(E1 and E2). These envelope glycoproteins play a crucial role in facilitating the binding and entry of the virus into hepatocytes [23,24]. The seven nonstructural (NS) proteins are designated p7, NS2, NS3, NS4A, NS4B, NS5A, and NS5B [25]. The NS3, NS4, and NS5 proteins play an important role in viral replication, so various classes of DAAs directly target them [26]. Additionally, assessing antibodies against these nonstructural proteins helps to confirm HCV exposure and evaluate acute and chronic infections [27].

Ultrastructural analysis of the HCV particle reveals heterogeneous sizes ranging between 40 and 100 nm in diameter [24,28]. The genetic material is surrounded by a nucleocapsid consisting of the HCV C protein and E1/E2 heterodimers [24,28,29]. Anchored by these E1/E2 heterodimers is the viral lipid membrane derived from the host endoplasmic reticulum (ER) [24]. The lipid bilayer incorporates high amounts of cholesterol, resembling the composition of very-low-density lipoprotein (VLDL) and distinguishing it from human host cells and other viral envelopes [30–33]. The major targets of anti-HCV neutralizing antibodies (nAb)s are the structural envelope glycoproteins E1, E2, and their E1/E2 heterodimer (with a vast majority targeting E2 due to its direct role in host cell entry) [34,35].

3. Biomarkers and Diagnostic Testing

The key biomarkers that the diagnostic assay targets include the HCV RNA, HCV core antigen, and anti-HCV antibodies. The initial two weeks after infection are characterized by the previremic phase in which the HCV RNA levels gradually increase in blood, which can only be targeted by highly sensitive diagnostic assays [21]. Detection during the acute stage is unreliable, given that the RNA levels may fluctuate [21,36,37]. Nucleic acid testing (NAT) offers the gold standard approach for detection during this stage; however, it is limited by its high cost and high turnaround time [38]. The RNA levels peak at a million copies per mL within 6–10 weeks [21]. The RNA levels can drop to undetectable levels for self-resolving cases and patients undergoing DAA therapy after 6 months [22]. For such cases, viral load monitoring tests become necessary to evaluate the condition of the disease. The expression of the HCV core antigen is similar to that of the HCV-RNA but with a slight delay. Therefore, HCV core antigen has been shown to be an alternative to RNA testing [39]. The expression of anti-HCV antibodies, however, significantly lags. The serologic window period characterized by the initial infection until the seroconversion can take up to 8 weeks [21,36]. Regardless of acute or chronic infections, the anti-HCV antibody levels may remain detectable after this stage. These factors can cause problems with diagnosis, as anti-HCV-based tests can miss the patients who are acute HCV and cannot differentiate between patients who are recovered or have a chronic infection [22,39].

The traditional approach to establishing an HCV diagnosis is an initial Ab test to document exposure, followed by a reflex polymerase chain reaction (PCR) HCV RNA test [40]. Serological exams are widely used to detect HCV exposure due to their cost-effectiveness, availability in the POC setting, and simplicity (e.g., storage and handling) compared to molecular tests. The presence of HCV Abs warrants screening for HCV RNA and a basic assessment for any signs of liver disease. Additional testing for other virus infections, including HBV and HIV, is also recommended. Practically, however, that is not always the case. The CDC notes that one-third of patients have incomplete testing [41]. Incomplete testing is characterized by a reactive HCV antibody test, which is not followed by an HCV RNA test. To combat this, the CDC has updated guidelines to ensure all screening sites do single-visit sample collection, allowing automatic RNA testing on all samples that are reactive to the HCV antibody [41]. WHO has recommended adopting point-of-care HCV viral load testing as an alternative to centralized lab testing to make HCV diagnosis more accessible. This is important to reach marginalized populations with whom it may be difficult to follow up [42]. To achieve this, an ideal test should work with capillary blood, have integrated sample preparation, have a low limit of detection (<3000 IU/mL) with a clinical sensitivity of >95%, have a low turnaround time of under 30 min, and be under USD 10 per test [43].

4. Current Detection Methods

4.1. Serological Assays

4.1.1. Enzyme Immunoassay (EIA)

The duration of acute HCV infection averages 8 to 11 weeks but has been reported to be from 2 weeks to 6 months [44,45]. Four generations of immunoassays have been developed [46]. The first generation of viral antigen-targeting enzyme immunoassays detected NS4 with a window period of 4–6 months [46]. The second generation detected core, NS3, and NS4 with a window period of 10–24 weeks [46]. The third generation detected the previously mentioned viral proteins utilized in the second-generation test with the addition of NS5, improving its window period to 7–8 weeks [46]. Finally, the fourth-generation test utilized the same viral targets but improved the window period to as early as 26 days [46].

The first antibody assay was developed by Kuo et al. in 1989 when they first discovered HCV [6]. They created a recombinant yeast clone that expressed the polypeptide c100-3 of NS4, which was utilized to capture anti-NS4 Abs, which were subsequently measured qualitatively [6,46]. Their c100-3 bound Ab was detected using a radioactive secondary antibody [6]. To test the sensitivity, they had seven samples of HCV serum from chimpanzees, and they found that all but one had a high signal for the anti-HCV antibodies [6]. However, a major limitation of the test developed by Kuo et al. was that it could not detect Abs in the acute phase of an infection competently [47].

The ORTHO HCV second-generation ELISA test, by Ortho Diagnostic Systems, was created in 1992 and expanded on its first-generation counterpart by detecting both structural (HCV core) and non-structural proteins (NS3/NS4) [47]. In the second-generation test, non-structural antigens c100-3 and c33c, along with a recombinant antigen c22-3, were employed. However, as mentioned earlier, the first-generation test solely relied on c100-3 [47]. The second-generation ELISA platform exhibited higher sensitivity than the first-generation version, achieving 80% detection in acute HCV cases and 88% in chronic HCV cases [47]. First-generation testing only achieved a sensitivity of 60% in acute HCV and 72% in chronic HCV cases [47]. Both tests showed 99% specificity [47]. During another study involving Saudi Arabian blood donors, the application of the second-generation anti-HCV test revealed a 38% higher positivity rate compared to the first-generation test [48].

The third-generation tests, like the ORTHO EIA-3.0 and the Chiron RIBA-3 prototype, expanded on the second-generation tests by adding non-structural regions, including NS3, NS4, and NS5 [49]. Furthermore, these third-generation tests were able to reduce the false positive results that arose from c100-3 and c22-3 reactions [49]. Vrielink et al. conducted a test that compared the sensitivities and specificities of three different third-generation tests: Abbott HCV EIA 3.0, Murex anti-HCV VK47, and ORTHO EIA-3.0 [50]. The study showed that Abbott and Ortho demonstrated 100% sensitivity, while Murex had a sensitivity of 99.7% [50]. The specificities of Abbott, Murex, and Ortho were 99.7, 99.3, and 99.9 percent, respectively [50]. A major limitation of the third-generation tests was that these tests provided low positive predictive values in populations with a low HCV prevalence [46].

HCV antigen and antibody were simultaneously detected using the fourth-generation HCV tests, which functioned as an antigen-antibody combo assay. This generation of testing proved to be more convenient as it allowed the identification of two HCV markers using a single test. Consequently, it became highly suitable for resource-limited settings [46].

The ability to detect an antigen and antibody combo reduced the window period to 26 days [46]. An example of such a fourth-generation enzyme immunoassay is the Murex Anti-HCV Version 4.0, which has mostly replaced the 3.0 version. This assay has shown robust performance and high throughput, making it a valuable tool for early HCV detection and blood donor screening [51].

In conclusion, enzyme immunoassays adequately detect HCV infection. Each generation has improved upon previous versions, and now, the fourth-generation tests have a window period as low as 26 days [46]. The tests are highly sensitive and specific, which can ensure appropriate diagnosis. A huge drawback is that it takes approximately 24 h to complete EIA, and trained personnel are needed. The availability of trained technicians may be limited in certain regions, which can diminish the utility of this test, which is further limited by the fact that it is not a POC diagnostic tool.

4.1.2. Rapid Immunoassays

Rapid testing is defined as having a turnaround of fewer than 30 min and a test that does not need specialized equipment [46,52,53]. Rapid immunoassays can be used in POC settings and can reduce time and costs for obtaining rigorous and clinically informative information.

The OraQuick HCV rapid antibody test (OraSure Technologies Inc., Bethlehem, PA, USA) detects antibodies against the recombinant HCV C protein using an indirect lateral immunoassay [54]. Furthermore, OraQuick can also detect NS3 and NS4 [54]. To administer the test, a finger-stick blood sample is taken [55]. The test has two lines, a T line and a C line [55]. The test is considered reactive if the line appears at both the C and T zones. It is not reactive if there is a line in the C zone but no line in the T zone [55]. An invalid test occurs with a line only at the C zone or partial lines in the C or T zone [55]. Results are available for interpretation after 20 to 40 min, which renders this OraQuick test fully amenable for use in the POC setting. The sensitivity of OraQuick in field studies has ranged from 88.3 percent to 99.3 percent in sera, while the specificity is usually 100 percent [54]. Recently, the WHO also prequalified the OraQuick self-test for HCV [56]. This test is an extension of the OraQuick HCV rapid antibody test, which means that it offers similar testing performance in terms of sensitivity and specificity [57]. Although this is a great step in increasing access to diagnostics, the drawbacks of antigen testing, coupled with problems associated with user interpretation errors and limited data available on real-world effectiveness, necessitate ongoing evaluation to ensure its reliability across diverse populations and settings [58].

Another rapid immunoassay awaiting FDA approval that can be used to detect antibodies against HCV (anti-HCV), hepatitis B, and HIV 1 and 2 is MedMira's Miriad HBc/HIV/HCV rapid test, which does not require complex laboratory equipment or highly trained personnel, making it suited for resource-limited settings [59]. The ARCHITECT HCV Ag assay is also a fourth-generation chemiluminescent microparticle immunoassay (CMIA) that enables earlier detection of HCV infections due to its dual detection of HCV core antigens as well as anti-HCV antibodies, making it more cost-effective and potentially suitable for point-of-care settings [60].

Rapid Ab tests can be both cost-effective and time-effective in diagnosing someone with exposure to HCV. If a person tests Ab positive, per CDC guidelines, they are then given an HCV RNA test. A drawback of rapid tests is that they are not as sensitive as their enzyme immunoassay counterparts, which are also lower in cost per assay and can be used in settings where high-throughput testing is needed. Rapid tests, not conducted by well-trained technicians, can also be incorrectly performed or interpreted, giving someone a false positive or negative test result.

4.2. Molecular and Nucleic Acid-Based Detection

Nucleic acid amplification tests (NAATs) are a family of molecular diagnostics that detect viral RNA/DNA. These assays can be categorized as either qualitative or quantitative. NAATs exhibit high levels of sensitivity and specificity, enabling the detection of the virus during the acute phase of the infection [61,62]. To ensure accuracy and comparability, all HCV assays are calibrated utilizing international units (IU). According to the European Association for the Study of the Liver (EASL) guidelines as of April 2019, it is recommended to utilize assays that have a lower limit of detection (LLOD) of under 15 IU/mL, despite the vast majority of patients with HCV having viral RNA serum/plasma levels over 50,000 IU/mL [63].

A significant limitation of molecular diagnostics for HCV diagnosis is the expense of the test and their reliance on specialized laboratories [64]. This can pose a barrier for populations without access to capable healthcare facilities, such as developing nations, prisoners, sex workers, and migrants [65]. For certain assays and regions of the world, confirmatory HCV RNA assays can be more costly than the antiviral treatment itself [64]. This precludes the use of molecular testing in the initial diagnostic screening for the virus.

4.2.1. Polymerase Chain Reaction (PCR) Based Tests

PCR, developed in the 1980s, is a method of exponentially multiplying a target DNA strand through thermocycling, giving 2^n copies (where n is the number of cycles performed) [66]. PCR methods can be employed to amplify RNA samples by initially generating complementary DNA (cDNA) through reverse transcription (RT-PCR). The use of RT-PCR offers many benefits in the diagnosis and treatment of HCV. RT-PCR relies on the presence of HCV RNA in peripheral blood and not on the formation of anti-HCV Abs, making it the preferred method for both the acute and chronic phases of infection [67]. On the other hand, anti-HCV antibodies signify past or present infection, and the presence of serum HCV RNA is specific to ongoing viral replication [67]. In 1998, Krarup et al. developed the first successful assay for quantitative RT-PCR for HCV detection, which has remained the gold standard for confirmation of acute infection and viral load [68–70]. Real-time RT-PCR employs the same principles as traditional PCR, with the added ability to quantify the sample DNA/cDNA, as the process takes place in real-time using fluorescent reporter dyes or probes (Figure 2) [71,72]. In this assay, a fluorescent signal is emitted during every replication cycle and measured proportionally to the amount of DNA/cDNA produced at that moment [72]. Multiple probes can target multiple genes simultaneously (multiplex real-time PCR) [72].

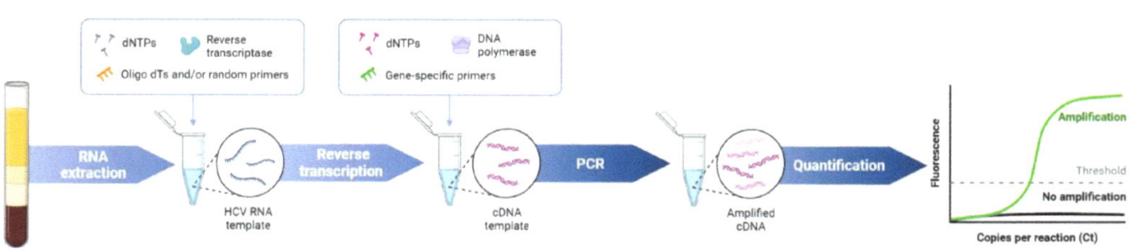

Figure 2. Depiction of real-time RT-PCR. Viral RNA extracted from peripheral blood is converted to cDNA via reverse transcription. cDNA then undergoes PCR amplification and quantification to determine viral load. Created with BioRender.com, accessed on 13 December 2022.

The two main real-time RT-PCR-based assays commonly utilized in HCV testing are the COBAS AmpliPrep/COBAS TaqMan (CAP/CTM) assay and the Abbott RealTime HCV test (Abbott) [73,74]. Both assays are very similar, basing their techniques on automated sample preparation followed by real-time RT-PCR [75]. Following a 12-week course of HCV antiviral therapy, both the CAP/CTM assay and the Abbott RealTime HCV test were compared and exhibited comparable performance. CAP/CTM has an LLOD of 15 IU/mL with a sensitivity and specificity of 96% and 49%, respectively [76,77]. Abbott has an LLOD of 12 IU/mL with a sensitivity and specificity of 95% and 46%, respectively [76,77]. Version 1 (CAP/CTM v1.0) of the CAP/CTM assay was known to sporadically under-quantify HCV genotype 4 (GT4), though this has since been resolved with the release of the version 2 assay (CAP/CTM v2.0) [74]. A significant drawback of real-time RT-PCR is its cost. While a traditional PCR instrument costs approximately USD 5000, the price of a real-time RT-PCR instrument ranges between USD 15,000 and USD 90,000 [78].

4.2.2. Branched DNA Assays (bDNA)

Branched DNA (bDNA) assays employ bDNA amplifier molecules, which serve as a hybridization site for linear amplification of the target as opposed to exponential amplification [79,80]. In this assay, target-specific probes known as capture extenders (CEs) are used to capture targeted nucleic acids onto a microtiter well plate [79–82]. Then, the second set of probes, termed label extenders (LE), hybridizes to the target, allowing the bDNA amplifiers to bind [82]. Alkaline phosphatase and a chemiluminescent substrate are then added to the mixture, allowing for luminescence production to be measured as a direct proportion of starting HCV RNA [83]. The VERSANT HCV RNA 3.0 Assay (VERSANT 3.0 bDNA assay) is one such assay used for HCV detection. This assay has a reported LLOD of 615 IU/mL with a specificity of 98.2% [84]. The assay also has a high dynamic range of between 615 and 7,690,000 IU/mL [83]. It was also shown to be an improvement to the Quantiplex HCV RNA 2.0, where the latter required 100 μL of serum compared to the VERSANT 3.0 bDNA assay, which only uses 50 μL of serum [84]. In contrast to other molecular assays, bDNA incorporates an in-assay mechanism to isolate HCV RNA and does not necessitate separate RNA purification steps, which makes the workflow more streamlined. It is also less prone to contamination and limits false positive results [83–85].

4.2.3. Transcription-Mediated Amplification (TMA)

TMA is an isothermal method that imitates retroviral RNA replication. It involves the use of RNA polymerase and reverse transcriptase to amplify RNA [86]. Since RNA amplicons are more labile than PCR products, the risk for carryover contamination and false positives is quite low [87]. The TMA test used for HCV detection is the VERSANT HCV RNA TMA assay (VERSANT TMA). This is a qualitative assay offering 99.6% specificity, detecting >95% of clinical samples with HCV RNA at 50 copies/mL, including patients infected with HCV genotypes 1a, 1b, 2a, 2c, 3a, 4a, 5a, and 6a (genotype 2b showed detection of 88.4% at the same concentration) [88]. One of the main benefits of the VERSANT TMA assay is that it maintains specificity even in clinical RNA samples exposed to long storage durations, multiple freeze-dry cycles, various collection tubes, prescription drugs, and microorganisms [88]. The LLOD for genotype 1 ranges from 5.3 to 9.6 IU/mL, while for genotype 2b, it is 14.4 IU/mL [83]. The assay has proven more effective than RT-PCR for the detection of HCV RNA in liver tissue (p-value = 0.032) [89]. A drawback of the VERSANT TMA assay is its relatively high labor demand and bench space requirement compared to other qualitative assays [83]. Another TMA-based assay is the Aptima® HCV Quant Dx Assay, which has determined its LOD for plasma to be 3.9 IU/mL and 3.4 IU/mL in serum [90]. This assay removes the need for batch processing and condenses the automation of nucleic acid testing into a single step [91]. The Procleix® Ultrio Assay is an in vitro supplemental multiplex nucleic acid test (NAT) using TMA to detect HCV RNA and a few other viral diseases like HIV and HBV [92]. However, according to the FDA, this test is not meant to be used for diagnosis but as a supplemental test [92].

4.3. Non-Invasive and Point-of-Care Testing

4.3.1. Dried Blood Tests

Dried blood testing originated a century ago after Christian Bang studied glucose levels from dried blood spots (DBS) eluates [93]. DBS has four inherent advantages: (1) less blood volume is required compared to conventional venipuncture, (2) blood collection is not complex and expensive, (3) bacterial infection risk is minimal, and (4) DBS is stabilized for longer time periods without any significant damage to the sample [93]. The process of obtaining blood for DBS is quite simple and does not require trained personnel. The technician punctures the subject's finger via a contact-activated lancet. Capillary blood is then collected on filter paper (Figure 3) [93]. The blood is dried, after which the card can be transported to centralized testing labs [93]. In the labs, technicians punch out the sample from the card and incubate it with a buffer to elute the sample [93]. The sample is then used for downstream analysis for HCV markers, including the anti-HCV Ab and the HCV C antigen [93,94]. The process (Figure 3) is promising for at-home self-collection, which makes HCV testing accessible to a broader population with limited access.

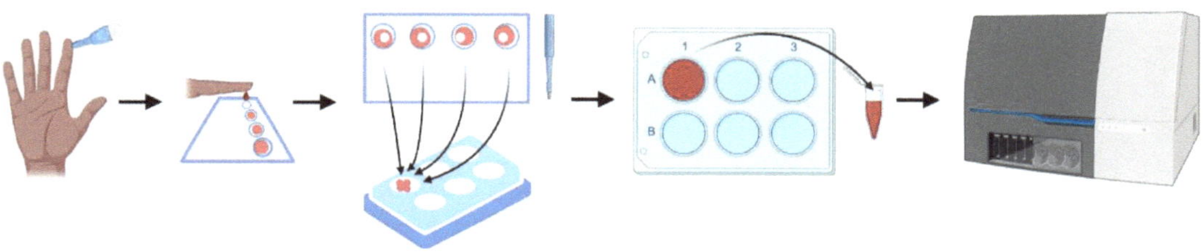

Figure 3. Depiction of dried blood spot (DBS)-based testing. Capillary blood is acquired via finger-stick and blotted onto a filter paper-based DBS card. The DBS card can be transported to a centralized lab facility for infectious disease screening. The filter paper with the sample is then incubated with a buffer. The resulting supernatant can be used to analyze viral proteins, genetic material, and Abs. Created with BioRender.com, accessed on 13 December 2022.

Biondi et al. determined the effect of freezing temperatures on DBS sensitivity [94]. The sensitivity of the HCV C antigen assay was 94% (−80 °C), 94% (4 °C), 91% (21 °C), 93% (37 °C), and 93% (37 °C/4 °C), while the sensitivity of the anti-HCV Ab tests was 100% (−80 °C), 100% (4 °C), 100% (21 °C), 98.6% (37 °C), and 98.6% (37 °C/4 °C) [94]. The study showed that the temperature change had little effect on the ability to test for HCV [94]. Their study also demonstrated that the sensitivity of DBS was 94%, which was higher than that reported in other studies [94].

Public health officials in Scotland implemented more DBS sampling as part of their community drug services to diagnose individuals infected with HCV. Following the implementation of DBS, there was a 3-fold increase in testing and a 12-fold increase in positive results. This demonstrates that DBS can detect more cases, particularly in high-risk populations [95]. DBS testing should be considered an alternative to other HCV testing methods as it is cheaper, simpler to run, and does not require trained personnel [94]. However, DBS is limited by the lack of standardized testing protocols. Temperature, blood drying time, and other related conditions often vary between testing sites. Furthermore, the assay used can make a difference in both sensitivity and specificity.

4.3.2. Point-of-Care NAAT Testing

With the importance of rapid HCV RNA detection in the diagnosis and treatment of acute and chronic infections, the development of a POC molecular diagnostic test offers great value. The first such test developed for HCV detection is the Xpert HCV Viral Load test (a real-time RT-PCR) designed in 2015 and manufactured by Cepheid [96]. This test combines all steps of real-time RT-PCR (sample preparation, DNA/RNA extraction, amplification, and detection of targets) into a single cartridge leveraging microfluidics, allowing it to fit on a small benchtop [97]. This assay has an LLOD of 10 IU/mL (similar to that of the Abbott test) with a sensitivity and specificity of 94.4% and 100%, respectively. A new version, called the Xpert HCV Viral Load Finger-Stick assay (Xpert HCV VL FS), which does not use venipuncture, has reported even higher levels of sensitivity and specificity [98]. The Xpert HCV test and its associated GeneXpert Express System have recently been approved by the FDA for operations under a CLIA (Clinical Laboratory Improvement Amendments) Certificate Waiver [99]. However, reported drawbacks to this assay have been associated with the cost of both the assay kit and the GeneXpert instrument needed for its use [96]. There are other similar assays, including the Genedrive HCV ID (98.6% sensitivity, 100% specificity), which received prequalification by WHO in 2020, and the TrueNAT HCV RNA assay, which had reported sensitivity and specificity of 95% and 99%, respectively [96,100]. Sharma et al. successfully developed an automated reverse-transcription loop-mediated isothermal amplification (RT-LAMP) test designed for HCV detection. The system they created comprises a disposable microfluid chip that is automated, a reusable magnetic actuation platform, and a compact surface heater [101–103]. The plasma samples were processed in multiple chambers within the microfluidic chip. SYBR green dye is employed to enable the visual detection of the amplification product without the need for specialized equipment [101]. Human plasma samples spiked with HCV virions were employed to evaluate the microfluid chip's performance. The observed limit of detection (LOD) was determined to be 500 virions/mL, achieved within a timeframe of 45 min [101]. Although developing a fully automated setup for rapid HCV detection using RT-LAMP is a promising advancement, there are still areas for improvement, particularly in terms of automation. Currently, the system requires a plasma sample to be prepared before testing, which can be time-consuming and may limit its practicality in point-of-care settings. To further streamline and increase the practical use of this technology in POC settings, efforts should focus on incorporating whole blood isolates into the system. Comprehensive data about key characteristics of the various diagnostic techniques discussed that have been clinically tested and conventionally used in managing HCV testing are summarized in Table 1.

Table 1. Data for current HCV diagnostic tests along with their key features and shortcomings.

Name	Method	Sample	Target	LOD	Time	Sensitivity	Specificity	Status	Strengths	Limitations	Reference
Vitros Anti-HCV, Ortho Clinical Diagnostics	CLIA	Serum/Plasma	Anti-HCV/Antigen; Core, NS3, NS4, NS5			100.00%	99.85%	FDA approved	High throughput; automated processing; good sensitivity and specificity	Longer processing time compared to other CLIA methods; requires specialized instruments	[104]
ARCHITECT HCV Ag/Ab Combo Assay	CMIA	Serum/Plasma	Anti-HCV/Antigen			93.40%	98.80%	Unknown	Combines antigen and antibody detection; reduces diagnostic window period; high throughput	Requires specialized equipment; higher cost compared to antibody-only tests	[61,105]
Alinity s Anti-HCV	CMIA	Serum/Plasma	Anti-HCV			100.00%	99.92%	FDA approved	High throughput; suitable for blood donor screening	Not intended for diagnostic confirmation; requires specialized equipment	[106,107]
Alinity s Anti-HCV II assay	CMIA	Serum/Plasma	Anti-HCV			100.00%	99.96%	FDA approved	High sensitivity and specificity, automated, high throughput,	Not intended for diagnostic confirmation; requires specialized equipment	[108]
Abbot Architect Anti-HCV	CMIA	Serum/Plasma	Anti-HCV			93.40%	98.92%	FDA approved	Can be used as a screening assay because of its high sensitivity, high throughput, and short turnaround time	Prone to false positives	[61,109]
Abbott PRISM HCV	ChLIA	Serum/Plasma	Anti-HCV			100.00%	99.89%	FDA approved	Qualitative detection of antibodies to HCV, suitable to donor screening	Not intended for diagnostic confirmation; requires specialized equipment	[110]
Abbott Anti-HCV 3.0	ELISA	Serum/Plasma	Anti-HCV/Antigen; Core, NS3, NS4, NS5				99.70%	FDA approved	Widely validated, sensitive as RNA detection techniques	Expensive, requires specialized equipment for processing	[50,111]
ORTHO EIA-3.0	ELISA	Serum/Plasma	Anti-HCV/Antigen; Core, NS3, NS4, NS5				99.90%	FDA approved	Established method with high sensitivity; suitable for blood donor screening	Requires specific equipment; requires confirmatory testing	[50,112]
Murex Anti-HCV 4.0	ELISA	Serum/Plasma	Anti-HCV			100.00%	99.80%	WHO prequalified	High sensitivity and specificity; detects all major HCV genotypes; suitable for high-throughput settings	Requires laboratory infrastructure; cannot detect acute infections during the window period	[113–115]
OraQuick HCV Rapid Antibody Test	Lateral Flow Assay	Fingerstick and Venipuncture Whole Blood/Serum/Plasma/Oral Fluid	Anti-HCV	20 IU/mL	20–40 min	Serum: 100.00%/Oral Fluid: 97.80%	100.00%	FDA approved	Rapid results, suitable for point of care for mass screening, clinical performance of the OraQuick HCV Test is comparable to that of laboratory-based tests with both serum and oral fluid, simple, non-instrumented	Higher chance of false-negative results	[54,116,117]

Table 1. *Cont.*

Name	Method	Sample	Target	LOD	Time	Sensitivity	Specificity	Status	Strengths	Limitations	Reference
OraQuick HCV Self-Test	Lateral Flow Assay	Oral Fluid	Anti-HCV		20 min	85.10%	99.80%	FDA approved	Only approved self-test, can be done at-home	high cost makes it difficult to deploy in low-resource areas, additional RNA testing required to validate results	[118]
UltraQual Multiplex PCR Assay	PCR	Serum/Plasma	RNA			93.70%	100.00%	FDA approved	High sensivitivty and specificity	Requires trained staff	[119]
Xpert HCV Viral Load test by Cepheid	RT-PCR	Plasma	RNA	10 IU/mL	2 h	94.40%	100.00%,	FDA approved	High specificity, suitable for smaller labs	Requires specialized platform to run tests	[97,98]
Xpert HCV Viral Load Finger-Stick assay (Xpert HCV VL FS)	RT-PCR	100 µL Whole Blood	RNA	>40 IU/mL	1 h	98.00%	100.00%	FDA approved	Accurately detect active infection from a finger-stick sample in 1 h allowing single-visit HCV diagnosis	Requires trained staff	[99]
TrueNAT HCV RNA assay	RT-PCR	Whole Blood/Serum/Plasma	RNA	Blood: 1153.94 IU/mL/Serum: 260.42 IU/mL/Plasma: 204.71 IU/mL	35 min	95.00%	99.00%	FDA approved	Small sample required, reusable chips, rapid results, easy to use	Not suitable for early infection detection	[120–122]
COBAS® AmpliPrep/COBAS® TaqMan® HCV Test, v2.0	RT-PCR	650 µL Serum/Plasma	RNA	15 IU/mL			100.00%	FDA approved	Fully automated, provides precise viral load measurements for effective treatment monitoring, high specificity	High cost, slow, specialized equipment and lab facilities required	[123–126]
Abbott Realtime HCV	RT-PCR	500 µL Serum/Plasma	RNA	12 IU/mL		100.00%	99.74%	FDA approved	High sensitivity and specificity; suitable for monitoring viral load during therapy	Not intended for blood donor screening; requires specialized equipment	[126–128]
Genedrive HCV ID	RT-PCR	30 µL Plasma	RNA	2362 IU/mL	90 min	98.60%	100.00%	CE-IVD	Ideal for low throughput, decentralised laboratories	Specialized equipment is needed, large sample volume required	[65,120, 129–131]
MedMira Miriad rapid HBc/HIV/HCV test	Rapid Immunoassay	Blood/Serum	Anti-HCV					Awaiting FDA approval	Rapid detection of multiple infectious markers; no complex infrastructure required	Lower sensitivity in early HCV infection	[132]
VERSANT HCV RNA TMA	TMA	Serum	RNA	Genotype 1: 5.3-9.6 IU/mL/Genotype 2b: 14.4 IU/mL			99.60%	FDA approved	No nucleic acid extraction is needed, and the process can be fully automated	Laborious process and bench space requirement when compared to other qualitative assays	[84,89,133, 134]
Aptima® HCV Quant Dx Assay	TMA	Serum/Plasma	RNA	4.3 IU/mL	2.5 h for first 5 samples then 5 min for every sample		98.60%	FDA approved	Detects and quantitates HCV RNA genotypes 1-6, is rapid, sensitive, and reproducible and accurately quantifies HCV RNA in serum samples from patients with chronic HCV infection	Requires expensive automation systems and is not approved for use as a screening test for the presence of HCV RNA in blood or blood products	[91,92, 135]

Table 1. *Cont.*

Name	Method	Sample	Target	LOD	Time	Sensitivity	Specificity	Status	Strengths	Limitations	Reference
Procleix® Ultrio Assay	TMA	2.5 mL Serum/Plasma	RNA			99.70%	100.00%	FDA approved	High sensitivity and specificity; simultaneous detection of multiple viruses (HIV-1, HCV, HBV); suitable for high-throughput screening	Requires specialized equipment and trained personnel; not intended for diagnostic purposes	[136]
VERSANT HCV RNA 3.0 Assay	bDNA	50 µL Serum	RNA	615 IU/mL			98.20%	FDA approved	Low risk of carryover contamination, enhanced branched design leads to more specificity	Requires trained staff and is expensive	[85,137]

5. Emerging and Future Detection Methods

5.1. Isothermal Amplification Based Tests

Isothermal amplification is a molecular testing method where amplification of the nucleic acids of interest is achieved utilizing a constant temperature instead of the thermocycling required of traditional PCR [138–140]. Rapid temperature cycling requires more complex power circuitry and precise temperature controllers. Isothermal tests simplify the equipment requirements by requiring basic incubators that are smaller, lighter, and consume less power [138]. These features, along with enhanced specificity, sensitivity, and shorter analysis time, make isothermal amplification techniques a promising avenue for decentralized testing as required by WHO recommendations [7]. Isothermal amplification has evolved tremendously since its initiation in the early 1990s. Numerous diverse isothermal amplification methods have been created, providing high sensitivity and commercial accessibility [141,142]. Some of the relevant isothermal amplification methods used for HCV detection are described here [143]. These isothermal amplification methods include Rolling Circle Amplification (RCA), Nucleic Acid Sequence-Based Amplification (NASBA), Recombinant polymerase amplification (RPA), Loop-mediated isothermal amplification (LAMP), and transcription-mediated amplification (TMA).

5.1.1. Loop-Mediated Isothermal Amplification (LAMP)

The technique of loop-mediated isothermal amplification (LAMP) was initially described in 2000. The LAMP method utilizes auto-cycling strand displacement of DNA, enabling the rapid accumulation of up to 10^9 copies of the target DNA/RNA within an hour [144]. The incorporation of reverse transcriptase allows for the amplification of RNA sequences (RT-LAMP). In the LAMP method, a DNA polymerase and four primers (inner and outer primers) are utilized, designed to recognize six specific target DNA sequences. During the initial stage of LAMP, two inner primers facilitate the synthesis of a stem-loop structure from the target DNA. This stem-loop structure acts as the starting point for the subsequent amplification cycles in LAMP [144]. In the second stage of LAMP, the primers bind to the loop region of the initial product, initiating displacement DNA synthesis. This procedure produces both the initial stem-loop DNA and a fresh stem-loop DNA strand twice the original length [144,145].

LAMP provides commercial and hospital laboratories with increased specificity, simplicity, and timeliness. The sole equipment necessary for this reaction is a heat block or a water bath maintained at a consistent temperature range of 62–65 °C (Figure 4) [144–146]. The convenience of this process allows it to be used in POC screening for targeted populations at higher risk for virus infection that often remain asymptomatic, as is the case with HCV [142]. This assay also has a high tolerance to biological substrate contamination [70]. The LAMP assays' drawbacks include the primer design complexity and their inability to perform multiplex amplification [70]. LAMP has also been used to successfully identify multiple viruses, including influenza virus, SARS-CoV-2, mumps virus, West Nile virus, hepatitis B (HBV), human immunodeficiency virus 1 (HIV-1), hepatitis A virus (HAV), and hepatitis E virus (HEV) [147–154].

5.1.2. AP-LAMP

The use of LAMP in the detection of HCV, which has traditionally been complicated by the complex secondary structure of the 5′ untranslated region (5′-UTR), was achieved through a modified method by Yang et al. in 2011 [155]. In their method, termed AP-LAMP, they utilized three additional primers: two loop primers (LF and LB) and an acceleration primer (AP) [155]. Here, the AP is particularly important to the modified reaction as it adds a starting DNA synthesis site, binding between the active sites of primers F1 and B1. SYBR

Green I cyanine dye was added to the assay to allow easier detection of the nucleic acids without specialized equipment, turning the sample from orange to green upon positive AP-LAMP reactions [155]. AP-LAMP showed a sensitivity of 84 IU/mL [155]. They also reported an average threshold time (Tt) for positive assay signal detection of 17.99 $\pm$ 0.62 min (mean $\pm$ SD) for a 5×10^5 IU RNA sample and 31.70 $\pm$ 0.43 min (mean $\pm$ SD) for a sample containing 5×10^2 IU of HCV RNA [155].

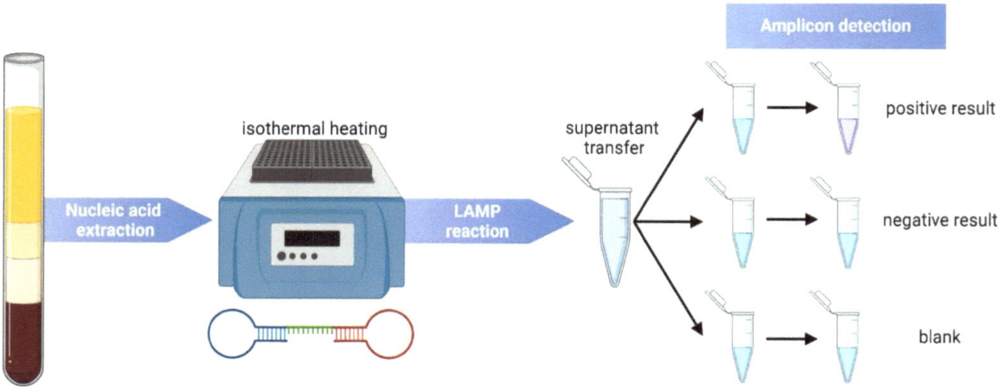

Figure 4. LAMP process. The figure illustrates the LAMP reaction that is used for the amplification of DNA. The process begins with the binding of the primers to the target DNA sequence. The primers then initiate the strand displacement amplification, where the target DNA is amplified at a constant temperature. Visual detection can be achieved by adding an appropriate reagent. Created with BioRender.com, accessed on 13 December 2022.

5.1.3. Other LAMP Assays

Additionally, LAMP assay variations have also been developed to detect HCV. In 2015, Nyan et al. published a rapid fluorogenic multiplex isothermal amplification assay allowing for naked-eye visualization of a positive test under UV light and quantitative measurability with a fluorospectrophotometer [156]. Their assay showed an impressive 97% sensitivity and 100% specificity with no viral cross-reactions observed [156]. In 2016, Nyan and Swinson published an RT-LAMP method for simultaneous HCV detection and identification of genotypes 1–6 in under 60 min [156]. Their assay had a 91.5% diagnostic sensitivity and detection rates of 50% and 100% at 50 and 10^2 IU of HCV RNA, respectively [157]. In 2018, Chen et al. published a method called BEAMing LAMP, which combines emulsion microreactors and single-molecule magnetic capture with on-bead LAMP [158]. This assay first immobilizes FIP primers onto magnetic beads and incubates with an HCV cDNA sample [158]. The cycling process is initiated once the beads are washed and resuspended in a mixture containing LAMP reagents and primers. This method demonstrates significant potential for the future diagnosis of HCV, boasting a detection limit of 300 RNA copies. However, it still faces challenges related to its intricate workflow and primer design [158].

5.2. Surface Plasmon Resonance Based Testing

Surface plasmon resonance (SPR) is a highly sensitive and label-free detection technique utilized to measure biomolecular interactions in real-time (Figure 5) [159]. Since its development in the 1990s, there have been multiple advancements in SPR-type technology. SPR finds several biomedical applications, including the analysis of molecular interactions, investigations into conformational changes, mutation detection, and the primary screening of potentially druggable molecules [159]. Raman spectroscopy (RS) is an example of a technology similar to SPR that has been employed in the detection and diagnosis of infectious diseases. RS relies on the inelastic scattering of light photons following interaction with molecular bonds within a given sample. This provides valuable information regarding the molecular composition of a sample; however, RS is not without its own shortcomings. Differentiating the spectra of pathological samples from normal ones with the naked eye is challenging due to the complex nature of Raman spectra [160]. This is where other technological developments may come into play in the future when considering increasing the utility of this method.

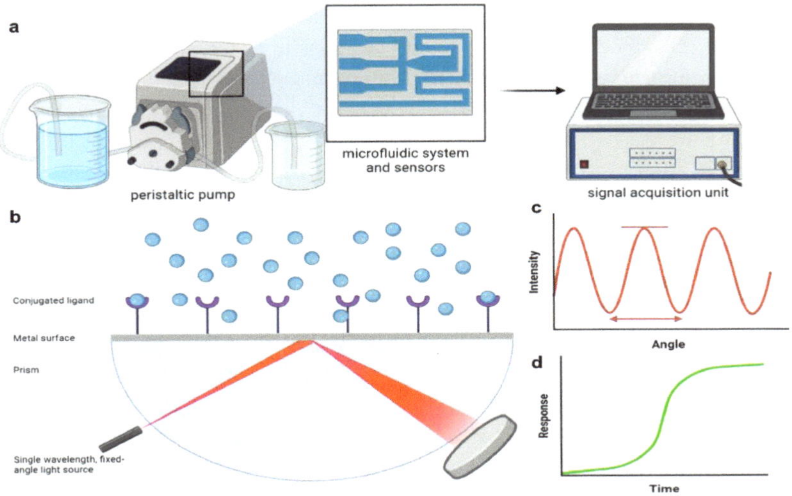

Figure 5. (**a**) Schematic of SPR sensor integrated with microfluidics and other peripherals. (**b**) Prototypical SPR biosensor. Analyte (blue) binds ligand (purple), causing a change in the refractive index of the surrounding solution. (**c**,**d**) Differences in single-wavelength light reflection, absorbance, and refraction are detected using surface plasmon resonance. Created with BioRender.com, accessed on 13 December 2022.

Another specific example of an SPR-type technology that has been used in the study of HCV is surface-enhanced Raman spectroscopy (SERS). This technique increases the detection signal in comparison with Raman spectroscopy by detecting absorbed particles on a metal surface. Noble metal nanoparticles (NPs) are required to enable high detection sensitivity. These NPs should be of the proper shape and size for the SERS platform [161]. The metallic nanostructures amplify the Raman scattering signals, which has been shown to increase sensitivity by 10–400 fold [162]. Additionally, using different Raman-active labels, Shi et al. have shown multiplex detection. This is important in HCV diagnostics because it offers comprehensive antigen detection and simultaneously tests for HBV and HIV coinfections [163]. The ability to minimize the autofluorescence of the sample helps to enhance the clarity of the specific signals, improving the sensitivity of the assay since background fluorescence can obscure specific signals.

In one study, SERS was used for the detection of HCV from human serum samples. SERS resulted in a peak detected at 785 cm^{-1} (ring breathing modes in the RNA base/uracil). This SERS signal is related to RNA present in the virus, as uracil is present only in the RNA (not DNA) [164]. This feature is of utmost importance, given that HCV is an RNA virus. This study observed that the primary distinguishing SERS characteristics are absent in the control (uninfected) sample while being present in the HCV-positive samples [164]. Therefore, the spectral features mentioned with SERS in the HCV RNA could be used for diagnostic purposes and further employed for qualitative and quantitative analysis of HCV from patient blood samples [165].

Researchers have developed another method utilizing polypyrrole-peptide chips and surface plasmon imaging (Figure 5) [166]. One peptide was derived from ovalbumin, while 11 peptides were derived from the HCV virus, encompassing both structural and non-structural proteins [166]. These peptides were functionalized and immobilized on the chip's gold surface (as 300 and 500 μm spots) (Figure 5b). A p-polarized LED beam was used to illuminate the gold sensor chip, and the light reflected is recorded by a CCD camera, enabling simultaneous analysis of binding events on all spots [166]. This method allowed the detection of antibodies even at low concentrations in serum [166]. This technique has shown promise to be highly specific in studying and screening biological samples in label-free, real-time conditions [166].

5.3. Microfluidics

Microfluidics relies on two main factors: micrometric size and the handling of nanoliter quantities of fluids [167]. Microfluidic chip devices provide precise fluid control, a high surface-to-volume ratio, low sample requirements, and high integration with functional components. Several microfluidic-based HCV testing methods have been developed, including microfluidic DNA/RNA amplification, rapid immunoassay systems, and sensors. The immunoassay system comprises lateral flow assays (LFAs) and immuno-filtration assays (IFAs) that detect specific antigens or antibodies in samples. LFAs detect the target in a liquid sample that migrates laterally across a test strip via capillary action. The detection is made when the target analyte binds with the labeled antibodies, providing qualitative results in the form of a visible colored line [168]. Guo et al. developed a single-line flow assay platform that is based on orthogonal emissive upconversion nanoparticles. Their single-line platform combines the test and control lines on traditional LFAs, where one emission is used as a reporting signal and the other as a calibrating signal [169]. Since the diffusion distance of the sample is limited on the chip, this method reduces the size of the strip or allows the testing of multiple targets in a sample [169]. Tang et al. demonstrated a signal enhancement technique for LFAs by integrating a sponge shunt to decrease the fluid flow rate. Their idea was to allow an extended time for the analyte to bind to immobilized antibodies, resulting in a higher number of detectable complexes. They demonstrated a 10-fold increase in sensitivity over unmodified LFA by detecting down to 10^3 copies/mL of HBV DNA [170]. This technique highlights the potential for point-of-care application in various disease diagnostics, including HCV [170].

IFA, on the other hand, is known as a flow-through assay, in which a porous filtration membrane is used where specific antigens are immobilized so that specific HCV antibody binding can take place along with filtration [167]. IFAs are constricted in their clinical diagnostic capabilities and are qualitative or semi-qualitative. Zhang et al. devised an immunofluorescence assay (IFA) using quantum dots (QDs) as fluorescent labels, which were coated with polyethylene glycol (PEG) and glutathione. This IFA was designed specifically for quantitatively detecting C-reactive proteins, a commonly utilized diagnostic indicator for acute viral and bacterial infections [167].

Furthermore, microfluidic paper-based analytic devices (μPAD) use paper as an emerging substrate material, which is less expensive [171]. Its intrinsic capillary force has the ability to move liquids; as a result, it eliminates the need for external power sources [171]. Nitrocellulose is a patterned structure at 100 °C to create multiple test zones [171]. The antigen or antibody is diluted to specific concentrations using phosphate-buffered saline (PBS) with a pH of 7.4 [171]. Then, 0.5 μL of the solutions is pipetted onto each detection zone of the patterned paper [171]. The paper is left to air dry for 30 min, and then it is subjected to blocking in a solution of PBS containing 5% BSA and 0.05% Tween-20 for 60 min [171]. A total of 0.3 µL of positive and negative control and diluted patient serum are pipetted into the blocked detection zone for 1 min to detect anti-HCV. Subsequently, the detection zones are washed [171]. The patient's serum is diluted (1:50) in PBS containing 10% BSA [171]. The patterned paper is subsequently exposed to a solution containing HRP-labeled anti-human IgG (diluted at a ratio of 1:50,000) for 2 min. After the incubation period, the paper is carefully washed. A total of 250 µL of mixed chemiluminescence substrate is poured into the patterned paper after separating enzyme-labeled antibodies [171]. A minute later, the majority of the liquid is aspirated out, followed by detection [171]. The modulus micro-plate multimode reader detects the chemiluminescence of the commercial ELISA kit [171].

A novel lab-on-disk (LOD) system utilizing LAMP was specifically developed to enable the concurrent detection of cytomegalovirus (CMV), hepatitis B (HBV), and (HCV) infections [172]. This system offers a highly sensitive and specific one-step nucleic acid amplification process in the microfluidic-based LOD system [172]. The LAMP-based LOD test results are determined by observing turbidity using the SPR lamp detection system [172]. Chang et al. developed a fully automated LAMP-based LOD system that enables rapid diagnostics in less than one hour. This system is capable of detecting hepatitis B virus (HBV), cytomegalovirus (CMV), and hepatitis C virus (HCV) infections [172]. The Chang et al. system has key advantages: it requires less sample volume and time for sample processing than conventional LAMP [172]. These features can make it a POC technology used in resource-limited areas. However, the test takes longer to report results than an ideal POC test, so future research should focus on reducing the time to obtain results.

The advantage of using the microfluid technique is that it can work with a small sample size, which helps in reducing the overall cost [173]. Other advantages are in the potential applications in the POC setting [173]. Sensing or sample pretreatment modules used by microfluidic systems significantly increase efficiency and decrease the chances of cross-contamination [173].

5.4. Electrochemical-Based Sensing

Electrochemical sensing has been used to detect viruses and other pathogens. This technique utilizes conducting and semiconducting materials as an electrode. The binding between the biorecognition element and the pathogen produces chemical energy, which is then converted to electrical energy [174]. The different methods utilizing electrochemical energy for pathogen detection can be categorized as amperometric, conductometric, ion-charge/field effect, impedimetric, and potentiometric [175]. Electrochemical genosensor technology used to detect HCV facilitates obtaining results with higher sensitivity. However, it is essential to note that replication of cDNA requires PCR [176].

Another type of electrochemical-based sensing that has been used in the study of HCV is electrochemical immunosensors. In a recent study, a biosensor was created employing graphitized mesoporous carbon-methylene blue as an electrode modification material. At the same time, a secondary antibody layer was formed using horseradish peroxidase-DNA-coated carboxyl multi-wall carbon nanotubes [177]. The immunosensor exhibited excellent performance, demonstrating a low detection limit of 0.01 pg/mL [177]. The future of this technology appears promising.

Electrochemical sensors have even been integrated with microfluidics for the detection of viral RNA from HCV. A 2016 study showed that a DNA-grafted multiwall carbon nanotube (MWCNT) biosensor in a microfluidic device with enhanced flow protocol demonstrated promising sensitivity. For HCV, this study demonstrated an enhanced dynamic range from one per second to six per second compared to macroscale systems [178].

5.5. CRISPR

Clustered regularly interspaced short palindromic repeats (CRISPR) systems can potentially be extended into diagnosing HCV. CRISPR is a gene-editing technology that has many applications in addition to diagnostics. CRISPR has two components: an endonuclease, most commonly CAS9, and a guide RNA that matches the gene target [179]. The endonuclease causes a break in the DNA genome, allowing it to be modified in many ways. Some uses include modifying genes that underlie genetic disorders, treatment of HIV, and engineering somatic stem cells as novel therapeutic approaches to treat malignancies [179].

Recently CRISPR has been used to detect HCV and also to inhibit the virus. Weiss et al. developed the ability to target HCV within eukaryotic cells using the endonuclease from Francisella novicida [180]. They also used FnCas9 proteins to inhibit viral protein production during HCV infection within the infected cells [180]. Furthermore, Jain et al. used CRISPR-Cas12a complexes to detect HCV [181]. In addition, they also developed a platform with crRNAs and optimized conditions to detect various clinically significant nucleic acid targets in the femtomolar range [181]. CRISPR is an emerging technology being used to detect viral infection; however, additional advances will be needed before it can be developed into a routinely utilized technology to detect HCV RNA. The characteristics of the various diagnostic techniques discussed above that show promising use in HCV testing in the future are highlighted (Table 2).

Table 2. Summary of future diagnostic techniques for HCV, their strengths and limitations.

	Strengths	Limitations	References
LAMP	Isothermal technique does not require expensive bulky thermocyclers, making it suitable for low-resource settings. Tests for viral nucleic acid, which makes it more sensitive than immunoassays.	Is known to have higher false positive rates. Utilizes 4–6 primers, which makes primer designing complex.	[138,144,156]
Surface Plasmon Resonance	Real-time quantification with high sensitivity. Precise measurement of binding kinetics. High multiplexing capacity. Label-free method.	Requires instruments that are not currently point-of-care friendly. Performance can be affected by non-specific binding. Needs extensive sample preparation for effective analysis.	[159,165,182]
Microfluidics	Minimizes reagent and sample volumes, reducing costs. Facilitates the combination of multiple analytical steps on a single chip. Enables high-throughput analysis with faster turnaround times.	Developing and manufacturing microfluidic devices can be intricate and expensive. Susceptible to blockages and issues with sample flow control.	[173,183]
Electrochemical Sensors	Capable of detecting low concentrations of analytes. Potential for compact, point-of-care devices. Generally lower production costs compared to optical systems. Label-free.	Electrochemical signals can be affected by impurities. Electrode surfaces may degrade over time, impacting performance. Requires regular calibration for accurate results.	[177,178,184]
CRISPR	Utilizes CRISPR-Cas systems for precise target recognition, offering high specificity. Potential to be point-of-care friendly.	Is still under development, with limited widespread clinical validation. Pending comprehensive regulatory endorsements for clinical use.	[185,186]

6. Future Directions and Conclusions

In conclusion, HCV is a viral infection that is associated with significant mortality and morbidity globally. HCV prevalence is estimated to be around 50 million people. Early detection of HCV infection through testing is crucial in preventing long-term complications such as cirrhosis, hepatocellular carcinoma, and decompensated liver disease. Despite the limitations of testing methods, early detection of HCV remains a crucial step in the clinical management of the infection and facilitates the initiation of antiviral therapy.

The most common testing methods, as stated earlier, are PCR and EIA. The most widely used approach for testing is an EIA to test for the presence of HCV Abs, which indicates exposure. If the EIA is positive, a PCR test is subsequently performed to confirm active viral infection. EIA can produce false-negative results if conducted too soon after exposure to the virus and the inability to differentiate between those with active infections, those who have spontaneously cleared the virus, or those who have been cured through antiviral therapy. PCR, on the other hand, is more expensive and requires specialized laboratory equipment and trained personnel, which hinders its ability to be used in resource-limited areas. Additionally, the two-step testing approach is not feasible since it results in incomplete testing when patients do not return for confirmatory molecular testing. There is a dire need for single-step sample collection and dried blood spot testing to be adopted globally. In the long term, testing needs to be decentralized, for which technologies such as LAMP, SPR, microfluidics, electrochemical-based sensing, and CRISPR are looking to bridge the gap and cut the cost of traditional molecular tests that leverage PCR. If developed for HCV, these technologies can be used for the detection of other viral diseases.

The emerging technologies being developed are paramount in improving affordability and sensitivity. POC rapid RNA detection can detect HCV when an active infection occurs, and antibodies are yet to be produced. However, POC rapid RNA detection methods may require more extensive sample preparation, which is a significant challenge. Ideally, new technologies will facilitate the development of a low-cost automated sample preparation process that can take whole blood without extensive preprocessing and create a more amenable analyte to enable HCV detection on the same platform/device in under an hour. If successful, this would be a significant advance in HCV diagnosis, particularly in resource-limited settings, making sure that undiagnosed patients could be linked with appropriate antiviral therapy.

Funding: We acknowledge research support from the National Institute of Health (NIH), awards—RAI154643B, R61AI154643, and the National Science Foundation (NSF) CAREER, award—1942487. Also, R35GM124915 for ET.

Institutional Review Board Statement: Not applicable.

Informed Consent Statement: Not applicable.

Data Availability Statement: Not applicable.

Conflicts of Interest: Authors declare no conflicts of interest.

References

1. Hoofnagle, J.H. Course and Outcome of Hepatitis C. *Hepatology* **2002**, *36*, s21–s29. [CrossRef] [PubMed]
2. Rantala, M.; van de Laar, M.J. Surveillance and Epidemiology of Hepatitis B and C in Europe—A Review. *Eurosurveillance* **2008**, *13*, 18880. [CrossRef] [PubMed]
3. Centers for Disease Control and Prevention (U.S.). The ABCs of Hepatitis—for Health Professionals. Available online: https://stacks.cdc.gov/view/cdc/130187 (accessed on 29 November 2024).
4. Ohto, H.; Terazawa, S.; Sasaki, N.; Sasaki, N.; Hino, K.; Ishiwata, C.; Kako, M.; Ujiie, N.; Endo, C.; Matsui, A.; et al. Transmission of Hepatitis C Virus from Mothers to Infants. *N. Engl. J. Med.* **1994**, *330*, 744–750. [CrossRef] [PubMed]
5. Choo, Q.-L.; Kuo, G.; Weiner, A.J.; Overby, L.R.; Bradley, D.W.; Houghton, M. Isolation of a CDNA CLone Derived from a Blood-Borne Non-A, Non-B Viral Hepatitis Genome. *Science* **1989**, *244*, 359–362. [CrossRef]
6. Kuo, G.; Choo, Q.-L.; Alter, H.J.; Gitnick, G.L.; Redeker, A.G.; Purcell, R.H.; Miyamura, T.; Dienstag, J.L.; Alter, M.J.; Stevens, C.E.; et al. An Assay for Circulating Antibodies to a Major Etiologic Virus of Human Non-A, Non-B Hepatitis. *Science* **1989**, *244*, 362–364. [CrossRef]
7. World Health Organization. *Global Hepatitis Report 2024: Action for Access in Low- and Middle-Income Countries*; World Health Organization: Geneva, Switzerland, 2024.

8. Kwo, P.Y.; Poordad, F.; Asatryan, A.; Wang, S.; Wyles, D.L.; Hassanein, T.; Felizarta, F.; Sulkowski, M.S.; Gane, E.; Maliakkal, B.; et al. Glecaprevir and Pibrentasvir Yield High Response Rates in Patients with HCV Genotype 1–6 without Cirrhosis. *J. Hepatol.* **2017**, *67*, 263–271. [CrossRef]
9. Guntipalli, P.; Pakala, R.; Kumari Gara, S.; Ahmed, F.; Bhatnagar, A.; Endaya Coronel, M.-K.; Razzack, A.A.; Solimando, A.G.; Thompson, A.; Andrews, K.; et al. Worldwide Prevalence, Genotype Distribution and Management of Hepatitis C. *Acta Gastro Enterol. Belg.* **2021**, *84*, 633–652. [CrossRef]
10. Clinicalinfo.HIV.gov. Hepatitis C Virus. Available online: https://clinicalinfo.hiv.gov/en/guidelines/hiv-clinical-guidelines-adult-and-adolescent-opportunistic-infections/hepatitis-c-virus?utm_source=chatgpt.com (accessed on 4 December 2024).
11. Manns, M.P.; Buti, M.; Gane, E.; Pawlotsky, J.-M.; Razavi, H.; Terrault, N.; Younossi, Z. Hepatitis C Virus Infection. *Nat. Rev. Dis. Primers* **2017**, *3*, 17006. [CrossRef]
12. Hoofnagle, J.H. Hepatitis C: The Clinical Spectrum of Disease. *Hepatology* **1997**, *26*, 15S–20S. [CrossRef]
13. Hoofnagle, J. Fulminant Hepatic Failure: Summary of a Workshop*1. *Hepatology* **1995**, *21*, 240–252. [CrossRef]
14. Meshram, R.J.; Kathwate, G.H.; Gacche, R.N. Progress, Evolving Therapeutic/Diagnostic Approaches, and Challenges in the Management of Hepatitis C Virus Infections. *Arch. Virol.* **2022**, *167*, 717–736. [CrossRef] [PubMed]
15. Baber, A.S.; Suganthan, B.; Ramasamy, R.P. Current Advances in Hepatitis C Diagnostics. *J. Biol. Eng.* **2024**, *18*, 48. [CrossRef] [PubMed]
16. Hayes, C.N.; Imamura, M.; Tanaka, J.; Chayama, K. Road to Elimination of HCV: Clinical Challenges in HCV Management. *Liver Int.* **2022**, *42*, 1935–1944. [CrossRef] [PubMed]
17. Centers for Disease Control and Prevention Clinical Screening and Diagnosis for Hepatitis C. Available online: https://www.cdc.gov/hepatitis-c/hcp/diagnosis-testing/index.html (accessed on 29 November 2024).
18. Alaama, A.S.; Khattabi, H.; Mugisa, B.; Atta, H.; Hermez, J.; Hutin, Y.J. Progress towards Elimination of Viral Hepatitis by 2030 in the WHO Eastern Mediterranean Region, 2019. *Lancet Gastroenterol. Hepatol.* **2022**, *7*, 862–870. [CrossRef] [PubMed]
19. Niepmann, M.; Gerresheim, G.K. Hepatitis C Virus Translation Regulation. *Int. J. Mol. Sci.* **2020**, *21*, 2328. [CrossRef]
20. Bajpai, P.S.; Collignon, L.; Sølund, C.; Madsen, L.W.; Christensen, P.B.; Øvrehus, A.; Weis, N.; Holmbeck, K.; Fahnøe, U.; Bukh, J. Full-Length Sequence Analysis of Hepatitis C Virus Genotype 3b Strains and Development of an *in Vivo* Infectious 3b CDNA Clone. *J. Virol.* **2023**, *97*, e0092523. [CrossRef]
21. Glynn, S.A.; Wright, D.J.; Kleinman, S.H.; Hirschkorn, D.; Tu, Y.; Heldebrant, C.; Smith, R.; Giachetti, C.; Gallarda, J.; Busch, M.P. Dynamics of Viremia in Early Hepatitis C Virus Infection. *Transfusion* **2005**, *45*, 994–1002. [CrossRef]
22. Mulrooney-Cousins, P.M.; Michalak, T.I. Molecular Testing in Hepatitis Virus-Related Disease. In *Diagnostic Molecular Pathology*; Elsevier: Amsterdam, The Netherlands, 2024; pp. 63–77.
23. Moradpour, D.; Penin, F. Hepatitis C Virus Proteins: From Structure to Function. *Curr. Top. Microbiol. Immunol.* **2013**, *369*, 113–142.
24. Catanese, M.T.; Uryu, K.; Kopp, M.; Edwards, T.J.; Andrus, L.; Rice, W.J.; Silvestry, M.; Kuhn, R.J.; Rice, C.M. Ultrastructural Analysis of Hepatitis C Virus Particles. *Proc. Natl. Acad. Sci. USA* **2013**, *110*, 9505–9510. [CrossRef]
25. Fusco, D.N.; Chung, R.T. Novel Therapies for Hepatitis C: Insights from the Structure of the Virus. *Annu. Rev. Med.* **2012**, *63*, 373–387. [CrossRef]
26. Martinello, M.; Naggie, S.; Rockstroh, J.K.; Matthews, G. V Direct-Acting Antiviral Therapy for Treatment of Acute and Recent Hepatitis C Virus Infection: A Narrative Review. *Clin. Infect. Dis.* **2023**, *77*, S238–S244. [CrossRef] [PubMed]
27. Sillanpaa, M.; Melen, K.; Porkka, P.; Fagerlund, R.; Nevalainen, K.; Lappalainen, M.; Julkunen, I. Hepatitis C Virus Core, NS3, NS4B and NS5A Are the Major Immunogenic Proteins in Humoral Immunity in Chronic HCV Infection. *Virol. J.* **2009**, *6*, 84. [CrossRef] [PubMed]
28. Popescu, C.-I.; Riva, L.; Vlaicu, O.; Farhat, R.; Rouillé, Y.; Dubuisson, J. Hepatitis C Virus Life Cycle and Lipid Metabolism. *Biology* **2014**, *3*, 892–921. [CrossRef]
29. Falson, P.; Bartosch, B.; Alsaleh, K.; Tews, B.A.; Loquet, A.; Ciczora, Y.; Riva, L.; Montigny, C.; Montpellier, C.; Duverlie, G.; et al. Hepatitis C Virus Envelope Glycoprotein E1 Forms Trimers at the Surface of the Virion. *J. Virol.* **2015**, *89*, 10333–10346. [CrossRef]
30. Aizaki, H.; Morikawa, K.; Fukasawa, M.; Hara, H.; Inoue, Y.; Tani, H.; Saito, K.; Nishijima, M.; Hanada, K.; Matsuura, Y.; et al. Critical Role of Virion-Associated Cholesterol and Sphingolipid in Hepatitis C Virus Infection. *J. Virol.* **2008**, *82*, 5715–5724. [CrossRef]
31. Gastaminza, P.; Dryden, K.A.; Boyd, B.; Wood, M.R.; Law, M.; Yeager, M.; Chisari, F.V. Ultrastructural and Biophysical Characterization of Hepatitis C Virus Particles Produced in Cell Culture. *J. Virol.* **2010**, *84*, 10999–11009. [CrossRef]
32. Merz, A.; Long, G.; Hiet, M.-S.; Brügger, B.; Chlanda, P.; Andre, P.; Wieland, F.; Krijnse-Locker, J.; Bartenschlager, R. Biochemical and Morphological Properties of Hepatitis C Virus Particles and Determination of Their Lipidome. *J. Biol. Chem.* **2011**, *286*, 3018–3032. [CrossRef]
33. Yamamoto, M.; Aizaki, H.; Fukasawa, M.; Teraoka, T.; Miyamura, T.; Wakita, T.; Suzuki, T. Structural Requirements of Virion-Associated Cholesterol for Infectivity, Buoyant Density and Apolipoprotein Association of Hepatitis C Virus. *J. Gen. Virol.* **2011**, *92*, 2082–2087. [CrossRef]

34. Cashman, S.B.; Marsden, B.D.; Dustin, L.B. The Humoral Immune Response to HCV: Understanding Is Key to Vaccine Development. *Front. Immunol.* **2014**, *5*, 550. [CrossRef]
35. Brasher, N.A.; Adhikari, A.; Lloyd, A.R.; Tedla, N.; Bull, R.A. Hepatitis C Virus Epitope Immunodominance and B Cell Repertoire Diversity. *Viruses* **2021**, *13*, 983. [CrossRef]
36. Busch, M.P.; Shafer, K.A.P. Editorial Commentary: Acute-Phase Hepatitis C Virus Infection: Implications for Research, Diagnosis, and Treatment. *Clin. Infect. Dis.* **2005**, *40*, 959–961. [CrossRef] [PubMed]
37. Nübling, C.M.; Unger, G.; Chudy, M.; Raia, S.; Löwer, J. Sensitivity of HCV Core Antigen and HCV RNA Detection in the Early Infection Phase. *Transfusion* **2002**, *42*, 1037–1045. [CrossRef] [PubMed]
38. Tharakan, S.; Faqah, O.; Asghar, W.; Ilyas, A. Microfluidic Devices for HIV Diagnosis and Monitoring at Point-of-Care (POC) Settings. *Biosensors* **2022**, *12*, 949. [CrossRef]
39. Wang, Y.; Jie, W.; Ling, J.; Yuanshuai, H. HCV Core Antigen Plays an Important Role in the Fight against HCV as an Alternative to HCV-RNA Detection. *J. Clin. Lab. Anal.* **2021**, *35*, e23755. [CrossRef]
40. Feld, J.J. Hepatitis C Virus Diagnostics: The Road to Simplification. *Clin. Liver Dis.* **2018**, *12*, 125–129. [CrossRef]
41. Cartwright, E.J.; Patel, P.; Kamili, S.; Wester, C. Updated Operational Guidance for Implementing CDC's Recommendations on Testing for Hepatitis C Virus Infection. *MMWR Morb. Mortal. Wkly. Rep.* **2023**, *72*, 766–768. [CrossRef]
42. Trickey, A.; Fajardo, E.; Alemu, D.; Artenie, A.A.; Easterbrook, P. Impact of Hepatitis C Virus Point-of-Care RNA Viral Load Testing Compared with Laboratory-Based Testing on Uptake of RNA Testing and Treatment, and Turnaround Times: A Systematic Review and Meta-Analysis. *Lancet Gastroenterol. Hepatol.* **2023**, *8*, 253–270. [CrossRef]
43. Ivanova Reipold, E.; Shilton, S.; Donolato, M.; Fernandez Suarez, M. Molecular Point-of-Care Testing for Hepatitis C: Available Technologies, Pipeline, and Promising Future Directions. *J. Infect. Dis.* **2024**, *229*, S342–S349. [CrossRef]
44. Thomson, E.C.; Nastouli, E.; Main, J.; Karayiannis, P.; Eliahoo, J.; Muir, D.; McClure, M.O. Delayed Anti-HCV Antibody Response in HIV-Positive Men Acutely Infected with HCV. *AIDS* **2009**, *23*, 89–93. [CrossRef]
45. Vanhommerig, J.W.; Thomas, X.V.; van der Meer, J.T.M.; Geskus, R.B.; Bruisten, S.M.; Molenkamp, R.; Prins, M.; Schinkel, J.; Arends, J.; van Baarle, D.; et al. Hepatitis C Virus (HCV) Antibody Dynamics Following Acute HCV Infection and Reinfection Among HIV-Infected Men Who Have Sex With Men. *Clin. Infect. Dis.* **2014**, *59*, 1678–1685. [CrossRef]
46. Warkad, S.D.; Song, K.-S.; Pal, D.; Nimse, S.B. Developments in the HCV Screening Technologies Based on the Detection of Antigens and Antibodies. *Sensors* **2019**, *19*, 4257. [CrossRef] [PubMed]
47. Lee, S.; McHutchinson, J.; Francis, B.; DiNello, R.; Polito, A.; Quan, S.; Nelles, M. Improved Detection of Antibodies to Hepatitis C Virus Using a Second Generation Elisa. *Adv. Exp. Med. Biol.* **1992**, *312*, 183–189. [PubMed]
48. Bernvil, S.S.; Andrews, V.J.; Sasich, F. Second-Generation Anti-HCV Screening in a Saudi Arabian Donor Population. *Vox Sang.* **1994**, *66*, 33–36. [CrossRef]
49. Uyttendaele, S.; Claeys, H.; Mertens, W.; Verhaert, H.; Vermylen, C. Evaluation of Third-Generation Screening and Confirmatory Assays for HCV Antibodies. *Vox Sang.* **1994**, *66*, 122–129. [CrossRef]
50. Vrielink, H.; Zaaijer, H.L.; Reesink, H.W.; van der Poel, C.L.; Cuypers, H.T.M.; Lelie, P.N. Sensitivity and Specificity of Three Third-Generation Anti-Hepatitis C Virus ELISAs. *Vox Sang.* **1995**, *69*, 14–17. [CrossRef]
51. Jiang, X.; Chang, L.; Yan, Y.; Ji, H.; Sun, H.; Guo, F.; Wang, L. A Study Based on Four Immunoassays: Hepatitis C Virus Antibody against Different Antigens May Have Unequal Contributions to Detection. *Virol. J.* **2021**, *18*, 137. [CrossRef]
52. Hawkins, R.C. Laboratory Turnaround Time. *Clin. Biochem. Rev.* **2007**, *28*, 179–194.
53. Smith, B.D.; Jewett, A.; Drobeniuc, J.; Kamili, S. Rapid Diagnostic HCV Antibody Assays. *Antivir. Ther.* **2012**, *17*, 1409–1413. [CrossRef]
54. Cha, Y.J.; Park, Q.; Kang, E.-S.; Yoo, B.C.; Park, K.U.; Kim, J.-W.; Hwang, Y.-S.; Kim, M.H. Performance Evaluation of the OraQuick Hepatitis C Virus Rapid Antibody Test. *Ann. Lab. Med.* **2013**, *33*, 184–189. [CrossRef]
55. Step-by-Step Instructions For OraQuick® HCV Rapid Antibody Test. Available online: https://www.health.ny.gov/diseases/communicable/hepatitis/hepatitis_c/docs/oraquick_step_by_step.pdf (accessed on 29 November 2024).
56. World Health Organization. WHO Prequalifies the First Self-Test for Hepatitis C Virus. Available online: https://www.who.int/news/item/10-07-2024-who-prequalifies-the-first-self-test-for-hepatitis-c-virus (accessed on 9 December 2024).
57. OraQuick OraQuick HCV Self Test. Available online: https://global.oraquick.com/media/wysiwyg/hcv/ART-3001-3729-70_V1.0.pdf (accessed on 9 December 2024).
58. Fajardo, E.; Watson, V.; Kumwenda, M.; Usharidze, D.; Gogochashvili, S.; Kakhaberi, D.; Giguashvili, A.; Johnson, C.C.; Jamil, M.S.; Dacombe, R.; et al. Usability and Acceptability of Oral-Based HCV Self-Testing among Key Populations: A Mixed-Methods Evaluation in Tbilisi, Georgia. *BMC Infect. Dis.* **2022**, *22*, 510. [CrossRef]
59. Medmira Multiplo Rapid HBc/HIV/HCV Antibody Test. Available online: https://medmira.com/multiplex/ (accessed on 9 December 2024).

60. Freiman, J.M.; Tran, T.M.; Schumacher, S.G.; White, L.F.; Ongarello, S.; Cohn, J.; Easterbrook, P.J.; Linas, B.P.; Denkinger, C.M. Hepatitis C Core Antigen Testing for Diagnosis of Hepatitis C Virus Infection. *Ann. Intern. Med.* **2016**, *165*, 345. [CrossRef] [PubMed]
61. Kabir, M.A.; Zilouchian, H.; Younas, M.A.; Asghar, W. Dengue Detection: Advances in Diagnostic Tools from Conventional Technology to Point of Care. *Biosensors* **2021**, *11*, 206. [CrossRef]
62. Scott, J.D.; Gretch, D.R. Molecular Diagnostics of Hepatitis C Virus Infection. *JAMA* **2007**, *297*, 724. [CrossRef] [PubMed]
63. Pawlotsky, J.-M.; Negro, F.; Aghemo, A.; Berenguer, M.; Dalgard, O.; Dusheiko, G.; Marra, F.; Puoti, M.; Wedemeyer, H. EASL Recommendations on Treatment of Hepatitis C 2018. *J. Hepatol.* **2018**, *69*, 461–511. [CrossRef]
64. Shahid, I.; Alzahrani, A.R.; Al-Ghamdi, S.S.; Alanazi, I.M.; Rehman, S.; Hassan, S. Hepatitis C Diagnosis: Simplified Solutions, Predictive Barriers, and Future Promises. *Diagnostics* **2021**, *11*, 1253. [CrossRef]
65. Fourati, S.; Feld, J.J.; Chevaliez, S.; Luhmann, N. Approaches for Simplified HCV Diagnostic Algorithms. *J. Int. AIDS Soc.* **2018**, *21*, e25058. [CrossRef]
66. Mullis, K.B.; Faloona, F.A. Specific Synthesis of DNA in Vitro via a Polymerase-Catalyzed Chain Reaction. *Methods Enzymol.* **1987**, *155*, 335–350. [CrossRef]
67. Laurent, F.; Li, J.S.; Vitvitski, L.; Berby, F.; Lamelin, J.P.; Alonso, C.; Trepo, C. Importance of PCR in the Diagnosis of Hepatitis C. *Rev. Fr. Transfus. Hemobiol.* **1992**, *35*, 211–224. [CrossRef]
68. Krarup, H.B.; Drewes, A.M.; Madsen, P.H. A Quantitative HCV-PCR Test for Routine Diagnostics. *Scand. J. Clin. Lab. Investig.* **1998**, *58*, 415–422. [CrossRef]
69. Shen, F.; Sun, B.; Kreutz, J.E.; Davydova, E.K.; Du, W.; Reddy, P.L.; Joseph, L.J.; Ismagilov, R.F. Multiplexed Quantification of Nucleic Acids with Large Dynamic Range Using Multivolume Digital RT-PCR on a Rotational SlipChip Tested with HIV and Hepatitis C Viral Load. *J. Am. Chem. Soc.* **2011**, *133*, 17705–17712. [CrossRef]
70. Zaghloul, H.; El-Shahat, M. Recombinase Polymerase Amplification as a Promising Tool in Hepatitis C Virus Diagnosis. *World J. Hepatol.* **2014**, *6*, 916–922. [CrossRef] [PubMed]
71. Singh, C.; Roy-Chowdhuri, S. Quantitative Real-Time PCR: Recent Advances. *Methods Mol. Biol.* **2016**, *1392*, 161–176. [CrossRef] [PubMed]
72. Nolan, T.; Hands, R.E.; Bustin, S.A. Quantification of MRNA Using Real-Time RT-PCR. *Nat. Protoc.* **2006**, *1*, 1559–1582. [CrossRef] [PubMed]
73. Marins, E.G.; Bodinaidu, K.; Lin, M.; Deforest, A. Evaluation of the COBAS® AmpliPrep/COBAS® TaqMan® HCV Test v2.0 for HCV Viral Load Monitoring Using Dried Blood Spot Specimens. *J. Virol. Methods* **2017**, *247*, 77–80. [CrossRef] [PubMed]
74. Vermehren, J.; Colucci, G.; Gohl, P.; Hamdi, N.; Abdelaziz, A.I.; Karey, U.; Thamke, D.; Zitzer, H.; Zeuzem, S.; Sarrazin, C. Development of a Second Version of the Cobas AmpliPrep/Cobas TaqMan Hepatitis C Virus Quantitative Test with Improved Genotype Inclusivity. *J. Clin. Microbiol.* **2011**, *49*, 3309–3315. [CrossRef]
75. Michelin, B.D.A.; Muller, Z.; Stelzl, E.; Marth, E.; Kessler, H.H. Evaluation of the Abbott RealTime HCV Assay for Quantitative Detection of Hepatitis C Virus RNA. *J. Clin. Virol.* **2007**, *38*, 96–100. [CrossRef]
76. Bossler, A.; Gunsolly, C.; Pyne, M.T.; Rendo, A.; Rachel, J.; Mills, R.; Miller, M.; Sipley, J.; Hillyard, D.; Jenkins, S.; et al. Performance of the COBAS® AmpliPrep/COBAS TaqMan® Automated System for Hepatitis C Virus (HCV) Quantification in a Multi-Center Comparison. *J. Clin. Virol.* **2011**, *50*, 100–103. [CrossRef]
77. Halfon, P.; Bourlière, M.; Pénaranda, G.; Khiri, H.; Ouzan, D. Real-Time PCR Assays for Hepatitis C Virus (HCV) RNA Quantitation Are Adequate for Clinical Management of Patients with Chronic HCV Infection. *J. Clin. Microbiol.* **2006**, *44*, 2507–2511. [CrossRef]
78. Johnson, M. PCR Machines. *Mater. Methods* **2013**, *3*, 193. [CrossRef]
79. Collins, M.L.; Irvine, B.; Tyner, D.; Fine, E.; Zayati, C.; Chang, C.; Horn, T.; Ahle, D.; Detmer, J.; Shen, L.P.; et al. A Branched DNA Signal Amplification Assay for Quantification of Nucleic Acid Targets below 100 Molecules/Ml. *Nucleic Acids Res.* **1997**, *25*, 2979–2984. [CrossRef]
80. Hendricks, D.A.; Stowe, B.J.; Hoo, B.S.; Kolberg, J.; Irvine, B.D.; Neuwald, P.D.; Urdea, M.S.; Perrillo, R.P. Quantitation of HBV DNA in Human Serum Using a Branched DNA (BDNA) Signal Amplification Assay. *Am. J. Clin. Pathol.* **1995**, *104*, 537–546. [CrossRef] [PubMed]
81. Elbeik, T.; Markowitz, N.; Nassos, P.; Kumar, U.; Beringer, S.; Haller, B.; Ng, V. Simultaneous Runs of the Bayer VERSANT HIV-1 Version 3.0 and HCV BDNA Version 3.0 Quantitative Assays on the System 340 Platform Provide Reliable Quantitation and Improved Work Flow. *J. Clin. Microbiol.* **2004**, *42*, 3120–3127. [CrossRef] [PubMed]
82. Nolte, F.S. Branched DNA Signal Amplification for Direct Quantitation of Nucleic Acid Sequences in Clinical Specimens. *Adv. Clin. Chem.* **1998**, *33*, 201–235. [CrossRef] [PubMed]
83. Holland, C.A.; Pribyl, T.M. Molecular Diagnostics for the Hepatitis C Virus. In *Molecular Diagnostics*; Elsevier: Amsterdam, The Netherlands, 2010; pp. 263–275.

84. Trimoulet, P.; Halfon, P.; Pohier, E.; Khiri, H.; Chêne, G.; Fleury, H. Evaluation of the VERSANT HCV RNA 3.0 Assay for Quantification of Hepatitis C Virus RNA in Serum. *J. Clin. Microbiol.* **2002**, *40*, 2031–2036. [CrossRef]
85. Fuchs, T.C.; Truisi, G.L.; Hewitt, P.G. Toxicogenomics in Preclinical Development. In *A Comprehensive Guide to Toxicology in Nonclinical Drug Development*; Elsevier: Amsterdam, The Netherlands, 2017; pp. 893–920.
86. Shen, C.-H. Amplification of Nucleic Acids. In *Diagnostic Molecular Biology*; Academic Press: Cambridge, MA, USA, 2019; pp. 215–247.
87. Warkad, S.D.; Nimse, S.B.; Song, K.-S.; Kim, T. HCV Detection, Discrimination, and Genotyping Technologies. *Sensors* **2018**, *18*, 3423. [CrossRef]
88. Gorrin, G.; Friesenhahn, M.; Lin, P.; Sanders, M.; Pollner, R.; Eguchi, B.; Pham, J.; Roma, G.; Spidle, J.; Nicol, S.; et al. Performance Evaluation of the VERSANT HCV RNA Qualitative Assay by Using Transcription-Mediated Amplification. *J. Clin. Microbiol.* **2003**, *41*, 310–317. [CrossRef]
89. Hofmann, W.P.; Dries, V.; Herrmann, E.; Gärtner, B.; Zeuzem, S.; Sarrazin, C. Comparison of Transcription Mediated Amplification (TMA) and Reverse Transcription Polymerase Chain Reaction (RT-PCR) for Detection of Hepatitis C Virus RNA in Liver Tissue. *J. Clin. Virol.* **2005**, *32*, 289–293. [CrossRef]
90. Hologic Aptima® HCV Quant Dx Assay. Available online: https://www.hologic.com/hologic-products/molecular-diagnostics/aptima-hcv-quant-dx-assay?utm_source=google&utm_medium=cpc&utm_term=aptima%20hcv&utm_campaign=2023_Brand_Virology&gad_source=1&gclid=CjwKCAiA6t-6BhA3EiwAltRFGBftVUiHGQ5sBrlgZWQ06fT9IiaatOqdoAAeUjsrAfZLBXuIKfFdeRoCTaEQAvD_BwE (accessed on 9 December 2024).
91. Chevaliez, S.; Dubernet, F.; Dauvillier, C.; Hézode, C.; Pawlotsky, J.-M. The New Aptima HCV Quant Dx Real-Time TMA Assay Accurately Quantifies Hepatitis C Virus Genotype 1–6 RNA. *J. Clin. Virol.* **2017**, *91*, 5–11. [CrossRef]
92. U.S. Food and Drug Administration. Procleix Ultrio Elite Assay. Available online: https://www.fda.gov/vaccines-blood-biologics/blood-blood-products/procleix-ultrio-elite-assay (accessed on 9 December 2024).
93. Grüner, N.; Stambouli, O.; Ross, R.S. Dried Blood Spots–Preparing and Processing for Use in Immunoassays and in Molecular Techniques. *J. Vis. Exp.* **2015**, *97*, 52619. [CrossRef]
94. Biondi, M.J.; van Tilborg, M.; Smookler, D.; Heymann, G.; Aquino, A.; Perusini, S.; Mandel, E.; Kozak, R.A.; Cherepanov, V.; Kowgier, M.; et al. Hepatitis C Core-Antigen Testing from Dried Blood Spots. *Viruses* **2019**, *11*, 830. [CrossRef]
95. McLeod, A.; Weir, A.; Aitken, C.; Gunson, R.; Templeton, K.; Molyneaux, P.; McIntyre, P.; McDonald, S.; Goldberg, D.; Hutchinson, S. Rise in Testing and Diagnosis Associated with Scotland's Action Plan on Hepatitis C and Introduction of Dried Blood Spot Testing. *J. Epidemiol. Community Health* **2014**, *68*, 1182–1188. [CrossRef] [PubMed]
96. Grebely, J.; Applegate, T.L.; Cunningham, P.; Feld, J.J. Hepatitis C Point-of-Care Diagnostics: In Search of a Single Visit Diagnosis. *Expert Rev. Mol. Diagn.* **2017**, *17*, 1109–1115. [CrossRef] [PubMed]
97. Gupta, E.; Agarwala, P.; Kumar, G.; Maiwall, R.; Sarin, S.K. Point-of-Care Testing (POCT) in Molecular Diagnostics: Performance Evaluation of GeneXpert HCV RNA Test in Diagnosing and Monitoring of HCV Infection. *J. Clin. Virol.* **2017**, *88*, 46–51. [CrossRef] [PubMed]
98. Lamoury, F.M.J.; Bajis, S.; Hajarizadeh, B.; Marshall, A.D.; Martinello, M.; Ivanova, E.; Catlett, B.; Mowat, Y.; Marks, P.; Amin, J.; et al. Evaluation of the Xpert HCV Viral Load Finger-Stick Point-of-Care Assay. *J. Infect. Dis.* **2018**, *217*, 1889–1896. [CrossRef]
99. U.S. Food and Drug Administration. FDA Permits Marketing of First Point-of-Care Hepatitis C RNA Test. Available online: https://www.fda.gov/news-events/press-announcements/fda-permits-marketing-first-point-care-hepatitis-c-rna-test (accessed on 9 December 2024).
100. Llibre, A.; Shimakawa, Y.; Mottez, E.; Ainsworth, S.; Buivan, T.-P.; Firth, R.; Harrison, E.; Rosenberg, A.R.; Meritet, J.-F.; Fontanet, A.; et al. Development and Clinical Validation of the Genedrive Point-of-Care Test for Qualitative Detection of Hepatitis C Virus. *Gut* **2018**, *67*, 2017–2024. [CrossRef]
101. Sharma, S.; Thomas, E.; Caputi, M.; Asghar, W. RT-LAMP-Based Molecular Diagnostic Set-Up for Rapid Hepatitis C Virus Testing. *Biosensors* **2022**, *12*, 298. [CrossRef]
102. Coarsey, C.; Coleman, B.; Kabir, M.A.; Sher, M.; Asghar, W. Development of a Flow-Free Magnetic Actuation Platform for an Automated Microfluidic ELISA. *RSC Adv.* **2019**, *9*, 8159–8168. [CrossRef]
103. Kabir, M.A.; Zilouchian, H.; Sher, M.; Asghar, W. Development of a Flow-Free Automated Colorimetric Detection Assay Integrated with Smartphone for Zika NS1. *Diagnostics* **2020**, *10*, 42. [CrossRef]
104. Improved Clinical Specificity of the VITROS® Anti-HCV Assay. Available online: https://www.orthoclinicaldiagnostics.com/assets/pdf/Poster-ISBT-2021-HCV-PR-11277-V2.pdf (accessed on 10 December 2024).
105. WHO. Prequalification of In Vitro Diagnostics PUBLIC REPORT. Available online: https://extranet.who.int/prequal/sites/default/files/whopr_files/PQDx_0374-130-00_ARCHITECT-HCV_v1.0.pdf (accessed on 10 December 2024).
106. Alinity s Anti-HCV. Available online: https://www.fda.gov/vaccines-blood-biologics/blood-blood-products/alinity-s-anti-hcv (accessed on 10 December 2024).

107. Alinity Anti-HCV Reagent Kit. Available online: https://www.versiti.org/getmedia/2086cb9d-867f-4c83-b5ed-2f7d41bb12c3/alinity-hcv.pdf (accessed on 10 December 2024).
108. Alinity s Anti-HCV II Assay. Available online: https://www.fda.gov/vaccines-blood-biologics/alinity-s-anti-hcv-ii-assay (accessed on 10 December 2024).
109. Jonas, G.; Pelzer, C.; Beckert, C.; Hausmann, M.; Kapprell, H.-P. Performance Characteristics of the ARCHITECT® Anti-HCV Assay. *J. Clin. Virol.* **2005**, *34*, 97–103. [CrossRef]
110. Hepatitis C Virus Encoded Antigens (Recombinant C100-3, HCr43, NS5). Available online: https://www.fda.gov/media/73334/download?attachment (accessed on 10 December 2024).
111. HEPATITIS C VIRUS ENCODED ANTIGEN (RECOMBINANT C100-3, HC-31, AND HC-34) ABBOTT HCV EIA 2.0. Available online: https://www.fda.gov/media/72001/download#:~:text=Unbound%20enzyme%20conjugate%20is%20then,is%20bound%20to%20the%20bead (accessed on 10 December 2024).
112. Hepatitis C Virus Encoded Antigen (Recombinant C22-3, C200 and NS5) ORTHO® HCV Version 3.0 ELISA Test System. Available online: https://www.fda.gov/media/77425/download?attachment (accessed on 10 December 2024).
113. Murex Anti-HCV (Version 4.0). Available online: https://kimhung.vn/wp-content/uploads/2020/03/Test-elisa-Murex-Anti-HCV-V4-Murex-Diasorin-2.pdf (accessed on 10 December 2024).
114. DiaSorin Australia Pty Ltd—Murex Anti-HCV (Version 4.0)—Hepatitis C Virus Total Antibody IVD, Kit, Enzyme Immunoassay (EIA) (301860). Available online: https://www.tga.gov.au/resources/artg/301860 (accessed on 10 December 2024).
115. Ré, V.; Gallego, S.; Treviño, E.; Barbás, G.; Domínguez, C.; Elbarcha, O.; Bepre, H.; Contigiani, M. Evaluation of Five Screening Tests Licensed in Argentina for Detection of Hepatitis C Virus Antibodies. *Mem. Inst. Oswaldo Cruz* **2005**, *100*, 303–307. [CrossRef]
116. OraSure Technologies. OraQuick® HCV Rapid Antibody Test. Available online: https://orasure.com/products/OraQuick-HCV.html (accessed on 30 November 2024).
117. Hepatitis C Point-of-Care Testing: What Is Its Impact on Testing and Linkage to Care? Available online: https://www.catie.ca/prevention-in-focus/hepatitis-c-point-of-care-testing-what-is-its-impact-on-testing-and-linkage-0#:~:text=In%20comparison%20to%20standard%20laboratory,Xpert%20HCV%20Viral%20Load%20Fingerstick (accessed on 10 December 2024).
118. OraSure OraQuick HIV In-Home Self Test Oral Swab Rapid Antibody CLIA Waived. Available online: https://transmedco.com/oraquick-hiv-rapid-antibody-test-clia-waived-25-box/ (accessed on 10 December 2024).
119. Summary Basis for Regulatory Action—NGI Ultraqual Multiplex PCR Assay. Available online: https://www.fda.gov/files/vaccines,%20blood%20&%20biologics/published/May-25--2018-Summary-Basis-for-Regulatory-Action---NGI-Ultraqual-Multiplex-PCR-Assay-for-HCV--HIV-1-HIV-2--and-HBV.pdf (accessed on 10 December 2024).
120. Page, K.; Feinberg, J. What Hepatitis C Virus (HCV) Diagnostic Tools Are Needed to Advance Diagnosis of Current HCV Infection in Outreach Settings and in a Nonclinical Setting? *J. Infect. Dis.* **2024**, *229*, S328–S333. [CrossRef] [PubMed]
121. Truenat® HCV. Available online: https://www.molbiodiagnostics.com/product_details.php?id=22 (accessed on 10 December 2024).
122. True® Nat HCV. Available online: https://www.molbiodiagnostics.com/uploads/product_download/20240919.145137~Truenat-HCV-packinsert-V-06.pdf (accessed on 10 December 2024).
123. COBAS® AmpliPrep/COBAS® TaqMan® HCV Test, v2.0. Available online: https://www.aphl.org/programs/infectious_disease/Documents/CAP_CTM%20HCV%20v2%20US-IVD%20PI%20rev4%20(Dx%20claim).PDF (accessed on 10 December 2024).
124. Chevaliez, S.; Bouvier-Alias, M.; Rodriguez, C.; Soulier, A.; Poveda, J.-D.; Pawlotsky, J.-M. The Cobas AmpliPrep/Cobas TaqMan HCV Test, Version 2.0, Real-Time PCR Assay Accurately Quantifies Hepatitis C Virus Genotype 4 RNA. *J. Clin. Microbiol.* **2013**, *51*, 1078–1082. [CrossRef] [PubMed]
125. Pas, S.; Molenkamp, R.; Schinkel, J.; Rebers, S.; Copra, C.; Seven-Deniz, S.; Thamke, D.; de Knegt, R.J.; Haagmans, B.L.; Schutten, M. Performance Evaluation of the New Roche Cobas AmpliPrep/Cobas TaqMan HCV Test, Version 2.0, for Detection and Quantification of Hepatitis C Virus RNA. *J. Clin. Microbiol.* **2013**, *51*, 238–242. [CrossRef]
126. REALTIME HCV VIRAL LOAD. Available online: https://www.molecular.abbott/us/en/products/infectious-disease/realtime-hcv-viral-load (accessed on 10 December 2024).
127. Wiesmann, F.; Naeth, G.; Sarrazin, C.; Berger, A.; Kaiser, R.; Ehret, R.; Knechten, H.; Braun, P. Variation Analysis of Six HCV Viral Load Assays Using Low Viremic HCV Samples in the Range of the Clinical Decision Points for HCV Protease Inhibitors. *Med. Microbiol. Immunol.* **2015**, *204*, 515–525. [CrossRef]
128. Abbott RealTime HCV. Available online: https://www.molecular.abbott/content/dam/add/molecular/products/infectious-disease/realtime-hcv-viral-load/realtime-hcv-package-insert.pdf (accessed on 15 December 2024).
129. Genedrive®. Available online: https://www.sysmex-egypt.com/products/products-detail/genedriver/ (accessed on 10 December 2024).
130. Padhi, A.; Gupta, E.; Singh, G.; Agarwal, R.; Sharma, M.K.; Sarin, S.K. Evaluation of the Point of Care Molecular Diagnostic Genedrive HCV ID Kit for the Detection of HCV RNA in Clinical Samples. *Epidemiol. Infect.* **2020**, 1–23. [CrossRef]
131. Lamoury, F.M.J.; Njouom, R.; Amougou-Atsama, M.; Yiagnigni Mfopou, E.; Berishvili, N.; Sologashvili, M.; Fajardo, E.; Malobela, A.; Macé, A.; Chirehwa, M.; et al. Diagnostic Performance and Usability of the Genedrive® HCV ID Kit in Two Decentralized Settings in Cameroon and Georgia. *Diagnostics* **2021**, *11*, 746. [CrossRef]

132. Miriad Rapid HBc/HIVHCV Antibody Test. Available online: https://medmira.com/wp-content/uploads/2018/01/ADAICUVZIS0001EN-Rev-0_1-8-x-14-Miriad-HBcHIVHCV-Package-Insert-English.pdf (accessed on 15 December 2024).
133. VERSANT HCV RNA Qualitative Assay (TMA). Available online: https://www.siemens-healthineers.com/nl/molecular-diagnostics/molecular-diagnostics-in-vitro-diagnostics/versant-hcv-rna-qualitative-assay (accessed on 10 December 2024).
134. Saludes, V.; González, V.; Planas, R.; Matas, L.; Ausina, V.; Martró, E. Tools for the Diagnosis of Hepatitis C Virus Infection and Hepatic Fibrosis Staging. *World J. Gastroenterol.* **2014**, *20*, 3431–3442. [CrossRef]
135. Hepatitis C Virus HCV Quantitative NAAT. Available online: https://www.eurofins-viracor.com/test-menu/33257-hepatitis-c-virus-hcv-quantitative-naat/ (accessed on 10 December 2024).
136. Procleix Ultrio® Assay. Available online: https://www.fda.gov/media/85280/download (accessed on 10 December 2024).
137. VERSANT HCV RNA 3.0 Assay (BDNA). Available online: https://www.siemens-healthineers.com/nl/molecular-diagnostics/molecular-diagnostics-in-vitro-diagnostics/versant-hcv-rna-3-assay (accessed on 10 December 2024).
138. He, H.; Luo, G.; Zhang, J.; Tang, L.; Zhou, Y.; Hu, B.; Dai, J.; Huang, Z. Signal Extraction, Transformation, and Magnification for Ultrasensitive and Specific Detection of Nucleic Acids. *Anal. Chem.* **2021**, *93*, 10611–10618. [CrossRef]
139. Xue, C.; Luo, M.; Wang, L.; Li, C.; Hu, S.; Yu, X.; Yuan, P.; Wu, Z.-S. Stimuli-Responsive Autonomous-Motion Molecular Machine for Sensitive Simultaneous Fluorescence Imaging of Intracellular MicroRNAs. *Anal. Chem.* **2021**, *93*, 9869–9877. [CrossRef]
140. Xu, J.; Qiu, X.; Hildebrandt, N. When Nanoworlds Collide: Implementing DNA Amplification, Nanoparticles, Molecules, and FRET into a Single MicroRNA Biosensor. *Nano Lett.* **2021**, *21*, 4802–4808. [CrossRef]
141. Craw, P.; Balachandran, W. Isothermal Nucleic Acid Amplification Technologies for Point-of-Care Diagnostics: A Critical Review. *Lab Chip* **2012**, *12*, 2469. [CrossRef] [PubMed]
142. Chang, C.-C.; Chen, C.-C.; Wei, S.-C.; Lu, H.-H.; Liang, Y.-H.; Lin, C.-W. Diagnostic Devices for Isothermal Nucleic Acid Amplification. *Sensors* **2012**, *12*, 8319–8337. [CrossRef]
143. Zanoli, L.M.; Spoto, G. Isothermal Amplification Methods for the Detection of Nucleic Acids in Microfluidic Devices. *Biosensors* **2013**, *3*, 18–43. [CrossRef] [PubMed]
144. Notomi, T.; Okayama, H.; Masubuchi, H.; Yonekawa, T.; Watanabe, K.; Amino, N.; Hase, T. Loop-Mediated Isothermal Amplification of DNA. *Nucleic Acids Res.* **2000**, *28*, E63. [CrossRef]
145. Nagamine, K.; Hase, T.; Notomi, T. Accelerated Reaction by Loop-Mediated Isothermal Amplification Using Loop Primers. *Mol. Cell. Probes* **2002**, *16*, 223–229. [CrossRef]
146. Kabir, M.A.; Zilouchian, H.; Caputi, M.; Asghar, W. Advances in HIV Diagnosis and Monitoring. *Crit. Rev. Biotechnol.* **2020**, *40*, 623–638. [CrossRef]
147. Poon, L.L.M.; Leung, C.S.W.; Chan, K.H.; Lee, J.H.C.; Yuen, K.Y.; Guan, Y.; Peiris, J.S.M. Detection of Human Influenza A Viruses by Loop-Mediated Isothermal Amplification. *J. Clin. Microbiol.* **2005**, *43*, 427–430. [CrossRef]
148. Yoshida, N.; Fujino, M.; Miyata, A.; Nagai, T.; Kamada, M.; Sakiyama, H.; Ihara, T.; Kumagai, T.; Okafuji, T.; Okafuji, T.; et al. Mumps Virus Reinfection Is Not a Rare Event Confirmed by Reverse Transcription Loop-mediated Isothermal Amplification. *J. Med. Virol.* **2008**, *80*, 517–523. [CrossRef]
149. Parida, M.; Posadas, G.; Inoue, S.; Hasebe, F.; Morita, K. Real-Time Reverse Transcription Loop-Mediated Isothermal Amplification for Rapid Detection of West Nile Virus. *J. Clin. Microbiol.* **2004**, *42*, 257–263. [CrossRef]
150. Yoneyama, T.; Kiyohara, T.; Shimasaki, N.; Kobayashi, G.; Ota, Y.; Notomi, T.; Totsuka, A.; Wakita, T. Rapid and Real-Time Detection of Hepatitis A Virus by Reverse Transcription Loop-Mediated Isothermal Amplification Assay. *J. Virol. Methods* **2007**, *145*, 162–168. [CrossRef]
151. Lan, X.; Yang, B.; Li, B.Y.; Yin, X.P.; Li, X.R.; Liu, J.X. Reverse Transcription-Loop-Mediated Isothermal Amplification Assay for Rapid Detection of Hepatitis E Virus. *J. Clin. Microbiol.* **2009**, *47*, 2304–2306. [CrossRef] [PubMed]
152. Cai, T.; Lou, G.; Yang, J.; Xu, D.; Meng, Z. Development and Evaluation of Real-Time Loop-Mediated Isothermal Amplification for Hepatitis B Virus DNA Quantification: A New Tool for HBV Management. *J. Clin. Virol.* **2008**, *41*, 270–276. [CrossRef] [PubMed]
153. Makler-Disatham, A.; Caputi, M.; Asghar, W. Development of a LAMP-Based Diagnostic for the Detection of Multiple HIV-1 Strains. *Biosensors* **2024**, *14*, 157. [CrossRef]
154. Sharma, S.; Caputi, M.; Asghar, W. Development of a Diagnostic Microfluidic Chip for SARS-CoV-2 Detection in Saliva and Nasopharyngeal Samples. *Viruses* **2024**, *16*, 1190. [CrossRef]
155. Yang, J.; Fang, M.; Li, J.; Lou, G.; Lu, H.; Wu, N. Detection of Hepatitis C Virus by an Improved Loop-Mediated Isothermal Amplification Assay. *Arch. Virol.* **2011**, *156*, 1387–1396. [CrossRef]
156. Nyan, D.-C.; Swinson, K.L. A Novel Multiplex Isothermal Amplification Method for Rapid Detection and Identification of Viruses. *Sci. Rep.* **2015**, *5*, 17925. [CrossRef]
157. Nyan, D.-C.; Swinson, K.L. A Method for Rapid Detection and Genotype Identification of Hepatitis C Virus 1–6 by One-Step Reverse Transcription Loop-Mediated Isothermal Amplification. *Int. J. Infect. Dis.* **2016**, *43*, 30–36. [CrossRef]
158. Chen, J.; Xu, X.; Huang, Z.; Luo, Y.; Tang, L.; Jiang, J.-H. BEAMing LAMP: Single-Molecule Capture and on-Bead Isothermal Amplification for Digital Detection of Hepatitis C Virus in Plasma. *Chem. Commun.* **2018**, *54*, 291–294. [CrossRef]

159. Nguyen, H.; Park, J.; Kang, S.; Kim, M. Surface Plasmon Resonance: A Versatile Technique for Biosensor Applications. *Sensors* **2015**, *15*, 10481–10510. [CrossRef]
160. Sohail, A.; Khan, S.; Ullah, R.; Qureshi, S.A.; Bilal, M.; Khan, A. Analysis of Hepatitis C Infection Using Raman Spectroscopy and Proximity Based Classification in the Transformed Domain. *Biomed. Opt. Express* **2018**, *9*, 2041. [CrossRef]
161. Wang, C.M.; Roy, P.K.; Juluri, B.K.; Chattopadhyay, S. A SERS Tattoo for in Situ, Ex Situ, and Multiplexed Detection of Toxic Food Additives. *Sens. Actuators B Chem.* **2018**, *261*, 218–225. [CrossRef]
162. He, W.; Wang, M.; Cheng, P.; Liu, Y.; You, M. Recent Advances of Upconversion Nanoparticles-Based Lateral Flow Assays for Point-of-Care Testing. *TrAC Trends Anal. Chem.* **2024**, *173*, 117641. [CrossRef]
163. Shi, W.; Li, K.; Zhang, Y. The Advancement of Nanomaterials for the Detection of Hepatitis B Virus and Hepatitis C Virus. *Molecules* **2023**, *28*, 7201. [CrossRef] [PubMed]
164. Kashif, M.; Majeed, M.I.; Hanif, M.A.; Rehman, A.U. Surface Enhanced Raman Spectroscopy of the Serum Samples for the Diagnosis of Hepatitis C and Prediction of the Viral Loads. *Spectrochim. Acta A Mol. Biomol. Spectrosc.* **2020**, *242*, 118729. [CrossRef]
165. Nasir, S.; Majeed, M.I.; Nawaz, H.; Rashid, N.; Ali, S.; Farooq, S.; Kashif, M.; Rafiq, S.; Bano, S.; Ashraf, M.N.; et al. Surface Enhanced Raman Spectroscopy of RNA Samples Extracted from Blood of Hepatitis C Patients for Quantification of Viral Loads. *Photodiagnosis Photodyn. Ther.* **2021**, *33*, 102152. [CrossRef]
166. Cherif, B.; Roget, A.; Villiers, C.L.; Calemczuk, R.; Leroy, V.; Marche, P.N.; Livache, T.; Villiers, M.-B. Clinically Related Protein-Peptide Interactions Monitored in Real Time on Novel Peptide Chips by Surface Plasmon Resonance Imaging. *Clin. Chem.* **2006**, *52*, 255–262. [CrossRef]
167. Narayanamurthy, V.; Jeroish, Z.E.; Bhuvaneshwari, K.S.; Samsuri, F. Hepatitis C Virus (HCV) Diagnosis via Microfluidics. *Anal. Methods* **2021**, *13*, 740–763. [CrossRef]
168. Dey, M.K.; Iftesum, M.; Devireddy, R.; Gartia, M.R. New Technologies and Reagents in Lateral Flow Assay (LFA) Designs for Enhancing Accuracy and Sensitivity. *Anal. Methods* **2023**, *15*, 4351–4376. [CrossRef]
169. Guo, X.; Yuan, Y.; Liu, J.; Fu, S.; Zhang, J.; Mei, Q.; Zhang, Y. Single-Line Flow Assay Platform Based on Orthogonal Emissive Upconversion Nanoparticles. *Anal. Chem.* **2021**, *93*, 3010–3017. [CrossRef]
170. Tang, R.; Yang, H.; Gong, Y.; Liu, Z.; Li, X.; Wen, T.; Qu, Z.; Zhang, S.; Mei, Q.; Xu, F. Improved Analytical Sensitivity of Lateral Flow Assay Using Sponge for HBV Nucleic Acid Detection. *Sci. Rep.* **2017**, *7*, 1360. [CrossRef]
171. Mu, X.; Zhang, L.; Chang, S.; Cui, W.; Zheng, Z. Multiplex Microfluidic Paper-Based Immunoassay for the Diagnosis of Hepatitis C Virus Infection. *Anal. Chem.* **2014**, *86*, 5338–5344. [CrossRef]
172. Chang, H.-C.; Chao, Y.-T.; Yen, J.-Y.; Yu, Y.-L.; Lee, C.-N.; Ho, B.-C.; Liu, K.-C.; Fang, J.; Lin, C.-W.; Lee, J.-H. A Turbidity Test Based Centrifugal Microfluidics Diagnostic System for Simultaneous Detection of HBV, HCV, and CMV. *Adv. Mater. Sci. Eng.* **2015**, *2015*, 306708. [CrossRef]
173. Xing, Y.; Zhao, L.; Cheng, Z.; Lv, C.; Yu, F.; Yu, F. Microfluidics-Based Sensing of Biospecies. *ACS Appl. Bio Mater.* **2021**, *4*, 2160–2191. [CrossRef]
174. Cesewski, E.; Johnson, B.N. Electrochemical Biosensors for Pathogen Detection. *Biosens. Bioelectron.* **2020**, *159*, 112214. [CrossRef]
175. Thévenot, D.R.; Toth, K.; Durst, R.A.; Wilson, G.S. Electrochemical Biosensors: Recommended Definitions and Classification. *Biosens. Bioelectron.* **2001**, *16*, 121–131. [CrossRef] [PubMed]
176. Uliana, C.V.; Riccardi, C.S.; Yamanaka, H. Diagnostic Tests for Hepatitis C: Recent Trends in Electrochemical Immunosensor and Genosensor Analysis. *World J. Gastroenterol.* **2014**, *20*, 15476–15491. [CrossRef] [PubMed]
177. Ma, C.; Liang, M.; Wang, L.; Xiang, H.; Jiang, Y.; Li, Y.; Xie, G. MultisHRP-DNA-Coated CMWNTs as Signal Labels for an Ultrasensitive Hepatitis C Virus Core Antigen Electrochemical Immunosensor. *Biosens. Bioelectron.* **2013**, *47*, 467–474. [CrossRef]
178. Zribi, B.; Roy, E.; Pallandre, A.; Chebil, S.; Koubaa, M.; Mejri, N.; Gomez, H.M.; Sola, C.; Korri-Youssoufi, H.; Haghiri-Gosnet, A.-M. A Microfluidic Electrochemical Biosensor Based on Multiwall Carbon Nanotube/Ferrocene for Genomic DNA Detection of *Mycobacterium tuberculosis* in Clinical Isolates. *Biomicrofluidics* **2016**, *10*, 014115. [CrossRef]
179. Redman, M.; King, A.; Watson, C.; King, D. What Is CRISPR/Cas9? *Arch. Dis. Child. Educ. Pract. Ed.* **2016**, *101*, 213–215. [CrossRef]
180. Price, A.A.; Sampson, T.R.; Ratner, H.K.; Grakoui, A.; Weiss, D.S. Cas9-Mediated Targeting of Viral RNA in Eukaryotic Cells. *Proc. Natl. Acad. Sci. USA* **2015**, *112*, 6164–6169. [CrossRef]
181. Nguyen, L.T.; Smith, B.M.; Jain, P.K. Enhancement of Trans-Cleavage Activity of Cas12a with Engineered CrRNA Enables Amplified Nucleic Acid Detection. *Nat. Commun.* **2020**, *11*, 4906. [CrossRef] [PubMed]
182. Schlücker, S. SERS Microscopy: Nanoparticle Probes and Biomedical Applications. *ChemPhysChem* **2009**, *10*, 1344–1354. [CrossRef] [PubMed]
183. Wang, X.; Hong, X.-Z.; Li, Y.-W.; Li, Y.; Wang, J.; Chen, P.; Liu, B.-F. Microfluidics-Based Strategies for Molecular Diagnostics of Infectious Diseases. *Mil. Med. Res.* **2022**, *9*, 11. [CrossRef]
184. Ma, J.; Li, X.; Lou, C.; Lin, X.; Zhang, Z.; Chen, D.; Yang, S. Utility of CRISPR/Cas Mediated Electrochemical Biosensors. *Anal. Methods* **2023**, *15*, 3785–3801. [CrossRef]

185. Azimzadeh, M.; Mousazadeh, M.; Jahangiri-Manesh, A.; Khashayar, P.; Khashayar, P. CRISPR-Powered Microfluidics in Diagnostics: A Review of Main Applications. *Chemosensors* **2021**, *10*, 3. [CrossRef]
186. Wei, X.; Shen, Y.; Yuan, M.; Zhang, A.; Duan, G.; Chen, S. Visualizing In-Field Detection of HCV Using a One-Pot RT-RAA-CRISPR/Cas12a Platform. *Anal. Methods* **2024**, *16*, 7484–7493. [CrossRef]

chemosensors

MDPI

Review

Recent Advancements in Multimodal Chemically Powered Micro/Nanorobots for Environmental Sensing and Remediation

Natarajan Vijay [1,2,†], Sampathkumar Jeevanandham [3], Subramaniyan Ramasundaram [1,4,†], Tae Hwan Oh [1,*] and Subramanian Tamil Selvan [5,*]

1 School of Chemical Engineering, Yeungnam University, Gyeongsan 38541, Republic of Korea; jmcvijay@gmail.com (N.V.); ramasundaram79@hotmail.com (S.R.)
2 Department of Interdisciplinary Sciences, National Institute of Food Technology and Entrepreneurship Management, Kundli, Sonipat 131028, Haryana, India
3 Molecular Science and Engineering Laboratory, Amity Institute of Click Chemistry Research and Studies, Amity University, Noida 201313, Uttar Pradesh, India; sampathkumarj4@gmail.com
4 Saveetha School of Engineering, Saveetha Institute of Medical and Technical Sciences (SIMATS), Chennai 602105, Tamil Nadu, India
5 Azion Global Pte. Ltd., 622 Bukit Batok Central, #11-504, Singapore 650622, Singapore
* Correspondence: taehwanynu@gmail.com (T.H.O.); selvanst02@gmail.com (S.T.S.)
† These authors contributed equally to this work.

Abstract: Chemically powered micro/nanorobots (CPMNRs) are self-propelling artificially engineered materials or machines designed with micro-to-nano precision, inspired by the self-migration of biomolecules and microorganisms. CPMNRs convert chemical or external energy into mechanical motion, overcoming forces like Brownian diffusion and viscosity. They are created using top-down or bottom-up approaches for applications in chemo-/biosensing, environmental remediation, molecular imaging, and drug delivery. As self-mixing of contaminated water accelerates the remediation process, CPMNRs are preferred as an ideal choice for environmental applications. Recent advancements in multimodal propulsion technologies, material engineering, and surface modifications have significantly enhanced the capabilities of CPMNRs, enabling them to navigate complex environments and interact with contaminants at the molecular level. This review highlights the latest developments in chemical-driven CPMNRs, focusing on their use in environmental monitoring, pollutant detection, and remediation of heavy metals, microplastics, and organic contaminants in water and soil. It also discusses prospects, sustainability of chemical fuels, environmental biocompatibility, and scalability for large-scale deployment.

Keywords: micro/nanorobots; chemo-/biosensing; chemical propulsion; nanotechnology; environmental remediation; contaminant removal

1. Introduction

Micro/nanorobots (MNRs) are assemblies of materials at the micro/nanoscale, capable of autonomous movement in a liquid medium, effectively overcoming the Brownian motion and viscosity constraints. In a liquid medium, the autonomous movement of MNRs induces flow-induced mixing. MNRs are either powered by chemical fuel or physical energy sources such as magnetic, light, electrical, ultrasound, and thermal energy. MNRs convert fuel and physical energy forms into kinetic energy [1,2]. In conventional magnetic stirring, both functional materials and targets rotate in the same direction, resulting in a less mixing effect than the self-propelled MNRs. By attaching the component capable of energy conversion, multiple types of MNRs have been designed to perform specified tasks.

The applications of MNRs include chemical synthesis, drug delivery, and environmental monitoring and remediations. Initially relying on inorganic materials, MNRs now integrate organic molecules, enzymes, and sensitive biomolecules such as motor proteins to facilitate the active detection and capture of microbes [3]. The accelerated removal of pollutants by MNRs is due to self-propulsion-induced improved mixing and mass transfer in the fluid while they are swimming. The self-movement can also be accelerated by controlling the structure. MNRs with asymmetric structures facilitate easy self-propulsion [4]. Hybrids, core–shell, and self-assembled MNRs have been developed for different applications. Different nanoparticles (NPs), nanofibers, nanorods, nanotubes, and nanobeads have been used to tune the collective motion and direction of MNRs. Both bottom-up growth, and template-assisted methods have been used for the preparation of MNRs. Porous silica, metal–organic framework (MOF), graphene oxide (GO), natural fibers, and plant components with hierarchical porous structures have been used as templates [5]. To equip the MNRs for certain specific applications, they have been additionally functionalized with components enabling tracking, movement control, responsivity to external stimuli, and separation. These are called multifunctional MNRs, where components with magnetic properties, such as Fe_3O_4 NPs, are attached to aid magnetic tracking, separation, and reuse. Integration of polymeric hydrogels with MNRs imparts thermal responsivity via the temperature-induced orientation of polymer chains. As they combine a variety of materials with different functional properties, multicomponent MNRs are considered more advantageous than single-component MNRs [6].

Chemical reactions that generate bubbles offer a rapid method for self-propulsion and mixing. The thrust from these bubbles propels MNRs, enhancing micro-mixing and mass transfer. In chemically powered MNRs (CPMNRs), commonly used fuels are hydrogen peroxide (H_2O_2), citric acid, glucose, urea, alkali, alcohols, acetylene, halogens, water, sodium borohydride, and hydrazine. Oxygen (O_2) bubbles generated from the catalyzed decomposition of H_2O_2 are widely used for the self-propulsion of CPMNRs. Catalysts such as platinum (Pt), silver (Ag), manganese oxide (MnO_2), and enzymes are often used for the decomposition of H_2O_2. Additionally, hydrogen (H_2) and carbon dioxide (CO_2) bubbles can also be used for the self-propulsion of CPMNRs. Metals such as Zinc (Zn), gallium (Ga), and magnesium (Mg) are commonly used for the generation of H_2. Bubble generation and propulsion within a liquid medium enhance mass diffusion [7–9], making CPMNRs ideal for pollutant sensing and remediation. Multifunctional CPMNRs with magnetic tracking and thermal and light responsivities have been developed. These features enable easy separation, reuse, and on/off sensing properties. CPMNRs have been effectively explored for the removal and sensing of organic contaminants, oil droplets, microorganisms, micro/nanoplastics, heavy metals, toxins, explosives, chemical, and biowarfare agents [9].

Motion-induced mixing is crucial for environmental remediation, where rapid pollutant removal and monitoring are essential. In a liquid medium, motion-induced mixing occurs as soon as fuel molecules come into contact with CPMNRs. There is no need for additional equipment to deliver light, magnetic, or thermal stimuli. Compared to other types of MNRs, CPMNRs can be easily obtained via a single-step preparation. Asymmetric deposition of metals such as Pt, Ag, and Au, which decompose H_2O_2 on almost any type of nano- or microparticle, resulting in CPMNRs. The O_2 bubbles generated by CPMNRs are used for both propulsion and replenishing O_2 consumed during the degradation of organic pollutants. There is no performance fading due to light- or heat-induced degradation or weathering-induced loss of magnetic properties.

Based on the working environment, CPMNRs can be designed to work with compatible fuels. For example, biomolecules like glucose can be used as a fuel in CPMNR sensors required to operate in biologically sensitive environments. H_2O_2-based CPMNRs can be used to decontaminate water containing complex organic pollutants. Cost-effective CPMNRs can be achieved by choosing suitable fuel decomposition catalysts, for instance replacing Pt with MnO_2. Therefore, CPMNRs are the ideal choice for accelerating chemical reactions in environmental applications, particularly in water treatment. Self-mixing of pollutants in contaminated water accelerates the decontamination process. Multifunctional CPMNRs have been extensively used in both sensing and remediation applications [7–10]. The number and nature of contamination is increasing due to rapid urbanization and industrialization. It necessitates the identification of lethal chemical contaminants. CPMNRs are being utilized for sensing toxins, explosives, bio and chemical warfare agents, and microorganisms. Toxic organic contaminants such as dyes and organic waste are removed by degradation and mineralization. Heavy metals, organic micropollutants, and oils are removed via adsorption. CPMNRs with photocatalysts such as titanium dioxide (TiO_2) mineralize organic pollutants into CO_2 and H_2O. CPNMRs with Fenton catalysts (iron catalyst, Fe^{2+} or Fe^{3+}/H_2O_2) have also been widely studied for oxidative degradation of organic pollutants. The use of H_2O_2 enhances the generation of reactive oxygen species (ROS) that are responsible for the oxidative degradation of organic compounds. Unlike photocatalysts, Fenton processes can occur in dark conditions. Photo-Fenton- and electro-Fenton-type CPMNRs have been developed to enhance water remediation efficiency. CPMNRs have also been used for disinfection of water contaminated with microorganisms [11–13].

Interestingly, CPMNRs have been explored for non-traditional environmental remediation processes, particularly for emerging pollutants such as micro- and nanoplastics. CPMNRs have been used for the on-the-fly capturing of micro- and nanoplastics, which are plastic debris generated by slow environmental erosion and degradation. Due to their size, their occurrence in water bodies is largely unknown. Analytical techniques such as pyrolysis, gas chromatography–mass spectrometry are tools widely used for measuring the concentration of micro- and nanoplastics [14,15]. Engineered CPMNRs are developed for simple dye staining-based colorimetric autonomous detection and quantification of pathogens. Conventional microbial detection involves the use of sampling, cell-culture, and demand equipment (PCR and optical devices). As microorganisms are motile in nature, self-propelled CPMNRs are suitable for their rapid detection. CPMNRs functionalized with specific receptors can be used to detect, capture, and release particular microorganisms [16,17]. In relevance to environmental remediation, recent reviews have focused on the design aspects of MNRs used in water purification, advancements in MNRs for improving the pollutant removal efficiency, sensing of toxic contaminants, soil decontamination, and solid waste removal [5,18–20]. To the best of our knowledge, there are no recent reviews focusing on the application of CPMNRs for water purification. Therefore, this review specifically focuses on recent developments in CPMNRs used in environmental sensing and remediation. We emphasize the salient features of synthesis strategies and the role of chemical fuels in inducing autonomous movement and improving the efficiency of CMMNRs. To enhance clarity, we have dedicated separate sections to each type of CPMNR, including photocatalysts, Fenton reactions, adsorption, and sensors. We also provide insights into the future directions and practical applications of CPMNRs for monitoring and mitigating water contamination.

2. Mechanistic Overview of CPMNRs

Synthetic CPMNRs have attracted greater interest for their precise motion control behavior, functional mobility, and tunability. Inspired by Feynman's breakthrough speech "There's Plenty of Room at the Bottom" in 1959 [21] and Eric Drexler's book "*Engines of creation: The coming era of nanotechnology*" in 1987 [22], the design of micro-/nanomachines that can be controlled at molecular scales or even by atom-by-atom arrangements for desired functionalities has progressed rapidly. Generally, the motion of micro-/nanoscale machines often requires unconventional approaches based on physical and chemical principles. Like rocket propulsion systems, these machines have three main components: fuel, oxidizer, and combustion chamber. Mimicking those platforms, CPMNRs have the advantage of harnessing energy from the chemical fuels surrounding them in the liquid or solid media and self-propagate like tiny catalytic rockets autonomously until the fuel is exhausted [23]. Emphasizing the significance of such desirable small dimensions, active targeting abilities, and controllable speed, CPMNRs can revolutionize the micro-/nanoengineering field focusing on sustainability and environmental remediation [24].

CPMNRs can be designed with diverse shapes/dimensions and specific structures such as catalytic materials, biocompatible materials, hybrid materials, etc. Such synthetic parts are most commonly in asymmetric orientation like Janus structures with various shapes like spherical, tubular, and thin nanosheet morphology (e.g., 2D porous nanostructures), which can directly harvest energy from surrounding chemical environment (e.g., glucose, urea, H_2O_2, etc.) and autonomously create movements via chemical reactions [25]. The speed of CPMNRs defines the extent of micro-mixing. Thus, higher speed renders highly efficient CPMNRs for pollutant degradation, capture, and sensing. The size and shape of CPMNRs significantly affect their speed. The magnitude of interfacial tension between the bubbles generated by the chemical fuel and water determines their speed. The extent of interfacial tension differs with respect to their shape. For example, in the case of the crescent- and hemispherical-shaped CPMNRs, bubbles generated by a catalyst particle (Ag) attached to the functional component (Fe_3O_4) stay around the concave surface. As the bubbles grow in number, CPMNRs are propelled forward when the bubbles continuously move out of the concave surface. However, the high interfacial tension between the bubble and water restricts bubble movement, slowing down CPMNR motion. Surfactants and additional fuels are required to increase the speed of CPMNRs. In bowl-shaped CPMNRs, larger bubbles prevent the catalyst particles from accessing the fuel molecules, trapping bubbles on the concave surface. It is very difficult to alleviate the interfacial tension even with the addition of surfactants [26].

Insufficient energy flow and uncontrollable direction of motion are significant drawbacks in precisely activating CPNMRs toward specific target trajectories as per preassigned tasks [27]. The shape of CPMNRs determines their hydrodynamics and mobility in liquid media with localized chemical microenvironments. Complex shapes with rough surfaces or porous structures increase the active surface area for pollutant interaction, promoting efficient adsorption and degradation. Asymmetric shapes like nanotubes facilitate the trapping of specific pollutants due to their structural properties. Meanwhile, helical [28] and corkscrew-shaped [29] CPMNRs are better suited for navigation in complex or viscous environments, such as wastewater or soil, as their design mimics the movement of natural microorganisms like bacteria.

Surface area-to-volume ratio, propulsion kinetics, and target accessibility are critical parameters in designing size-tunable CPMNRs that can adapt their dimensions based on environmental conditions. Robust shapes of CPMNRs like spheres [30,31] or tubes perform better in turbulent or high-flow environments, while helical designs are advantageous in stagnant or viscous media [2,7]. The propulsion of CPMNRs typically relies on asymmetric reactions at their surface, generating forces that drive motion, as well as other external environmental factors (pH, light, thermal, electrical, magnetic, acoustic, etc.) that can directly or indirectly influence catalytic propulsion mechanisms and reaction pathways (Scheme 1) [32–35]. Based on their self-propulsion mechanism, they can be categorized into four methods, such as self-electrophoresis, non-electrolyte diffusiophoresis, electrolyte diffusiophoresis, and bubble propulsion.

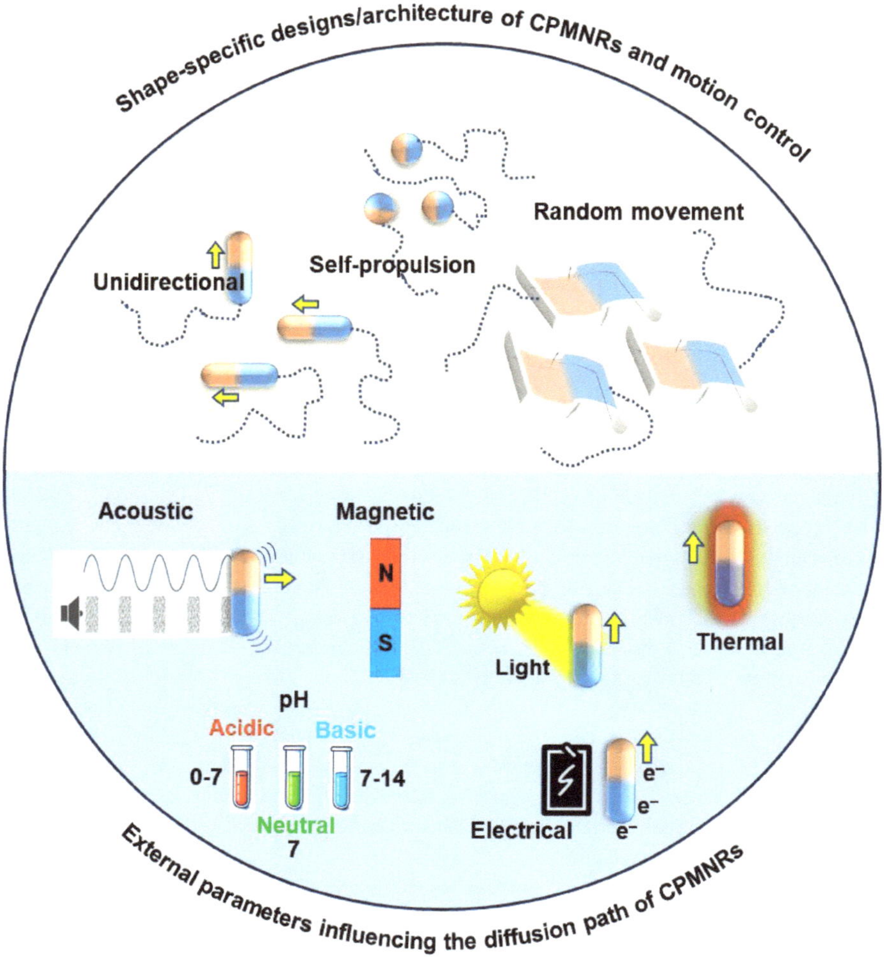

Scheme 1. Graphical illustration of CPMNRs depicting diverse shape-specific designs/architectures influencing motion control and diffusion pathways affected by external environmental factors.

Fundamentally, CPMNRs are mostly asymmetric structures employing catalytic materials (e.g., Pt, Au, Ag, etc.) to decompose chemical fuels such as H_2O_2, O_2, etc. [36,37]. For instance, Pt catalyzes the breakdown of H_2O_2 into water and O_2, generating a thrust force due to O_2 bubble propulsion. Firstly, in the case of the self-electrophoresis mechanism, CPMNRs utilize active redox surfaces, exploiting the local environment for electrochemical-based gradient zone separation created via ionic diffusion processes. Such preferentially asymmetric reactions generate differential concentration gradients around the particle surface consuming the ions and establishing a local electric field that can drive/propel the particle motion. In some cases, like semiconductor-based CPMNRs, self-electrophoresis is responsible for electron-hole separation influenced by the light traveling in the proper matched wavelength and further migrates them in redox-half reactions to drive the reaction. Secondly, self-diffusiophoresis can also be the driving principle for CPMNRs, wherein one side of the asymmetric/Janus structures remains unreactive, leaving the other side with propulsive chemical reactions. Depending on the nature of such reactions (i.e., presence and absence of electric field), it can be further categorized into two categories such as electrolyte and non-electrolyte diffusiophoresis. Finally, the bubble-propulsion technique is one of the most significant mechanisms driven by the gas bubbles (e.g., O_2 and CO_2) generated through chemical reactions. For instance, Mg is an extremely attractive material in terms of high stability, biocompatibility, and eco-friendly parameters [38]. Such active Mg metal can form a passive layer of $Mg(OH)_2$ when rapidly dissolved in $NaHCO_3$ aqueous solution, forming soluble $MgCO_3$ [39]. Eventually, continuous H_2 bubbles are released from the catalyst surface and reaction environment to propel CPMNRs. Recently, CPMNRs with multimodal propulsion capabilities have also been developed. These multimodal propulsions enable CPMNRs to operate in diverse physicochemical and biological environments [40].

3. Photocatalyst-Type CPMNRS for Environmental Remediation

Photocatalysis is an advanced oxidation process used for treating both domestic and industrial effluents. It has been proven highly effective in removing a broad spectrum of water contaminants, including dyes, pesticides, pharmaceuticals, and toxins. When exposed to light (ultraviolet, visible, or direct sunlight) at specific wavelengths, ROS such as hydroxyl ($\bullet OH$), superoxide ($O_2\bullet^-$), and perhydroxyl ($HO_2\bullet^-$) radicals are generated. These ROS facilitate the mineralization of organic pollutants through non-selective oxidation.

These photocatalyst-type CPMNRs can utilize both light and chemical energy for self-propulsion in micromotors, enabling potential environmental remediation [34,41,42]. For example, a highly efficient, light-driven photocatalytic TiO_2-Au Janus micromotor (~1.0 μm in diameter) has been developed by Dong et al. for efficient pollutant degradation [43] (Figure 1a,b). The Janus micromotor consists of a catalytic TiO_2 particle (~1.0 μm in diameter), with one hemisphere coated with a 40 nm thick layer of Au metal. When exposed to UV light, the TiO_2 surface activates the self-electrophoretic propulsion mechanism, driving the micromotor in pure water. UV irradiation causes charge separation within the TiO_2, with electrons transferred from the TiO_2 conduction band to the Au hemisphere. This triggers water oxidation at the TiO_2 surface, producing protons (H^+), while the electrons reduce H^+ at the Au hemisphere. The resulting proton flux generates fluid flow toward the Au hemisphere, creating a slip velocity that propels the micromotor forward with the TiO_2 side leading. The micromotor achieves efficient propulsion, moving at over 25 body lengths/s under extremely low UV light intensity (40×10^{-3} W/cm^2) in pure water. Its velocity can be further enhanced by increasing light intensity or adding low concentrations of chemical fuel, such as H_2O_2. Akhavan et al. reported a remotely controllable graphite-based swimmer powered by a graphene jet nanomotor [44]. These swimmers self-exfoliate in water after sodium intercalates between graphene layers, causing graphene flakes to eject at speeds of up to 7000 m/s. This jet propulsion generated a force (~0.7 pN) that enabled the swimmer to move at the speed of 17–40 μm/s. The swimmers are made by attaching TiO_2 NPs (~15 nm) to pyramidal graphite particles, followed by sodium intercalation. When exposed to water, a sodium–water reaction led to the generation of gaseous H_2, which caused nanobubble explosions and propelled the nanomotors. The motion, enhanced by UV light, can be controlled by a magnetic field. An increase in the intensity of UV irradiation accelerated the movement of nanomotors due to an increase in the production of H_2 nanobubbles.

A glucose-fueled visible-light active cuprous oxide@N-doped carbon nanotube (Cu_2O@N-CNT) micromotor was also explored for water remediation [45] (Figure 1c,d). These micromotors are fabricated by the facile one-pot method. Briefly, a certain ratio of N-CNTs, copper acetate, sodium dodecyl sulfate (SDS), sodium hydroxide, and glucose was dissolved in an aqueous ethanol solution and heated to 73 °C for 30 min. The asymmetric surface chemical reaction on Cu_2O@N-CNT particles is the driving force for the propulsion of the micromotors. Briefly, with exposure of the micromotor to visible light on one side, a charge separation within Cu_2O occurred, which resulted in the migration of electrons from a conduction band of Cu_2O to N-CNT. The holes (h^+) and charges formed during this process led to the photocatalytic degradation of glucose, which produces a product gradient around the surface of the micromotors and propelled the micromotors to the opposite direction of the light source (negative phototaxis). The Cu_2O@N-CNT micromotors displayed promising propulsion with a maximum speed of 18 μm/s in a glucose solution under visible light. The velocities of these micromotors were tuned by either regulating the composition of N-CNT and glucose or changing the intensities of the light source.

Synthetic dyes find applications in textile, leather, pharmaceutical, and food processing industries. It was reported that around 80% of dye-contaminated water is discharged into waterways meant for domestic and agricultural use. Untreated synthetic dyes are detrimental to ecosystems and human health. Some of the dyes are designated as potential carcinogens, and toxic to plants and animals [46]. Photocatalytic CPMNRs capable of degrading representative dyes such as Rhodamine B (RB dye) and methylene blue (MB dye) were developed. Nickel (Ni) nanowire-filled TiO_2-noble metal (Pt, and PtPd) nanotube nanomotors were prepared for photocatalytic water remediation under both UV, visible, and natural sunlight [47]. These multicomponent nanostructures were fabricated using an electrochemical synthesis route, specifically through sequential template-assisted electrodeposition. The bimetallic Pt-Pd nanotubes exhibited 1.7 times higher photocatalytic efficiency compared to monometallic Pd nanotubes. TiO_2-PtPd-Ni nanotubes achieved 100% degradation of the organic pollutant, RB dye, within 50 min (the rate k = 0.071 min^{-1}) under visible light, and within 30 min under natural sunlight. To enable precise control and reusability, these nanomotors were designed to respond to external fields. The novel architecture of these coaxial nanotubes, coupled with Ni nanowires, allowed their operation under three different propulsion mechanisms: wireless magnetic, acoustic fields, and self-propulsion. Under a rotational magnetic field, the hybrid nanotubes could be accurately guided along a preplanned trajectory. A single, self-propelled Ni-TiO_2-PtPd nanotube motor demonstrated autonomous movement in 5% H_2O_2 solution, where the PtPd nanotube catalyzed the decomposition of H_2O_2, and self-propelled the motor by the ejecting O_2 bubbles. The dual propulsion modes, the H_2O_2 fuel-based propulsion, and wireless magnetic field guidance enabled precise control over the movement of these nanomotors.

Visible-light-driven micromotors based on iron phthalocyanine (FePc) and gelatin were developed and used as an eco-friendly photocatalyst for the removal of organic pollutants [48]. The spherical micromotors, composed of FePc and gelatin, were fabricated using an emulsion method. Under visible light, these FePc-based micromotors rapidly move toward the light source through a self-diffusiophoresis mechanism, achieving a maximum speed of 47 μm/s at a light intensity of 1.2 W/cm. Upon light exposure, charge separation occurred in FePc, where electrons in the conduction band reduced molecular oxygen, forming $O_2\bullet^-$. Simultaneously, h^+ in FePc oxidized the water to produce H^+ and •OH. The resulting ionic species create an electric field on the FePc surface, propelling the micromotors toward the light source via self-diffusiophoresis. The micromotors demonstrated significant potential for organic pollutant degradation under visible light, degrading the RB dye within 9 min with a normalized rate constant of 2.49×10^{-2} L/m^2s. An effort was also made to develop a simple strategy for the continuous fabrication of MOF-integrated photocatalytic micromotors for the efficient degradation of organic contaminants [49] (Figure 1e,f). Zeolite imidazolate framework-8@ZnO NPs (ZIF-8-ZnO NPs), serving as potential photocatalysts, and Fe_3O_4@Ag NPs, acting as nanoengines, were integrated into emulsion microdroplets to produce porous micromotors. These micromotors were decorated with ZIF-8@ZnO NPs on the surface and Fe_3O_4@Ag NPs at the base. The resultant micromotors exhibited a synergistic effect in the photocatalytic degradation of organic pollutants, with bubble-propelled motion contributing to the process. Upon UV exposure, the ZIF-8@ZnO NPs generate electron-hole pairs (e^- and h^+), and the interaction of h^+ with water leads to the formation of •OH, which efficiently organic contaminants. Meanwhile, the Fe_3O_4@AgNPs at the base acted as the nanoengines facilitated the asymmetric decomposition of H_2O_2 into O_2 bubbles, enabling negative axial self-propelled motion (motion opposite to the direction of the light source). The speed of the micromotors was controlled by adjusting the concentration of H_2O_2 and SDS. At 30% H_2O_2, varying the SDS concentration from 0.01% to 2% resulted in velocities ranging from ~204 to ~1109 μm/s. With a fixed SDS concentration of 1.5%, increasing the H_2O_2 concentration from 5% to 30% increased the micromotor velocity from ~75 to ~1063 μm/s. The combined effect of the micromotor components achieved a maximum RB dye degradation efficiency of 98% within 60 min of UV exposure.

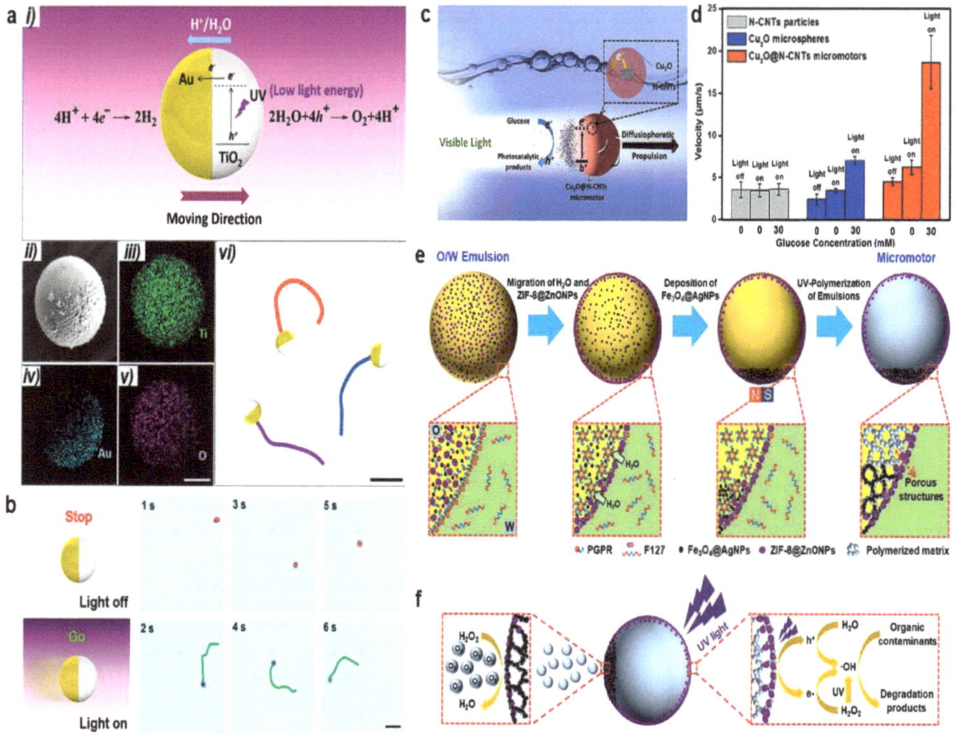

Figure 1. Hybrid photocatalytic CPMNRs for environmental remediation: (**a**) Schematic representation of (*i*) catalytic TiO_2-Au Janus micromotors powered by UV light in water, (*ii–v*) SEM images of spherical TiO_2-Au Janus micromotors with corresponding EDS mapping for Ti, Au, O, respectively, (Scale bar: 0.5 μm) and (*vi*) tracking lines showing distance traveling by three sample motors in water (over 1 s, Scale bar: 10 μm). (**b**) Cyclic "on" and "off" UV light activation of TiO_2-Au Janus micromotor with time-lapse moving status in pure water, respectively. (**c**) Propulsion mechanism of light-driven Cu_2O@N-CNT sphere micromotors. (**d**) Comparison of the velocities of N-CNT particles, Cu_2O spheres, and Cu_2O@N-CNT micromotors in different glucose concentrations and under varying conditions (with or without green light). (**e**) Fabrication process of MOF-integrated photocatalytic micromotors from O/W emulsion droplets. (**f**) Bubble-propulsion technique of micromotors for enhanced photocatalytic degradation of organic contaminants in water. Figures reproduced with permission from [43,45,49].

Decoration of Au NPs on soft-oxometalate (SOM)-based TiO_2 (TiO_2-{Mo_7}-Au) also rendered the visible-light-driven photocatalytic nanomotor capable of degrading organic pollutants [50]. The TiO_2 NPs synthesized by incorporating ammonium heptamolybdate ({Mo_7}), a polyoxometalate (POM), and Au NPs were used to create the SOM-based nanomotor. When exposed to visible light, the TiO_2-{Mo_7}-Au nanomotor was propelled via diffusiophoresis at a speed of 10 μm/s in water, demonstrating excellent photocatalytic performance. Upon light exposure, the nanomotor induces the simultaneous generation of O_2, •OH, and H^+ through water splitting, and oxidation of organic pollutants by the newly formed •OH. This reaction creates a concentration gradient of the photogenerated products on the illuminated side of the nanomotor, driving its autonomous motion. Due to the asymmetric surface reactions, the concentrations of •OH, H^+, $O_2{\bullet}^-$, and O_2 were higher on the irradiated part of TiO_2-{Mo_7}-Au, inducing self-diffusiophoresis, which propelled the nanomotor. This concentration gradient causes the nanomotors to move away from the light source, exhibiting negative phototaxis. The motion of the nanomotors can also be controlled by rapid light On/Off mechanism. The continuous production of photogenerated species (•OH, H^+, O_2•$^-$, and O_2) enables the nanomotors to operate for up to 3 h. These nanomotors significantly enhance the photocatalytic removal of MB dye and benzyl bromide under visible light. Around 73% MB dye degradation was noticed in 30 min, and the benzyl bromide was completely removed within 12 min.

Military activities release potentially toxic organic contaminants used in warfare. Eco-friendly remediation methods such as photocatalysis lower the risk of further chemical pollution [51]. Li et al. reported a groundbreaking innovation that may reshape how we address acute biological and chemical warfare agents (CBWAs) [52]. (Figure 2a–g) They introduced water-driven micromotors-tiny, autonomous systems capable of rapidly degrading harmful substances without the need for external fuels or chemicals. These micromotors consist of magnesium (Mg) NPs at their core, which are coated with a layer of TiO_2 embedded with Au (Au) NPs. This unique structure allows them to harness the photocatalytic properties of TiO_2, while their movement is powered by a simple reaction: when Mg comes into contact with water, it generates H_2 bubbles that propel the micromotors autonomously. This propulsion occurs naturally in water, without any mechanical interference. The H_2 bubbles propelled these micromotors with an average speed of ~80 µm/s, which corresponds to a relative speed of nearly four body lengths/s. In the fabrication process, first, Mg NPs (20 nm) were spread onto a glass slide. Using a modified sputtering technique, these particles are coated with Au NPs. Then, the outer TiO_2 shell was deposited via atomic layer deposition (ALD), a method that ensures an even coating while leaving a small opening where the sphere contacts the glass slide. As these micromotors move through water, their UV-activated TiO_2 surface generates highly reactive species (•OH, O_2•$^-$, and HO_2•). These reactive species play a crucial role in the photocatalytic degradation process, swiftly neutralizing CBWAs and leading to effective decontamination. Without forced convection or external mixing, the micromotors ensured thorough interaction with their environment, and maximized the cleaning efficiency. Within just 10 min of UV irradiation, the micromotors achieved an 86% inactivation of *Bacillus globigii* spores, demonstrating significant antispore activity. They also displayed impressive efficiency in neutralizing persistent organophosphate nerve agents such as bis(4-nitrophenyl) phosphate and methyl paraoxon, achieving 95.7% and 95% degradation, respectively, within the same timeframe. The application of these micromotors can be extended for broader environmental applications. These peroxide-free, autonomous micromotors introduce a new paradigm in photocatalytic decontamination, offering a swift and effective solution to some of the most stable environmental pollutants.

Nitroaromatic compounds are potentially toxic and mutagenic in nature, they are used as an intermediate in the production of explosives, dyes, pharmaceuticals, and pesticides [53]. Noble metal-free, single-component, light-powered WO_3 micromotors were developed for the photocatalytic degradation of nitroaromatic pollutants [54]. These WO_3 micromotors were fabricated through a simple hydrothermal process (200 °C for 20 h) using a tungsten precursor and glucose, followed by calcination at 550 °C. Asymmetric light illumination enables fuel-free self-actuation of the micromotors in pure water, with remote control capability via on/off switching of UV light. When exposed to photons with energies higher than the optical bandgap of WO_3, the micromotors generate e^--h^+ pairs. The resulting e^- decomposes water or H_2O_2 into H^+, while the photogenerated h^+ breaks down water or H_2O_2 into •OH, O_2, and additional H^+. The uneven light exposure creates an asymmetrical distribution of these chemical species, generating a product gradient that propels the micromotors through self-phoresis. The micromotors achieved a speed of 26 ± 2 µm/s in 1% H_2O_2 and degraded 70% of p-nitroaniline and 40% of 4-nitrophenol in water without external agitation. Phenol is the most important chemical intermediate used in fine chemical, plastic, and pharmaceutical industries. Commercial synthesis of phenol involves the use of corrosive acids, and has serious environmental complications [55]. Photocatalyst-type CPMNRs are used to alleviate environmental complications and offer an eco-friendly route for the synthesis of phenol. Dual-responsive rod-like nanomotors have been reported for the photocatalytic conversion of benzene to phenol [56], the typical example for converting water-immiscible hydrophobic pollutants into hydrophilic. This research explored the intricate interplay between optical and magnetic fields in actuating TiO_2/NiFe photocatalytic nanomotors. (Figure 2h–j) The rod-shaped nanomotors were fabricated using a combination of hydrothermal and metal deposition methods. Initially, TiO_2 rods were grown on FTO (fluorine-doped tin oxide) substrates via hydrothermal treatment of TiO_2 seeds. After calcination, a 50 nm Ni/Fe alloy cap was deposited onto the TiO_2 rods using magnetron sputtering. Finally, the TiO_2/NiFe nanomotors were released into water by mechanical scratching. The motion mechanism of these nanomotors is driven by light-induced self-electrophoresis. Upon light irradiation, excitons were generated within the TiO_2 component, followed by electron transfer from TiO_2 to the NiFe alloy, while h^+ accumulated in the semiconductor region. These photogenerated carriers react with fuel to produce O_2 molecules and a proton flux toward the metallic side, creating an imbalance in product formation on each side of the nanomotor. The resultant product gradient caused self-propulsion toward the semiconductor end. The nanomotors maintained motion for up to 2 h under constant light irradiation, achieving speeds of 13.3 ± 0.8 μm/s with light and a weak magnetic field, and 17.0 ± 1.0 μm/s with a strong magnetic field. Additionally, the photocatalytic oxidation of benzene to phenol was investigated in the presence of the oxidant H_2O_2. Upon photoactivation, the TiO_2/NiFe nanomotors generate e^--h^+ pairs, which then react with H_2O_2 or surface-adsorbed hydroxyl groups to produce •OH. These radicals attack benzene, forming a hydroxyl cyclohexadienyl radical, which subsequently yields phenol after losing a proton. The presence of a magnetic field resulted in a 100% increase in photocatalytic phenol production compared to light alone.

In day-to-day life, microplastics are generated from cosmetics, clothes, and packing materials. Microplastics largely harm humans and marine animals. Tackling microplastic pollution is considered the second most serious environmental problem [57]. Photocatalytic CPMNRs were also used for treating water contaminated with microplastics. A water and H2O2-powered photocatalytic Au@Ni@TiO_2-based micromotor was developed for the removal of microparticles and microplastics [58]. These magnetically active Au@mag@TiO_2 micromotors were fabricated by first coating a layer of TiO_2 NPs (10 nm) on Ni or Fe, followed by a 30 nm Au coating. Upon UV-light photoexcitation, conduction band e^- and valence band h^+ were generated on the TiO_2 NP's surface, initiating water oxidation at the TiO_2 hemisphere, which left the h^+. Meanwhile, the e^- migrates to the metal cap, facilitating h^+ reduction at the metal hemisphere. The h^+ consumption induced fluid flow toward the metal cap and caused photocatalytic propulsion. As a result, the micromotors achieved self-propulsion at a speed of 14.72 μm/s in water and 65.52 μm/s in 0.1% H_2O_2 solution under UV light. The self-propelled micromotors employed two distinct strategies for removing microplastics and suspended particles. Individual micromotors achieved the removal of particles via phoretic interactions, while magnetic micromotor chain assemblies relied on shoveling or pushing actions. Remarkably, 67% of microplastics were removed via phoretic interactions in pure water within 40 s. In 0.1% H_2O_2, 77% removal efficiency of suspended particles was achieved within 120 s through shoveling interactions, and 71% removal of microplastics occurred in 0.2% H_2O_2 via the same mechanism. These light-driven micromotors demonstrated potential applications in removing various suspended particles, irrespective of their material composition and shape.

Pathogenic microorganisms are primarily responsible for the outbreak of diseases. Photocatalytic water disinfection has been preferred over traditional chlorination and UV disinfection. The former leads to the generation of carcinogenic byproducts and the latter allows the regrowth of bacteria and viruses [59]. In this regard, light-propelled CPM-NRs are also utilized for the eradication of bacterial films and disinfection of pathogens. Single-component, star-shaped $BiVO_4$ micromotors capable of autonomous movement under visible light were studied for microbial disinfection [60] (Figure 2k,l). The micromotors were synthesized via a hydrothermal method, where aqueous solutions of bismuth and vanadium precursors were initially mixed at room temperature in the presence of ethylenediaminetetraacetic acid (EDTA), a capping agent that promotes the formation of star-shaped $BiVO_4$ particles. Upon visible-light exposure, the asymmetric generation of reactive chemical species on the multifaceted $BiVO_4$ surface drives the self-propulsion of the micromotors through a self-diffusiophoretic mechanism, achieving speeds up to 5 ± 1 µm/s at the H_2O_2 concentration of 0.025 wt%. Under visible light, self-propulsion was observed from the low concentration of H_2O_2 (0.01 wt%). In fuel-free conditions, these micromotors selectively targeted yeast cells, suggesting a promising fungicidal potential under visible light. Micromotor–yeast cell interactions in light on/off conditions over 40 min confirmed the minimal cell death in the dark, and nearly complete yeast cell death under light. This biocidal effect is attributed to the photocatalytic generation of highly oxidizing ROS (HO•, $O_2{\bullet}^-$, and H_2O_2) on the micromotor surface, which disrupts microbial cell membranes and ultimately leads to their disinfection. The chemical gradient around the activated $BiVO_4$ micromotors created phoretic attraction, and enabled cargo loading and transport of polystyrene (PS) particles. Repeated loading and release of PS particles was also controlled by light on/off. Self-propelled mesoporous SiO_2/Au nanomotors driven by near-infrared (NIR) light were explored for the eradication of *Pseudomonas aeruginosa* biofilms [61]. The outer Au shell was sputtered on the SiO_2 base. Upon NIR irradiation, the photothermal effect of the Au component initiates their motion. Au absorbs NIR light and converts it into heat, creating an asymmetric temperature gradient around the SiO_2/Au nanomotors. This gradient causes differential mobility of water molecules to generate thermophoretic force that is converted into motion. The nanomotors show faster movement at higher laser power, reaching a maximum velocity of approximately 86 µm/s at 57.5 mW, irrespective of the specific wavelength within the NIR range. The self-propulsion allowed their penetration deep inside the biofilm matrix and dispersed and eradicated the film via the photothermal effect rendered by Au. This rapid movement enables effective penetration into bacterial biofilms and gradual biofilm destruction. NIR exposure reduced the bacterial biomass by 20% within 30 s, and a 30 min exposure resulted in a 71% reduction. These nanomotors hold significant potential for future biomedical applications, particularly due to the high drug-loading capacity within the mesoporous SiO_2 framework.

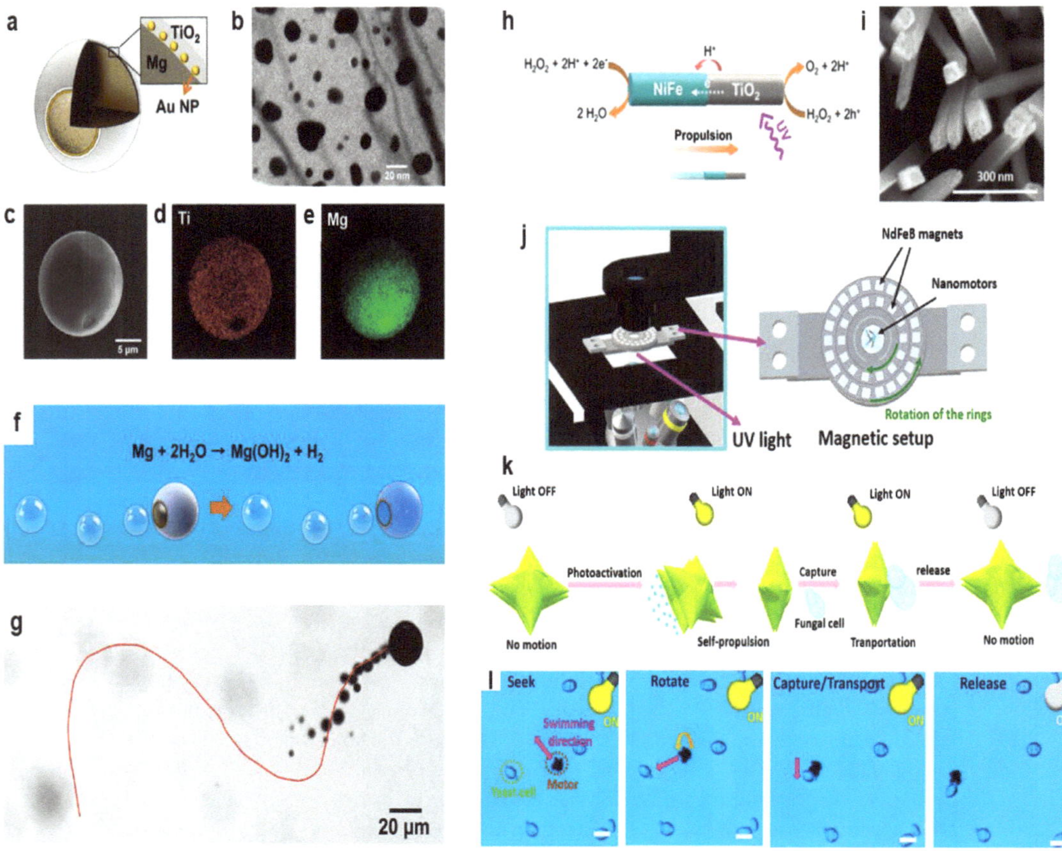

Figure 2. CPMNRs showing self-propulsion and photocatalytic degradation of biological and chemical agents: (**a**) Graphical illustration of photoactive TiO_2/Au/Mg motor design depicting the Mg core, Au NPs, and shell TiO_2 layer. (**b**) TEM images of Au NPs embedded inside TiO_2 surface. (**c**) SEM image of single TiO_2/Au/Mg motor with (**d**,**e**) corresponding EDS images of Mg core and TiO_2 shell, respectively. (**f**) Propulsion scheme of TiO_2/Au/Mg motor. (**g**) Tracking the motion path of motor's propulsion over 3 s period in 90% seawater (Surfactant level: 0.075% Triton X-100). (**h**) Photocatalytic motion activation mechanism of TiO_2/NiFe nanomotors and its (**i**) FESEM image. (**j**) Scheme depicting the optical/magnetic setup used for motion activation of nanomotors. (**k**) Mechanism of visible-light-driven photoactivated $BiVO_4$ micromotors for controlled cargo transportation. (**l**) Diverse stages of $BiVO_4$ micromotors interaction with yeast cells under visible-light activation. Figures reproduced with permission from [52,56,60].

4. Fenton-Type CPMNRs for Environmental Remediation

The Fenton process is also an advanced oxidation process that relies on the reaction between Fe^{2+} or Fe^{3+} ions and H_2O_2 to generate •OH. This process is particularly effective for treating water contaminated with stable, non-biodegradable organic compounds. Unlike photocatalysis, which requires light, Fenton oxidation occurs in the dark. The use of H_2O_2 as both a reagent and a propellant, along with the magnetic properties of iron catalysts, makes Fenton-type CPMNRs highly adaptable for water remediation. To minimize sludge formation, Fenton processes are sometimes combined with light irradiation (photo-Fenton).

Both classical and photo-Fenton-type heterogenous catalysis-based CPMNRs were investigated for removing various water contaminants. MB dye was predominantly used as the target pollutant. In a few cases, RB dye and methyl orange dye (MO dye) were also used as target pollutants. Soler et al. fabricated Fe-Pt tubular micromotors, in which Fe formed an outer layer and Pt formed an inner layer [62] (Figure 3a–d). The nanomembranes of Fe and Pt were rolled up. This micromotor enables Fenton-reaction-mediated oxidation. This micromotor degraded RB dye at a rate of 12 times faster than the typical Fenton reaction. H_2O_2 was used as a reagent as well as propellent for moving the micromotor. The efficient oxidation capability of this micromotor can be used for designing new and faster water remediation strategies meant for removing organic contaminants. With the objective of preparing a micromotor at the kilogram scale, instead of H_2O_2, Teo et al. used eco-friendly citric acid for bubble-propelled zerovalent iron (ZVI) nanomotors [63]. Upon reacting with metallic iron, acids release H_2 bubbles. These bubbles are used for the propulsion of ZVI (100–400 nm), and synthesized by the thermally induced solid-state method. ZVI was stabilized by the natural oxide (iron oxide) shell. When observed under optical microspore, bubble generation was noticed from 0.42 wt.% concentration of citric acid, and movement (7–20 μm/s) for ZVI was noticed from 3.38 wt.%. Up to 27.1%, the velocity of ZVI remained unaltered. For water remediation studies, MO and MB dyes were used as model pollutants. When compared with controls, the ZVI–citric acid mixture led to high pollutant degradation due to the asymmetric propulsion of ZVI. Bubble ejection and propulsion set the continuous movement of ZVI and resulted in an effect similar to mechanical mixing. Accelerated pollutant removal shown by ZVI nanomotors was suggested as being useful for practical water decontamination. Large-scale synthesis of ZVI offered by the solid-state method was considered advantageous for practical applications.

MNRs with large functional areas are preferred for coating with a higher amount of catalyst particles, which facilitate bubble formation via H_2O_2 decomposition and an increase in propulsion. Li et al. used magnetic mesoporous SiO_2 as a matrix to prepare a micromotor capable of degrading pollutants via the Fenton process [64]. The matrix was prepared using an emulsion template-based microfluidics method. On the top of the template, a hemispherical polydopamine (PDA) coating was formed. (Figure 3e). This allowed the subsequent coating of Ag NPs via PDA-induced reduction of the $AgNO_3$ precursor. The hemispherical PDA resulted in a magnetic SiO_2 matrix coated with Ag on one side, and the other side had Fe_3O_4. This asymmetric structure is suitable for bubble-based propulsion of micromotor via the Ag NP-catalyzed decomposition of H_2O_2. The •OH produced by the Fenton reaction degraded the water pollutant. Directional O_2 bubbles generated by the Ag NP-catalyzed cyclic decomposition of H_2O_2 propelled the locomotion of micromotors. The addition of 30% (*w*/*v*) H_2O_2 enhanced the velocity of this micromotor to 566.9 μm/s (Figure 3f). When tested for the degradation of MB dye, this micromotor demonstrated 56.15% higher efficiency than the mesoporous magnetic SiO_2. The enhanced mass transfer and large surface area associated with Ag-catalyzed magnetic mesoporous SiO_2 were attributed to the higher pollutant degradation efficiency. Lee et al. prepared a bubble-propelled ZVI micromotor, where Pt was deposited by electron beam evaporation [65]. The stripping of ZVI coated on a glass substrate rendered a hemispherical Pt coating. ZVI acted as an autonomously movable heterogenous Fenton catalyst. In the presence of 5% H_2O_2, the ZVI/Pt micromotors were propelled at a velocity of over 200 μm/s. The spontaneous decomposition of H_2O_2 surrounding asymmetric ZVI-Pt, generated O_2 bubbles, induced strong momentum, and propelled the micromotors forward. Due to mixing-induced mass transfer at a given condition, ZVI-Pt exhibited the complete degradation of MB dye, while only 12% MB dye removal was achieved by ZVI microspheres. In ZVI microspheres, local production of •OH alone was used for dye removal. As H_2O_2 did not propel ZVI microspheres, it remained static and caused lower dye removal efficiency. ZVI-Pt can be tracked by the magnet and separated for reuse. In the fourth cycle, 82% MB dye degradation efficiency was retained. Electron beam deposition and solution phase stripping processes restrict the large-scale preparation of multifunctional ZVI-Pt.

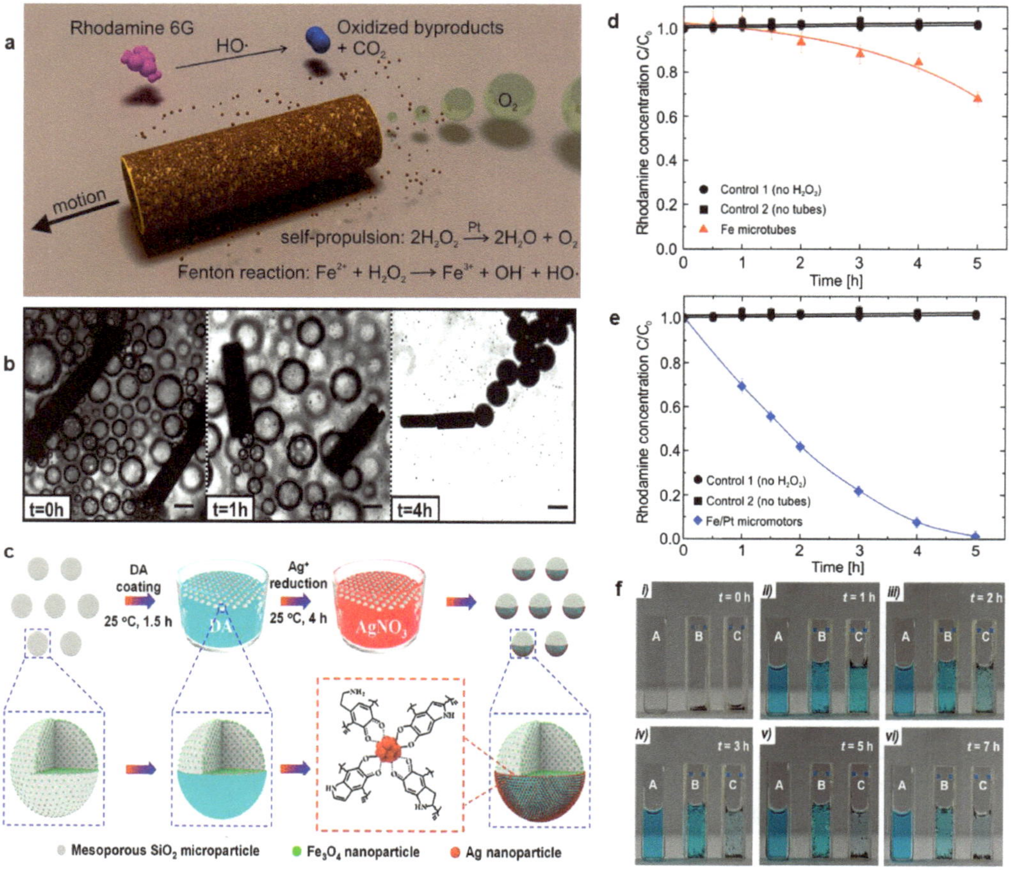

Figure 3. Schematic representation: (**a**) The process of degrading polluted water (RB6G dye as a model contaminant) into inorganic products with the help of multifunctional micromotors is illustrated. The micromotors achieve self-propulsion through an inner catalytic Pt layer, enabling movement in H_2O_2 solutions. Polluted water remediation is facilitated by the interaction of Fe^{2+} ions with peroxide, producing hydroxyl (•OH) radicals that break down organic pollutants. (**b**) Rapid motion of Fe/Pt micromotors vs. time (Scale bar: 125 μm). (**c**) Schematic illustration of fabricating bubble-propelled nanocatalyst-carrying micromotors, initially Fe_3O_4 NP-containing mesoporous SiO_2 microparticles were selectively DA coated in hemispherical fashion, later decorated with Ag NPs, and finally nanocatalyst-carrying micromotors containing Fe_3O_4 NPs were synthesized like Janus nanomotors. (**d**,**e**) Quantitative analysis comparing the degradation of RB6G dye by pure iron (Fe) tubes, represented by red triangles, and catalytically active Fe/Pt tubes, denoted by blue diamonds, over a duration of 5 h. Experimental conditions: pH = 2.5, initial concentration (C_0) RB6G dye = 45 mg/L, H_2O_2 = 15%, SDS = 0.5%, and ~441 ± 10 microtubes dispersed in 1 mL. Control tests, both without H_2O_2 and without microtubes, were included for comparison. (**f**) Micromotors carrying nanocatalysts for water purification. (*i*–*vi*) Optical images depict the degradation of MB dye in aqueous solutions. In samples A–C, 25% (*w*/*v*) H_2O_2 is used. Sample B includes mesoporous SiO_2 microparticles containing Fe_3O_4 NPs, while sample C incorporates nanocatalyst-loaded micromotors (Scale bar: 1 cm). Figures reproduced with permission from [62,64].

Liu et al. fabricated the tubular poly(3,4-ethylenedioxythiophene) (PEDOT)-Fe-MnO_2 micromotors with fish-scale-like intercalated structure, where an active layer of Fe_2O_3, MnO_2, and Mn_2O_3 was deposited via electrodeposition [66]. The Fe layer was formed by cathodic electrodeposition. Electropolymerization was used to generate the outer PEDOT layer. The inner MnO_2 layer was formed by anodic deposition. The surface and structure of bubble-generating MnO_2 can be tuned or designed on-demand by modulating the electrodeposition process. In 5% H_2O_2, the FSI structure enabled the movement of the micromotor at the speed of 111 μm/s. When tested for the degradation of MB dye, PEDOT/Fe−MnO_2 resulted in 97.5% degradation. A hierarchically rough Fe_2O_3 surface and nanoscale MnO_2 provided a large surface area. Thereby improving accessibility of H_2O_2, propulsion, and dye removal efficiency. A high surface area and Fenton reaction rendered higher dye removal efficiency. The O_2 bubbles produced a recoil effect and propelled the micromotor in various modes including linear, helical and flower, rotary, and orbital modes. These motions led to violent mixing and enhanced the efficiency of water decontamination. The bilayer PEDOT/MnO_2 micromotors led to 72% MB dye degradation and the speed was significantly low (65 μm/s). The authors suggested that this method is suitable for mass-scale production and PEDOT/Fe−MnO_2 can be extended to practical applications. However, the multicomponent system and use of the moisture-sensitive PEDOT layer make this system expensive and lacks stability. Ren et al. developed shape- and size-controllable micromotors for water remediation applications [67]. These micromotors were fabricated via phase separation and UV-induced polymerization. Spherical, hemispherical, and crescent-shaped micromotors were fabricated by adjusting the ratio of ethoxylated trimethylolpropane triacrylate and paraffin oil. The size was controlled by fluid flow parameters. Fe_3O_4 and MnO_2 NPs were loaded on the symmetric structure of the polymer matrix, and this resulted in Janus micromotors. Fe_3O_4 and MnO_2 NPs were used as catalysts for the Fenton reaction and H_2O_2 decomposition induced directional formation of O_2 bubbles. The 20% (w/w) H_2O_2 concentration propelled the micromotor with a velocity of about 127 μm/s. The use of Janus micromotors rendered 46.4% higher MB dye degradation than the microparticles only coated with Fe_3O_4. The self-propelled movement of Janus micromotors not only promoted the efficiency of the Fenton reaction but also facilitated its post-separation using an external magnet. Post-separation is helpful for reusing the Janus micromotors and the recovery of pollutants such as dyes and heavy metals, if adsorbed. Magnetic post-separation and high pollutant removal efficiency make this Janus micromotor a potential multifunctional system for water remediation.

With the objective of replacing Pt- and Ag NP-induced propulsion, Liu et al. used MnO_3-induced bubbling for the self-propulsion of a heterogenous Fenton catalyst bearing Janus micromotor [68]. Pt is costly, while there was concern over the toxicity of Ag. Visible-light responsive and chemically stable Fe^+ doped BiOBr with a direct band gap was used as support. The average velocity of solvothermally synthesized FeBiOBr/Fe_3O_4/Mn_3O_4 in the aqueous medium with 5% H_2O_2 was 214.7 ± 19.4 μm/s. At higher H_2O_2 concentration (15%), a random motion (353.6 ± 10.4 μm/s) induced by bubbles released at one end propelled the micromotor. In the lower H_2O_2 concentration (3%), a circular motion (186.7 ± 9.58 μm/s) pattern was noticed. Under these conditions, the non-micromotor, FeBiOBr/Fe_3O_4, remained static. In the solar-Fenton water remediation studies, FeBiOBr/Fe_3O_4 without stirring (static), mechanically stirred FeBiOBr/Fe_3O_4 and FeBiOBr/Fe_3O_4/Mn_3O_4 exhibited 69%, 82%, and 98% MB dye degradation. In addition, the micromotor resulted in 85% total organic carbon (TOC) removal due to the deep oxidation process. The presence of Fe_3O_4 allows the post-separation of micromotors. The autonomous propulsion of micromotors induced convection flow and effective mass transfer, and accelerated the degradation of MB dye. The use of a visible-light-active BiOBr photocatalyst and MB dye target allows for a reasonable comparison between FeBiOBr/Fe_3O_4/Mn_3O_4 photo-Fenton catalysis and traditional stir-mixed BiOBr visible-light photocatalysis. After 240 min, 0.01 g of BiOBr nanobelts (NBs) prepared by Li et al. degraded 65% of MB dye (5 mg/L, 50 mL) under visible light [69]. The degradation efficiency of MB dye (10 mg/L, 100 mL, 3 mL 30% H_2O_2) using FeBiOBr/Fe_3O_4/Mn_3O_4 (0.1 g) was 98% after 50 min exposure to natural sunlight. To maintain the velocity of CPMNRs, a sufficient dosage of H_2O_2 was continually added to maintain its concentration throughout the reaction period. Although the efficiency of FeBiOBr/Fe_3O_4/Mn_3O_4 CPMNRs appears slightly higher, even without stir mixing, the multicomponent structure and the addition of a strong oxidizing agent (H_2O_2) make photo-Fenton CPMNRs more complicated than traditional photocatalysis.

GO can facilitate the easy dispersion of Fe_3O_4 and function as a supporting matrix for Fe_3O_4. Shi et al. prepared a Fe_3O_4-rGO-Pt microjet for Fenton-based heterogeneous oxidation-based environmental remediation [70]. First, on GO, reduced GO (rGO) was coated and made into a tubular structure, where the inside was coated with Pt, and Fe_3O_4 was deposited outside. The fuel concentration and motion thrust were estimated at H_2O_2 concentrations of 1.5% (200 μm/s) and 10% (1300 μm/s). The velocity of the microjets was unaffected by the quantity of the Fe_3O_4 coating. This microjet was studied for the degradation of MB dye. In the presence of 1.5% H_2O_2, 71% MB dye degradation was noticed, whereas no significant degradation was noticed with single components (Fe_3O_4 and rGO). These microjets can be separated by an external magnet and used for diverse environmental applications. On the fifth reuse cycle, 62% degradation efficiency was retained. The process followed for fabricating microjets was tedious and may not be suitable for large-scale and cost-effective application.

Chen et al. used naturally abundant kapok fiber as a template for the fabrication of a bubble-propelled micromotor, where MnO_2 was used as the bubble-generating catalyst via decomposition of H_2O_2 [71]. MnO_2 was generated by dip-coating $KMnO_4$ on the Kapok fiber, and subsequent in situ reduction at ambient temperature. Cellulose present in the fiber cell wall reduced the $KMnO_4$ into MnO_2. The Fe_3O_4 NPs were deposited by stirring MnO_2-coated kapok fiber with Fe_3O_4 NPs suspension. MnO_2 was coated on both the outer and inner cell wall of the Kapok fiber. In 2.5% H_2O_2, the motion speed of the micromotor reached 615 μm/s. When tested for the degradation of MB dye, the micromotor exhibited higher efficiency than the Fe_2O_4 and MnO_2-coated kapok fiber due to self-propulsion, Fe^{2+}-triggered, and MnO_2-induced Fenton reaction. In wastewater and D.I water medium, the MB dye degradation was 89.5%, and 77%, respectively. This is attributed to the velocity of kapok fiber-MnO_2-Fe_2O_4 in D.I water (1027.76 μm/s) and wastewater (283.96 μm/s). This micromotor can also be navigated and separated by an external magnet. A cost-effective preparation method and the efficiency of these micromotors suggest its potential as an autonomous microcleaner for practical water remediation. Gao et al. developed a self-propelled nanomotor based on the combination of enzyme-nanozyme. Iron-1,3,5-benzenetricarboxylate (Fe-BTC) MOF was used as a support for preparing a hybrid nanomotor composed of natural multicopper oxidase enzyme - Laccase (Lac), NiFe-layered double hydroxide (NiFe-LDH) and MnO_2-loaded halloysite nanotubes (HNTs) [72]. H_2O_2 (5%) was used a fuel. This nanomotor exhibited peroxidase and Fenton-like catalytic activities, utilized for sensing and removal of minocycline (MC), an antibiotic. Further discussion on this hybird nanomotor was made in Section 6 focussed on CPMNRs based sensors for pollutant detection.

Like halloysite, several natural clays have been used to develop Fenton-type CPMNRs. These natural clay-based CPMNRs have emerged as an environmentally friendly alternative to fully synthetically fabricated CPMNRs, which often rely on stringent procedures often harmful to the environment. In addition to the inherent adsorption characteristics, due to the presence of Fe, the surface of microclays can induce Fenton catalysis reactions. Pt-deposited Cloisite displayed fast average autonomous motion (110 μm/s), in response to the addition of 5% H_2O_2. This CPMNR was proved to be useful for removing fenitrothion, which is used as a pesticide and improvised nerve agent [73]. Pelagic clays originating from the Indian Ocean possess high Fe and Mn content, and they function as Fenton catalysts and autonomous motion in the presence of H_2O_2 [74]. The main mineral constituents of Pelagic clays are illite/montmorillonite and amorphous ferromanganese nodules. In the absence of H_2O_2, the clay microparticles were static. In 10 wt.% H_2O_2, clay microparticles (2 mg) were moved with the highest average velocity of 183.0 μm/s and fully decolorized the RB dye (18 mL, 11.1 mg/L) via Fenton catalysis. Thus, naturally abundant clay resources can be used for preparing cost-effective and potential CPMNRS for water remediation.

Synergistic effects drawn from multi-metallic catalysts allow the operation of MOF-based micromotors across various environmental conditions. Cubic and sphere-shaped MOF structures based on CoMn-Prussian blue and its analog were developed by tuning the morphology and composition. They were set to move under light, bubble, and external magnetic fields [75]. Without H_2O_2 addition, sphere-shaped MOFs exhibited high mobility under UV and blue light. Cubic MOFs displayed motion upon H_2O_2 addition and immotile under light. The incorporation of Fe_3O_4 allowed spiral motion under an external magnetic field. With 3% H_2O_2 addition, sphere and cubic MOFs incorporated with Fe_3O_4 degraded 74.98%, and 99.99% of malachite green dye (30 ppm, 50 mL), respectively. These bimetallic MOFs were also shown to degrade chlortetracycline, a veterinary antibiotic. Magnetic recovery offered separation and reuse of these CPMNRs. However, CPMNRs with multi-component and complex structures require multi-step synthesis and are not suitable for large-scale practical environment remediation applications.

5. Adsorption-Type CPMNRs for Environmental Remediation

Adsorption is a simple yet effective method for removing both organic and inorganic contaminants from water. Materials with a high surface area, such as porous silica, clays, polymeric materials, and activated carbon, are typically employed as adsorbents. Recently, self-propelled CPMNRs with pollutant selectivity have been developed as dynamic platforms for the on-the-fly capture of various contaminants, ranging from dyes and microorganisms to explosives and heavy metals. Unlike photocatalysis and Fenton-type CPMNRs, adsorption-type CPMNRs have been studied for the removal of a broader range of pollutants, including dyes, antibiotics, heavy metals, herbicides, explosives, and microorganisms. Notably, pollutants like herbicides, which can severely impact aquatic ecosystems, and heavy metals such as mercury, lead, and arsenic, pose significant health risks even in trace amounts. CPMNRs designed for adsorption offer a rapid and efficient means of removing these non-biodegradable and persistent pollutants.

Unlike dyes, organic pollutants, which are more prone to oxidation, for the non-biodegradable and persisting pollutants mentioned above require advanced adsorption technology such as adsorption-type CPMNRs for efficient and rapid removal. MnO_2-based micromotors with combined catalytic degradation and adsorptive bubble separation were also explored for water remediation [76]. The synergistic action of MnO_2 microparticles achieved high decolorization rates of non-biodegradable organic dyes, reaching up to 90% within 1 h, without requiring external agitation or additional bubble generation (Figure 4a). These commercially available MnO_2 microparticles enable O_2 bubble-propelled motion, enhancing their potential for organic dye adsorption. MnO_2 microparticles catalyze the H_2O_2 decomposition and generate O_2 bubbles, which provide the necessary mechanical force for micromotor motion. In a solution containing 5% H_2O_2 and 0.1% SDS, the micromotors achieve rapid movement, reaching a maximum speed of 720 μm/s (Figure 4b).

The decomposition of H_2O_2 by MnO_2 micromotors generates oxygen bubbles along with ROS, which react with organic molecules, leading to efficient degradation of MB and RB dyes (Figure 4c). This combined effect enables MnO_2 micromotors to decolorize azo dyes over 90% within 1 h, progressing to nearly complete decolorization over extended periods without the need for external agitation.

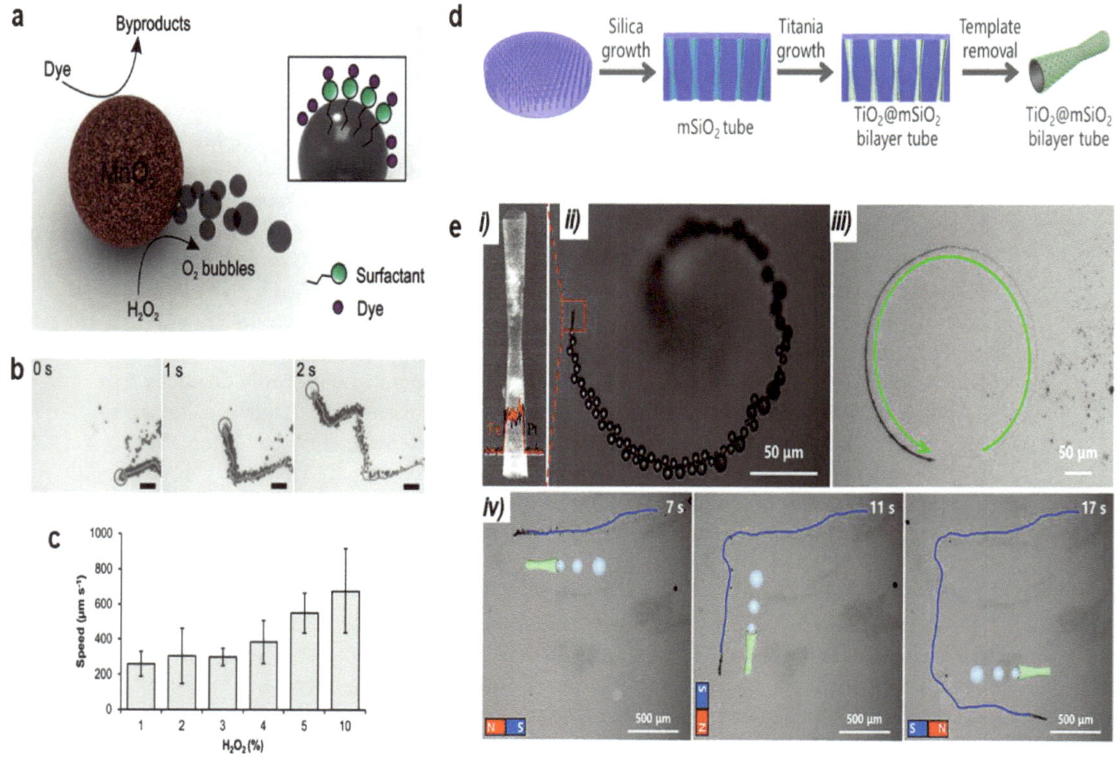

Figure 4. Adsorption-type CPMNRs for environmental remediation: (**a**) Schematic representation of water decolorization by MnO_2-based micromotors via catalytic degradation and adsorptive-type bubble separation of organic dyes. (Inset: adsorption of dye molecules at the bubble–air interface.) (**b**) Movement tracking of MnO_2 micromotors in the presence of 5% H_2O_2 as fuel and 0.1% SDS as surfactant. Scale bar 100 μm. (**c**) Average velocity of MnO_2 micromotors in different concentrations of H_2O_2 with 0.5% SDS as a surfactant (error bars = 1 SD; n = 7). (**d**) Graphical illustration of the synthesis of TiO_2@$mSiO_2$ bilayer tubes. (**e**) Corresponding (*i*) cross-section image after loading Pt and Fe_3O_4 NPs in bilayer tubular TiO_2@$mSiO_2$ motors, (*ii,iii*) video snapshots of its motion in aqueous solution, and (*iv*) trajectory of directional motion of a bubble-propelled micromotor guided by an external magnetic field. Figures reproduced with permission from [76,77].

A bubble-propelled bilayer tubular micromotor was developed, which consists of a mesoporous silica-coated titania (TiO_2@$mSiO_2$) structure, decorated with Pt and magnetic Fe_3O_4 NPs on the inner wall [77] (Figure 4d). The micromotors are fabricated using a template-assisted method. Initially, an $mSiO_2$ layer is grown on the inner surface of the micropores, followed by the addition of a TiO_2 layer to form TiO_2@$mSiO_2$ bilayer tubes. Pt and Fe_3O_4 NPs are then loaded onto the inner wall of the tubes. Then, the template was dissolved in DMF to yield the bilayer tubes. The outer mesoporous silica layer provides efficient pollutant adsorption, resulting in the TiO_2@$mSiO_2$ tube achieving threefold higher adsorption than the TiO_2 tubes. By applying an external magnetic field, the micromotors can be recovered to release collected pollutants for precise analysis. In an aqueous solution containing 2.5% H_2O_2 and 0.125% SDS, the micromotors efficiently generated O_2 bubbles, propelling them at an average speed of 970 ± 354 μm/s, with a maximum velocity of 1635 μm/s (Figure 4e). The motors effectively collect contaminants due to the strong pollutant adsorption of the $mSiO_2$ shell, aiding pollutant monitoring and removal. Using analytical techniques like SERS, the composition of model pollutants can be identified. These bilayer motors exhibited pollutant degradation capabilities, driven by the photocatalytic activity of the TiO_2 layer, self-propulsion-induced micro-mixing, and ROS generation from Pt-catalyzed H_2O_2 decomposition under solar irradiation. This system degraded nearly 98% of R6G within 30 min, demonstrating excellent degradation efficiency. Furthermore, the motors can be recovered by a magnetic field, minimizing secondary pollution and enhancing reusability and cost-effectiveness. Airborne carbon soot also was employed for the preparation of multifunctional micromotors via two different methods: physical deposition of catalytic Pt (110 nm) and magnetic Ni (100 nm) layers, and a chemical deposition of magneto-catalytic iron NPs onto carbon soot [78]. The fabrication process begins with depositing a layer of carbon soot on a glass slide using a paraffin candle, followed by thermal evaporation of a Ni nanofilm and sputtering of a Pt nanofilm on the soot-coated glass. The coated soot particles are dislodged from the glass slide, suspended in 50% ethanol, and sonicated to yield micrometer-sized "CARBOts". Alternatively, "iCARBOts" are fabricated by depositing iron NPs onto the soot surface via $NaBH_4$-assisted chemical reduction of $FeCl_3$ in the presence of soot particles. These carbon soot-based micromotors (CS micromotors) demonstrated dual capabilities: the oxidative degradation of MB dye and the potential removal of oil contaminants from seawater. With the catalytic reaction between Pt and H_2O_2-generated water and O_2, the continuous release of O_2 bubbles propelled the micromotors. CARBOts exhibit an average speed of ~2.8 μm/s in a 6% (v/v) H_2O_2 solution, which increases to ~47.5 μm/s in a 14% H_2O_2 solution. The micromotors facilitate the degradation of organic pollutants by forming photocatalytic products in H_2O_2 fuel, degrading approximately 60% of MB in 10 min and nearly 99.5% within ~40 min. Their self-propulsion enhances reactant diffusion and mixing, increasing MB dye degradation efficiency. The micromotors are also effective for the on-the-fly capture, transport, and removal of oil contaminants from water. The hydrophobic carbon soot, combined with a magnetically controllable Ni layer, allows remote-controlled oil removal from seawater. Upon contact with oil droplets, the micromotor surface immediately pins the droplets. After capturing oil, the micromotor can move from treated to untreated areas to capture additional oil. Finally, micromotors pinned with oil droplets are magnetically retrieved from the seawater, and the oil is removed by sonicating in ethanol for 20 min, followed by vacuum drying, which prepares the micromotors for another cycle. The use of 5 mg of micromotors removed 95% of surfactant-free oil and 70% of surfactant-stabilized oil.

An Fe_2O_3-decorated SiO_2/MnO_2 microjet was developed for the simultaneous removal of organic pollutants and heavy metals from contaminated water [79]. This microjet exhibits enhanced photocatalytic and adsorptive properties, enabling efficient degradation of specific organic contaminants like tetracycline (TC) and RB under visible-light irradiation, along with the removal of heavy metal ions such as Cd^{2+} and Pb^{2+}. Using a sol–gel method, the microjets were synthesized with a polycarbonate template to create multifunctional mesoporous SiO_2-based structures. These microjets feature MnO_2 on the tube's inner wall and magnetically active γ-Fe_2O_3 NPs on the outer surface. The MnO_2 catalytically decomposes H_2O_2 into water and O_2, generating microbubbles that propel the microjet. In a solution containing 7% H_2O_2 and 0.2% SDS, the microjets reach a maximum speed of 485 ± 32 μm/s. The decomposition of H_2O_2 not only provides propulsion but also enables the degradation of organic pollutants through a Fenton-like reaction. The reaction mechanism involves the generation of electron-hole pairs under visible light irradiation, which migrate to the surface and react with adsorbed molecules to produce radicals. These radicals, with high oxidation potential, effectively degrade organic molecules, TC, and RB dye into non-toxic products such as CO_2 and H_2O. Additionally, the microjets demonstrate an impressive ability to remove toxic heavy metals, achieving removal efficiencies of up to 98% for Cd^{2+} and 94% for Pb^{2+}. DNA-functionalized microtubes capable of self-propulsion through bubble generation were developed using electrodeposition and explored as micromachines for the potential removal of Hg(II) from water [80]. The microtube micromotors feature a catalytic Pt inner surface to drive self-propulsion by decomposing H_2O_2 fuel, and a Au outer surface for functionalization with DNA. The DNA sequence's strong affinity for Hg(II), via T-T mismatched pairing, enabled efficient adsorption of Hg(II) onto the microtubes. These tubular micromachines, fabricated through template-assisted electrodeposition, exhibited an average velocity of 244 μm/s in pure water with 3% H_2O_2, dropping to 179 μm/s when functionalized with DNA. Propulsion was sustained by continuous O_2 bubble thrust from the catalytic degradation of H_2O_2. In adsorption experiments, unmodified microtubes showed minimal influence on Hg(II), while DNA-functionalized microtubes achieved a 17% reduction in Hg(II) concentration. Further, in 3% H_2O_2 containing 0.3% SDS, DNA-functionalized microtubes removed 26% of Hg(II) within 20 min, demonstrating their effectiveness in Hg(II) removal from aqueous solutions. Zhang et al. used the electrospinning method for the scalable preparation of low-cost and large-scale preparation of MnO_2-based tubular micromotors capable of adsorbing heavy metal ions [81]. Various MnO_2-based tubular CPMNRs (MnO_2–TiO_2, MnO_2–SnO_2, and MnO_2–$MnWO_4$) were fabricated by hollowing the residual carbon in the electrospun metal oxide nanofibers during hydrothermal growth of MnO_2 from potassium permanganate. The MnO_2-catalyzed decomposition of H_2O_2 led to morphology-dependent motion. MnO_2–$MnWO_4$ exhibited the highest velocity (203.7 μm/s) in 5 wt.% H_2O_2. Morphology seriously influences the interaction between the bubbles and surrounding fluid. Changes in bubble–fluid interaction led to the movement of micromotors in the circular, linear, and spiral trajectories. Tubular MnO_2–$MnWO_4$@Fe_3O_4 micromotors demonstrated high Cu^{2+} (586.5 mg/g) and Pb^{2+} (156.4 mg/g) adsorption capacity. The electrospinning strategy reported in this work can pave the way for utilizing CPMNRs for practical heavy metal decontamination of water.

Pt-free, bio-inspired micromotors based on kapok fiber-derived ZIF-8 were also explored for efficient water remediation [82]. The micromotor design features an outer layer of ZIF-8 for pollutant adsorption, an inner catalytic component for photocatalytic H_2O_2 degradation to produce O_2 bubbles, and magnetic γ-Fe_2O_3 for magnetic control and retrieval after pollutant removal. To create these micromotors, kapok fibers served as templates to fabricate magnetic porous microtubes composed of mixed metal oxides (γ-Fe_2O_3/γ-Al_2O_3) and catalytic MnO_2 particles on both inner and outer tube surfaces. A suitable growth method was used to coat ZIF-8 onto the outer layer of the magnetic microtubes. In a solution of 5% H_2O_2 with 1% SDS, the micromotors demonstrated rapid movement, reaching speeds of up to 150 μm/s, driven by O_2 bubbles generated through MnO_2-catalyzed H_2O_2 decomposition. The Fe_2O_3 particles enabled magnetic control over the micromotors' movement direction and facilitated their recovery after pollutant capture. These bio-inspired ZIF-8-based micromotors exhibit excellent adsorption capacities for Congo red dye (394 mg/g) and doxycycline (242 mg/g), achieving nearly 100% removal efficiency for various contaminants within 1 h.

Various biotemplates were used as a sustainable, low-cost, and eco-friendly source for the preparation of MNRS. Biotemplates are rich in functional groups, and available with unique structures such as tubes, pollen, spherical, and spiral. These templates are non-toxic, eco-friendly, and can be volatilized to yield carbon without residue [83]. The biotemplate method was also used for the straightforward fabrication of Pt-free micromotors, and for temperature-controlled recognition, capture, and release of erythromycin (ERY) in water [84]. The micromotors exhibit precise temperature-dependent adsorption of ERY, enhanced by magnetic navigation and easy recovery. This was achieved through a two-step asymmetric modification: first, porous magnetic $Mn_3O_4/CoFe_2O_4$ (MMT) cores were prepared by heat-treating lotus pollen as a biotemplate. These MMT cores were then embedded in a poly(vinylpyrrolidone) (PVP) film on a glass substrate and coated with ERY-specific, hydrogel-based molecularly imprinted polymers (MIPs). Finally, the Janus-type micromotors (t-MIP-MMTs) were released from the substrate through a blade-scraping technique. When placed in an ERY solution with H_2O_2 fuel (2% H_2O_2 with 1.25% SDS), the micromotors demonstrated a mean velocity of 161 $\pm$ 9 μm/s. The velocity increased to 178 $\pm$ 6 μm/s and 191 $\pm$ 11 μm/s with H_2O_2 concentrations of 5 wt.% and 7 wt.%, respectively. In adsorption experiments, 50 mg of t-MIP-MMTs achieved 50% adsorption of ERY in 10 min, with nearly complete adsorption (98%) within 1 h. The temperature-controlled adsorption and release mechanism was attributed to the polymer's temperature-sensitive self-assembly. At temperatures above the lower critical solution temperature (LCST), the micromotors' linear polymer chains undergo a coil-to-globule transition, reducing hydrophilicity and shrinking the distance between the ERY molecules and the polymer matrix. This change increases the interaction between ERY and MAA through hydrogen bonding, enhancing ERY adsorption. For release, cooling below LCST causes the hydrogel layer to swell, weakening hydrogen bonds and releasing the captured ERY into the water. Additionally, the $CoFe_2O_4$ core enables magnetic navigation, facilitating directional control and rapid recovery of the micromotors post-ERY adsorption.

Substrate-free GO micromotors were fabricated using a simple microfluidic-based method for the rapid removal of antibiotics from wastewater [85]. In brief, GO sheets were encapsulated within droplets, subjected to thermal evaporation, and then compressed via capillary forces to form the desired micromotors. These micromotors are chemically propelled by O_2 generated through the decomposition of H_2O_2 in the presence of a Pt nanoflower catalyst. The motion direction can be controlled by applying a magnetic field due to the incorporation of Fe_3O_4 NPs into the micromotors. The propulsion is primarily driven by the imbalance in O_2 production on the micromotors' surface. At a fixed surfactant concentration (0.3% SDS), the speed of the micromotors increased from 72 $\pm$ 11.7 μm/s to 470 $\pm$ 36 μm/s as the H_2O_2 concentration was raised from 0.5% to 5%, respectively. The micromotors demonstrated high efficiency in removing TC from wastewater, achieving a removal rate of 96 $\pm$ 1.2% with active micromotors compared to just 8.7 $\pm$ 0.9% with static micromotors, at a TC concentration of 10 mg/L within 30 min. Additionally, the removal efficiency increased from 31.2 $\pm$ 1.09% to 99.2 $\pm$ 0.25% as the quantity of micromotors increased from 0.5×10^3 to 2.5×10^3, respectively. This high removal efficiency was attributed to the rapid movement of the micromotors, the abundant wrinkles and pores on their surface, and strong π–π interactions and cation–π bonding between GO and TC. The application of an external magnetic field further aids in controlling micromotor direction and facilitates their separation after remediation. In reusability tests, the micromotors maintained 96% efficiency after four cycles, highlighting their potential for repeated use. Pluronic tri-block copolymer (PTBC)-based thermosensitive magnetic nanorobots (TM nanorobots) were developed to enable efficient removal of pollutants from water [86]. These TM nanorobots utilized a temperature-controlled self-assembly process that facilitates the capture of pollutants like atrazine (ATZ) and Ar via a self-assembling mechanism. Each TM nanorobot consists of a hydrophobic core made from poly(propylene oxide) (PPO), and surrounded by a thermoresponsive hydrophilic shell of poly(ethylene oxide)

(PEO). Fe_3O_4 NPs were incorporated to enable propulsion under an external magnetic field. The PTBC exhibits a reversible, temperature-sensitive phase transition in water, dispersing below the critical micelle temperature (CMT) and precipitating above it. When the temperature rises above the CMT (~25 °C), PTBC undergoes dehydration and forms stronger intramolecular interactions, which trap pollutants within the PTBC matrix. A synergistic application of a rotating magnetic field enhances interactions among polymer blocks in the TM nanorobots, resulting in strong aggregation. Leveraging the magnetic sensitivity of Fe_3O_4, TM nanorobots can be guided to targeted areas by applying a magnetic field, reaching speeds of approximately 1.78 μm/s at 0.5 Hz, with a maximum velocity of 6.21 μm/s at 3 Hz. In pollutant removal experiments, the TM nanorobots demonstrated increasing efficiency, from 5.2% to 59.7%, when the TM nanorobot dosage increased from 3.1 mg to 18.6 mg over a 10 min period. In Ar removal studies, an extension of the movement time from 10 to 100 min increased efficiency from 59.7% to 65.2%. Under lower temperatures, the TM nanorobots achieved an Ar removal efficiency of 44.4%, while in a 100 min period of exposure to a rotating magnetic field, ATZ capture reached 61.5%. Pickup rates for Ar and ATZ were around 73% and 72% in tap water and approximately 65% and 63% in river water, respectively.

Commercially available, biocompatible, and low-cost Pt-decorated activated carbon (Pt-AC) was employed as a self-propelled micromotor for the rapid 'on-the-fly' capture of nitroaromatic compounds [87]. The motion of the micromotors is driven by O_2 bubble generation, resulting from the decomposition of H_2O_2 in the presence of Pt. As the concentration of H_2O_2 increases, the velocity of the micromotors also increases. At 1% H_2O_2, the average speed of the Pt-AC micromotors was 78 ± 32 μm/s, which rose to 382 ± 149 μm/s in a 10 wt% H_2O_2 solution. Activated carbon (AC), with its relatively large surface area, efficiently adsorbs organic contaminants; this was demonstrated using picric acid as a model nitroaromatic compound. The adsorption efficiency was evaluated both with and without micromotor motion over different adsorption times. Without motion, 84% adsorption efficiency was achieved in 30 min, whereas with micromotor motion, an enhanced adsorption efficiency of 87% was observed in just 10 min. This represents a threefold decrease in adsorption time, emphasizing the improved pollutant capture by the 'on-the-fly' adsorption process facilitated by the micromotors. Adsorbent materials are used for the passive sampling of contaminants from an aqueous medium. Passive sampling alleviates the need for active forces such as pumps. The same was used for the capture of pathogens, and it relies on a specific chemical interaction between the absorbent and pathogens [88]. CPMNRs were also developed for the trackable and rapid capture of pathogens. Magnetically controllable microrobots equipped with polymer "hands" were developed. These microrobots self-assembled under an applied magnetic field and effectively captured bacteria and microplastics on the fly, purifying aquatic environments [89]. The microrobots' cationic polymers are synthesized using reversible addition-fragmentation chain-transfer (RAFT) polymerization. The polymers, bearing negatively charged carboxyl groups, are immobilized on the surface of superparamagnetic Dynabeads via amide bonding, activated by EDC/NHS chemistry. When exposed to an external magnetic field, individual magnetic particles self-assemble into planar formations, which then propel under a rotating magnetic field. This motion significantly enhances the active capture of free-swimming Gram-negative bacteria and dispersed microplastics. Dynamic capture by these microrobotic planes proves more efficient than static polymer particles, with the integration of cationic polymers increasing their attraction to Gram-negative bacteria and microplastics, thereby improving overall capture. Additionally, the microrobots are recyclable; ultrasound sonication efficiently detaches the captured bacteria and microplastics from the microrobot surface, allowing for potential reuse.

GO/Pt NPs/Fe_2O_3 magnetic micromotors, modified with lantibiotic Nisin, were developed to capture and inactivate Gram-positive bacteria and biofilms [90]. These micromotors were self-propelled by both catalytic propulsion and magnetic actuation mode. Synthesis of these micromotors involved coating 20 μm PS spheres with a Au layer using sputtering, followed by incubation with sulfhydryl-modified graphene oxide (GO) to enable thiol linkages to the Au surface. Incubation conditions for GO were optimized to partially expose the Au, facilitating the Janus character by allowing selective growth of Pt and Fe_2O_3 NPs for directional propulsion. Subsequently, the micromotors were functionalized with Nisin through covalent immobilization. The GO layer was modified with thioglycolic acid, introducing a high density of carboxylic groups. These were then activated with N-(3-Dimethylaminopropyl)-N′-ethyl carbodiimide hydrochloride to promote Nisin binding via amine group interactions. The specific interaction between Nisin and the Lipid II unit of *Staphylococcus aureus* significantly enhances the micromotors' movement, leading to a two-fold increase in capture and bactericidal efficacy compared to free peptides or static adsorbents. The micromotors achieved a speed of over 55 ± 25 μm/s, demonstrating an 83% capture efficiency for *Staphylococcus aureus* and prolonged contact for rapid bacterial inactivation.

6. CPMNR-Based Sensors for Pollutant Detection

The self-propelling nature of CPMNRs also makes them ideal for environmental sensing applications, where traditional mixing or analytical tools may face limitations. These CPMNRs offer a simple and rapid detection method, leveraging colorimetric changes or changes in their speed due to interactions with target molecules. Bio and non-bio hybrid CPMNRs have been developed for the selective detection of ions (e.g., metals), molecules (e.g., biomolecules, herbicides, explosives, toxins), and microorganisms (e.g., bacteria and viruses).

Moo et al. developed microfish robots to replace toxic biological assays for detecting heavy metals [91]. These Cu/Pt bimetallic microtubes were synthesized using a modified electrochemical deposition method with cyclopore polycarbonate as a template. The microfish robots selectively detect Pb^{2+}, mimicking the negative influence of Pb^{2+} on live fish activity. Pt-catalyzed H_2O_2 decomposition led to the formation of O_2 bubbles, enabling the autonomous movement of microfish robots. This innovation offers a safer alternative for heavy metal detection. The poisoning of Pt by heavy metals affects its catalytic efficiency, which was used as a model. Studies showed that $Pb(NO_3)_2$ decreased the velocity of microfish robots more than $Cd(NO_3)_2$. In 3% H_2O_2, the average velocity of microfish robots was 310 μm/s, decreasing to 196 μm/s with 0.96 mM of $Pb(NO_3)_2$ and further to 110 μm/s at 1.92 mM $Pb(NO_3)_2$. Microfish robots can be used for continuous monitoring of Pb^{2+} in water bodies via optical visualization.

A graphene-based bubble-propelled micromotor was developed for detecting ricin, one of the deadliest plant-derived poisons, which leads to rapid death [92]. For recognizing ricin B, the rGO-Pt micromotors were developed and modified with the aptamer-dye component. In this case, fluorescein-amidine dye was used to facilitate fluorescent on-off sensing of ricin. When the rGO in the micromotor interacted with ricin B toxin via π–π interactions, the fluorescence dye was quenched. Sensing was noticed across wide pH (2–7) and temperature (4–63 °C) conditions. The addition of propellent (H_2O_2) did not cause fluorescence quenching. The speed of the micromotor was 0, 155, 380, and 860 μm/s, at the H_2O_2 concentration of 0%, 0.5%, 1%, and 2%, respectively. Optimal recognition was observed at the ricin B concentration of 10 μg/mL and 3 min incubation time. The signal recovery rate was 90%, and 10% in the case of self-propelled and static micromotors, respectively. This micromotor can be extended for high-speed detection of bio and chemical warfare agents and toxins.

Pt nanomotors and a cellphone combination were used for the detection of Zikavirus (ZIKV), which causes fatal infections in newborns. Draz et al. conjugated Pt NPs with monoclonal anti-Zika virus antibody (anti-ZIKV mAb), loaded on poly(styrene) (3 μm) beads, and transferred to a single-channel microchip [93]. When in contact with ZIKV, Pt conjugate forms a 3D immunocomplex. This system was moved by the addition of H_2O_2. The movement was captured by a cellphone enabled with an optical tracking unit and relevant mobile cellphone application. Thus, the speed of the nanomotor was quantitatively correlated with the ZIKV concentration. When there were 10^6 virus particles/μL, 10% H_2O_2 propelled the bead at an average velocity of 1.199 μm/s, which was ~5.2 times greater than the velocity of ZIKV-free samples. The detection limit was 1 particle/μL. This system was suggested for on-site diagnostic applications meant for pathogen detection and disease management.

Three-dimensional printing is used for constructing components with simple-to-complex designs and is a powerful tool for cost-effective and customized engineering fabrications. Lue et al. designed a self-propelled minimotor (SPM) using 3D printing for monitoring underwater pollutants [94]. They tried to combine 3D-printing with nano-analytical technology. Acrylonitrile butadiene styrene was used for fabricating a submarine-shaped SPM (2 cm in length and 1 cm in height). Hallow space was designated in the SPM, which allowed the filing of chemicals that were used as a fuel for self-propulsion. The mixture of tartaric acid and sodium bicarbonate was used as a fuel, and CO_2 generated from this mixture was used for bubble-induced self-propulsion. Cruising speed was maintained by optimizing the size of the outlet (hole) in the SPM. A small piece of cotton was stuck on the SPM, and on it, acetylcholinesterase (AChE) and RB dye-Au NPs were drop-cast. The fluorescence of RB dye molecules became weak when integrated with Au NPs. The addition of AChE makes RB dye detach from Au NPs and thereby recover its fluorescence. This change was accompanied by a red-to-blue color change. The said phenomena were used for the calorimetric detection of pesticides. A hollow space was designated in the SPM, which allowed the filing of chemicals that were used as a fuel for self-propulsion. The functionalized SPM was placed in the simulated river and allowed to sink. The depth of the SPM submerging was controlled by adjusting the weight of the metal ballast on the SPM. The minimum detection limit for ethodan, endosulfan, and acephate by the UV–Vis spectroscopy/fluorescent signal was 0.32/0.38, 0.18/0.29, and 0.18/0.32 μg/L, respectively. The RB dye-Au NPs colorimetric assay was used to replace the traditional pesticide sensing routes requiring spot samples and expensive instruments.

Similar to natural photosynthesis, Villa et al. developed micromotors capable of harvesting light and utilized them for their propulsion [95]. They developed a graphitic carbon nitride ($g\text{-}C_3N_4$)-based tubular micromotor, which is free from metal, and responsive to light-source-based on/off sensing. A simple template-free synthesis method was used. This enabled mass production and yielded low-cost micromotors. In a metal or enzyme catalyst containing micromotors, bubble propulsion usually occurs via H_2O_2 decomposition, and the motion cannot be controlled. There is no stop-and-go mechanism. The $g\text{-}C_3N_4$ is stable and a biocompatible visible-light photocatalyst that is used for H_2 generation, water remediation, CO_2 activation, and sensing applications. Earlier, $g\text{-}C_3N_4$ was used for constructing Janus spheres with Pt (for decomposing H_2O_2). The micromotors were propelled by visible-light photocatalysis-induced bubbling. Heavy metal enhanced the speed of $g\text{-}C_3N_4$ micromotors. Under visible light, $g\text{-}C_3N_4$ micromotors and 10 wt.% of H_2O_2 were required to witness the movement. In the presence of heavy metals, the speed was accelerated, and the speeds witnessed for 5 wt.% of H_2O_2 addition were 100, 31, 22,

14, 9, and 5 μm/s in the presence of Cu, Cr, Ni, Co, Cd, and Pb, respectively. There was a 30% speed increase in the case of Cu. In the presence of Cu, 0.5% of H_2O_2 moved the micromotor 20 times faster than in the absence of heavy metals. The g-C_3N_4 micromotors act as a label-free tool for simultaneous monitoring and adsorption of heavy metals. This phenomenon is used for detecting and removal of heavy metals. In addition to inherent adsorptive and fluorescence capabilities, the translucent tubular structure visualized the formation and migration of O_2 bubbles. This micromotor led to the development of a bubble-propelled non-metal-based detection system for water contaminant monitoring and remediation. Visible-light-induced propulsion of g-C_3N_4 can make use of sunlight and enables the development of sustainable water remediation technologies.

In a biological environment, nanomotors can effectively navigate and perform assigned tasks. Nanomotors, having a size > 200 nm, usually do not interfere with the regular activities of the immune system [96]. By ligand exchange, surfactants were replaced by thiolated analog stealthy to the immune system of living organisms. Plasmonic core–shell (Au-Ag) nanomotors were prepared by Novotny et al. via a seeded growth route. These wet chemical methods allowed higher scalability (10^{10} ppm to Liters) than the plain substrate-based methods. High yield and greater control of submicron-scale monodispersed nanorod shapes were achieved via this wet chemical synthesis. Catalysis-driven plasmonic nanomotors exhibited enhanced diffusion with the use of low fuel (H_2O_2) concentration. High nanomotor diffusion was found even at a 0.1% concentration of H_2O_2. Au-Ag nanomotors detected a trace of picric acid, a nitroaromatic explosive, via surface-enhanced Raman spectroscopy (SERS). The lowest picric acid detection limit was 100×10^{-9} M, when compared with the SERS detection without nanomotors, the detection limit was two-fold higher (100×10^{-6} M). Au-Ag nanomotors worked as an effective moveable single-particle SERS platform. These nanomotors were suggested for the practical on-time detection of dangerous explosives. Yang et al. developed a CoNi-$Zn(OH)_2/MnO_2$ micromotor capable of sensing and degradation of phenolic pollutants [97]. The natural plant ramie was used as a template for the synthesis of this ternary structured material by a multi-step synthesis route comprising hydrothermal, coprecipitation, and ion doping processes. CoNi-$Zn(OH)_2/MnO_2$ displayed an enzyme-like catalytic activity. MnO_2 catalyzed H_2O_2 fuel and generated O_2 bubbles propelling CoNi-$Zn(OH)_2/MnO_2$, 5 wt.% H_2O_2-induced maximum velocity (77.504 ± 5.19 μm/s), and calorimetrically detected the phenolic compounds, catechol (CC), and hydroquinone (HQ). The lowest detection limits toward CC and HQ were 3.9×10^{-7} M and 4.21×10^{-7} M, respectively. Under neutral pH, within 30 min, CoNi-$Zn(OH)_2/MnO_2$ degraded CC (98%) and HQ (96.5%). Synergistic detection and degradation of phenolic pollutants were facilitated by the use of H_2O_2 and peroxomonosulfate as the catalytic substrates generating ROS including •OH, O_2•$^-$, singlet-linear oxygen ($1O^2$), and sulfate radicals (SO•$^{-4}$). While multiple metal ions enhanced the activation of H_2O_2, the large number of active sites on the surface of CoNi-$Zn(OH)_2/MnO_2$ rendered higher interaction with the target molecules. O_2 generated upon the degradation of H_2O_2 replenished O_2 consumed upon degradation of phenolic compounds. The CC degradation efficiency of CoNi-$Zn(OH)_2/MnO_2$ remained above 92% even after five reuse cycles. Tubular CoNi-$Zn(OH)_2/MnO_2$ micromotors are expected to find potential use in water sensing and detoxification.

Zhao et al. utilized a motion-capture lighting strategy for the fabrication of micromotors applied for bacterial detection and capturing [98]. They have integrated motion-enhanced capture and associated fluorescence. On the surface of electrospun flexible fiber rods subjected to cryocutting, the enzymes catalase and mannose were immobilized on opposite sides. The former catalyzed the H_2O_2 decomposition and bubble-induced movement of the micromotor, while the latter was used for the specific recognition of bacterial protein.

The average speed of the micromotor in 7.5% H_2O_2 was 1–2 μm/s. The micromotor with an aspect ratio of two exhibited a higher magnitude of displacement, an increase in bacterial capture, and maximized the changes in fluorescence intensity. Fluorescence was caused by an aggregation-induced emission effect. Under UV light, micromotors incubated with *E. coli* of 10^2 and 10^5 CFU/mL turned blue to bluish-green and green, respectively. The capture-lighting strategy offers rapid and visual detection of bacteria without expensive instruments and sample pretreatment complexities. Yuan et al. developed a capsule-type micromotor for detection of an explosive, 2,4,6-trinitrotoluene (TNT) [99]. On the silica microparticles (of 5 μm), eight bilayers of poly(allylamine hydrochloride) and poly(styrene sulfonate) PAH/PSS were self-assembled, and mixed with amine-functionalized upconversion NPs (UCNPs) in a 1:10 ratio. After making a Pt coating on this, the SiO_2 core was removed to obtain the capsule-type micromotor. The Pt-catalyzed H_2O_2 decomposition (10%) resulted in the self-movement micromotors with a speed of 110 μm/s. TNT quenched the luminescence of UCNPs and paved its detection. When the microcapsules self-propelled for 3 min, 0.2 μg m/L TNT, it immediately led to luminescent quenching. This was not obvious in the case of UCNPs and unpropelled capsules. The lowest detection limit was lower than 2.4 ng/mL. These microcapsules also adsorbed TNT. This detection limit was 3.5 times greater than the static UCNPs. The self-propulsion-induced dictation and adsorption properties of microcapsules can be effectively used for the detection and adsorptive removal of explosives from water.

Local convection in a liquid brings the analyte to be determined to the proximity of the probe, and decreases the reagent consumption and overall duration of sensing or analysis. The integration of probe molecules into CPMNRs can result in miniaturized and on-the-move analytical platforms and sensing assays. Asuncion-Nadal et al. explored the bubble-propelled WS_2/Pt micrometer for fluorescent detection of biomolecules [100]. They used lipopolysaccharides as a model endotoxin target. Lipopolysaccharides are known to be associated with the sepsis shock and inflammatory process. Tetramethylrhodamine (TMRho)-labeled peptide was used as an "on/off" fluorescent probe. The peptide loading/release, surface roughness, and catalytic performance of the WS_2-Pt and MoS_2-Pt were given importance. The authors suggested the use of WS_2-Pt micromotors for the clinical detection of biomolecules. In a typical microliter sensing experiment, 4% H_2O_2 spiked as a fuel. Spiking H_2O_2 in tap water, serum, saliva, and lysogeny broth accelerated the microlites in 110 ± 50, 60 ± 30, 19 ± 4, and 130 ± 70 μm/s, respectively. WS_2-Pt also exhibited satisfactory results obtained for sensing Cholera toxin units and various bacterial cultures. The endotoxins released by real bacterial stains (S. aureus, and E. coli) showed fluorescence signals. When E. coli was present, the fluorescence recovered, enabling peptide selectivity. When compared with static and stirred WS_2, WS_2-Pt micromotors exhibited high sensitivity (90 s) toward endotoxins in water, serum, saliva, and bacteria. The high surface area of WS_2-Pt resulted in 3.5 times higher sensitivity than the MoS_2-Pt. WS_2-Pt was termed a powerful sensing tool for microliter samples with a detection time of 60 s and a negligible amount of reagent use. Via an interfacial super-assembly strategy (Figure 5), asymmetric multilayer-mesoporous silica nanobottles (MMSNBs) were prepared and used as nanomotors for the detection and removal of heavy metals [101]. Fe_3O_4 NPs and mesoporous silica with a surface area of 613.4 m^2/g were self-assembled on the silica nanobottles. Fe_3O_4 layers magnetized the entire assembly to the extent of 8.5 emu/g. This magnetized assembly was integrated with an enzyme catalase (Cat-MMSNBs), which decomposes the fuel, H_2O_2. Use of 1.5% H_2O_2 enabled the self-propulsion of this assembly at a velocity of 7.59 μm/s. The applicability of this nanomotor in the detection and removal of heavy metals was studied using Cu^{2+} as a model pollutant. The inactivation of catalase by Cu^{2+} was identified as a detection mechanism. Upon addition of 50 mg/L of Cu, within

3 min, the movement of the nanomotor slowed down due to the Brownian motion. The same trend was noticed with Pb^{2+} and Cd^{2+}, and this confirmed the applicability of this nanomotor in detecting a wide range of heavy metals. These heavy metal ions changed the speed of the nanomotors and inhibited the activity of the catalase integrated with the nanomotor assembly. Abundant hydroxyl groups in the surface of mesoporous silica (3.6 nm), provided a high surface area for adsorption. The nanomotors (1 mg/mL) removed 80% of Cu from 20 mg/L Cu solution; 60% of Cu was removed within 5 min. The decrease in the rate of Cu removal confirms the occurrence of the surface adsorption process. This self-assembly can be tracked by an external magnet, magnetically separated for reuse.

Bioinspired magnetically derived nanomotor functioning like peroxidase was developed for the simultaneous detection and removal of Glyphosate (N-(phosphonomethyl) glycine) [102]. Glyphosate is a widely used non-selective organophosphorus herbicide. Hierarchical $ZrO_2/MnFe_2O_4$/FeZr-MOF nanomotors were constructed and studied under complex environmental conditions. ZrO_2 microtubes and $MnFe_2O_2$ were used as support and catalyst-cum-magnetic guide, respectively. Cynanchum seed fibers having a natural tubular structure were used as a template. H_2O_2 was used as the fuel for bubble-powered propulsion. In 5% H_2O_2, this nanomotor moves with the speed of 101.6 ± 10.2 μm/s. The electronic absorbance of nanomotors at 652 nm was dropped, and the color turned from blue to pale due to the specific Lewis acid-base interaction between Zr–O and the phosphate group. The lowest glyphosate detection limit was 0.05 mg/mL. These interactions were powerful enough to bind the organophosphates and decontaminate water via adsorptive removal. At neutral pH, the maximum adsorption capacity was 313.5 mg/g. The hierarchical structure provided greater active sites for binding glyphosate. Magnetic tracking allowed for easy separation and reuse. Thus, this nanomotor appeared to be multifunctional and useful for the simultaneous detection and removal of organic contaminants from water. As mentioned in Section 4, Lac/Fe-BTC-@NiFe-LDH@MnO_2/HNTs hybrid nanomotor combinining enzyme and nonozyme was utilized for both detection and degradation of MC [72]. In 5% H_2O_2, this hybrid nanomotor (Figure 6), was propelled at the speed of 2.65 $\mu m^2/s$. The motion pathway of nanomotor was circular to directional. Higher H_2O_2 concentration produced O_2 bubbles. The bubbles dislodged from nanomotor created friction and propelled it in the opposite direction. The outer layer was Lac/Fe-BTC-@NiFe-LDH@ MnO_2/HNTs, which acted as a catalytic functional unit, and exhibited peroxide-like enzyme activity. The outer layer also had an abundant host site for Lac. This nanomotor also selectively detected MC. A clear color change was noticed when nanomotor and H_2O_2 were added to the water containing 0–100 μM of MC (Figure 7). H_2O_2 adsorbed on the surface of nanozyme broken down, leading to the generation of •OH and O_2•$^-$. In the presence of chromogenic agent, 3,3′,5,5′-tetramethyl benzidine (TMB), the solution turned from colorless to blue. The ROS generated in this system oxidized TMB (colorless) to ox-TMB (blue). This change facilitated the colorimetric detection of MC. Furthermore, MC was shown to be mineralized by oxidation mediated by ROS. Under optimized conditions, this hybrid nanomotor exhibited 87.1% MC removal efficiency. When reused, at the fourth cycle, 78.1% MC removal efficiency was observed. These findings suggest that Lac/Fe-BTC-@NiFe-LDH@MnO_2/HNTs hybrid nanomotor can be explored for sensing and removal of other organic pollutants.

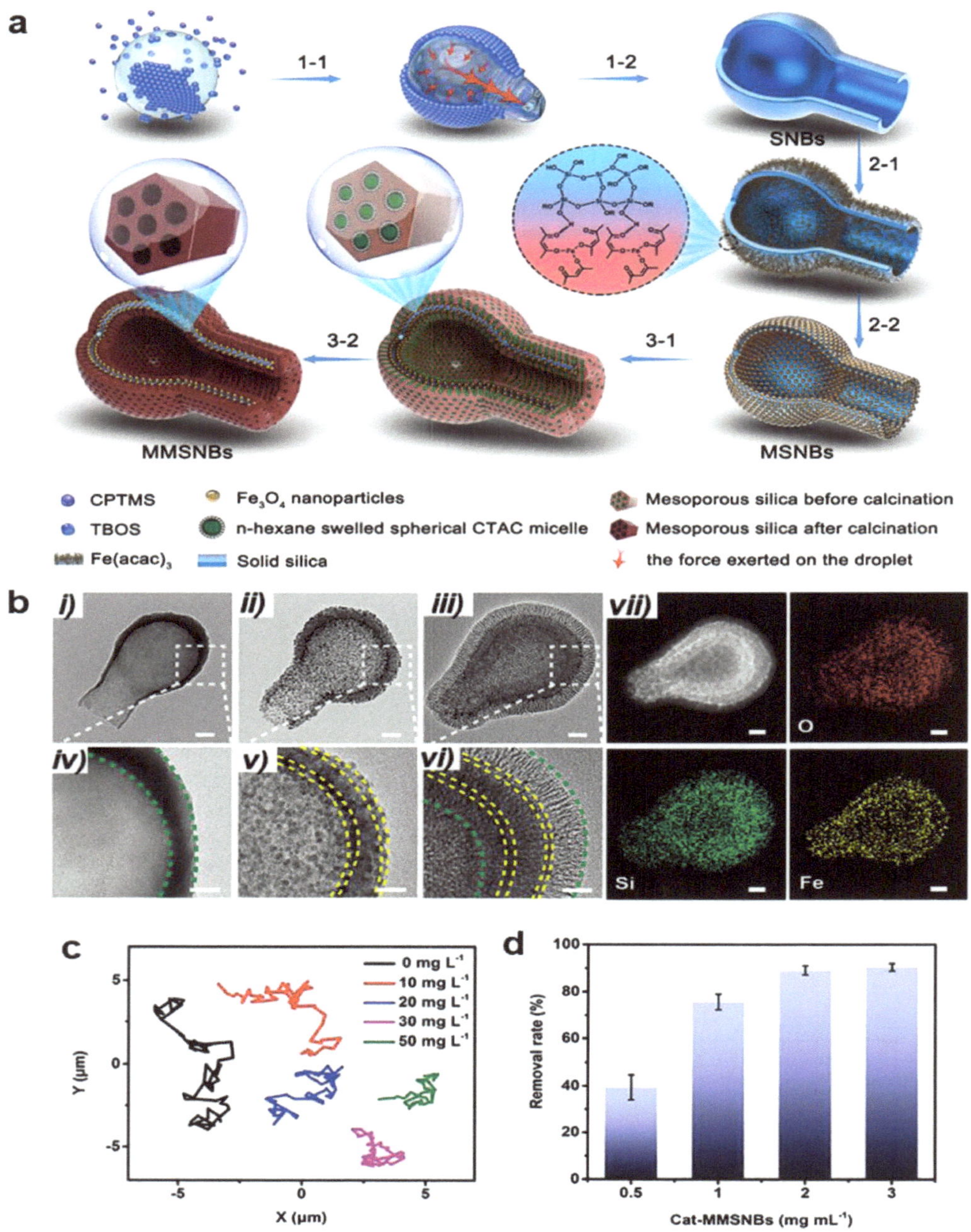

Figure 5. CPMNRs grown sequentially using interfacial super-assembly strategy: (**a**) Synthetic procedure for growing MMSNBs. (**b**) TEM images of different growth stages of (*i,iv*) SNBs, (*ii,v*) MSNBs, (*iii,vi*) MMSNBs, and their corresponding EDS mapping of (*vii*) MMSNBs. Scale bar: 50 nm. (**c**) Pathway for tracking trajectories versus fuel concentration taken over a 10 s period. (**d**) Comparative removal rate of 20 mg/L Cu^{2+} for different concentrations of MMSNBs of 0.5, 1, 2, 3 mg/mL after 30 min duration, respectively. Figures reproduced with permission from [94].

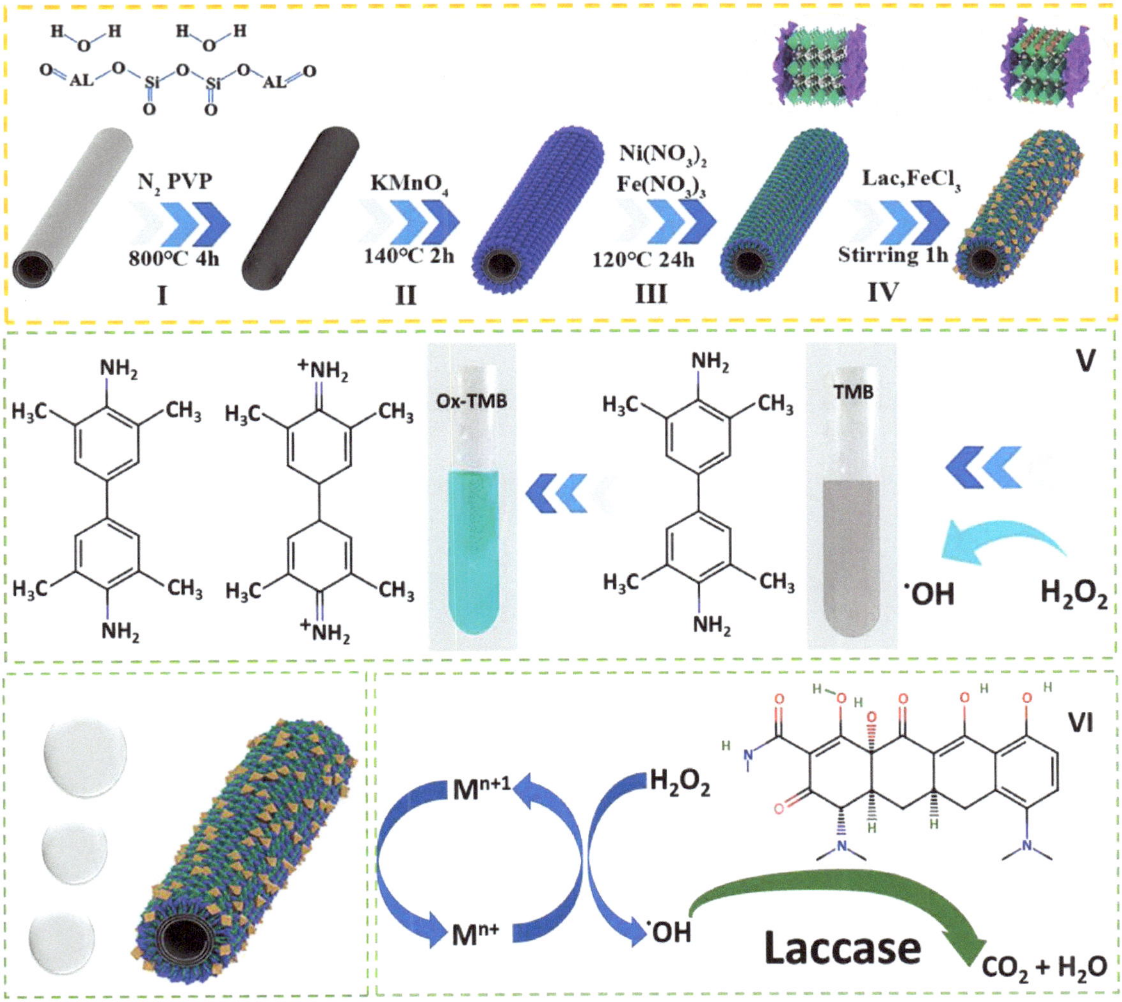

Figure 6. Hybrid dual-function nanomotors for environmental remediation: Schematic demonstration of synthetic procedure for Lac/Fe-BTC@NiFe-LDH@MnO_2/HNT NPs and application of dual function for detection and degradation. (I) HNTs modified after calcination; (II) growth of MnO_2 nanosheets on the surface; (III) surface growth of NiFe-LDH nanosheets; (IV) padding of laccase on nanosheets; (V) NP-catalyzed TMB mechanism; and (VI) NP-catalyzed MC degradation mechanism. Figures reproduced with permission from [72].

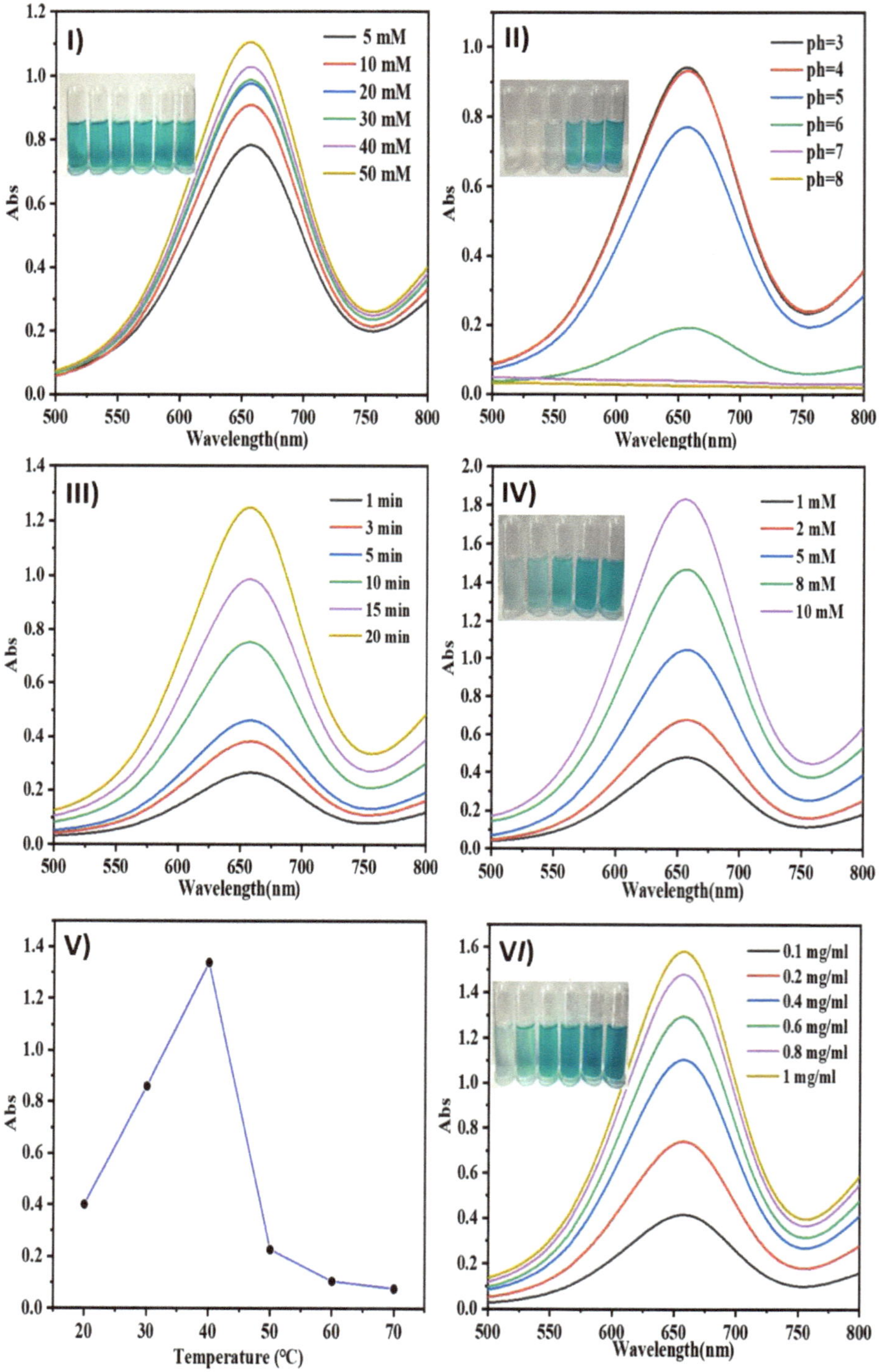

Figure 7. Hybrid dual-function nanomotors for environmental remediation: Study on the effects of (**I**) different H_2O_2 concentrations, (**II**) pH values, (**III**) times, (**IV**) TMB concentrations, (**V**) catalyst concentrations, and (**VI**) temperatures. Figures reproduced with permission from [72].

Nanoplastics are plastic fragments, a part of plastic pollution, and are considered a higher hazard due to their easy diffusion. Urso et al. used multilayered TiO_2 photocatalysts derived from $Ti_3C_2T_x$ MXene by thermal annealing for fabricating microrobots for the trapping and detection of nanoplastics [103]. On these multilayered TiO_2, Pt was deposited and magnetic γ-Fe_2O_3 NPs were immobilized. MXene was used as UV-light-driven fuel-free micromotors due to the Pt-mediated formation of superficial TiO_2 in water. Under UV light, γ-Fe_2O_3/Pt/TiO_2 microrobots exhibited a negative photogravitactic behavior, which led to powerful three-dimensional self-propulsion. The surface charge of microrobots can be programmed via adjusting pH, changing the electrostatic interaction between the nanoplastics and microrobots. Using electrochemical impedance spectroscopy and screen-printed electrodes, microrobots detected the nanoplastics dispersed in water. Microrobots captured a 47% higher amount of nanoplastics than the static multilayered TiO_2. Due to their superparamagnetic behavior, the microrobots were collected from water. These microrobots were suggested for the on-site tracking, capture of nanoplastics, and photocatalytic degradation of organic pollutants. Spherical magnetite NPs were also used for the direct detection and capturing of nanoplastics in water [104]. Detection and quantification experiments were conducted using spectrofluorimetric techniques, with Nile Red dye used to stain nanoplastics for fluorescence tracking. Nanorobots enable real-time monitoring and the capture of nanoplastics, effectively aiding water purification. Activated wirelessly by a rotating magnetic field, the nanorobots exhibit increased movement speeds as the magnetic field frequency is adjusted from 0 to 5 Hz. For quantifying nanoplastics, Nile Red staining generates a fluorescence signal, where higher concentrations of stained nanoplastics yield stronger fluorescence signals. This technique enables the quantification of nanoplastic concentrations in water within the range of 10^8 to 10^{10} beads/mL. To facilitate nanoplastic removal, nanorobots and nanoplastics were mixed under a rotating magnetic field at various time intervals, from 0 to 120 min. Captured nanoplastics adhering to the nanorobots' surfaces were then removed using a permanent neodymium magnet. The supernatant was treated with Nile Red to assess residual nanoplastic concentrations. Initial mixing and immediate removal achieved a 30% nanoplastic removal efficiency, which increased to 90% with extended mixing over 120 min.

7. Future Advancements and Challenges

While CPMNRs have shown tremendous promise in environmental sensing and remediation, several challenges remain that must be addressed to unlock their full potential. The future development of CPMNRs can be directed toward addressing limitations related to propulsion mechanisms, materials design, scalability, and real-world deployment. Below, we highlight key research directions and actionable goals for the advancement of CPMNRs.

Sustainable catalysts: Replacing toxic catalysts with biocompatible alternatives, such as magnesium (Mg) or zinc (Zn), will improve the environmental friendliness of CPMNRs, especially in aqueous environments. Research should explore novel catalyst formulations that combine catalytic, magnetic, and antimicrobial properties to enhance the multifunctionality of CPMNRs for pollutant degradation and microbial inactivation.

Non-toxic and eco-friendly fuels: A critical challenge for the practical deployment of CPMNRs in natural environments is their reliance on chemical fuels such as H_2O_2. To make CPMNRs more sustainable and adaptable to real-world conditions, eco-friendly propulsion mechanisms inspired by biological systems should be developed.

Large-scale production: One of the most significant challenges for the widespread adoption of CPMNRs is their scalability and deployment in real-world polluted environments. Achieving the mass production of CPMNRs with high uniformity, stability, and functionality is crucial for practical deployment. More attention should be given to fabrication techniques that allow for large-scale fabrication of nanomaterials assembly such as electrospinning, electrospraying, microfabrication, 3D printing, or self-assembly processes.

Testing in real-world polluted water systems: While CPMNRs have been tested in controlled laboratory environments, their performance in complex, real-world polluted systems such as industrial effluents, oil spills, and municipal wastewater remains unproven. Future studies should focus on the deployment of CPMNRs in these environments to evaluate their effectiveness in remediating diverse pollutants under realistic conditions.

Targeted carbon capture and greenhouse gas mitigation: CPMNRs could play a crucial role in addressing greenhouse gas emissions in water bodies and assist in carbon capture and sequestration strategies. Research should explore how CPMNRs can be optimized for capturing CO_2 or other greenhouse gases from polluted aquatic systems and contributing to climate change mitigation.

Salinity gradient-driven propulsion: Harnessing natural salinity gradients in marine environments for propulsion can reduce reliance on chemical fuels. Research should focus on optimizing the efficiency and scalability of salinity-driven propulsion, with a goal to integrate this mechanism in CPMNRs for long-term, eco-friendly deployment in marine ecosystems.

Glucose metabolism: Another promising approach is utilizing glucose metabolism in polluted water bodies to power CPMNRs. Developing bio-inspired metabolic pathways that allow CPMNRs to extract energy from organic pollutants would significantly enhance their sustainability in polluted water bodies.

Solar-powered systems: Advancements in solar-driven propulsion can decrease the amount of fuel required to drive CPMNRs. By incorporating materials with hybrid nanostructured photocatalysts, future CPMNRs could use sunlight to drive internal photochemical reactions or photothermal effects for propulsion and simultaneous pollutant degradation. Research should aim to improve the efficiency and stability of such light-sensitive nanomotors under variable environmental conditions.

Hybrid propulsion mechanisms: Integration of magnetic and thermal stimuli with CPMNRs could significantly enhance the mixing and environmental remediation efficiency. Future work should focus on integrating multiple propulsion strategies into a single CPMNR platform, allowing for dynamic propulsion control in challenging and changing environments, such as turbulent water and pollutant dense zones.

Biodegradable polymers: The use of biodegradable materials such as polylactic acid (PLA) or alginate can minimize the environmental impact of CPMNRs after deployment. Future studies should focus on optimizing the degradation rates of these polymers in various environmental conditions to ensure that CPMNRs perform efficiently before breaking down safely.

Self-healing polymers: Incorporating self-healing polymers into CPMNRs will extend their operational lifespan, especially in harsh environments. This can be achieved by embedding self-repairing mechanisms within the materials to ensure continuous functionality, particularly for long-term environmental remediation tasks.

Artificial intelligence (AI)-driven on-board data processing: Embedding CPMNRs with AI algorithms will enable real-time pollutant detection, hotspot identification, and autonomous optimization of remediation strategies. Machine learning models should be developed to predict contamination patterns and guide CPMNRs or robot swarms for maximum efficiency. Future work should focus on the integration of these AI algorithms into miniaturized, energy-efficient platforms to allow for autonomous decision-making without external intervention.

Swarm intelligence for large-scale applications: Coordinating CPMNRs using advanced communication protocols could transform environmental monitoring and remediation on a large scale. Research should focus on developing protocols for swarm coordination that allow CPMNRs to self-organize and allocate their activities dynamically based on pollutant concentrations and environmental conditions. This would enable efficient remediation of complex, and large-scale pollution scenarios.

Self-powered sensing systems: To enable continuous, long-term operation in the field, CPMNRs could integrate miniaturized energy harvesters (e.g., from vibrations, light, or thermal gradients) with embedded sensors for pollutants such as heavy metals or organic compounds. Future research should prioritize the development of hybrid energy harvesting technologies to power the sensors and ensure that CPMNRs can operate indefinitely, transmitting real-time data for environmental monitoring.

8. Conclusion and Outlook

In conclusion, CPMNRs have demonstrated significant potential for a wide range of environmental applications, including pollutant remediation and sensing. A particular strength of CPMNRs in sensing applications lies in their ability to detect and simultaneously remove a variety of contaminants, such as toxins, microorganisms, and organic pollutants. In environmental remediation, advanced oxidation processes (AOPs), including photocatalysis and Fenton oxidation, are key methods for degrading organic pollutants through non-selective oxidation, with the generation of reactive oxygen species (ROS) playing a crucial role. Both processes benefit from the use of H_2O_2, which acts as both a fuel and a contributor to ROS generation.

Comparison of photo-Fenton-type CPMNRs and traditional photocatalysis can bring an adequate understanding of the potential of using CPMNRs in practical environmental remediation. In this regard, MB dye degradation efficiency of suspension-type photocatalysis performed using Degussa (Evonik) P25 TiO_2, nitrogen-doped TiO_2 (N-TiO_2), and BiOBr-based solar-Fenton-type CPMNRs were taken into consideration. Degussa P25 is a well-known bench-mark UV-active photocatalyst, and N-TiO_2 is a well-recognized visible-light-active version of TiO_2. BiOBr is active under visible light. In a conventional stir-mixed photocatalysis, under UV light, in the time span of 90 min, 0.04 g of P25 fully degraded 20 mL of MB dye (12 mg/L) [105]. The efficiency of BioBr nanomaterials and N-TiO_2 NPs under stir mixing and visible light are as follows: (i) in 75 min, BioBr NPS (0.03g) degraded 67.25% of 50 mL of MB dye (6.3 mg/L or 2×10^{-5} M) [106]; (ii) in 240 min, 0.01 g of BiOBr NBs degraded 65% of MB dye (50 mL, 5 mg/L); (iii) in 240 min, 0.01 g of BiOBr nanosheets (NSs) degraded 35% of MB dye (50 mL, 5 mg/L); and in 240 min, 0.01g of N-TiO_2 NPs degraded 23% of MB dye (50 mL, 5 mg/L) [69]. The MB dye (10 mg/L, 100 mL, 3 mL 30% H_2O_2) degradation efficiency of the typical chemically powered solar Fenton micromotor, FeBiOBr/Fe_3O_4/Mn_3O_4 (0.1 g), at various conditions are as follows: (i) 69% of MB dye degradation at static condition (no stirring, and propulsion); (ii) 82% MB dye degradation at stir-mixed condition; and (iii) 98% MB dye degradation under chemical propulsion (3 mL 30 wt.% H_2O_2). The time span was 50 min [68]. Although the light source in each work depended on the type of photo-Fenton catalyst or photocatalyst used, the mass fraction of MB dye degraded per minute was estimated to allow for reasonable comparison. Table 1 provides the mass fraction (mg) of MB dye degraded per minute in the aforementioned systems. FeBiOBr/Fe_3O_4/Mn_3O_4 exhibited the highest MB dye removal efficiency compared to conventional stir-mixed photocatalysis.

The use of biodegradable polymers in CPMNRs is of significant importance. Recent studies [30,89,107] have elaborated different nanorobotic strategies for effectively using biodegradable polymers and their composites/conjugates as active and targeted cargos for environmental remediation. However, those biohybrid-based CPMNRs are sensitive to environmental factors like moisture, pH, and temperature, causing the premature degradation of micro/nanorobots before achieving their targeted operational lifespan. Also, other parameters include variable degradation kinetics, strength and durability of polymers, restricted functionalization options (limited exposure of active sites of catalysts in micro/nanobots), localized degradation products (byproduct formation during the remediation activities), and limited temperature range due to their easy biodegradable nature. In addition, biodegradable polymer nanorobots typically rely on embedded catalysts or external energy sources for propulsion. In environmental remediation, these fuels (e.g., H_2O_2) might not always be available in sufficient amounts, or they may require additional energy inputs, which increases operational complexity. The soft and flexible nature of biodegradable polymers often leads to lower propulsion efficiency compared to rigid materials, reducing the overall effectiveness of pollutant targeting and transport in dynamic environments. In the case of bio-hybrid-based CPMNRs, achieving multifunctionality—such as combining pollutant detection, targeted removal, and degradation—is more complex with biodegradable polymers. This is due to their limited capacity to incorporate diverse functional components while maintaining structural integrity. In enzyme-functionalized biodegradable polymer nanorobots, enzymes may lose activity due to harsh environmental conditions, further limiting the remediation capability.

Table 1. Comparison of MB dye degradation efficiency by conventional stir-mixed photocatalysis and solar-Fenton catalysis by CPMNRs.

Name of the Catalyst	Quantity of Catalyst Used (g)	Type of Mixing	Light Source	Mass Fraction (mg) of MB Degraded/min	Reference
P25 TiO_2 NPs	0.04	Stirring	UV	0.0027	[105]
N-TiO_2 NPs	0.01	Stirring	Visible	0.0002	[69]
BiOBr NPs	0.03	Stirring	Visible	0.0028	[106]
BiOBr NS	0.01	Stirring	Visible	0.0007	[69]
BiOBr NB	0.01	Stirring	Visible	0.0004	[69]
FeBiOBr/Fe_3O_4/Mn_3O_4	0.1	Static	Solar	0.0138	[68]
FeBiOBr/Fe_3O_4/Mn_3O_4	0.1	Stirring	Solar	0.0164	[68]
FeBiOBr/Fe_3O_4/Mn_3O_4	0.1	H_2O_2 Propulsion	Solar	0.0196	[68]

Looking forward to the practical application, the development of CPMNRs for environmental remediation requires further attention to overcoming issues related to sludge formation, magnetic property degradation, and the optimization of self-propulsion mechanisms. Additionally, integrating CPMNRs with other technologies, such as membrane filtration and bioremediation, could enhance their effectiveness and cost-efficiency. The use of photocatalysts in the degradation of dye and non-dye organic compounds, particularly under UV and visible light, is well-established, but practical challenges persist, such as the need for easy separation of powder-type materials and the optimization of self-propulsion behavior, especially when surfactants are involved. One of the major limitations is the use of H_2O_2 as the primary fuel for self-propulsion and oxidation processes. While H_2O_2 is effective in generating ROS for pollutant degradation, its toxicity and safety concerns must be carefully considered, particularly in large-scale applications. The potential for residual H_2O_2 to pose environmental or health risks requires the development of alternative and safer fuels. Non-toxic fuels such as glucose, tannic acid, or tartaric acid could offer more eco-friendly options, but further research is needed to assess their efficiency in driving CPMNRs' motion and their compatibility with existing catalytic systems.

Another significant limitation is the scalability of CPMNRs, especially in large-scale environmental remediation. Many studies focus on small-scale, laboratory-based applications, where issues related to the size, complexity, and multicomponent nature of CPMNRs are manageable. However, scaling these systems to industrial levels presents challenges in maintaining the efficiency of the catalysts, ensuring uniform light exposure on complex structures, and addressing the loss of material stability over multiple reuse cycles. The aggregation of nanomaterials during reuse reduces their surface area and, consequently, their catalytic and propulsion efficiency, highlighting the need for robust regeneration strategies to restore their activity. Current methods for the regeneration of CPMNRs are not yet optimized, and more research is needed to develop efficient and cost-effective approaches for their reuse without compromising performance. Moreover, the synthesis of CPMNRs often involves the use of precious metals such as Pt, Au, Ag, and Pd as catalysts for bubble generation, which adds to the cost and complexity of their production. Developing alternative, less expensive catalysts and simplifying the deposition techniques for these materials could help reduce the overall cost and make CPMNRs more accessible for widespread use. Additionally, the reliance on surfactants in many systems increases organic loading and can lead to higher total organic carbon (TOC) levels in the water, which in turn could reduce the efficiency of the photocatalytic processes. Minimizing or avoiding the use of surfactants is essential to improve the environmental friendliness and efficiency of CPMNRs, but alternative approaches for propulsion and catalytic activity without surfactants need further exploration.

Future research should also focus on the development of more cost-effective and environmentally friendly materials, such as substrates for immobilizing photocatalysts, and improving the long-term stability and reusability of CPMNRs. For sensing applications, the selectivity, accuracy, and resolution of CPMNRs need further refinement to enable reliable and efficient detection in real-world environments. Finally, while the integration of CPMNRs with other technologies, such as membrane filtration and bioremediation, shows promise for improving efficiency, the compatibility and cost-effectiveness of these hybrid systems require thorough investigation. Overall, while significant progress has been made, addressing the challenges associated with fuel toxicity, scalability, catalyst cost, and material stability will be crucial for advancing CPMNRs from laboratory studies to practical, large-scale environmental remediation and sensing applications.

Author Contributions: Conceptualization, S.R. and S.J.; writing—original draft preparation, S.T.S. and N.V.; writing—review and editing, T.H.O. All authors have read and agreed to the published version of the manuscript.

Funding: This study was supported by the National Research Foundation of Korea grant funded by the Korean Government (MSIT) (No. 2022R1A2C1004283) and by Korea Basic Science Institute (National research Facilities and Equipment Center) grant funded by the Ministry of Education. (2019R1A6C1010046).

Conflicts of Interest: Author Subramanian Tamil Selvan was employed by the company Azion Global Pte. Ltd. The remaining authors de-clare that the research was conducted in the absence of any commercial or financial relationships that could be construed as a potential conflict of interest.

References

1. Teo, W.Z.; Pumera, M. Motion Control of Micro-/Nanomotors. *Chem.–A Eur. J.* **2016**, *22*, 14796–14804. [CrossRef]
2. Tu, Y.; Peng, F.; Wilson, D.A. Motion manipulation of micro-and nanomotors. *Adv. Mater.* **2017**, *29*, 1701970. [CrossRef] [PubMed]
3. Yang, M.; Guo, X.; Mou, F.; Guan, J. Lighting up micro-/nanorobots with fluorescence. *Chem. Rev.* **2022**, *123*, 3944–3975. [CrossRef]
4. Lyu, X.; Liu, X.; Zhou, C.; Duan, S.; Xu, P.; Dai, J.; Chen, X.; Peng, Y.; Cui, D.; Tang, J. Active, yet little mobility: Asymmetric decomposition of H_2O_2 is not sufficient in propelling catalytic micromotors. *J. Am. Chem. Soc.* **2021**, *143*, 12154–12164. [CrossRef] [PubMed]
5. Urso, M.; Ussia, M.; Pumera, M. Smart micro-and nanorobots for water purification. *Nat. Rev. Bioeng.* **2023**, *1*, 236–251. [CrossRef]
6. Parmar, J.; Vilela, D.; Villa, K.; Wang, J.; Sánchez, S. Micro-and nanomotors as active environmental microcleaners and sensors. *J. Am. Chem. Soc.* **2018**, *140*, 9317–9331. [CrossRef] [PubMed]
7. Sánchez, S.; Soler, L.; Katuri, J. Chemically powered micro-and nanomotors. *Angew. Chem. Int. Ed.* **2015**, *54*, 1414–1444. [CrossRef] [PubMed]
8. Wang, W. Open questions of chemically powered nano-and micromotors. *J. Am. Chem. Soc.* **2023**, *145*, 27185–27197. [CrossRef]

9. Panda, S.K.; Kherani, N.A.; Debata, S.; Singh, D.P. Bubble-propelled micro/nanomotors: A robust platform for the detection of environmental pollutants and biosensing. *Mater. Adv.* **2023**, *4*, 1460–1480. [CrossRef]
10. Ferreira, V.R.; Azenha, M. Advancements in Visible Light-Driven Micro/nanomotors for Photodegradation of Environmental Pollutants. *Environ. Sci. Adv.* **2024**, *3*, 1474–1499. [CrossRef]
11. Dong, R.; Cai, Y.; Yang, Y.; Gao, W.; Ren, B. Photocatalytic micro/nanomotors: From construction to applications. *Acc. Chem. Res.* **2018**, *51*, 1940–1947. [CrossRef]
12. Eskandarloo, H.; Kierulf, A.; Abbaspourrad, A. Nano-and micromotors for cleaning polluted waters: Focused review on pollutant removal mechanisms. *Nanoscale* **2017**, *9*, 13850–13863. [CrossRef]
13. Liu, X.-Y.; Li, R.-F.; Jia, J.; Yu, Z.-L. Antibacterial micro/nanomotors: Current research progress, challenges, and opportunities. *Theranostics* **2024**, *14*, 1029. [CrossRef]
14. Li, W.; Wang, J.; Xiong, Z.; Li, D. Micro/nanorobots for efficient removal and degradation of micro/nanoplastics. *Cell Rep. Phys. Sci.* **2023**, *4*, 101639. [CrossRef]
15. Wang, L.; Villa, K. Self-propelled micro/nanomotors for removal of insoluble water contaminants: Microplastics and oil spills. *Environ. Sci. Nano* **2021**, *8*, 3440–3451. [CrossRef]
16. Zhang, Y.; Yuan, K.; Zhang, L. Micro/nanomachines: From functionalization to sensing and removal. *Adv. Mater. Technol.* **2019**, *4*, 1800636. [CrossRef]
17. Cai, L.; Xu, D.; Zhang, Z.; Li, N.; Zhao, Y. Tailoring functional micromotors for sensing. *Research* **2023**, *6*, 0044. [CrossRef] [PubMed]
18. Preetam, S. Nano Revolution: Pioneering the Future of Water Reclamation with Micro/Nanorobots. *Nanoscale Adv.* **2024**, *6*, 2569–2581. [CrossRef]
19. Wang, Q.; Yang, S.; Zhang, L. Untethered micro/nanorobots for remote sensing: Toward intelligent platform. *Nano-Micro Lett.* **2024**, *16*, 40. [CrossRef]
20. Hou, J.-Y.; Liu, H.-T.; Huang, L.-T.; Wu, S.-B.; Zhang, Z.-L. Recent advances in micro/nano-robots for environmental pollutant removal: Mechanism, application, and prospect. *Chem. Eng. J.* **2024**, *498*, 155135. [CrossRef]
21. Feynman, R.P. An invitation to enter a new field of physics. *Int. J. Eng. Sci.* **1960**, *23*, 22–36.
22. Drexler, E. *Engines of Creation: The Coming Era of Nanotechnology*; Anchor books, Doubleday: New York, NY, USA, 1987.
23. Li, J.; Rozen, I.; Wang, J. Rocket science at the nanoscale. *ACS Nano* **2016**, *10*, 5619–5634. [CrossRef]
24. Gao, W.; Wang, J. The environmental impact of micro/nanomachines: A review. *ACS Nano* **2014**, *8*, 3170–3180. [CrossRef]
25. Xu, L.; Mou, F.; Gong, H.; Luo, M.; Guan, J. Light-driven micro/nanomotors: From fundamentals to applications. *Chem. Soc. Rev.* **2017**, *46*, 6905–6926. [CrossRef]
26. Chen, A.; Ge, X.-h.; Chen, J.; Zhang, L.; Xu, J.-H. Multi-functional micromotor: Microfluidic fabrication and water treatment application. *Lab. A Chip* **2017**, *17*, 4220–4224. [CrossRef] [PubMed]
27. Pal, M.; Somalwar, N.; Singh, A.; Bhat, R.; Eswarappa, S.M.; Saini, D.K.; Ghosh, A. Maneuverability of magnetic nanomotors inside living cells. *Adv. Mater.* **2018**, *30*, 1800429. [CrossRef] [PubMed]
28. Dong, Y.; Wang, L.; Iacovacci, V.; Wang, X.; Zhang, L.; Nelson, B.J. Magnetic helical micro-/nanomachines: Recent progress and perspective. *Matter* **2022**, *5*, 77–109. [CrossRef]
29. Hu, N.; Ding, L.; Wang, A.; Zhou, W.; Zhang, C.; Zhang, B.; Yin, R. Comprehensive modeling of corkscrew motion in micro-/nano-robots with general helical structures. *Nat. Commun.* **2024**, *15*, 7399. [CrossRef]
30. Peng, X.; Oral, C.M.; Urso, M.; Ussia, M.; Pumera, M. Active Microrobots for Dual Removal of Biofilms via Chemical and Physical Mechanisms. *ACS Appl. Mater. Interfaces* **2025**, *17*, 3608–3619. [CrossRef]
31. Li, B.; Yang, J.; Lu, S.; Zhao, J.; Du, Y.; Cai, Y.; Dong, R. Chlorella-Based Biohybrid Microrobot for Removing Both Nutrient and Microalgae toward Efficient Water Eutrophication Treatment. *Nano Lett.* **2025**, *25*, 48–55. [CrossRef]
32. Wang, X.; Sridhar, V.; Guo, S.; Talebi, N.; Miguel-López, A.; Hahn, K.; van Aken, P.A.; Sánchez, S. Fuel-free nanocap-like motors actuated under visible light. *Adv. Funct. Mater.* **2018**, *28*, 1705862. [CrossRef]
33. Tang, S.; Zhang, F.; Zhao, J.; Talaat, W.; Soto, F.; Karshalev, E.; Chen, C.; Hu, Z.; Lu, X.; Li, J. Structure-dependent optical modulation of propulsion and collective behavior of acoustic/light-driven hybrid microbowls. *Adv. Funct. Mater.* **2019**, *29*, 1809003. [CrossRef]
34. Kong, L.; Mayorga-Martinez, C.C.; Guan, J.; Pumera, M. Photocatalytic micromotors activated by UV to visible light for environmental remediation, micropumps, reversible assembly, transportation, and biomimicry. *Small* **2020**, *16*, 1903179. [CrossRef]
35. Renfeng, D.; Yan, H.; Yefei, W.; Wei, G.; Biye, R.; Qinglong, W.; Yuepeng, C. Visible-Light-Driven BiOI-Based Janus Micromotor in Pure Water. *J. Am. Chem. Soc.* **2017**, *139*, 1722–1725.
36. Dai, B.; Wang, J.; Xiong, Z.; Zhan, X.; Dai, W.; Li, C.-C.; Feng, S.-P.; Tang, J. Programmable artificial phototactic microswimmer. *Nat. Nanotechnol.* **2016**, *11*, 1087–1092. [CrossRef]
37. Chen, C.; Ding, S.; Wang, J. Materials consideration for the design, fabrication and operation of microscale robots. *Nat. Rev. Mater.* **2024**, *9*, 159–172. [CrossRef]

38. Xiong, K.; Xu, L.; Lin, J.; Mou, F.; Guan, J. Mg-based micromotors with motion responsive to dual stimuli. *Research* **2020**, *2020*, 6213981. [CrossRef]
39. Mou, F.; Chen, C.; Ma, H.; Yin, Y.; Wu, Q.; Guan, J. Self-propelled micromotors driven by the magnesium-water reaction and their hemolytic properties. *Angew. Chem. Int. Ed.* **2013**, *52*, 28. [CrossRef]
40. Wu, C.; Li, X.; Shum, H.C. Micro/nanomotors from single modal to multimodal propulsion. *Nano Res.* **2024**, *19*, 94907105. [CrossRef]
41. Ochiai, T.; Fujishima, A. Photoelectrochemical properties of TiO_2 photocatalyst and its applications for environmental purification. *J. Photochem. Photobiol. C Photochem. Rev.* **2012**, *13*, 247–262. [CrossRef]
42. Daghrir, R.; Drogui, P.; Robert, D. Modified TiO_2 for environmental photocatalytic applications: A review. *Ind. Eng. Chem. Res.* **2013**, *52*, 3581–3599. [CrossRef]
43. Dong, R.; Zhang, Q.; Gao, W.; Pei, A.; Ren, B. Highly efficient light-driven TiO_2–Au Janus micromotors. *ACS Nano* **2016**, *10*, 839–844. [CrossRef] [PubMed]
44. Akhavan, O.; Saadati, M.; Jannesari, M. Graphene jet nanomotors in remote controllable self-propulsion swimmers in pure water. *Nano Lett.* **2016**, *16*, 5619–5630. [CrossRef] [PubMed]
45. Wang, Q.; Dong, R.; Wang, C.; Xu, S.; Chen, D.; Liang, Y.; Ren, B.; Gao, W.; Cai, Y. Glucose-fueled micromotors with highly efficient visible-light photocatalytic propulsion. *ACS Appl. Mater. Interfaces* **2019**, *11*, 6201–6207. [CrossRef] [PubMed]
46. Lanjwani, M.F.; Tuzen, M.; Khuhawar, M.Y.; Saleh, T.A. Trends in photocatalytic degradation of organic dye pollutants using nanoparticles: A review. *Inorg. Chem. Commun.* **2024**, *159*, 111613. [CrossRef]
47. Mushtaq, F.; Asani, A.; Hoop, M.; Chen, X.Z.; Ahmed, D.; Nelson, B.J.; Pané, S. Highly efficient coaxial TiO_2-PtPd Tubular nanomachines for photocatalytic water purification with multiple locomotion strategies. *Adv. Funct. Mater.* **2016**, *26*, 6995–7002. [CrossRef]
48. Tong, J.; Wang, D.; Wang, D.; Xu, F.; Duan, R.; Zhang, D.; Fan, J.; Dong, B. Visible-light-driven water-fueled ecofriendly micromotors based on iron phthalocyanine for highly efficient organic pollutant degradation. *Langmuir* **2019**, *36*, 6930–6937. [CrossRef]
49. Chen, L.; Zhang, M.-J.; Zhang, S.-Y.; Shi, L.; Yang, Y.-M.; Liu, Z.; Ju, X.-J.; Xie, R.; Wang, W.; Chu, L.-Y. Simple and continuous fabrication of self-propelled micromotors with photocatalytic metal–organic frameworks for enhanced synergistic environmental remediation. *ACS Appl. Mater. Interfaces* **2020**, *12*, 35120–35131. [CrossRef] [PubMed]
50. Mallick, A.; Roy, S. Visible light driven catalytic gold decorated soft-oxometalate (SOM) based nanomotors for organic pollutant remediation. *Nanoscale* **2018**, *10*, 12713–12722. [CrossRef]
51. Fernandez-Lopez, C.; Posada-Baquero, R.; Ortega-Calvo, J.-J. Nature-based approaches to reducing the environmental risk of organic contaminants resulting from military activities. *Sci. Total Environ.* **2022**, *843*, 157007. [CrossRef] [PubMed]
52. Li, J.; Singh, V.V.; Sattayasamitsathit, S.; Orozco, J.; Kaufmann, K.; Dong, R.; Gao, W.; Jurado-Sanchez, B.; Fedorak, Y.; Wang, J. Water-driven micromotors for rapid photocatalytic degradation of biological and chemical warfare agents. *ACS Nano* **2014**, *8*, 11118–11125. [CrossRef]
53. Kovacic, P.; Somanathan, R. Nitroaromatic compounds: Environmental toxicity, carcinogenicity, mutagenicity, therapy and mechanism. *J. Appl. Toxicol.* **2014**, *34*, 810–824. [CrossRef]
54. Peng, X.; Urso, M.; Pumera, M. Metal oxide single-component light-powered micromotors for photocatalytic degradation of nitroaromatic pollutants. *npj Clean. Water* **2023**, *6*, 21. [CrossRef]
55. Xie, J.; Li, X.; Guo, J.; Luo, L.; Delgado, J.J.; Martsinovich, N.; Tang, J. Highly selective oxidation of benzene to phenol with air at room temperature promoted by water. *Nat. Commun.* **2023**, *14*, 4431. [CrossRef]
56. Ferrer Campos, R.; Bakenecker, A.C.; Chen, Y.; Spadaro, M.C.; Fraire, J.; Arbiol, J.; Sánchez, S.; Villa, K. Boosting the Efficiency of Photoactive Rod-Shaped Nanomotors via Magnetic Field-Induced Charge Separation. *ACS Appl. Mater. Interfaces* **2024**, *16*, 30077–30087. [CrossRef] [PubMed]
57. Chellasamy, G.; Ramasundaram, S.; Veerapandian, M.; Chandran, M.; Dhanasekaran, B.; Oh, T.H.; Govindaraju, S.; Yun, K. Systematic review on fate and behavior of microplastics towards the environment. *TrAC Trends Anal. Chem.* **2023**, *169*, 117390. [CrossRef]
58. Wang, L.; Kaeppler, A.; Fischer, D.; Simmchen, J. Photocatalytic TiO_2 micromotors for removal of microplastics and suspended matter. *ACS Appl. Mater. Interfaces* **2019**, *11*, 32937–32944. [CrossRef]
59. Wang, W.; Huang, G.; Jimmy, C.Y.; Wong, P.K. Advances in photocatalytic disinfection of bacteria: Development of photocatalysts and mechanisms. *J. Environ. Sci.* **2015**, *34*, 232–247. [CrossRef] [PubMed]
60. Villa, K.; Novotný, F.; Zelenka, J.; Browne, M.P.; Ruml, T.S.; Pumera, M. Visible-light-driven single-component $BiVO_4$ micromotors with the autonomous ability for capturing microorganisms. *ACS Nano* **2019**, *13*, 8135–8145. [CrossRef]
61. Maric, T.; Løvind, A.; Zhang, Z.; Geng, J.; Boisen, A. Near-Infrared Light-Driven Mesoporous SiO_2/Au Nanomotors for Eradication of Pseudomonas aeruginosa Biofilm. *Adv. Healthc. Mater.* **2023**, *12*, 2203018. [CrossRef]

62. Soler, L.; Magdanz, V.; Fomin, V.M.; Sanchez, S.; Schmidt, O.G. Self-propelled micromotors for cleaning polluted water. *ACSNano* **2013**, *7*, 9611–9620. [CrossRef] [PubMed]
63. Teo, W.Z.; Zboril, R.; Medrik, I.; Pumera, M. Fe0 nanomotors in ton quantities (1020 units) for environmental remediation. *Chem. –A Eur. J.* **2016**, *22*, 4789–4793. [CrossRef]
64. Li, Z.-L.; Wang, W.; Li, M.; Zhang, M.-J.; Tang, M.-J.; Su, Y.-Y.; Liu, Z.; Ju, X.-J.; Xie, R.; Chu, L.-Y. Facile fabrication of bubble-propelled micromotors carrying nanocatalysts for water remediation. *Ind. Eng. Chem. Res.* **2018**, *57*, 4562–4570. [CrossRef]
65. Lee, C.-S.; Gong, J.; Oh, D.-S.; Jeon, J.-R.; Chang, Y.-S. Zerovalent-iron/platinum Janus micromotors with spatially separated functionalities for efficient water decontamination. *ACS Appl. Nano Mater.* **2018**, *1*, 768–776. [CrossRef]
66. Liu, W.; Ge, H.; Chen, X.; Lu, X.; Gu, Z.; Li, J.; Wang, J. Fish-scale-like intercalated metal oxide-based micromotors as efficient water remediation agents. *ACS Appl. Mater. Interfaces* **2019**, *11*, 16164–16173. [CrossRef]
67. Ren, M.; Guo, W.; Guo, H.; Ren, X. Microfluidic fabrication of bubble-propelled micromotors for wastewater treatment. *ACS Appl. Mater. Interfaces* **2019**, *11*, 22761–22767. [CrossRef]
68. Liu, Y.; Li, J.; Li, J.; Yan, X.; Wang, F.; Yang, W.; Ng, D.H.; Yang, J. Active magnetic Fe^{3+}-doped BiOBr micromotors as efficient solar photo-fenton catalyst. *J. Clean. Prod.* **2020**, *252*, 119573. [CrossRef]
69. Li, H.; Liu, J.; Hu, T.; Du, N.; Song, S.; Hou, W. Synthesis of belt-like BiOBr hierarchical nanostructure with high photocatalytic performance. *Mater. Res. Bull.* **2016**, *77*, 171–177. [CrossRef]
70. Shi, H.; Chen, X.; Liu, K.; Ding, X.; Liu, W.; Xu, M. Heterogeneous Fenton ferroferric oxide-reduced graphene oxide-based composite microjets for efficient organic dye degradation. *J. Colloid. Interface Sci.* **2020**, *572*, 39–47. [CrossRef]
71. Chen, L.; Yuan, H.; Chen, S.; Zheng, C.; Wu, X.; Li, Z.; Liang, C.; Dai, P.; Wang, Q.; Ma, X. Cost-effective, high-yield production of biotemplated catalytic tubular micromotors as self-propelled microcleaners for water treatment. *ACS Appl. Mater. Interfaces* **2021**, *13*, 31226–31235. [CrossRef]
72. Gao, S.; Liu, C.; Yang, X.; Lan, Z.; Zuo, M.; Yang, P.; Li, J. New synthetic strategy toward a natural enzyme–nanozyme hybrid dual-function nanomotor and its application in environmental remediation. *Catal. Sci. Technol.* **2024**, *14*, 1239–1254. [CrossRef]
73. Maric, T.; Nasir, M.Z.M.; Mayorga-Martinez, C.C.; Rosli, N.F.; Budanović, M.; Szokolová, K.I.; Webster, R.D.; Sofer, Z.; Pumera, M. Cloisite microrobots as self-propelling cleaners for fast and efficient removal of improvised organophosphate nerve agents. *ACS Appl. Mater. Interfaces* **2019**, *11*, 31832–31843. [CrossRef]
74. Zhang, P.; Sun, X.; Guo, J.; Wang, Y.; Zhang, W.; Ning, W.; Li, W.; Wei, C.; Shi, X.; Miao, S. Deep-sea clays using as active Fenton catalysts for self-propelled motors. *J. Am. Ceram. Soc.* **2022**, *105*, 3797–3808. [CrossRef]
75. Lin, J.; Zhou, W.; Wu, Q.; Li, K.; Ying, Y.; Wang, S. Shape, morphology, and components-dependent motion and water purification performance study of multi-metal–organic frameworks based micromotors. *Sep. Purif. Technol.* **2025**, *11*, 131559. [CrossRef]
76. Wani, O.M.; Safdar, M.; Kinnunen, N.; Jänis, J. Dual effect of manganese oxide micromotors: Catalytic degradation and adsorptive bubble separation of organic pollutants. *Chem. A Eur. J.* **2016**, *22*, 1244–1247. [CrossRef]
77. Liang, C.; Zhan, C.; Zeng, F.; Xu, D.; Wang, Y.; Zhao, W.; Zhang, J.; Guo, J.; Feng, H.; Ma, X. Bilayer tubular micromotors for simultaneous environmental monitoring and remediation. *ACS Appl. Mater. Interfaces* **2018**, *10*, 35099–35107. [CrossRef] [PubMed]
78. Singh, A.K.; Bhuyan, T.; Maity, S.; Mandal, T.K.; Bandyopadhyay, D. Magnetically actuated carbon soot nanoparticle-based catalytic CARBOts coated with Ni/Pt nanofilms for water detoxification and oil-spill recovery. *ACS Appl. Nano Mater.* **2020**, *3*, 3459–3470. [CrossRef]
79. Villa, K.; Parmar, J.; Vilela, D.; Sánchez, S. Metal-oxide-based microjets for the simultaneous removal of organic pollutants and heavy metals. *ACS Appl. Mater. Interfaces* **2018**, *10*, 20478–20486. [CrossRef]
80. Wang, H.; Khezri, B.; Pumera, M. Catalytic DNA-functionalized self-propelled micromachines for environmental remediation. *Chem* **2016**, *1*, 473–481. [CrossRef]
81. Zhang, J.; Fang, Y.; Lin, J.; Du, W.; Feng, Z.; Lin, Y.; Xu, L.; Liu, L.; Guan, J.; Mou, F. Generalized and Scalable Synthesis of Manganese Dioxide-Based Tubular Micromotors for Heavy Metal Ion Removal. *ACS Nano* **2024**, *18*, 29248–29260. [CrossRef] [PubMed]
82. Liu, J.; Li, J.; Wang, G.; Yang, W.; Yang, J.; Liu, Y. Bioinspired zeolitic imidazolate framework (ZIF-8) magnetic micromotors for highly efficient removal of organic pollutants from water. *J. Colloid. Interface Sci.* **2019**, *555*, 234–244. [CrossRef] [PubMed]
83. Chen, T.; Cai, Y.; Ren, B.; Sánchez, B.J.; Dong, R. Intelligent Micro/nanorobots Based on Biotemplate. *Mater. Horiz.* **2024**, *11*, 2986. [CrossRef]
84. Li, J.; Ji, F.; Ng, D.H.; Liu, J.; Bing, X.; Wang, P. Bioinspired Pt-free molecularly imprinted hydrogel-based magnetic Janus micromotors for temperature-responsive recognition and adsorption of erythromycin in water. *Chem. Eng. J.* **2019**, *369*, 611–620. [CrossRef]
85. Dong, Y.; Yi, C.; Yang, S.; Wang, J.; Chen, P.; Liu, X.; Du, W.; Wang, S.; Liu, B.-F. A substrate-free graphene oxide-based micromotor for rapid adsorption of antibiotics. *Nanoscale* **2019**, *11*, 4562–4570. [CrossRef]

86. Vaghasiya, J.V.; Mayorga-Martinez, C.C.; Matějková, S.; Pumera, M. Pick up and dispose of pollutants from water via temperature-responsive micellar copolymers on magnetite nanorobots. *Nat. Commun.* **2022**, *13*, 1026. [CrossRef]
87. Oral, C.M.; Ussia, M.; Pumera, M. Self-Propelled Activated Carbon Micromotors for "On-the-Fly" Capture of Nitroaromatic Explosives. *J. Phys. Chem. C* **2021**, *125*, 18040–18045. [CrossRef]
88. Hayes, E.K.; Gagnon, G.A. From capture to detection: A critical review of passive sampling techniques for pathogen surveillance in water and wastewater. *Water Res.* **2024**, *261*, 122024. [CrossRef] [PubMed]
89. Ussia, M.; Urso, M.; Oral, C.M.; Peng, X.; Pumera, M. Magnetic Microrobot Swarms with Polymeric Hands Catching Bacteria and Microplastics in Water. *ACS Nano* **2024**, *18*, 13171–13183. [CrossRef] [PubMed]
90. Yuan, K.; Jurado-Sánchez, B.; Escarpa, A. Dual-Propelled Lanbiotic Based Janus Micromotors for Selective Inactivation of Bacterial Biofilms. *Angew. Chem. Int. Ed.* **2021**, *60*, 4915–4924. [CrossRef]
91. Moo, J.G.S.; Wang, H.; Zhao, G.; Pumera, M. Biomimetic artificial inorganic enzyme-free self-propelled microfish robot for selective detection of Pb2+ in water. *Chem.–A Eur. J.* **2014**, *20*, 4292–4296. [CrossRef]
92. Esteban-Fernández de ávila, B.; Lopez-Ramirez, M.A.; Báez, D.F.; Jodra, A.; Singh, V.V.; Kaufmann, K.; Wang, J. Aptamer-modified graphene-based catalytic micromotors: Off–on fluorescent detection of ricin. *ACS Sens.* **2016**, *1*, 217–221. [CrossRef]
93. Draz, M.S.; Lakshminaraasimulu, N.K.; Krishnakumar, S.; Battalapalli, D.; Vasan, A.; Kanakasabapathy, M.K.; Sreeram, A.; Kallakuri, S.; Thirumalaraju, P.; Li, Y. Motion-based immunological detection of Zika virus using Pt-nanomotors and a cellphone. *ACS Nano* **2018**, *12*, 5709–5718. [CrossRef] [PubMed]
94. Luo, Q.; Yu, F.; Yang, F.; Yang, C.; Qiu, P.; Wang, X. A 3D-printed self-propelled, highly sensitive mini-motor for underwater pesticide detection. *Talanta* **2018**, *183*, 297–303. [CrossRef]
95. Villa, K.; Manzanares Palenzuela, C.L.; Sofer, Z.k.; Matejková, S.; Pumera, M. Metal-free visible-light photoactivated C_3N_4 bubble-propelled tubular micromotors with inherent fluorescence and on/off capabilities. *ACS Nano* **2018**, *12*, 12482–12491. [CrossRef]
96. Novotný, F.; Plutnar, J.; Pumera, M. Plasmonic Self-Propelled Nanomotors for Explosives Detection via Solution-Based Surface Enhanced Raman Scattering. *Adv. Funct. Mater.* **2019**, *29*, 1903041. [CrossRef]
97. Yang, X.; Lan, Z.; Wang, G.; Li, J. Dynamic activation of PMS by CoNi-Zn $(OH)_2/MnO_2$ micromotors for efficient degradation of phenolic pollutants. *Sep. Purif. Technol.* **2025**, *361*, 131507. [CrossRef]
98. Zhao, L.; Xie, S.; Liu, Y.; Liu, Q.; Song, X.; Li, X. Janus micromotors for motion-capture-lighting of bacteria. *Nanoscale* **2019**, *11*, 17831–17840. [CrossRef] [PubMed]
99. Yuan, Y.; Gao, C.; Wang, D.; Zhou, C.; Zhu, B.; He, Q. Janus-micromotor-based on–off luminescence sensor for active TNT detection. *Beilstein J. Nanotechnol.* **2019**, *10*, 1324–1331. [CrossRef]
100. la Asunción-Nadal, V.c.d.; Pacheco, M.; Jurado-Sánchez, B.; Escarpa, A. Chalcogenides-based tubular micromotors in fluorescent assays. *Anal. Chem.* **2020**, *92*, 9188–9193. [CrossRef] [PubMed]
101. Qiu, B.; Xie, L.; Zeng, J.; Liu, T.; Yan, M.; Zhou, S.; Liang, Q.; Tang, J.; Liang, K.; Kong, B. Interfacially super-assembled asymmetric and H_2O_2 sensitive multilayer-sandwich magnetic mesoporous silica nanomotors for detecting and removing heavy metal ions. *Adv. Funct. Mater.* **2021**, *31*, 2010694. [CrossRef]
102. Yang, W.; Lyu, Y.; Lan, Z.; Li, J.; Ng, D.H. Biomass-derived 3D hierarchical Zr-based tubular magnetomotors with peroxidase-like properties for selective colorimetric detection and specific decontamination of glyphosate at neutral pH. *Environ. Sci. Nano* **2023**, *10*, 1676–1688. [CrossRef]
103. Urso, M.; Ussia, M.; Novotný, F.; Pumera, M. Trapping and detecting nanoplastics by MXene-derived oxide microrobots. *Nat. Commun.* **2022**, *13*, 3573. [CrossRef]
104. Velikov, D.I.; Jancik-Prochazkova, A.; Pumera, M. On-the-Fly Monitoring of the Capture and Removal of Nanoplastics with Nanorobots. *ACS Nanosci. Au* **2024**, *4*, 243–249. [CrossRef] [PubMed]
105. Nawi, M.; Zain, S.M. Enhancing the surface properties of the immobilized Degussa P-25 TiO_2 for the efficient photocatalytic removal of methylene blue from aqueous solution. *Appl. Surf. Sci.* **2012**, *258*, 6148–6157. [CrossRef]
106. Shih, K.-Y.; Kuan, Y.-L.; Wang, E.-R. One-step microwave-assisted synthesis and visible-light photocatalytic activity enhancement of BiOBr/RGO nanocomposites for degradation of methylene blue. *Materials* **2021**, *14*, 4577. [CrossRef]
107. Abal, C.C.; Escarpa, A.; Sánchez, B.J. Micromotors for antimicrobial resistance bacteria inactivation in water systems: Opportunities and challenges. *Environ. Sci. Nano* **2025**, *12*, 967–978. [CrossRef]

MDPI AG
Grosspeteranlage 5
4052 Basel
Switzerland
Tel.: +41 61 683 77 34

Chemosensors Editorial Office
E-mail: chemosensors@mdpi.com
www.mdpi.com/journal/chemosensors